LUNG IMAGING
and
COMPUTER-AIDED DIAGNOSIS

LUNG IMAGING and COMPUTER-AIDED DIAGNOSIS

EDITED BY
AYMAN EL-BAZ
AND
JASJIT S. SURI

CRC Press
Taylor & Francis Group
Boca Raton London New York

CRC Press is an imprint of the
Taylor & Francis Group, an **informa** business

CRC Press
Taylor & Francis Group
6000 Broken Sound Parkway NW, Suite 300
Boca Raton, FL 33487-2742

First issued in paperback 2017

ISBN-13: 978-1-4398-4557-8 (hbk)
ISBN-13: 978-1-138-07207-7 (pbk)

Library of Congress Cataloging-in-Publication Data

Lung imaging and computer aided diagnosis / editors, Ayman El-Baz, Jasjit S. Suri.
p. ; cm.
Includes bibliographical references and index.
ISBN 978-1-4398-4557-8 (hardcover : alk. paper)
I. El-Baz, Ayman S. II. Suri, Jasjit S.

[DNLM: 1. Lung Neoplasms--diagnosis. 2. Diagnostic Imaging--methods. 3. Early Diagnosis. 4. Image Processing, Computer-Assisted. WF 658]
616.99'424075--dc23 2011036048

Visit the Taylor & Francis Web site at
http://www.taylorandfrancis.com

and the CRC Press Web site at
http://www.crcpress.com

Contents

Editors

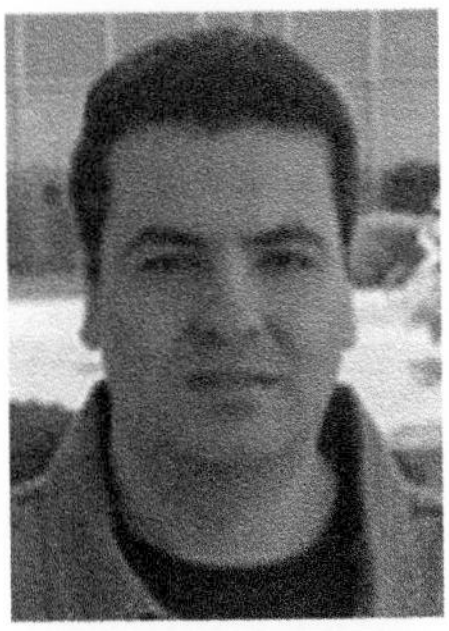

Ayman El-Baz received BSc and MS degrees in electrical engineering from Mansoura University, Egypt, in 1997 and 2000, respectively, and a PhD degree in electrical engineering from the University of Louisville, Louisville, KY. He joined the Bioengineering Department of the University of Louisville in August 2006. His current research is focused on developing new computer-assisted diagnosis systems for different diseases and brain disorders.

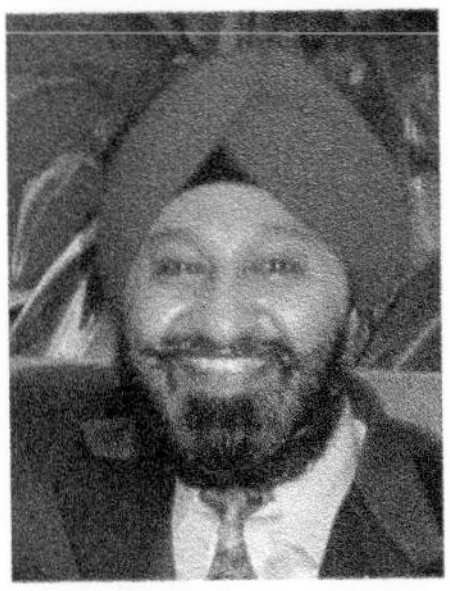

Jasjit S. Suri is an innovator, a scientist, a visionary, an industrialist, and an internationally known world leader in biomedical engineering. Dr. Suri has spent over 20 years in the field of biomedical engineering/devices and their management. He received his doctorate from the University of Washington, Seattle, and business management sciences degree from Weatherhead, Case Western Reserve University, Cleveland, Ohio. Dr. Suri was honored with the President's Gold Medal in 1980 and the Fellow of American Institute of Medical and Biological Engineering for his outstanding contributions.

Contributors

Til Aach
Institute of Imaging and Computer Vision
RWTH
Aachen University
Aachen, Germany

Xabier Artaechevarria
Center for Applied Medical Research
University of Navarra
Pamplona, Spain

Rahul Bhotika
GE Global Research
Niskayuna, New York

Mario Ceresa
Center for Applied Medical Research
University of Navarra
Pamplona, Spain

Paul Compton
School of Computer Science and Engineering
University of New South Wales
Sydney, Australia

Tessa Cook
Hospital of the University of Pennsylvania
Philadelphia, Pennsylvania

Marleen de Bruijne
Biomedical Imaging Group
Departments of Medical Informatics and Radiology
Erasmus MC–University Medical Center
Rotterdam, the Netherlands and
The Image Group
Department of Computer Science
University of Copenhagen
Copenhagen, Denmark

Ayman El-Baz
Bioimaging Laboratory
Bioengineering Department
University of Louisville
Louisville, Kentucky

Mohamed Abo El-Ghar
Urology and Nephrology Department
University of Mansoura
Mansoura, Egypt

Ahmed Elnakib
Bioimaging Laboratory
Bioengineering Department
University of Louisville
Louisville, Kentucky

Robert Falk
Medical Imaging Division
Jewish Hospital
Louisville, Kentucky

Aly Farag
Computer Vision and Image Processing Laboratory
University of Louisville
Louisville, Kentucky

Hiroshi Fujita
Graduate School of Medicine
Gifu University
Gifu, Japan

Mehrdad J. Gangeh
Pattern Analysis and Machine Intelligence (PAMI) Lab
Department of Electrical and Computer Engineering
University of Waterloo
Waterloo, Ontario, Canada

James Gee
University of Pennsylvania
Philadelphia, Pennsylvania

Warren B. Gefter
Hospital of the University of Pennsylvania
Philadelphia, Pennsylvania

Georgy Gimel'farb
Department of Computer Science
Tamaki Campus, University of Auckland
Auckland, New Zealand

Takeshi Hara
Graduate School of Medicine
Gifu University
Gifu, Japan

Celina Imielinska
Columbia University
New York, New York

Benjamin Irving
University College London
London, United Kingdom

Jens N. Kaftan
Institute of Imaging and Computer Vision
RWTH
Aachen University
Aachen, Germany

Robert Kaucic
GE Global Research
Niskayuna, New York

Fahmi Khalifa
Bioimaging Laboratory
Bioengineering Department
University of Louisville
Louisville, Kentucky

Patrick A. Kupelian
University of California, Los Angeles
Los Angeles, California

Yongbum Lee
Department of Radiological Technology
School of Health Sciences
Niigata University
Niigata, Japan

Paulo R. S. Mendonça
GE Global Research
Niskayuna, New York

Dimitris N. Metaxas
Center for Computational Biomedicine
Imaging and Modeling
Piscataway, New Jersey

Yugang Min
University of Central Florida
Orlando, Florida

Avishkar Misra
School of Computer Science and Engineering
University of New South Wales
Sydney, Australia

Arrate Muñoz-Barrutia
Center for Applied Medical Research
University of Navarra
Pamplona, Spain

Matthew Nitzken
Bioimaging Laboratory
Bioengineering Department
University of Louisville
Louisville, Kentucky

Kazunori Okada
Computer Science Department
San Francisco State University
San Francisco, California

Carlos Ortiz-de-Solorzano
Center for Applied Medical Research
University of Navarra
Pamplona, Spain

Rômulo Pinho
University of Antwerp
Antwerp, Belgium

Jannick P. Rolland
University of Rochester
Rochester, New York

Luca Saba
Department of Radiology
A.O.U. Cagliari – Polo di Monserrato
Monserrato, Italy

Anand P. Santhanam
Department of Radiation Oncology
University of California, Los Angeles
Los Angeles, California

Palaniappan Sethu
Bioengineering Department
University of Louisville
Louisville, Kentucky

Saher B. Shaker
Department of Respiratory Medicine
Gentofte University Hospital
Copenhagen, Denmark

Jan Sijbers
University of Antwerp
Antwerp, Belgium

Gang Song
University of Pennsylvania
Philadelphia, Pennsylvania

Lauge Sørensen
The Image Group
Department of Computer Science
University of Copenhagen
Copenhagen, Denmark

Arcot Sowmya
School of Computer Science and Engineering
University of New South Wales
Sydney, Australia

Jasjit Suri
Biomedical Technologies, Inc.
Roseville, California

Kenji Suzuki
Department of Radiology
The University of Chicago
Chicago, Illinois

Paul Taylor
University College London
London, United Kingdom

Andrew Todd-Pokropek
Medical Physics
University College London
London, United Kingdom

Drew Torigian
Hospital of the University of Pennsylvania
Philadelphia, Pennsylvania

Kurt G. Tournoy
Ghent University Hospital
Ghent, Belgium

DuYih Tsai
Department of Radiological Technology
School of Health Sciences
Niigata University
Niigata, Japan

Nicholas J. Tustison
University of Virginia
Charlottesville, Virginia

Eric Van Bogaert
Bioimaging Laboratory
Bioengineering Department
University of Louisville
Louisville, Kentucky

Jinghao Zhou
Flushing Radiation Oncology Services
Flushing, New York

1

A Novel Three-Dimensional Framework for Automatic Lung Segmentation from Low-Dose Computed Tomography Images

Ayman El-Baz, Georgy Gimel'farb, Robert Falk, and Mohamed Abo El-Ghar

CONTENTS

1.1 Introduction

Lung cancer remains the leading cause of cancer-related death in the United States. In 2006, there were approximately 174,470 new cases of lung cancer and 162,460 related deaths [1]. Early diagnosis of cancer can improve the effectiveness of treatment and increase the patient's chances of survival. Segmentation of the lung tissues is a crucial step for developing any computer-assisted diagnostic system for early diagnosis of lung cancer. Accurate segmentation of lung tissues from low-dose computed tomography (LDCT) images is a challenging problem because some lung tissues such as arteries, veins, bronchi, and bronchioles are very close to the chest tissues. Therefore, segmentation cannot be based only on image signals but should also account for spatial relationships between the region labels to preserve the details of the lung region.

In the literature, there are many techniques that have been developed for lung segmentation in CT images. Sluimer et al. [2] presented a survey on computer analysis of the lungs in CT scans. This survey addressed segmentation of various pulmonary structures, registration of chest scans, and their applications. Hu et al. [3] proposed an optimal gray level thresholding technique that is used to select a threshold value based on the unique characteristics of the data set. A segmentation-by-registration scheme was proposed by

Sluimer et al. [4] for automated segmentation of the pathological lung in CT. For more on lung segmentation techniques, refer to the survey by Sluimer et al. [2].

In this chapter, we describe LDCT images and the desired maps of regions (lung and the other chest tissues) by a joint Markov–Gibbs random field model (MGRF) of independent image signals and interdependent region labels but focus on most accurate model identification. To better specify region borders, each empirical distribution of signals is precisely approximated by a linear combination of discrete Gaussians (LCDG) with positive and negative components. Approximation of an empirical relative frequency distribution of scalar data with a particular probability density function is widely used in pattern recognition and image processing, e.g., for data clustering or image segmentation [5]. The basic problem is to accurately approximate, to within the data range, not only the peaks or modes of the probability density function for the measurements, but also its behavior between the peaks. This is most essential for a precise data classification because borders between data classes are usually formed by intersecting tails of the class distributions.

We propose a modification of the well-known expectation-maximization (EM) algorithm to approximate an empirical relative frequency distribution of the scalar data with an LCDG. The LCDG has both positive and negative components so that it approximates empirical data more accurately than a conventional mixture of only positive Gaussians [6]. At higher levels, the intraregion and interregion label co-occurrences are specified by a Markov–Gibbs model with the nearest eight-neighborhood of each pixel. Under assumed symmetric relationships between the neighboring labels, the model resembles the autobinomial ones. However, rather than use the predefined Gibbs potentials, we identify them using analytical estimates.

1.2 Joint Markov–Gibbs Model of LDCT Lung Images

Let $R = \{(i, j): 1 \le i \le I, 1 \le j \le J, 1 \le z \le Z\}$ denote a finite arithmetic grid supporting grayscale LDCT images $g: R \to Q$ and their region maps $m: R \to X$. Here, $Q = \{0,\ldots Q-1\}$ and $X = \{1,\ldots X\}$ are the sets of gray levels and region labels, respectively, where Q is the number of gray levels and X is the number of image classes to separate by segmentation. The MGRF model of images to segment is given by a joint probability distribution of LDCT images and desired region maps:

$$P(g, m) = P(m)P(g|m)$$

Here, $P(\mathrm{m})$ is an unconditional distribution of maps and $P(g|m)$ is a conditional distribution of images, given a map. The Bayesian MAP estimate of the map, given the image g, $m^* = \arg\max_{\mathrm{m}} L(g, m)$ maximizes the log-likelihood function:

$$L(g,m) = \log P(m) + \log P(g|m) \tag{1.1}$$

In this work, we focus on accurate identification of the spatial interaction between the lung pixels [$P(m)$] and the intensity distribution for the lung tissues [$P(g|m)$] as shown in Figure 1.1.

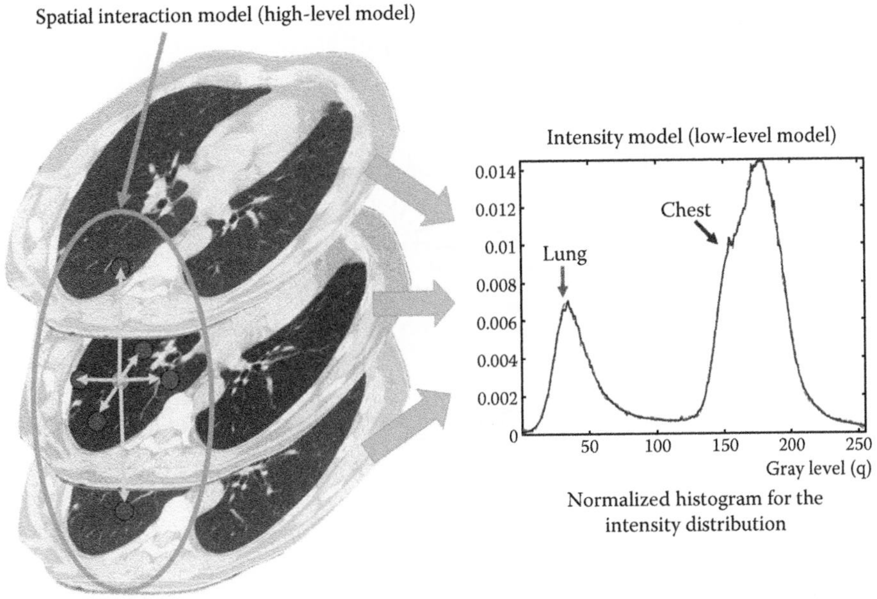

FIGURE 1.1
Illustration of joint Markov–Gibbs model of LDCT lung images.

1.2.1 Spatial Interaction Model of LDCT Images

The generic Markov–Gibbs model of region maps [7], which accounts for only pairwise interactions between each region label and its neighbors, generally has an arbitrary interaction structure and arbitrary Gibbs potentials identified from image data. For simplicity, we restrict the interactions to the nearest voxels (26-neighborhood system as shown in Figure 1.2) and assume, by symmetry considerations, that the interactions are independent of relative region orientation, are the same for all classes, and depend only on the intraregion or interregion positions of each voxel pair (i.e., whether the labels are equal or not). Under these restrictions, the model is similar to the conventional autobinomial ones [7] and differs only in that the potentials are not related to a predefined function and have analytical estimates.

The symmetric label interactions are threefold: the closest horizontal–vertical–diagonal in the current slice (hvdc), the closest horizontal–vertical–diagonal in the upper slice (hvdu), and the closest horizontal–vertical–diagonal in the lower slice (hvdl). The potentials of each type are bivalued because only coincidence or difference of the labels is taken into account. Let

$$\mathbf{V}_a = \{V_a(x,\chi) = V_{a,\text{eq}} \text{ if } x = \chi \text{ and } V_a = V_a(x,\chi) = V_{a,\text{ne}} \text{ if } x \neq \chi\}$$

denote bivalued Gibbs potentials describing symmetric pairwise interactions of type $a \in A = \{\text{hvdc, hvdu, hvdl}\}$ between the region labels. Let $N_{\text{hvdc}} = \{(1,0,0),(0,1,0),(-1,0,0),(0,-1,0)\}$, $N_{\text{hvdu}} = \{(0,0,1),(-1,-1,1),(-1,1,1),(1,-1,1),(1,1,1)\}$, and $N_{\text{hvdl}} = \{(0,0,-1),(-1,-1,-1),(-1,1,-1),(1,-1,-1),(1,1,-1)\}$ be

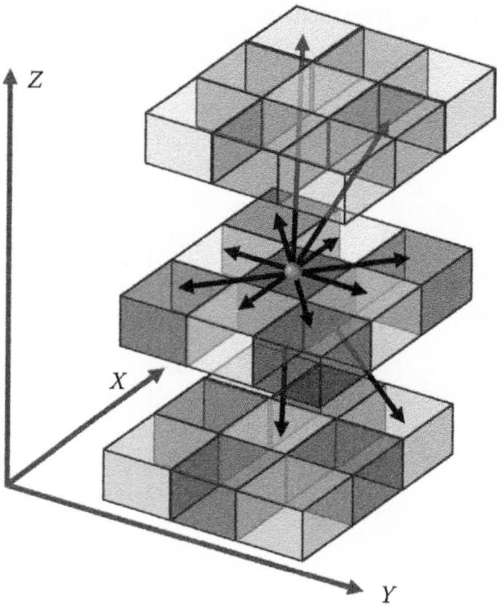

FIGURE 1.2
3D spatial interaction neighborhood system.

subsets of intervoxel offsets for the 26-neighborhood system. Then, the Gibbs probability distribution of region maps is as follows:

$$P(m)\alpha \exp \sum_{(i,j,z)\in R} \sum_{a\in A} \sum_{(\zeta,\eta,\xi)\in N_a} V_a\left(m_{i,j,z}, m_{i+\zeta,j+\eta,z+\xi}\right) \tag{1.2}$$

To identify the MGRF model described in Equation 1.2, we have to estimate the Gibbs potentials V. In this chapter, we introduce a new analytical maximum likelihood estimation for the Gibbs potentials.

$$\begin{aligned} V_{a,\mathrm{eq}} &= \frac{X^2}{X-1} f_a(m) - \frac{1}{X} \\ V_{a,\mathrm{ne}} &= \frac{X^2}{X-1} f_a(m) - 1 + \frac{1}{X} \end{aligned} \tag{1.3}$$

where $f_a(m)$ and $f_a(m)$ denote the relative frequency of the equal and nonequal pairs of the labels in all the equivalent voxel pairs $\{[(i, j, z), (i + \zeta, j + \eta, z + \xi)]: (i, j, z) \in R; (i + \zeta, j + \eta, z + \xi) \in R; (\zeta, \eta, \xi) \in N_a\}$, respectively.

1.2.2 Intensity Model of LDCT Lung Images

Let $q; q \in Q = \{0,1,\ldots,Q-1\}$ denote the Q-ary gray level. The discrete Gaussian (DG) is defined as the probability distribution $\psi_\theta = [\psi(q|\theta): q \in Q]$ on Q such that $\psi(q|\theta) = \phi_\theta(q + 0.5)$

$-\,\phi_\theta(q-0.5)$ for $q = 1,\ldots,Q-2$, $\psi(0|\theta) = \phi_\theta(0.5)$, $\psi(Q-1|\theta) = 1-\phi_\theta(Q-1.5)$, where $\phi_\theta(q)$ is the cumulative Gaussian probability function with a shorthand notation $\theta = (\mu,\sigma^2)$ for its mean, μ, and variance, σ^2.

We assume the number K of dominant modes, i.e., regions, objects, or classes of interest in a given LDCT image, is already known. In contrast with a conventional mixture of Gaussians and/or other simple distributions, one per region, we closely approximate the empirical gray level distribution for LDCT images with an LCDG having C_p positive and C_n negative components such that $C_p \geq K$:

$$p_{w,\Theta}(q) = \sum_{r=1}^{C_p} w_{p,r}\psi(q\,|\,\theta_{p,r}) - \sum_{l=1}^{C_n} w_{n,l}\psi(q\,|\,\theta_{n,l}) \tag{1.4}$$

under the obvious restrictions on the weights $w = (w_{p,.},w_{n,.})$: all the weights are nonnegative and

$$\sum_{r=1}^{C_p} w_{p,r} - \sum_{l=1}^{C_n} w_{n,l} = 1 \tag{1.5}$$

To identify the LCDG model, including the numbers of its positive and negative components, we modify the EM algorithm to deal with the LCDG.

First the numbers $C_p - K$, C_n and parameters w, Θ (weights, means, and variances) of the positive and negative DG components are estimated with a sequential EM-based initializing algorithm. The goal is to produce a close initial LCDG approximation of the empirical distribution. Then, under the fixed C_p and C_n, all other model parameters are refined with an EM algorithm that modifies the conventional one in ref. [8] to account for the components with alternating signs.

1.2.2.1 Sequential EM-Based Initialization

Sequential EM-based initialization forms an LCDG approximation of a given empirical marginal gray level distribution using the conventional EM algorithm [8] adapted to the DGs. At the first stage, the empirical distribution is represented with a mixture of K-positive DGs, each dominant mode being roughly approximated with a single DG. At the second stage, deviations of the empirical distribution from the dominant K component mixture are modeled with other, "subordinate" components of the LCDG. The resulting initial LCDG has K dominant weights, say, $w_{p,1},\ldots,w_{p,K}$ such that $\sum_{r=1}^{K} w_{p,r} = 1$, and a number of subordinate weights of smaller values such that

$$\sum_{r=K+1}^{C_p} w_{p,r} - \sum_{l=1}^{C_n} w_{n,l} = 0.$$

The subordinate components are determined as follows. The positive and negative deviations of the empirical distribution from the dominant mixture are separated and scaled up to form two new "empirical distributions." The same conventional EM algorithm is iteratively exploited to find the subordinate mixtures of positive or negative DGs that best approximate the scaled-up positive or negative deviations, respectively. The sizes $C_p - K$ and C_n of these mixtures are found by sequential minimization of the total absolute error between each scaled-up deviation and its mixture model by the number of the components. Then, the obtained positive and negative subordinate models are scaled down and then added to the dominant mixture yielding the initial LCDG model of the size $C = C_p + C_n$.

1.2.2.2 Modified EM Algorithm for LCDG

Modified EM algorithm for LCDG maximizes the log-likelihood of the empirical data by the model parameters assuming statistically independent signals:

$$L(w,\Theta) = \sum_{q\in Q} f(q)\log p_{w,\Theta}(q) \tag{1.6}$$

A local maximum of the log-likelihood in Equation 1.6 is given with the EM process extending the one in ref. [8] onto alternating signs of the components. Let $p(m)$ denote the current LCDG at iteration m, which is calculated as follows:

$$p_{w,\Theta}^{[m]}(q) = \sum_{r=1}^{C_p} w_{p,r}^{[m]}\psi(q\,|\,\theta_{p,r}^{[m]}) - \sum_{l=1}^{C_n} w_{n,l}^{[m]}\psi(q\,|\,\theta_{n,l}^{[m]})$$

Relative contributions of each signal $q \in Q$ to each positive and negative DG at iteration m are specified by the respective conditional weights.

$$\pi_p^{[m]}(r\,|\,q) = \frac{w_{p,r}^{[m]}\psi(q\,|\,\theta_{p,r}^{[m]})}{p_{w,\Theta}^{[m]}(q)}$$
$$\pi_n^{[m]}(l\,|\,q) = \frac{w_{n,l}^{[m]}\psi(q\,|\,\theta_{n,l}^{[m]})}{p_{w,\Theta}^{[m]}(q)} \tag{1.7}$$

such that the following constraints hold:

$$\sum_{r=1}^{C_p} \pi_p^{[m]}(r\,|\,q) - \sum_{l=1}^{C_n} \pi_n^{[m]}(l\,|\,q) = 1; \qquad q = 0,\ldots,Q-1 \tag{1.8}$$

The following two steps iterate until the log-likelihood changes become small:

E step $[m + 1]$: Find the weights of Equation 1.7 under the fixed parameters $w^{[m]},\Theta^{[m]}$ from the previous iteration m.

M step $[m + 1]$: Find conditional MLEs $w^{[m+1]},\Theta^{[m+1]}$ by maximizing $L(w,\Theta)$ under the fixed weights of Equation 1.7.

Considerations closely similar to those in ref. [8] show this process converges to a local log-likelihood maximum. Let the log-likelihood of Equation 1.6 be rewritten in the equivalent form with the constraints of Equation 1.8 as unit factors:

$$L(w^{[m]},\Theta^{[m]}) = \sum_{q=0}^{Q} f(q) \sum_{r=1}^{C_p} \pi_{\mathrm{p}}^{[m]}(r \mid q)\log p^{[m]}(q) - \sum_{l=1}^{C_n} \pi_{\mathrm{n}}^{[m]}(l \mid q)\log p^{[m]}(q) \tag{1.9}$$

Let the terms $\log p^{[m]}(q)$ in the first and second brackets be replaced with the equal terms $\log w_{\mathrm{p},r}^{[m]} + \log \psi(q \mid \theta_{\mathrm{p},r}^{[m]}) - \log \pi_{\mathrm{p}}^{[m]}(r \mid q)$ and $\log w_{\mathrm{n},l}^{[m]} + \log \psi(q \mid \theta_{\mathrm{n},l}^{[m]}) - \log \pi_{\mathrm{n}}^{[m]}(l \mid q)$, respectively, which follow from Equation 1.7. At the E step, the conditional Lagrange maximization of the log-likelihood of Equation 1.9 under the Q restrictions of Equation 1.8 results in only the weights $\pi_{\mathrm{p}}^{[m+1]}(r \mid q)$ and $\pi_{\mathrm{n}}^{[m+1]}(l \mid q)$ of Equation 1.7 for all $r = 1,\ldots,C_{\mathrm{p}}$; $l = 1,\ldots,C_{\mathrm{n}}$, and $q \in Q$. At the M step, the DG weights $w_{\mathrm{p},r}^{[m+1]} = \sum_{q \in Q} f(q)\pi_{\mathrm{p}}^{[m+1]}(r \mid q)$ and $w_{\mathrm{n},l}^{[m+1]} = \sum_{q \in Q} f(q)\pi_{\mathrm{n}}^{[m+1]}(l \mid q)$ follow from the conditional Lagrange maximization of the log-likelihood in Equation 1.9 under the restriction of Equation 1.5 and the fixed conditional weights of Equation 1.7. Under the latter, the conventional MLEs of the parameters of each DG stem from maximizing the log-likelihood after each difference of the cumulative Gaussians is replaced with its close approximation with the Gaussian density (in the following equations, c stands for p or n, respectively):

$$^{[m+1]}_{c,r} = \frac{1}{w_{c,r}^{[m+1]}} \sum_{q \in Q} q \cdot f(q)\pi_c^{[m+1]}(r \mid q)$$

$$\left(\sigma_{c,r}^{[m+1]}\right)^2 = \frac{1}{w_{c,r}^{[m+1]}} \sum_{q \in Q} \left(q - \, ^{[m+1]}_{c,r}\right)^2 \cdot f(q)\pi_c^{[m+1]}(r \mid q)$$

This modified EM algorithm is valid until the weights w are strictly positive. The iterations should be terminated when the log-likelihood of Equation 1.6 does not change or begins to decrease due to the accumulation of rounding errors.

The final mixed LCDG model $p_c(q)$ is partitioned into the K LCDG submodels $P_{[k]} = [p(q \mid k) : q \in Q]$, one per class $k = 1,\ldots, K$, by associating the subordinate DGs with the dominant terms so that the misclassification rate is minimal.

The whole iterative segmentation process is as follows:

1. Initialization: Find an initial map by the pixelwise Bayesian MAP classification of a given LDCT image after initial estimation of X from LCDG models of signals of each object class represented by one of the dominant modes (see Figure 1.3).
2. Iterative refinement: Refine the initial map by iterating the following two steps:
   - 2.1. Estimate the potential values for region map model using Equation 1.3.
   - 2.2. Recollect the empirical gray level densities for the current regions, reapproximate these densities, and update the map using the pixel-wise Bayesian classification as shown in Figure 1.3.

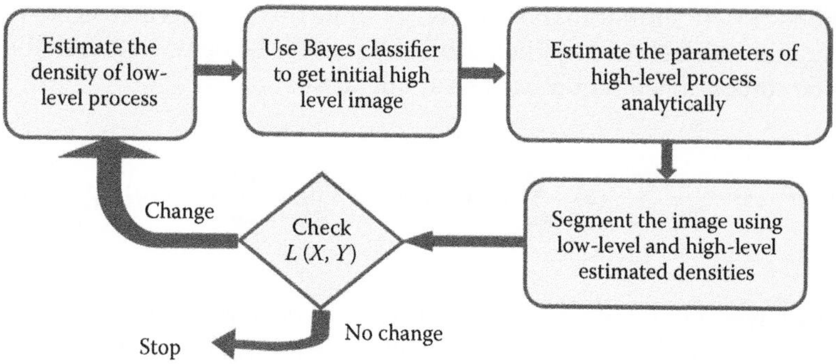

FIGURE 1.3
The proposed segmentation approach.

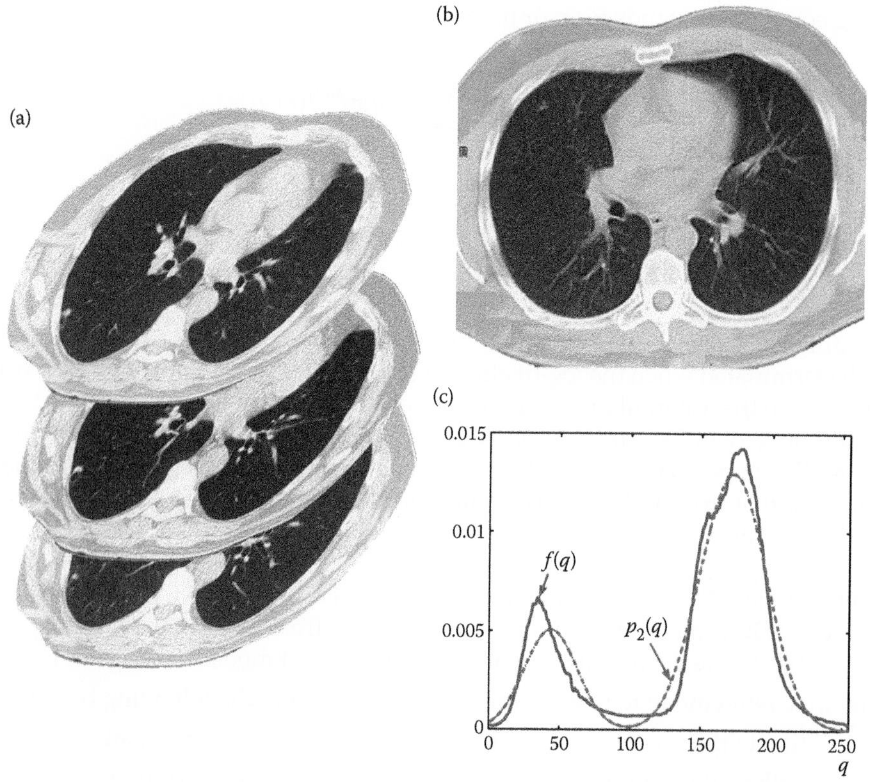

FIGURE 1.4
(a) Typical LDCT scan slices, (b) two-dimensional (2D) axial cross section picked up from the LDCT scan, and (c) the empirical distribution, $f(q)$, and the estimated two-dominant component mixture, $p_2(q)$.

1.3 Experimental Results and Validation

Experiments were conducted with the LDCT images acquired with a multidetector GE Light Speed Plus scanner (General Electric, Milwaukee, WI) with the following scanning parameters: slice thickness of 2.5 mm reconstructed every 1.5 mm, scanning pitch 1.5, pitch 1 mm, 140 kV, 100 mA, and field of view 36 cm. The size of each three-dimensional (3D) data set was 512 × 512 × 182. The LDCT images contain two classes ($K = 2$), namely, the darker lung tissues and the brighter chest region. A typical LDCT slice, its empirical marginal gray level distribution, $f(q)$, and the initial two-component Gaussian dominant mixture, $p_2(q)$, are shown in Figure 1.4. Figure 1.5 illustrates basic stages of our sequential EM-based initialization by showing the scaled-up alternating and absolute

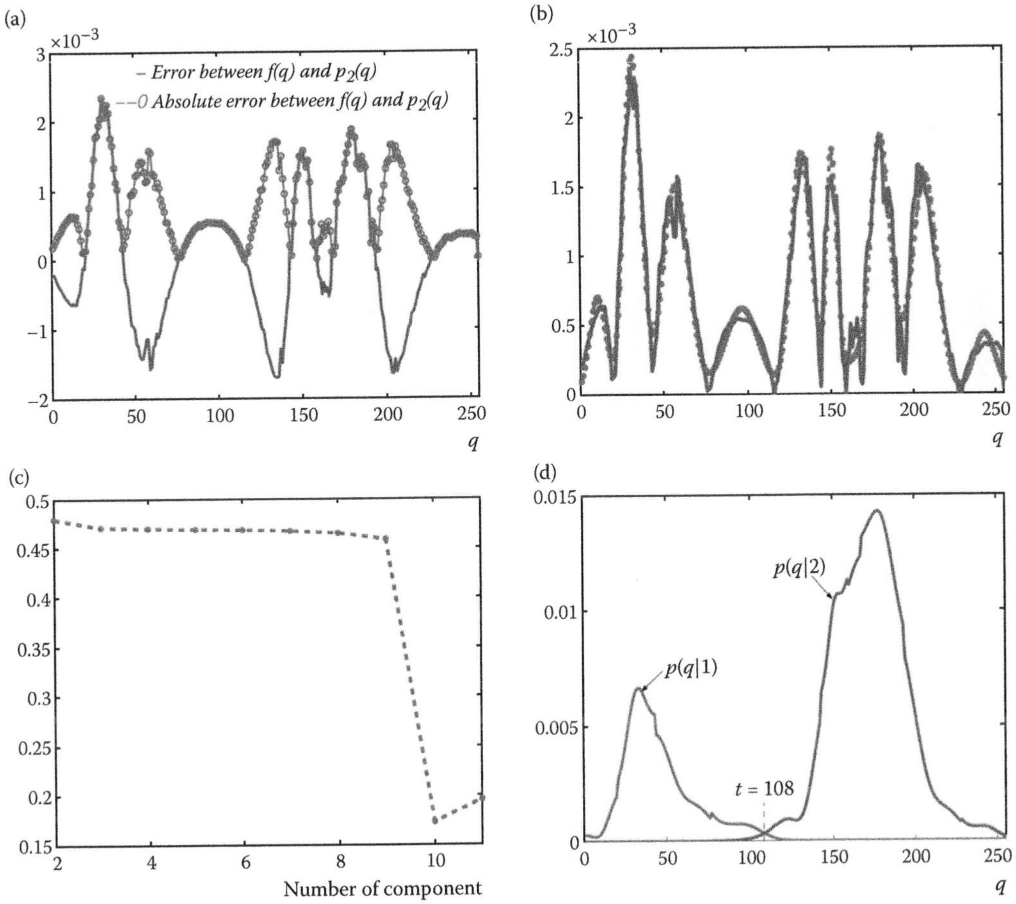

FIGURE 1.5
(a) Deviations and absolute deviations between $f(q)$ and $p_2(q)$, (b) the mixture model of the absolute deviations in (a), (c) the absolute error as a function of the number of Gaussians approximating the scaled-up absolute deviations in (a), and (d) the initial estimated LCDG models for each class.

deviations, $f(q) - p_2(q)$, the best mixture model estimated for the absolute deviations (these 10 Gaussian components give the minimum approximation error), and the initial LCDG models for each class.

Figure 1.6 presents the final LCDG model after refining the initial one with the modified EM algorithm and shows successive changes of the log-likelihood at the refinement iterations. The final LCDG of each class are obtained with the best separation threshold ($t = 109$). The first six refining iterations increase the log-likelihood from −5.7 to −5.2.

The region map obtained first with only the class LCDG models is further refined using the iterative segmentation algorithm. Changes in the likelihood, $L(g,m)$, become very small after 12 iterations. For this map, the initial estimated parameters are $V_{a,\mathrm{eq}} = -V_{a,\mathrm{ne}} = 1.02$, and the final estimated parameters are $V_{a,\mathrm{eq}} = -V_{a,\mathrm{ne}} = 1.67$. The final region map produced with these parameters using the Metropolis pixelwise relaxation is shown in Figure 1.7. For comparison, Figure 1.7 also presents the initial region map, the map refined with the

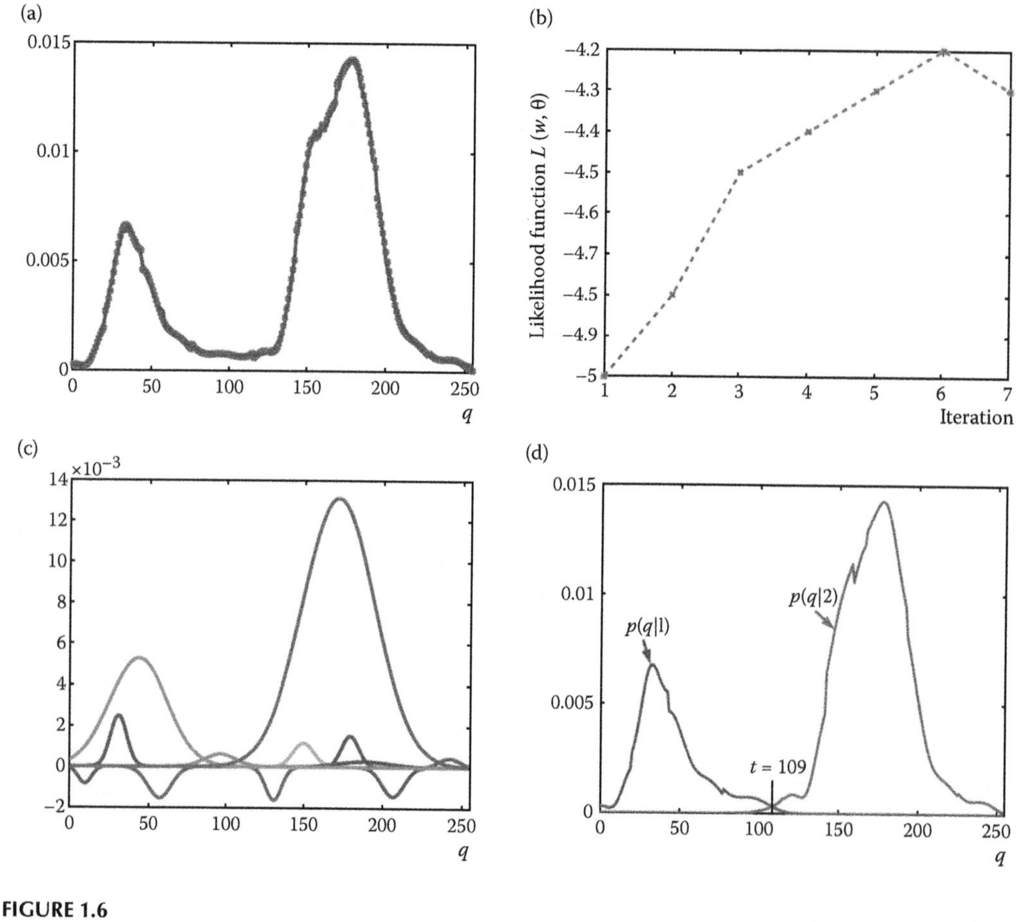

FIGURE 1.6
Final three-class LCDG model overlaying the (a) empirical density, (b) log-likelihood dynamics for the refining EM iterations, (c) refined model components, and (d) class LCDG models.

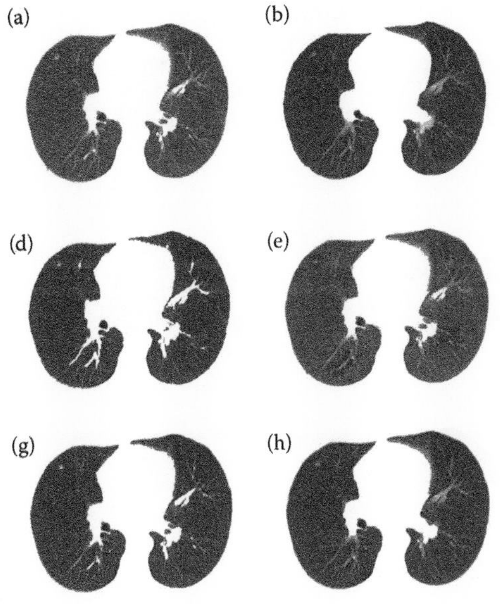

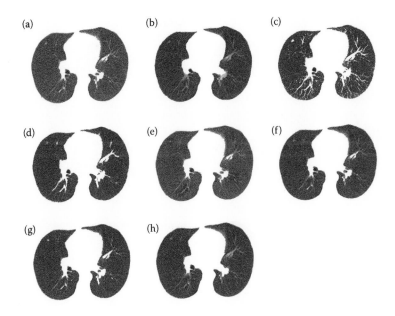

FIGURE 1.7
(a) Initial and (b) final segmentation by the proposed approach (final error, 1.1% compared with the ground truth); (c) initial and (d) final segmentation using the conventional normal mixture obtained by the EM algorithm (final error, 5.1%); (e) refined lung regions obtained from (a) using the randomly chosen Gibbs potentials of the map model (final error, 1.8%); (f) best segmentation obtained by the MRS algorithm with the potential values 0.3 and three levels of resolution (error, 2.3%); (g) best segmentation obtained by the ICM algorithm with the potential values 0.3 (error, 2.9%) and (h) the ground truth produced by a radiologist.

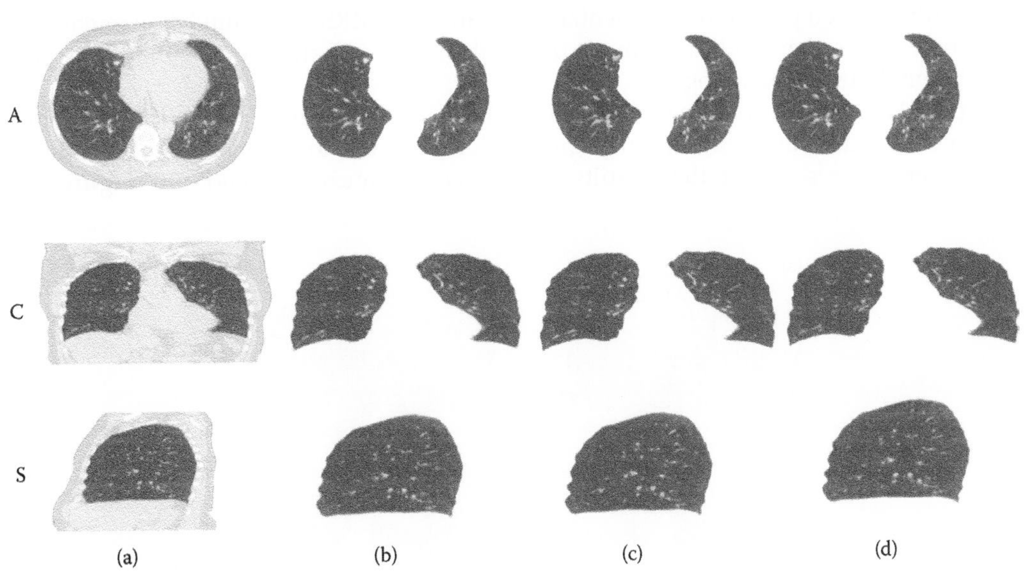

FIGURE 1.8
Results of 3D lung segmentation projected onto 2D (A) axial, (C) coronal, and (S) sagittal planes for visualization: 2D profiles of the (a) original LDCT images, (b) our segmentation, (c) IT segmentation, and (d) the radiologist's segmentation. Note that our segmentation errors are only around the outer edge (error, 0.79%) and the IT-based segmentation error is 4.57%.

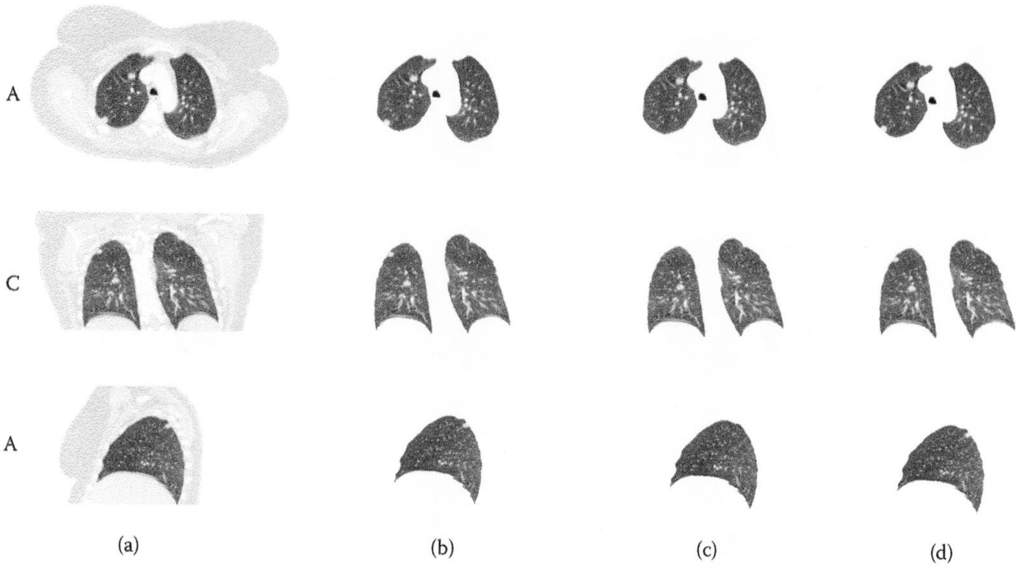

FIGURE 1.9
Results of 3D lung segmentation projected onto 2D (A) axial, (C) coronal, and (S) sagittal planes for visualization: 2D profiles of the (a) original LDCT images, (b) our segmentation, (c) segmentation by the approach proposed in ref. [40], and (d) the gold standard, the radiologist's segmentation. The segmentation errors, in comparison with the gold standard radiologist's segmentation. Note that our segmentation errors are minor (0.11%), appear only around the outer high-curvature edges, and are considerably smaller than the errors (2.49%) with the algorithm in ref. [9].

randomly selected potentials, segmentation obtained by MRS algorithm [9], segmentation obtained by iterative conditional mode (ICM) algorithm [10], and the "ground truth" segmentation done by a radiologist.

Figure 1.8 compares our segmentation with the iterative thresholding (IT) algorithm. In contrast with this method, our segmentation does not lose abnormal lung tissues. Moreover, more segmentation results are shown in Figures 1.9 and 1.10. Figure 1.11

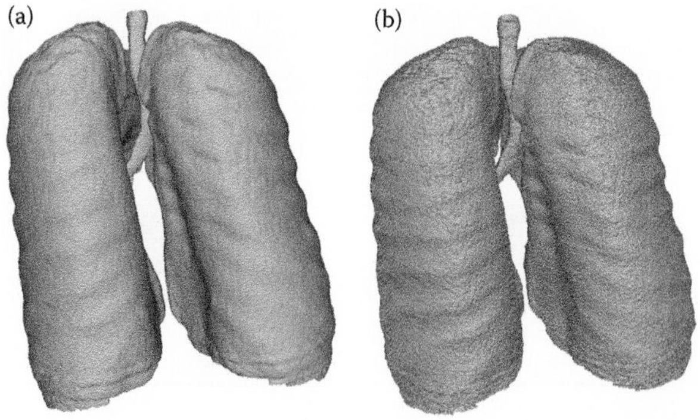

FIGURE 1.10
(See color insert.) 3D visualization of a healthy lung with no nodules: (a) our results and (b) result with the algorithm in ref. [9] (note that to be included in a software package usable at hospitals, the latter segmentation result based on the 2D algorithm still requires postprocessing for reconstruction of data in 3D space).

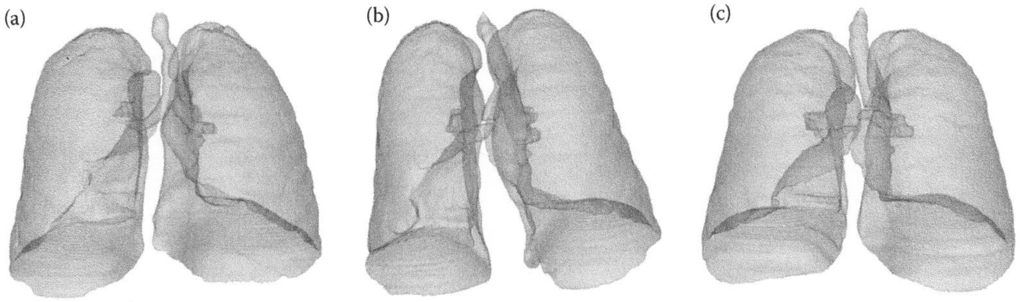

FIGURE 1.11
3D visualization of the segmented lung using the proposed approach.

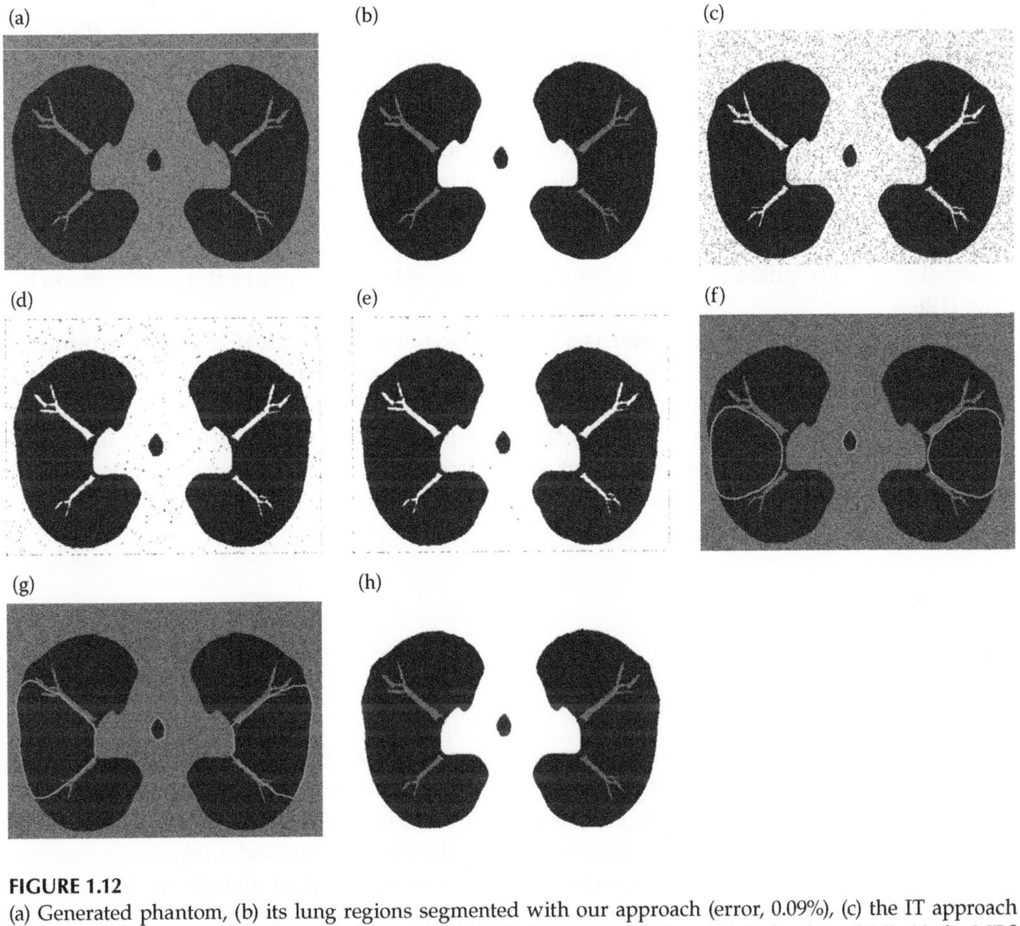

FIGURE 1.12
(a) Generated phantom, (b) its lung regions segmented with our approach (error, 0.09%), (c) the IT approach (error, 5.97%), (d) the ICM algorithm (least error, 2.91% obtained with the potential value of 0.3), (e) the MRS algorithm (error, 1.98% with the potential value of 0.3 and three resolution levels), (f) the deformable model using the traditional image gradient as an external force (error, 59.4%), the deformable model with the gradient vector field as an external force (g; error, 51.9%), and the ground truth (h).

TABLE 1.1

Comparison of Algorithm Accuracies

	Segmentation Algorithm					
Error (%)	**This Study**	**IT**	**MRS**	**ICM**	**DMG**	**GVF**
Minimum	0.1	2.81	1.9	2.03	10.1	4.10
Maximum	2.15	21.9	9.8	17.1	29.1	18.2
Mean	0.32	10.9	5.1	9.80	15.1	13.2
SD	0.71	6.04	3.31	5.11	7.77	4.81
Significance		<10–4	<10–3	<10–4	<10–4	<10–4

Note: The accuracy of our segmentation in comparison with five conventional algorithms (IT, MRS, ICM, the gradient-based deformable model DMG, and the deformable model based on the gradient vector flow; GVF).

demonstrates the 3D visualization of the segmented lung region using the proposed approach. In these and in preceding experiments, the errors are evaluated with respect to the ground truth produced by an expert. However, these prototypes may contain errors due to hand positioning instabilities during manual segmentation. To better measure the accuracy of our approach, we have created a 3D geometric phantom with the same gray level distribution in regions as in the CT slices at hand. An axial cross section in this synthetic phantom, its ideal region map, and the results of our segmentation are shown in Figure 1.12. The error between the found regions and ground truth (0.09%) confirms the high accuracy of the proposed segmentation techniques. For comparison, Figure 1.12 also shows the segmentation obtained with the IT approach, the ICM algorithm [10], the MRS algorithm [9], the deformable model that uses the traditional gradient-based external force [11], and the more advanced deformable model using the gradient vector flow [12].

The previous experiments, as well as additional experiments with 1820 different bimodal LDCT slices, have shown that our segmentation yields much better results than several more conventional algorithms. As indicated in Table 1.1, the most accurate algorithm among these latter algorithms, namely, the MRS [9], has the larger error range of 1.9% to 9.8%, a mean error of 5.1% with respect to the ground truth. Our segmentation has the notably smaller error range of 0.1% to 2.15% and its mean error of 0.32% is more than 15 times lower.

1.4 Conclusions

Our experiments show that the proposed accurate identification of the Markov–Gibbs random field model demonstrates promising results in segmenting the lung region from LDCT images. The main difference with respect to more conventional schemes is in the use of precise LCDG models to approximate signal distributions and analytical estimates of the MGRF parameters. The proposed segmentation techniques include (i) the accurate sequential initialization to form a starting LCDG model, (ii) the modified EM algorithm for refining the starting model, and (iii) the iterative map refinement using the identified conditional MGRF model. Our present implementation on C^{++} programming language on the Intel dual processor (3 GHz each) with 8-GB memory and 1.5-TB hard drive with RAID technology takes about 596 s for processing 182 LDCT slices of 512 × 512 pixels size each, i.e., about 3.27 s per slice.

References

1. American Cancer Society. 2006. *Cancer Facts and Figures.*
2. Sluimer, I., A. Schilham, M. Prokop, and B. van Ginneken. 2006. Computer analysis of computed tomography scans of the lung: A survey. *IEEE Transactions on Medical Imaging*, 25(4):385–405.
3. Hu, S., E. A. Hoffman, and J. Reinhardt. 2001. Automatic lung segmentation for accurate quantitation of volumetric x-ray CT images. *IEEE Transactions on Medical Imaging*, 20(6):490–498.
4. Sluimer, I., M. Prokop, and B. van Ginneken. 2005. Toward automated segmentation of the pathological lung in CT. *IEEE Transactions on Medical Imaging*, 24(8):1025–1038.
5. Duda, R.O., P.E. Hart, and D.G. Stork. 2001. *Pattern Classification*. 2nd ed. New York: Wiley.
6. Goshtasby, A., and W.D. O'Neill. 1999. Curve fitting by a sum of Gaussians. *CVGIP: Graphical Models and Image Processing*, 56(4):281–288.
7. Gimel'farb, G.L. 1999. *Image Textures and Gibbs Random Fields*. Dordrecht: Kluwer Academic.
8. Schlesinger, M.I., and V. Hlavac. 2002. *Ten Lectures on Statistical and Structural Pattern Recognition*. Dordrecht: Kluwer Academic.
9. Bouman, C., and B. Liu. 1991. Multiple resolution segmentation of textured images. *IEEE Transactions on Pattern Analysis and Machine Intelligence*, 13:99–113.
10. Besag, J.E. 1986. On the statistical analysis of dirty pictures. *Journal of the Royal Statistical Society. Series B, Statistical Methodology*, B48:259–302.
11. Kass, M., A. Witkin, and D. Terzopoulos. 1987. Snakes: Active contour models. *International Journal of Computer Vision*, 1:321–331.
12. Xu, C., and J.L. Prince. 1998. Snakes, shapes, and gradient vector flow. *IEEE Transactions on Pattern Analysis and Machine Intelligence*, 7:359–369.

2

Incremental Engineering of Lung Segmentation Systems

Avishkar Misra, Arcot Sowmya, and Paul Compton

CONTENTS

In recent decades, medical imaging has become an increasingly invaluable resource for physicians by providing them with a noninvasive view inside the patient, allowing them to diagnose diseases (Doi 2005), plan for surgical interventions (Archip et al. 2006), and evaluate the effectiveness of treatments (Pien et al. 2005). More than 95 million high-tech scans, including computed tomography (CT), magnetic resonance imaging, and positron emission tomography, are conducted in the United States each year (Kolata 2009). Automatic interpretation of medical images by computer-aided detection or diagnosis (CAD) systems have the potential not only to significantly reduce the burden on physicians to interpret a large number of medical scans in a timely manner, but also to improve their consistency in diagnosis across patient populations (Doi 2005). A fundamental component of any CAD system is medical image segmentation (Reinhardt et al. 2000; Sluimer et al. 2006).

The design and development of medical image segmentation systems is an extremely challenging task. A reasonably complex segmentation system has a number of components or processes intelligently combined to achieve the system goals. Computer vision experts, who develop these systems, must selectively apply various vision techniques and articulate the knowledge necessary to guide the image segmentation and interpretation tasks. In doing this, the expert articulates domain and control knowledge (Draper et al. 1996; Crevier and Lepage 1997; Clouard et al. 1999; Wangehheim et al. 2000). Image segmentation systems that segment lung regions in high-resolution CT (HRCT) scans require control knowledge about how to combine and apply the various computer vision algorithms appropriately, as well as knowledge about the medical domain itself, such as the anatomy or the appearance of anatomical structures under x-rays. The knowledge that experts attempt to encode in systems must address the complexities and intricacies of the domain.

Experts usually develop lung segmentation systems guided by their understanding of the segmentation techniques, the domain, as well as their intuitions. This naturally means that the quality of expertise available to develop these systems governs the quality of the resulting system. Considering that "the mental operations that we perform to interpret images lie almost totally beyond the threshold of consciousness" (Crevier and Lepage 1997), it is not surprising that experts find it so difficult to articulate the knowledge required. Vision experts therefore tend to be quasi experts, in the sense that they have a general understanding of how to interpret an image, but lack the specific knowledge of how the selection of algorithms and their parameters affect the interpretation of the image. Although pattern recognition and machine learning methods mitigate the influences of quasi-expertise by automatically deriving knowledge from the domain data (Duda et al. 2000), they do require a significant amount of labeled data. This would require medical experts to mark accurate ground truth for a large number of training instances, which can be difficult because of the demands on the expert's time. Even though some methods such as graph cut (Boykov and Kolmogorov 2004; Massoptier et al. 2009) eliminate the need for labeled data, they do require experts to design cost functions appropriate to the task and to tune their parameters. One can argue that defining a cost function is a skilled task, requiring significant domain and vision expertise, and this leaves systems yet again vulnerable to the influence of quasi-expertise. As Draper (2003) argues, vision researchers are "once again applying informal control policies under the guise of a theoretically sound system. Feature quality determines the quality of the image interpretation, but the features are selected heuristically."

In practice, experts discover the features appropriate for a specific segmentation task by trial-and-error, revising the features and tuning the parameters of the algorithms in a relatively ad hoc manner. The ad hoc incremental approach to engineering systems naturally introduces the risk in which changes made to correct errors for certain cases may unwittingly lead to errors for other cases that were correctly handled earlier. Furthermore, changes to one part of the system may adversely affect the performance of other parts of the system. The risk of system degradation because of well-intended changes grows in line with the size and complexity of the system. Yet, it is common practice for experts to tweak algorithms and tune the parameters of algorithms incrementally.

This chapter presents a framework called ProcessNet that helps experts to incrementally engineer a lung HRCT image segmentation system. ProcessNet allows experts to systematically revise existing algorithms, tune their parameters, or add newly developed algorithms in an image segmentation system. The framework enables experts to incrementally develop the system in a structured manner despite evolving expertise and incrementally available data. The incremental revisions also provide an opportunity for continual system improvement and adaptation for specific segmentation tasks. An expert developing a system using ProcessNet may continue to improve its components over time, even as it goes into production use.

A lung anatomy segmentation system built using ProcessNet demonstrates continual improvement in the segmentation of lung, spine, sternum, and shoulder blades, visible within a sparse HRCT study for a patient. Although the primary goal is the accurate segmentation of lung regions, the segmentation of other anatomical structures provides useful anatomical cues and partial registration to facilitate lung segmentation. Each of these anatomical structures must be segmented to sufficiently accurate levels and face their own segmentation challenges. ProcessNet mitigates the risks of incremental ad hoc revisions by the expert within the complex anatomy segmentation system.

This chapter is organized as follows. A background to some of the methods used in medical image segmentation systems along with the challenges they face appears in Section 2.1. A formulation of medical image systems as a network of processes is presented in Section 2.2. This forms the basis for the ProcessNet framework introduced in Section 2.3. A lung anatomy segmentation system that is incrementally developed using ProcessNet is introduced in Section 2.4. A discussion in Section 2.5 highlights the benefits and limitations of the ProcessNet system, followed by a summation in Section 2.6.

2.1 Background

Medical image segmentation systems attempt to partition an image into regions representing specific tissue or anatomical structures (Bankman 2008). To achieve these goals, several computer vision techniques have been applied to a range of medical imaging modalities. Regular reviews of the emerging challenges and techniques used in medical image analysis for various modalities have been conducted (Deklerck et al. 1993; Duncan and Ayache 2000; Frangi et al. 2001; Ginneken et al. 2001; Noble and Boukerroui 2006; Sluimer et al. 2006; Bankman 2008). The following sections present some of the approaches used to segment medical images and the challenges to accurately segment lungs in HRCT studies.

2.1.1 Approaches to Medical Image Segmentation

Over the years, experts have developed a plethora of methods to automatically segment medical images. Some of the common approaches to medical image segmentation include (Sluimer et al. 2006; Bankman 2008) classical image analysis, knowledge-based or syntactic techniques, deformable model-fitting, classification-based techniques, and atlas-based segmentation via registration.

Each of the approaches is described briefly and the challenges that experts face in using these techniques are highlighted. Although we focus on the segmentation of lungs in HRCT scans, relevant work highlighting novel techniques and applications in ultrasound and magnetic resonance imaging segmentation are also discussed. None of the applications, however, have thus far addressed the challenges of evolving quasi-expertise and labeled data, which are both encountered in developing medical imaging systems.

2.1.1.1 Classical Image Analysis

Classical image analysis techniques use standard image processing algorithms to segment an image into separate regions. Rogowska (2008) provides a good introduction to some of the fundamental imaging techniques used by medical image segmentation systems. These techniques use a variety of image processing algorithms such as thresholding, outlining, edge detection, morphological operators, and filters, with the objective of detecting regions or edges that define the boundaries between regions of anatomical structures (Ballard and Brown 1982). In almost all cases, a number of image processing algorithms are combined intelligently to develop a system that is capable of automatically segmenting the desired anatomy. Applications of classical image analysis techniques to the segmentation of CT and HRCT images have been reported (Ballard and Sklansky 1976; Giger et al. 1990; Duryea and Boone 1995; Armato et al. 1998; Hu et al. 2001; Zheng et al. 2003; Ukil and Reinhardt 2004; Zhou et al. 2006).

Almost all authors adapted similar approaches to segmenting anatomy within their specific imaging modalities and segmentation objectives. In the segmentation of the lung in HRCT images, the techniques used take advantage of the contrast between the air-filled lungs and the surrounding tissues. In normal circumstances, a fixed threshold value of −1000 Hounsfield units would provide a segmentation of regions filled with air. A single global threshold value, however, often does not lead to good separation between tissues and, therefore, locally adaptive thresholding methods are often used. Adaptive thresholding and region-growing have been used (Zheng et al. 2003) and a three-dimensional (3D) watershed algorithm to segment lung regions in CT images has been used (Kuhnigk et al. 2003). Despite best efforts, thresholding may result in noise or undesirable connection between tissues, especially because of the presence of disease or imaging artifacts. Therefore, morphological operators such as erosion and dilation are used to eliminate noise and improve segmentation. Spatial and frequency domain filtering is also used to eliminate noise and segment anatomical regions (Malik and Choi 2006).

Although most approaches attempt to segment a specific part of the anatomy, Zhou et al. (2006) segment multiple anatomical structures simultaneously. Their segmentation algorithm takes advantage of dense multidetector CT (MDCT) studies, in which more than 400 images provide better continuity between the slices, as compared with sparse HRCT studies with only 20 to 30 images. The proximity between the slices within MDCT studies makes it easier for algorithms to take advantage of continuity between images.

These techniques, however, are sensitive to noise, and because of the brittle nature of the algorithms, are seldom used in isolation. Instead, classical image analysis techniques are used in conjunction with other techniques, usually in preprocessing and segmentation stages. Classical image analysis techniques encode the required domain and control knowledge implicitly within the algorithms and the parameter values selected to control those algorithms. Experts develop classical image analysis–based systems by selecting intelligent combinations of the algorithms and their parameters.

2.1.1.2 Knowledge-Based or Syntactic Techniques

Knowledge-based or syntactic techniques represent knowledge in an explicit form independent of the image processing algorithms. The representations include rules (Matsuyama

1988; Levine and Nazif 1985), frames (McKeown et al. 1985), or semantic networks representing relationships (Freuder 1977; Paulus et al. 2000) and domain ontology (Maillot et al. 2004) between parts of the anatomy. By expressing characteristics about the anatomical structures and relationships between the structures, the vision system can gather support and reason about thus far unidentified objects within the scene. Rules also allow the expression of knowledge applicable under specific conditions, making it easier for experts to articulate the context-based applicability of a particular algorithm, parameter, or classification. Because these systems are closely related to expert systems for vision, they are commonly referred to as expert- or knowledge-based techniques.

Some examples of such systems include ANGY, a rule-based system to interpret angiograms (Stansfield 1986); IBIS, a rule and semantic network-based system to interpret magnetic resonance imaging (Vernazza et al. 1987); a system for 3D reconstruction of angiograms (Declaere et al. 1991); VISIPLAN, a hierarchical planning framework (Gong and Kulikowski 1994); a chest x-ray (radiography) segmentation system (Brown et al. 1998); a rule-based system to detect spinal cord in CT (Archip et al. 2002); and a multiagent system to segment intravascular ultrasound images (Bovenkamp et al. 2009).

The symbolic representations of objects within a semantic network offer a concise representation. However, as the complexity of the domain grows, describing and maintaining the relationships between the growing number of components becomes a challenge. The authors of the schema system (Draper et al. 1989) note that it took them over a month to develop and revise a relatively small semantic network. There may also be multiple relationships between the objects, according to different contexts. Bovenkamp et al. (2009) state that more than 450 rules were added to guide the image segmentation, yet no strategy was identified to ensure that the consistency and accuracy of the rules was maintained.

2.1.1.3 Deformable Model Fitting

Deformable model-fitting techniques represent expectations about an object being sought in a model, that is, fitted directly to the image data (McInerney and Terzopoulos 2009). In contrast with rigid pattern or template-matching techniques (Ballard and Brown 1982; Grimson 1990), deformable models allow the model to be deformed to fit the evidence within the images, albeit within certain limits. These techniques fit the model to the image data via optimization methods using energy or cost functions that evaluate the quality of the fit. The energy or cost function is often a composite of multiple terms, evaluating different aspects of the fit such as structural integrity of the boundary, the likely shape of the desired object, and the edges or regions in the image most likely to represent the object.

A variety of deformable models have been developed and applied to medical image segmentation, each of which attempts to find boundaries of regions or regions of homogeneity. These include active contours (Kass et al. 1988; McInerney and Terzopoulos 1996), active shape models (Cootes et al. 1995), active appearance models (Cootes et al. 2001), and level sets (Osher and Sethian 1988; Lin et al. 2004; Cremers et al. 2007).

He et al. (2008) provide a comparative study of various forms of deformable contour methods for medical image segmentation. Heimann and Meinzer (2009) provide a review of statistical shape models for 3D medical image segmentation. Lin et al. (2004) have incorporated region and boundary conditions in level sets.

The challenge in developing a deformable model-based solution is the high level of vision expertise required in defining the energy function and selecting its parameters. In addition, some techniques such as active contours must be initialized close to the target anatomical region; therefore, this requires either manual intervention or classical image analysis techniques to gain an initial estimate to automatically initialize the contours. Meanwhile, region growing or wave propagation techniques such as level sets (Osher and Sethian 1988) or T-snakes (McInerney and Terzopoulos 2000) may spill over the intended boundary in the absence of a sufficiently strong boundary condition, which therefore must be balanced by other terms within the energy function, such as shape information. Successful segmentation via deformable models rely on the weights for the terms within the energy function, which is a complex control problem understood poorly by the experts (Ozertem and Erdogmus 2007; He et al. 2008). Therefore, the definition of the energy function and the selection of its weights requires significant development effort via trial and error.

2.1.1.4 Classification-Based Techniques

Classification-based techniques attempt to label individual pixels or regions segmented using classical image analysis techniques with the labels of the anatomical structure of interest. These techniques derive numeric (continuous) or nominal (categorical) features from the pixel, a region, or the entire image, and use a classifier to predict the membership of specific classes. The classifier is developed using a variety of pattern recognition and machine learning techniques (Mitchell 1997; Duda et al. 2000; Jain et al. 2000). Factors such as similarity measures (e.g., clustering; Sutton 2010) or *k*-nearest neighbor (Jain et al. 1999), probabilistic support (e.g., Bayesian inference (MacKay 2003, p. 457), decision boundary (e.g., decision trees; Murthy 1998), support vector machines (Drucker et al. 1996), or neural networks (Wismueller 2010) are used by the classifier to perform class predictions.

McNitt-Gray et al. (1995) classified pixels into regions of the heart, lung, and axilla in chest radiographs. Zhang and Valentino (2001) used artificial neural networks to classify pixels within CT scans. Wei (2002) extracted frequency domain features from the image and used *k*-nearest neighbor clustering for segmentation. Ghosh and Mitchell (2006) have used genetic algorithms to evolve the level set function to segment the prostate in CT images. Sahba et al. (2007) have used reinforcement learning in the segmentation of ultrasound images. As mentioned previously, pattern recognition and machine learning techniques require experts to devise useful features and gather a sufficient amount of labeled data for training the classifier.

Recently, graph cuts (Boykov and Jolly 2001) were used in the segmentation of lung in HRCT (Massoptier et al. 2009). These techniques classify each pixel within the image as either belonging to the foreground representing the desired object or the background. These techniques have demonstrated good segmentation results without requiring large amounts of labeled data to induce the classifier. The expert constructs cost functions that consider the membership of a pixel to the foreground or background, whereas also taking into account the membership of its neighboring pixels. This involves considerable involvement from vision experts in defining and tuning a complex cost function, similar to the definition of the energy function used by deformable model-fitting techniques.

2.1.1.5 Atlas-Based Segmentation via Registration

Atlas-based segmentation techniques, also known as segmentation via registration, attempt to segment a new image by drawing a correspondence between the new image and a previously segmented atlas (Maintz and Viergever 1998). The atlas is often the representative or average of the variations in the anatomy. Once a correspondence between the pixels of the image and the atlas has been established, the labels from each pixel within the atlas can be applied to pixels in the image. The matching process is framed as an optimization process, looking to improve the level of similarity between corresponding pixels, whereas maintaining relational consistency between the aligned pixels.

Atlas-based segmentation has been used in segmenting magnetic resonance images of the brain and heart (Kikinis et al. 1996; Cuadra et al. 2004; Lorenzo-Valdes et al. 2002) as well as CT of the abdomen (Park et al. 2000) and lungs (Zhang and Reinhardt 2000; Li et al. 2002; Zhang et al. 2003; Sluimer et al. 2004). Sluimer et al. (2004) used classifier techniques to improve the quality of segmentation at the boundaries between regions, despite the presence of diseases.

Atlas-based segmentation techniques have the advantage of being robust in the presence of disease (Sluimer et al. 2004). However, to construct a statistically significant atlas, considerable effort is required in labeling pixels from a large number of training images, as well as aligning and deforming these in the process of generating the atlas.

2.1.2 Challenges to Segmenting Lungs in HRCT

In addition to the developmental challenges of quasi-expertise and incrementally available data, image segmentation systems face challenges specific to their domain. These challenges vary according to the nature of the anatomy and the imaging modality used. Interpretation of HRCT images, particularly in the presence of diffuse lung diseases (Webb 1990), faces a number of challenges that medical image segmentation systems must also contend with (Sluimer et al. 2006). These can be categorized as: (1) interpatient and intrapatient variations, (2) real and artificial artifacts, and (3) competing definitions of ground truth. Each of these challenges is briefly discussed.

2.1.2.1 Interpatient and Intrapatient Variations

There is a significant amount of natural variation in the expected anatomy, both within a patient and across patient groups. For example, the shape of the lung within the apical region (roughly top third) is circular, whereas the shape of the lung within the basal region (roughly bottom third) has a sickle-like shape. Therefore, a shape model or template to identify a lung must allow for a significant degree of variation across the images. Similarly, the lungs of a 68-year-old man would vary significantly in size, when compared with those of a 16-year-old girl.

2.1.2.2 Real and Artificial Artifacts

A range of real and artificial artifacts can affect the appearance of objects in the images. Artificial artifacts are those that are introduced in the process of acquiring the scans, and may not appear if scanned differently or at another time. Meanwhile, real artifacts are those that exist within the body and influence the appearance of the anatomy, and cannot be eliminated by changing the scanning protocol.

An example of an artificial artifact is the movement of a beating heart, which may appear as blurring of the boundaries, as shown in Figure 2.1a. CAD systems could mistake the high opacity of the motion artifact as abnormal lung tissue indicative of consolidation. Another example of an artificial artifact is the change in the density of the lung tissue because of gravity. This would show up in different parts of the lung, depending

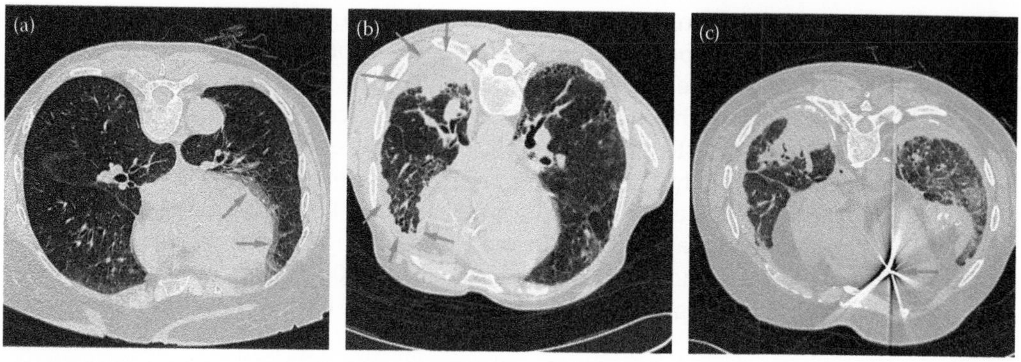

FIGURE 2.1
Three examples of real and artificial artifacts: (a) motion artifact because of a beating heart, (b) pleural plaques deforming lung tissue, and (c) metallic staples in the heart.

on whether the patient is lying on their stomach (i.e., prone) or back (i.e., supine) during the scan.

Similarly, real artifacts also complicate the task of automatic segmentation. Because medical scans are generally taken to facilitate diagnosis for a patient presenting with medical symptoms, the patient is more likely to have a disease of some kind. In many cases, the presence of disease may influence not just the anatomy or tissue that it affects, but also the adjacent structures, by deforming a structure's shape and position. A patient with severe pleural plaques in the right lung is shown in Figure 2.1b. The degradation of the pleural tissue of the lung gives it the appearance of muscle tissue outside the lung. Lung boundary segmentation may incorrectly segment the boundary at the edges of the darker air-filled regions, instead of the correct lung boundary marked by the blue arrows.

Another form of real artifact occasionally observed in scans is caused by the presence of implants, such as that shown in Figure 2.1c. The bright streaking effects, because of the metal staples embedded within the patient's heart, makes it difficult to segment the sternum, which may serve as an anatomical landmark for subsequent segmentation of other parts. The streaking effect also influences the appearance of the lung tissue.

2.1.2.3 Conflicting Ground Truth Definitions

Although ideally, one expects that all radiologists have the same notion of truth in defining anatomy, there are often differing perspectives among them, with disagreement on the delineation of an anatomical structure's boundary. For example, a radiologist may delineate the lung boundary by considering the region with the lung tissue as indicated by the green line in Figure 2.2a. Another radiologist may consider the bronchial tree at the hilum to be a part of the lung as shown by the blue line in Figure 2.2b.

Similarly, radiologists may disagree on the categorization of certain disease-affected tissue, and the ensuing differential diagnosis. This is particularly common when a patient has multiple pathologies or diseases and requires arbitration from more experienced radiologists. HRCT for diffuse lung diseases also tends to have a high level of variations in interobserver and intraobserver interpretations (Aziz et al. 2004). This is mainly because of the lack of standard criteria.

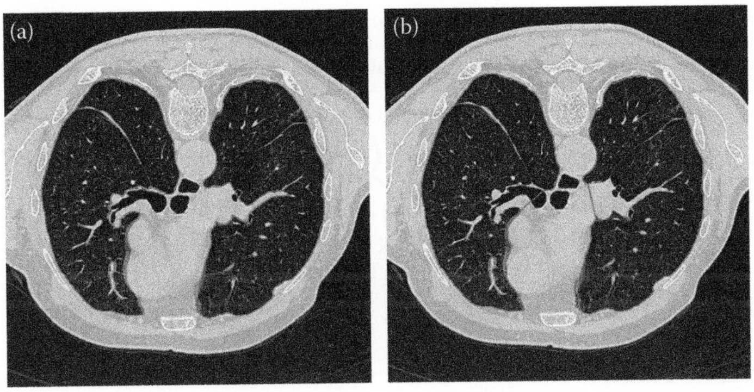

FIGURE 2.2
Differences in lung boundary delineation by experts: (a) marking by expert A and (b) marking by expert B.

2.2 ProcessNet as a Network of Processes

A lung HRCT image segmentation system can be formulated as a network of processes, wherein each process is responsible for a specific task. Each process produces an output and consumes the outputs from other processes as its input. All of the processes, in undertaking their specific task, collectively solve the overall system goals. The system can be represented as a directed graph in which each process is a node and a connection between them depicts the information flow between the processes. Note that only directed acyclic graphs are considered, so the system will have no circular dependencies between processes. A sorted topology of the system dependency graph provides the order in which the processes must be executed, such that data requirements for each process are satisfied. This sequence is called the process run order, which imposes no restriction on the parallel execution of processes and merely requires that if process B depends on the output of process A, then process B must only be executed after process A has produced the required data.

The algorithms within each process express domain and control knowledge to guide the various tasks. Over time, the expert might make changes to individual processes to improve the accuracy with which a process undertakes its task. Alternatively, the expert might introduce new processes to add new functionality to the system. The nature of a process and the types of changes that may affect the processes within the system are now discussed.

2.2.1 Internals of a Process

A process represents an arbitrarily complex algorithmic step. It may implement a simple image thresholding algorithm or apply the more sophisticated deformable models. Internally, a process may call on a machine learning algorithm or a decision tree to guide the selection of an algorithm, parameter values for the algorithm, or to classify a case. Such knowledge-based processes have the capacity to intelligently guide the processing appropriate to the circumstances of the input. Alternatively, a process may be a single processing algorithm, with no dynamic context-specific control.

In both scenarios, the process captures and applies the knowledge necessary to guide its specific task and contribute to the overall segmentation goals of the system. Considering

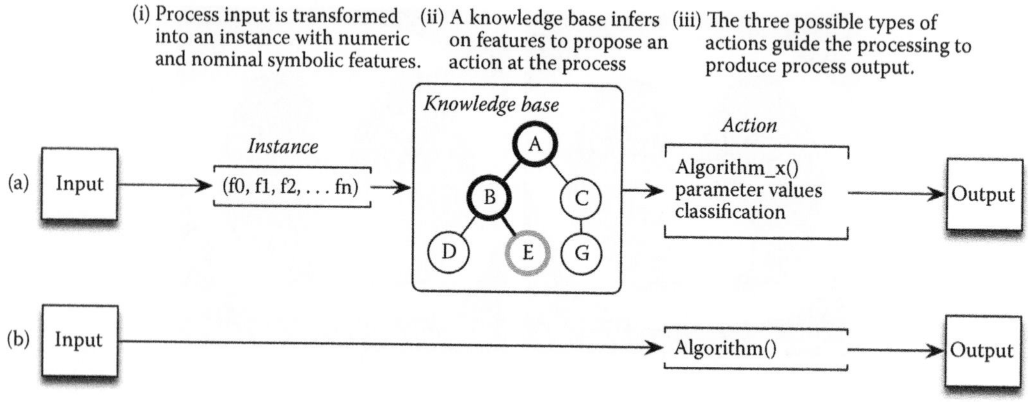

FIGURE 2.3
Internal processing steps for (a) a knowledge-based process and (b) a fixed algorithm.

the evolving nature of knowledge when developing such systems, it is reasonable to expect that even the single processing algorithm may undergo revisions, as problems or limits with the algorithm are detected.

The core functions of (a) a typical knowledge-based process and (b) a fixed algorithm process are shown in Figure 2.3. The knowledge-based process carries out three basic tasks:

i. Input data is transformed into features and represented as an inferable instance or case.
ii. The knowledge base infers on the instance or case to predict the action. The action may be the selection of an algorithm sequence, the parameters for an algorithm, or the class label to assign to the case.
iii. The actual processing as dictated by the action, generating the process output.

The internal functions of a machine learning–based process are similar to that of a knowledge-based process, with the inference system using a decision-making function defined by the machine learning algorithm used. The machine learning algorithm would also attempt to predict the action of the process, based on the features derived from the input data.

A process with a handcrafted vision algorithm may operate directly on the input data without deriving any features or inferring the correct algorithm, parameter, or label to assign. In such a process, the algorithm explicitly encodes the knowledge required to consume the process input and produce the output.

2.2.2 Changes Affecting a Process

The correct behavior of a process may be influenced by changes both external and internal to the process because of incremental revisions to the system. The four types of changes that may adversely affect process capacity to correctly carry out its task are changes to:

i. Raw input. Input data for a process may change if the output of other processes that serves as input to this process, changes. Alternatively, an expert may introduce new data sources, or remove redundant ones, that are no longer deemed to be useful for the process.

ii. Feature extraction. The derivation and expression of features that are used by an inference system may be revised, as the expressive limits of existing features are discovered. Experts often invent new features or project current features into new feature spaces, leading to changes in the derivation and expression of features.

iii. Control or inference knowledge. The decision-making mechanism that determines the actions of the process may change. These actions might be the selection of an algorithm, parameters to use, or the classification label. The inference system may be constructed using multiple machine learning techniques that guide the processing using different features. Improvements to the inference system may occur in the light of more labeled data becoming available for training, or revisions to the learning algorithms and its parameters. Examples include the induction of a decision tree from available data, and tuning of its pruning parameters.

iv. Algorithm, parameter mappings, and class labels. The actual processing algorithms, parameter mappings, and labels, which are used as actions of the process, may change. These algorithms may be improved independently of the control knowledge within the inference system.

A process representing a fixed algorithm may face changes to its input (i) and the algorithm itself (iv), whereas a knowledge-based vision process may encounter changes at any of the four levels. A method to help experts to manage these changes is presented in the following section.

2.3 ProcessNet Framework

The ProcessNet framework applies the concepts of incremental validated change management that have been successfully used by ripple-down rules (RDR) in addressing incremental ad hoc revision to knowledge in a variety of domains (Compton and Jansen 1988). Over the past two decades, RDRs have been successfully applied to a range of complex classification, control, and search problems. Richards (2009) presents an excellent review of RDR research during the last two decades. Although details about RDR are presented in Section 2.3.1, the key inspiration drawn from RDR is to ensure that any change made to knowledge is allowed only if the knowledge is maintained consistent to the evidence that has led to the knowledge thus far. Grounding of knowledge on evidence is fundamental to the process of scientific discovery (Popper 1963). In RDR, the knowledge is maintained within rules and the evidence is maintained in the form of cornerstone cases that act as support for the knowledge within the rule. Any changes to the rules are evaluated against the cornerstone cases of the rules potentially affected by the revision.

The ProcessNet framework generalizes the incremental case-based revision of RDR knowledge bases to system engineering in general. In ProcessNet, a segmentation system is represented as an acyclic network of processes, each of which may represent its internal knowledge in a form independent of other processes. The processes apply their knowledge and communicate the results to other processes. The knowledge within a ProcessNet processes may be represented within any arbitrary form. The ProcessNet framework offers strategies for:

i. Detecting changes and evaluating their effect on the processes within the ProcessNet, discussed in Section 2.3.2.
ii. Managing the impact of changes on processes within the ProcessNet, discussed in Section 2.3.3.

These two central tasks are critical for systematic incremental engineering of medical image segmentation systems, and form the change management mechanisms of ProcessNet. An example of validation of a ProcessNet system is demonstrated in Section 2.3.3. Details about an implementation of the ProcessNet framework used to build medical image segmentation system are presented in Section 2.3.4.

2.3.1 Ripple-Down Rules

RDRs are an incremental knowledge acquisition technique that recognizes the inability of experts to correctly and completely articulate the knowledge necessary when constructing knowledge- or expert-based systems (Compton and Jansen 1989). These are the same challenges encountered by quasi experts in vision domains, as they attempt to engineer medical image segmentation systems in light of evolving expertise and incrementally available data. RDRs provide decision-making support by classifying a given instance (or case) according to its characteristics or features. A case is defined in terms of the features that serve as input to the RDR and the predicted conclusion.

RDRs maintain knowledge in a nested hierarchy of rules and their exception rules. Each rule within the RDR knowledge base defines the context or conditions, which must be met in order for the rule to be applicable for a given case. A rule may have exception rules that override its conclusion, provided the context of the exception rules is also met by the case. Therefore, the inference process begins at a root rule and progresses down the rules and their exceptions until the last firing rule is reached. The conclusion of the last firing rule defines the conclusion for the given case. This conclusion represents a classification for a task given the context of the case interpreted by the knowledge base.

Recognizing the fact that knowledge within a knowledge base may not be complete, RDRs provide an easy way for experts to correct and update the incorrect knowledge. If the concluding RDR rule is incorrect and misclassifies a given case, the expert can correct the RDR knowledge base by adding a new exception rule to the misclassifying rule. In constructing the new rule, the expert merely has to justify his or her conclusion by defining the context of the new rule, such that it correctly applies to or "covers" the new case. A training event is initiated whenever a case or instance is incorrectly classified, prompting the expert to provide an exception rule to correct this behavior.

To ensure that a change to the knowledge base does not degrade existing knowledge, RDRs use validated change criteria that must be satisfied before the addition of a new exception rule. Each rule in an RDR knowledge base retains cornerstone cases, which are exemplars used to construct or modify the rule. A new exception rule must cover the training case, whereas not changing the conclusion of cornerstones of the parent and sibling rules within the neighborhood. The nested hierarchy of rules and their exceptions means that the expert has to consider only a small subset of cornerstone cases when attempting a revision to an existing knowledge base.

RDR knowledge bases are built incrementally, with each new rule added to resolve an error as it is discovered with new cases. Unlike batch mode learning systems, there is no distinction between the knowledge construction phase and knowledge application phase. They are equally part of the continuum of knowledge maintenance, where knowledge is used and corrected as and when issues are discovered. This makes RDR particularly effective in successfully operating in domains where data becomes available incrementally.

RDR are able to elicit even tacit knowledge that may not be consciously recognized by the domain experts, but used subconsciously in the application of their expertise to address complex tasks within the domain. The ease with which RDR facilitates changes to the knowledge base means that experts can quickly build large knowledge bases that eventually converge to describe the knowledge required to undertake the task. RDR have demonstratively addressed the knowledge acquisition bottleneck faced by expert-engineered knowledge-based systems in a number of applications including the interpretation of pathology results (Compton and Jansen 1988; Compton et al. 2006), very-large-scale-integration design (Bekmann and Hoffmann 2005), network security (Prayote 2007), and image analysis (Amin et al. 1996; Kerr and Compton 2003; Misra et al. 2004, 2006; Singh and Compton 2005; Park et al. 2008).

The cornerstone case-based validation of changes does not eliminate all risks of degradation of the knowledge base, and the consistency of the knowledge is contingent on the quality of the cornerstone cases used to cover the possible variations within the domain. In practice, however, it offers experts a reasonable means to evaluate the quality of their revisions. Over time, as sufficient cases are evaluated by RDR, limitations in knowledge are highlighted and provide experts with specific exemplars to assist in their efforts to revise the knowledge base.

2.3.2 Detecting Process Change via Cornerstone Shift

In keeping with RDR, a case is defined for each process in terms of its raw input data and the resulting output. This ensures that a process only considers the minimal set of data sources necessary to undertake its task. The input and output data at a process capture the process-specific behavioral requirements. Like RDR, any changes made to a process should be motivated by a case, and once the change is made, the case is captured as a cornerstone case for the process. Each process is considered a knowledge source, the consistency of which is evaluated against the set of cornerstone cases that influenced its construction.

The effect of the four types of changes on process consistency can be detected by evaluating the cornerstone cases for the process. Any difference to the output and input data for a cornerstone case highlights a potential effect as a consequence of changes at either the process itself or at other processes that this process depends on for its input data, respectively. These differences are called cornerstone shifts.

A cornerstone case for a process captures an example describing the requirements for that given process, but may not capture the implicit contract of expectation that other dependent processes have with the process. Therefore, although the correctness of a process can be validated against its own cornerstone cases, the responsibility of validating its effect on dependent processes lies with the latter. Each of the dependent processes should also be evaluated for changes to their input and subsequent output, by checking against their own set of cornerstone cases. This is because the original process may not have insight into how its dependent processes use its output.

This approach frees the expert from having to consider the whole system when revising a single process. An expert improves the correctness of a specific process with respect to its cornerstone cases, with the expectation that other dependent processes take responsibility for detecting and handling the cornerstone shifts relevant to them, which is discussed in the following section. The cornerstone validation process starts at the first process that is modified and continues in the process run order. The requirement of ProcessNet to allow only acyclic dependencies ensures that each process needs to be evaluated only once during a single validation check.

2.3.3 Managing Cornerstone Shifts

As discussed previously, cornerstone shifts are any deviation in the input and output data of a cornerstone case because of changes within the system. The key difference between RDR and ProcessNet is the handling of cornerstone shifts. In RDR, only changes to the conclusions of a cornerstone case are allowed. This means that only process outputs may change, whereas the inputs to the process, and the features used to infer against the knowledge base, do not change. In vision domains, however, even the inputs to a process may change. Therefore, ProcessNet allows changes to any aspect of the cornerstone case, as long as the resulting output of the cornerstone case agrees with ground truth for that case.

Furthermore, the notion of truth and the nature of data within the vision domain may change over time with evolving domain insight. This means that even the ground truth for a cornerstone case may change. To accommodate for this, ProcessNet allows for shifts in cornerstones as long as they are consistent with the present notion of truth and are deemed to be acceptable by the expert. If cornerstone shifts do not agree with the available ground truth or the expert's notion of truth, then the expert must either revert the changes that lead to the cornerstone shift or make further changes to ensure consistent operation of the system.

Cornerstone shifts such that they no longer support the knowledge defined using the cornerstone cases might be handled in one of two ways guided by the two perspectives on the nature of knowledge. One perspective is that because the knowledge no longer has any support of the cornerstone cases, it should be removed and new knowledge defined using the "corrected" cornerstone case be added. An alternative perspective is that the knowledge is still valid, albeit with no current support for it. There may be cases that the process has correctly handled using this knowledge and it may continue to be relevant. Such a view suggests that knowledge previously defined is still valid, and may be retained, with new evidence recorded for that knowledge as soon as it becomes available.

Although there are valid arguments in support of both approaches, the implementation of ProcessNet removes knowledge that no longer has the support of any cornerstone cases. This ensures that the knowledge within a process can shift and evolve in line with the concept drift in the underlying domain (Agnew et al. 1997; Clancey 1997).

Not all cornerstone shifts will lead to revisions. For example, minor deviations within the image pixels may not influence the high-level interpretations for the case, namely, the process output. Each of the shifted cornerstones that continue to be handled correctly by the process can be safely ignored. Cornerstone cases no longer handled correctly, however, require the expert to revise the process to handle these cases correctly.

The specific changes made to a process to handle the new versions of cornerstone cases are contingent on the internal nature of the processes and the expert's own assessment. For example, a process using an RDR knowledge base may require new rules added to the knowledge base, whereas a process implementing a handcrafted algorithm in source code would require the expert to make changes to the algorithm's source code. Once all of the cornerstones at a process are handled correctly, the validation process can continue onto validating other processes that are dependent on any revised processes.

Detecting cornerstone shifts and revising processes to handle these shifts may continue sequentially down the dependency graph of processes. The order in which the processes are validated and revised is determined by the system run order, which is the order in which processes are executed to satisfy the data requirements. All changes to cornerstone cases and processes must be considered tentative until the entire system of processes has been validated. Once all of the processes of the system have been validated and revised to handle any cornerstone shifts, the entire system can then be considered valid and the changes committed. Otherwise, the expert can wind back changes to any process and cornerstone case. This flexibility allows the expert to treat the system as an experimental sandbox to try different solutions, where the merits of each solution are evaluated by the cornerstone cases.

2.3.4 Change Validation in a ProcessNet

Consider an example of a ProcessNet system with processes A to F as shown in Figure 2.4. The arrows indicate the data flow between the processes. One process run order for the system is A, B, C, D, E, F. The run order of A, E, C, B, D, F is just as valid. Because there is no dependency between processes B, C, and E, they can be executed in parallel and interleaved in any order.

Consider a scenario in which process B is modified. The cornerstone cases at B would be used to validate B's consistent behavior against its existing cornerstone cases. After that, its direct dependents—in this case, process D—will also be validated against their own cornerstone cases. If process D handles any shifts in its cornerstone cases correctly, the validation process may terminate here. However, if process D requires further revisions leading to changes in its output, then its dependent process F must also be validated.

Consider an alternate scenario in which processes A and D are modified at the same time. The validation will start at process A, followed by its dependents (B, C, and E). Once these processes have been validated and/or modified to handle any cornerstone shifts, process D will be validated to check its own changes and those resulting from changes to outputs of processes B and C. The sequential validation in the process run order for the acyclic network of processes means that each process needs to be verified only once.

The incremental revision and validation of individual processes and, collectively, the entire system ensures that the system continues to adapt in the light of more labeled data and evolving expertise.

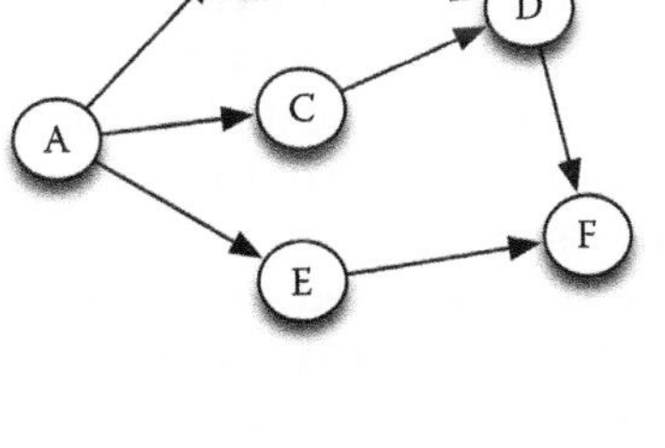

FIGURE 2.4
A typical ProcessNet system.

2.4 Lung Anatomy Segmentation Using ProcessNet

The ProcessNet framework has been used to incrementally develop an anatomy segmentation system that automatically segments multiple anatomical regions visible within sparse HRCT studies from real patients. Each HRCT study has an average of 15 images of 1 mm thickness, spaced every 15 mm along the axial plane of the body. The sparse HRCT studies lack the spatial continuity between images that was available within the MDCT studies used by Zhou et al. (2006). The sparse HRCT studies are, however, useful to detect a variety of diffuse diseases affecting the lung parenchyma. This is because they provide high spatial resolution while exposing patients to a lower dose of radiation as compared with MDCT studies. The studies were from real patients experiencing a variety of diffuse lung diseases that affected the parenchyma and pleura of the lung. A few patients had metallic implants within the body that introduced noisy artifacts in the scans, further complicating the segmentation task.

The anatomy segmentation system developed using ProcessNet segments the spine, sternum, shoulder blades, trachea, bronchi, esophagus, and lungs. Although the primary goal of the anatomy segmentation system is to correctly segment lung regions, the segmentation of the other anatomical structures provides useful spatial and anatomical cues. The expert incrementally introduces processes to undertake smaller tasks, which collectively operate to segment the anatomy. Each anatomical structure segmented relies on multiple processes. A process may implement an algorithm or call on a library of image processing functions available within the ImageJ library (Rasband 1997). A number of processes use RDR decision trees internally to guide classification.

The application of the ProcessNet framework to medical image segmentation evaluates three aspects of the framework and the developed system. First is an evaluation of ProcessNet in the development of the anatomy segmentation system in Section 2.4.1, which presents details about ProcessNet in operation. The capacity to continually revise and develop the anatomy segmentation system using ProcessNet means that it is never deemed finished. However, a snapshot of the anatomy segmentation system at the end of nine patient studies, denoted as PN9, is presented in Section 2.4.2. Finally, quantitative evaluation of the evolving anatomy segmentation system during various development stages is presented in Section 2.4.3.

2.4.1 Evaluation of ProcessNet in Operation

The anatomy segmentation system is developed incrementally in three training phases—A, B, and C. During each training phase, a vision expert introduces three patient studies, with an average of 15 images each, to the system and adapts the system to deal with them. Each image is first processed by the anatomy segmentation system and the results reviewed by the expert. If the expert notices any errors, the corresponding processes are determined and revised. Alternatively, the expert might introduce new processes to handle new segmentation tasks. Although system processing and revision occurs on a per image basis, a revision may involve multiple cases because of shifts in cornerstone cases requiring revisions to address more than one issue.

In the training phases, a process is added or modified as the need arises for better features or improved techniques to handle a specific task. Alternatively, processes that perform poorly or become redundant are removed from the system. In total, 61 revisions were made to the lung anatomy segmentation system across the three training phases. A

TABLE 2.1

Summary of Revisions during Training Phases A, B, and C

	A	B	C	Total
Studies	3	3	3	9
Images	59	47	58	164
System revisions	47	6	8	61
• Process additions	22	4	3	30
• Process modifications	147	51	23	221
• Process removal	0	1	3	4
Number of processes	22	25	25	25
Cornerstones added	52	45	38	135
Cornerstones shifted	21	28	55	104

summary of revisions undertaken during the training phases A, B, and C is presented in Table 2.1. Training phase B begins after revision number 47, and training phase C after revision number 53.

During training phase A, there were 47 system revisions/training events, in which a vision expert revised part of the system; these diminished to six and eight revisions by phases B and C, respectively. Each training event involved changes to one or more processes, as new processes were added and existing ones modified or removed.

In phase A, 22 new processes were added and later modified 147 times during the course of training, as issues were discovered in the light of new training data. The vision algorithms necessary for the system were introduced and later refined during this period. The processes implemented basic image-processing algorithms such as image filtering, thresholding, morphology, image subtraction, and region growing. By training phases B and C, the number of new processes added has decreased to 4 and 3, respectively, and the modifications made to processes also decreased to 51 and 23, respectively.

In phases B and C, one and three processes, respectively, were removed. This is because some processes were found not to perform well. The new processes added in lieu of these processes offered better algorithms to carry out specific tasks and achieve overall system goals. For example, the lungs detection processes evolved from a simple thresholding algorithm in phase A, to applying locally parameterized active contours in phase B, and was finally superseded by a statistical model and an RDR classifier using relational features defined with respect to spine, sternum, and left and right shoulders in phase C. This was driven by the expert's choice, but ProcessNet supported the decisions by providing for consistency checks on cornerstone cases.

At the end of phase C, the 164 images from nine patient scans available for training had been used to add 135 cornerstones to 25 processes within the system. Further analysis of the cornerstones shows that these 135 cornerstones came from 97 unique training images. Because each process maintains its own set of cornerstone cases, a new training image that results in revisions to multiple processes may lead to multiple cornerstone copies of the same case, stored against the process revised.

Figure 2.5 shows the number of processes added, modified, and removed during each of the 61 revisions across training phases A, B, and C. The x-axis represents the revision number and the start of each training phase is delineated by dashed vertical lines. In a similar format, the number of cornerstones added and the number of shifts in existing cornerstones are shown in Figure 2.6. The large number of cornerstone shifts tends to coincide with significant changes to the system, such as the removal of processes during training

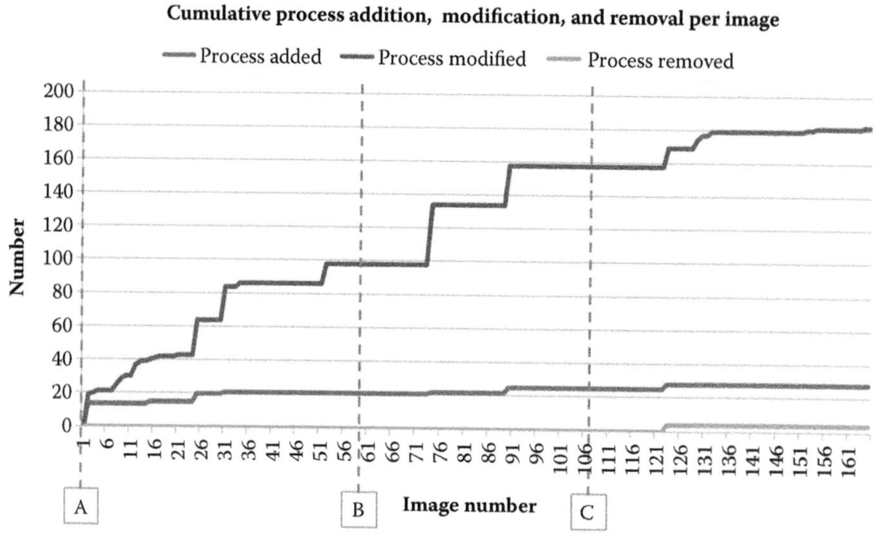

FIGURE 2.5
Number of processes removed, modified, or added for each system revision.

phases B and C. In total, there were 104 cornerstone shifts over the course of the training. A single cornerstone case at a process may shift with each revision made to the process.

In total, the vision expert made 221 revisions to the processes, in the form of either source code edits or the addition of new rules to process knowledge. Further analysis reveals that more than 70% of the modifications were source code edits, whereas the remaining 30% were revisions to the RDR knowledge bases used for classification within processes.

The number of cornerstone cases added does decrease with each training phase. This is not surprising because the cornerstone cases that are added during each training phase

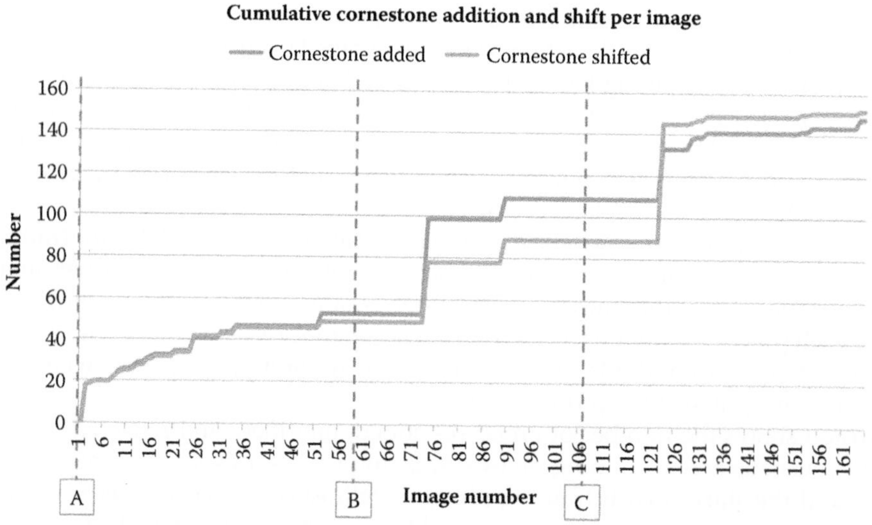

FIGURE 2.6
Number of cornerstone shifts and cornerstones added for each system revision.

represent noteworthy cases not previously encountered. As the cornerstone cases increasingly cover the variations in training data, the number of additions naturally decreases. Over the three training phases, an average of two cornerstone cases is added at each revision. This indicates that, on average, each revision required updates or changes to two processes.

The number of cornerstone cases that shift during revisions to the system increased during each training phase. As more cornerstone cases are added, changes to underlying processes would naturally affect an increasing number of other cornerstone cases. A change at a process that changes the output would naturally shift the cornerstone cases for the process, and the cornerstone cases of its dependents. It should also be noted that the majority of cornerstone cases shifted during the removal of existing processes. This is inevitable, as all cornerstone cases that previously covered the output of the deleted process must now be updated.

2.4.2 Analysis of the PN9 Anatomy Segmentation System

The incremental development using the ProcessNet framework means that the anatomy segmentation system can continue to evolve over time. The state of the system at the end of training phase C represents a snapshot of the knowledge within the system in the continuum of incremental development. This snapshot represents the knowledge acquired after nine patient studies and therefore is called PN9. The network of processes within the PN9 system is shown in Figure 2.7 and details about the processes and their dependencies are shown in Table 2.2. A short description of each process is also included in the table, identifying its role within the anatomy segmentation system.

An example of the segmentation results of the anatomy segmentation system is shown in Figure 2.8. The example shows the system correctly segmenting spine, sternum, shoulders, lung, and the left bronchus. It incorrectly identified the right bronchus as the esophagus. In ProcessNet, this represents an opportunity to revise the system and correct the knowledge responsible for identifying the bronchus, with the case serving as a cornerstone case for the relevant processes. The most likely candidates for revision would be *Bronchus Estimate, Bronchus Detection,* and *Sanity Check Bronchial Tree* processes.

The number of lines of Java source code for each process is listed in Table 2.3. The number of rules within the RDR knowledge bases used by processes is shown in Table 2.4. The ProcessNet framework automatically generates the source code in the *Main.java* class and the expert does not modify it. The expert introduces all the remaining classes, each representing a process within the system. Each process maintains an RDR knowledge base to capture knowledge within the form of rules. The expert modifies the source code within the class or adds rules to the knowledge base.

The complexity of the algorithm within a process may be roughly estimated by the number of lines of source code because it is indicative of the number of steps or method/function calls required to undertake the respective task. It is a commonly used metric in software engineering to define a module's complexity (Kaner and Bond 2004; Sommerville 1996, pp. 592–594). The smallest process is the *PrevKnownSternum* process, with only 113 lines of code, and it is responsible for simply loading the previously known sternum detected for the current HRCT study from the *results* directory.

The two largest processes are *ResultSaver* (802 lines of code) and *LungEstimate* (733 lines of code). The *ResultSaver* process captures the outputs of all other processes within the system and saves them to a results directory. Validating *ResultSaver* involves evaluating all the cases in the results directory to detect any shift in these cases. In essence, all the cases

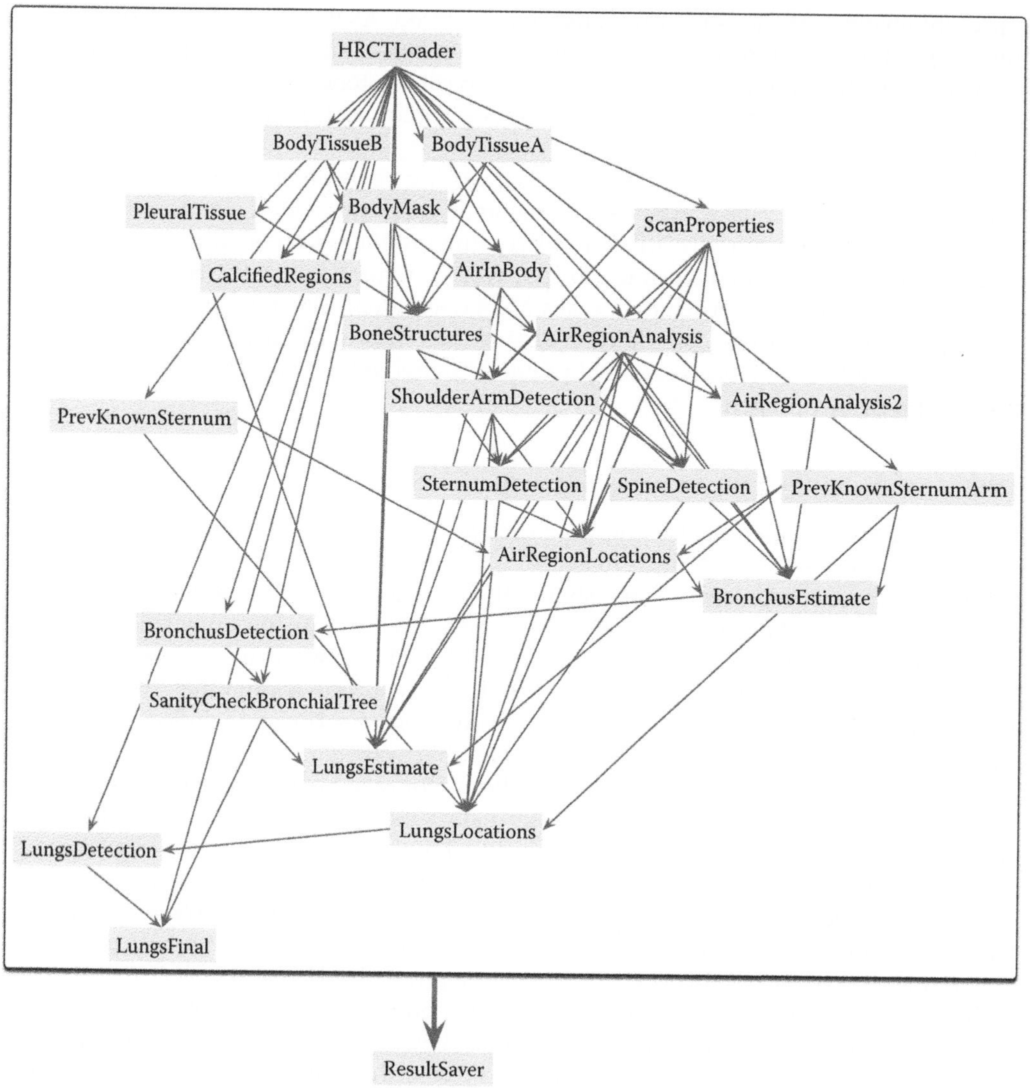

FIGURE 2.7
Data flow between processes of the anatomy segmentation system. ResultSaver gets data from all processes.

in the results directory form *ResultSaver's* cornerstone cases and record all cases processed by the system. This allows the expert to identify adverse effects on any case previously processed by the system, even if the case was not captured as a cornerstone case.

The *LungEstimate* process generates regions that are candidates for classification as lung or nonlung regions by the *LungsDetection* process. Because patients may experience diseases affecting the lung tissue, the volume of air present within the lungs may be significantly reduced. Therefore, the air-filled regions may not serve as a good estimate for lung regions. To handle these difficult cases, *LungEstimate* combines the air-filled regions with pleural regions detected by *PleuralTissue* process to generate candidate regions for lung regions. Of these, the regions that have already been labeled as trachea, bronchus, or esophagus by *SanityCheckBronchialTree* (and its predecessors—*BonchusEstimate* and

TABLE 2.2

Processes of the Anatomy Segmentation System, Their Purposes, and Dependencies

ID	Process	Purpose	Requires
1	HRCTLoader	Loads and enhances DICOM images	–
2	PrevKnownShoulderArm	Loads previously segmented shoulder regions	1
3	PleuralTissue	Segments pleural tissue	1
4	BodyTissueB	Segments fatty body tissue	1
5	BodyTissueA	Segments muscular body tissue	1
6	BodyMask	Generates a mask of the body	1, 4, 5
7	AirInBody	Detects air-filled regions within the body	1, 6
8	BoneStructures	Detects bone structures	3–7
9	CalcifiedRegions	Detects calcified regions	1, 6
10	PrevKnownSternum	Loads previously segmented sternum regions	1
11	ScanProperties	Extract scan information from DICOM header	1
12	AirRegionAnalysis	Measures structural features for air regions	1, 6, 7, 11
13	ShoulderArmDetection	Detects shoulder, arms, and shoulder blades	7, 8, 11, 12
14	SpineDetection	Detects the bone structures of the spine	8, 11–13
15	SternumDetection	Detects the bone structures of the sternum	8, 11, 12, 13
16	AirRegionLocations	Measures location-based features for air regions	1, 12
17	AirRegionAnalysis2	Measures textural features for air regions	2, 10–15
18	BronchusEstimate	Estimates bronchus, trachea, and esophagus	1, 2, 11–13, 16, 17
19	BronchusDetection	Labels bronchus, trachea, and esophagus	1, 18
20	SanityCheckBronchialTree	Resolve conflicts within bronchus regions	1, 19
21	LungsEstimate	Estimates regions likely to be lung	1–3, 6, 7, 11–13, 20
22	LungsLocation	Measures location-based features for lungs	2, 10–15, 21
23	LungsDetection	Labels lungs as left, right, or merged	1, 22
24	LungsFinal	Resolves conflicts between lung and bronchi	1, 20, 23
25	ResultSaver	Saves results of processes as XML and images	1–24

BronchusDetection) are eliminated. A 3D probability map of regions most likely to be lung is then used to score each candidate region's likelihood to be lung. The 3D map is generated using all previous lung segmentation results that have been verified by the expert. Each image that is being processed is aligned to the 3D map according to the position of the patient, the slice relative to the study and the pixel resolution. The 3D probability map

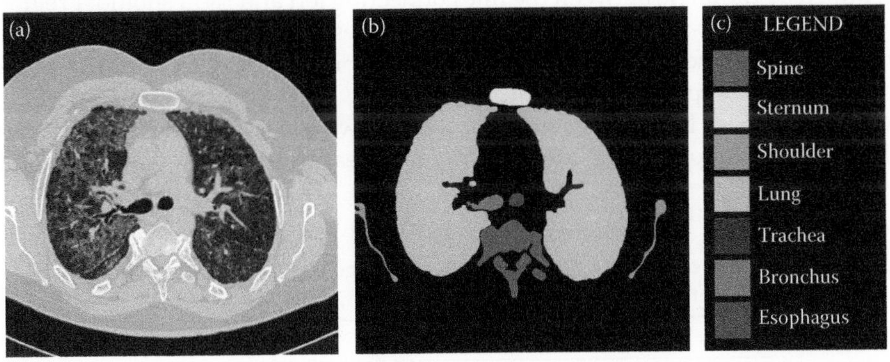

FIGURE 2.8
Anatomy segmentation results: (a) original HRCT image, (b) segmentation results, and (c) legend.

TABLE 2.3
Lines of Code for Processes of Anatomy Segmentation System

Source Code	Lines of Code (Includes Blank Lines for Readability)
HRCTLoader.java	272
PrevKnownShoulderArm.java	237
PleuralTissue.java	140
BodyTissueB.java	137
BodyTissueA.java	133
BodyMask.java	173
AirInBody.java	138
BoneStructures.java	169
CalcifiedRegions.java	144
PrevKnownSternum.java	113
ScanProperties.java	334
AirRegionAnalysis.java	353
ShoulderArmDetection.java	586
SpineDetection.java	547
SternumDetection.java	541
AirRegionLocations.java	428
AirRegionAnalysis2.java	187
BronchusEstimate.java	483
BronchusDetection.java	589
SanityCheckBronchialTree.java	348
LungsEstimate.java	733
LungsLocations.java	461
LungsDetection.java	588
LungsFinal.java	354
ResultSaver.java	802
Main.java	1012
Sum	**10,002**
Average	**389**

is scaled, rotated, and translated to match the image being interpreted. The body's rotation is determined by the angle between the line connecting left and right shoulder regions and the image horizontal x-axis. The 3D map can be represented as a sequence of 2D slices, as shown in Figure 2.9. Each image represents the probability density map for 10% of the lung region along the axial plane.

The RDR knowledge bases have only been used at two processes—*BronchusDetection* and *LungsDetection*. These processes infer on a range of features generated by other processes

TABLE 2.4
Number of Rules Within RDR Knowledge Bases for Processes of Anatomy Segmentation System

Process Using RDR	Rules
BronchusDetection.java	47
LungsDetection.java	25

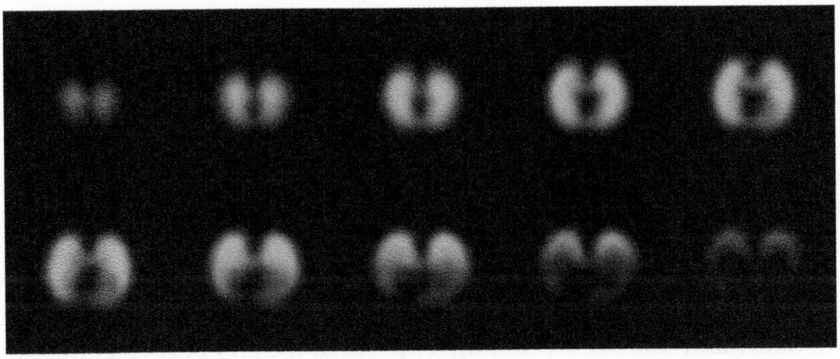

FIGURE 2.9
Lung probability map as slices, at 10% increments along the axial plane.

for extracted regions to classify them as trachea, bronchus, esophagus, lung, or unknown. The features include measurements on pixel intensity, image texture, structural features, as well as relational features that define a region's position relative to a number of anatomical landmarks detected by other processes. The anatomy landmarks used are the body, spine, sternum, and left and right shoulder regions. There are also a number of features that extract scan and patient information from the DICOM image header. Despite the range of features at the expert's disposal, the following features dominated the rule context within the resulting knowledge base of *LungsDetection*.

i. RELATIVE_DISTANCE_FROM_L2R_SHOULDERS: defines a value between 0.0 and 1.0, indicating the region's closest position on a line between left and right shoulders.
ii. RELATIVE_DISTANCE_ON_SPINE_STERNUM: defines a value between 0.0 and 1.0, indicating the region's closest position on a line between spine and sternum.
iii. DISTANCE_TO_BODY_CENTRE: defines the distance of the region to the body's centre in millimeters.
iv. LABEL_PROB_MODE: defines the mode score assigned by the 3D probability map to the pixels in the region within the *LungsEstimate* process.
v. LABEL_PROB_AVG: defines the average (mean) score assigned by the 3D probability map to the pixels in the region within the *LungsEstimate* process.
vi. AREA_REL_BODY: defines the ratio between the area of the region and the area of the body as measured for the given slice.
vii. Slice Location wrt Study: defines the relative position in terms of a percentage of the current slice within the study.
viii. PIXEL_VALUE_MODE: defines the mode of the pixel intensities on the original HRCT image bounded by the region.

A number of rules at *LungsDetection* were added with only slight changes in the boundary conditions for the same features. This indicates that the specific boundary cutoff values for a feature were not clear to the expert, leading to some duplication in the rules as the correct value is incrementally discovered with new cases. There is potential for inductive algorithms, such as Induct-RDR (Gaines and Compton 1995), to further revise the knowledge base once a sufficient number of cases have been gathered and the ground truth labeled.

2.4.3 Quantitative Evaluation of Anatomy Segmentation

ProcessNet's incremental validated change strategy should help the expert in ensuring that the performance of the anatomy segmentation system is either improved or maintained consistently, despite the frequent revisions by the expert as he or she attempts to expand the system's ability to segment new anatomical regions or improve its existing capability to segment an anatomical region. This means that the system performance is expected to ideally improve or conservatively remain consistent, despite system revisions.

To evaluate ProcessNet's ability to facilitate incremental engineering of vision systems, the anatomy segmentation system built using ProcessNet was quantitatively evaluated against ground truth data hand-marked by domain experts, at the end of each of the three training phases—A, B, and C. The accuracy of the system in segmenting anatomy was quantitatively evaluated on two independent test sets of hand-marked ground truth. The first test set, called Anatomy-20, contains ground truth image masks for lungs, spine, sternum, and shoulder regions for each of 342 images from 20 patient studies. The second test set, called Lungs-40, contains ground truth masks for only lung regions in 583 images from 40 patient studies. The 20 patient studies in the Anatomy-20 test set is a subset of the 40 patient studies in the Lungs-40 test set. These test sets were not used for training the system.

The segmentation results were compared against the hand-marked ground truth masks for spine, sternum, shoulder, and lung regions using the metrics of sensitivity and specificity defined below

$$\text{Sensitivity} = TP \,/\, (TP + FN)$$

$$\text{Specificity} = TN \,/\, (TN + FP)$$

where, in the case of lungs, TP is true positive, the number of pixels correctly labeled as lungs; TN is true negative, the number of the number of pixels correctly labeled as non-lung; FP is false positive, the number of pixels incorrectly labeled as lungs; FN is false negative, the number of pixels incorrectly labeled as non-lung.

A good segmentation system should have high sensitivity and specificity values. A sensitivity of 100% for the lung would indicate that all pixels within the image considered to be lung by the ground truth were detected as lung by the system. A specificity of 100% would indicate that all pixels identified as not belonging to lung by the ground truth were successfully excluded.

The mean sensitivity and specificity for lungs, spine, sternum, and shoulders across the three training phases are shown in Table 2.5. The high specificity values indicate that the

TABLE 2.5

Mean Sensitivity and Specificity as Percentages at the End of Phases A, B, and C

	A		B		C	
Test Set	**Sensitivity**	**Specificity**	**Sensitivity**	**Specificity**	**Sensitivity**	**Specificity**
Anatomy-20						
• Lungs	72.85	92.57	79.43	99.75	82.34	99.52
• Spine	40.90	99.81	88.28	99.59	88.28	99.59
• Sternum	7.58	99.95	40.72	99.85	46.98	99.79
• Shoulder	6.21	99.87	44.52	99.97	40.15	99.98
Lungs-40	88.40	99.80	93.90	99.70	95.90	99.40

processes are conservative in their detection and labeling of regions, hence, less likely to include regions that are not lung, spine, sternum, or shoulder. This is true for both Anatomy-20 and Lungs-40 data sets, with the mean specificity values around 99% across the three training phases. Only the lungs (in Anatomy-20) incorrectly include nonlung regions during phase A, as indicated by a specificity of 92.57%, which was improved in the subsequent training phases.

The sensitivity in segmenting lung regions saw an improvement across the three training phases for both the Anatomy-20 and the Lungs-40 data sets. The sensitivity for spine, sternum, and shoulder regions improves significantly during phase B and remains relatively consistent during phase C. The sensitivities for shoulders (at 40.15%) and sternum (at 46.98%) remain quite low even during phase C, but this must be evaluated in the context of their role within the system.

There are two reasons why this does not have an effect on lung segmentation. First, the intended purpose of shoulder and sternum segmentation is to acquire an approximation of landmarks to correctly align the 3D probability map used to segment lung regions. Even if all the pixels for the shoulder or sternum are not fully captured, even a partial segmentation is sufficient for their intended task. Second, *PrevKnownShoulderArm* and *PrevKnownSternum* help to compensate for regions missed by *ShoulderArmDetection* and *SternumDetection*, respectively, by retrieving the segmentation results for the preceding images for the same patient. Engineering a system as a network of processes allows limitations of an algorithm within one process to be compensated by algorithms in other processes. This means that the expert needed to ensure only a certain level of segmentation accuracy, around 40% sensitivity, to facilitate the remaining system.

Three examples of segmentation results from the Anatomy-40 test set are shown in Figure 2.10. The three columns represent segmentation performance for an image from three different patients—P34, P40, and P44—across the three training phases. The top row represents the original HRCT images and subsequent rows represent the segmentation results after training phases A, B, and C, respectively. As mentioned previously, the training and test sets contain patients with a variety of diffuse lung diseases. The lungs of patient P34 are affected by emphysema and honeycombing diseases patterns. The lungs of patient P40 are affected by ground-glass opacity. Patient P44 has normal lung tissue, albeit with pleural plaques affecting small parts of the lung wall.

At the end of training phase A, the anatomy segmentation system could correctly segment the healthy lung tissue in patient P44 but had difficulty segmenting lung regions in studies where the patient was severely affected by a variety of diffuse lung diseases, as in patients P34 and P40. In training phase B, revisions to the system led to an improvement in its ability to segment lung regions in patients affected by emphysema, as observable by the improvements in results for patient P34. It was also successful in segmenting shoulder regions missed previously by adjusting for the body's rotation as observed for patients P40 and P44. By the end of training phase C, the system correctly segments lungs severely affected by honeycombing (patient P34) and ground-glass opacity (patient P40). The segmentation for the sternum regions for patient P44 incorrectly includes other calcified regions and ribs. In patient P40, the sternum is fused with the ribs, thus making it difficult to separate them. Note that none of these cases from the test sets were used to train or revise the system. The improvements in these test cases were a result of improvements achieved on other training cases.

The erroneous cases in the test set denote the system's current limitation, and if used to revise the system, will become cornerstones for the processes of the anatomy segmentation system. Once captured as cornerstones, the validated change strategy of ProcessNet will

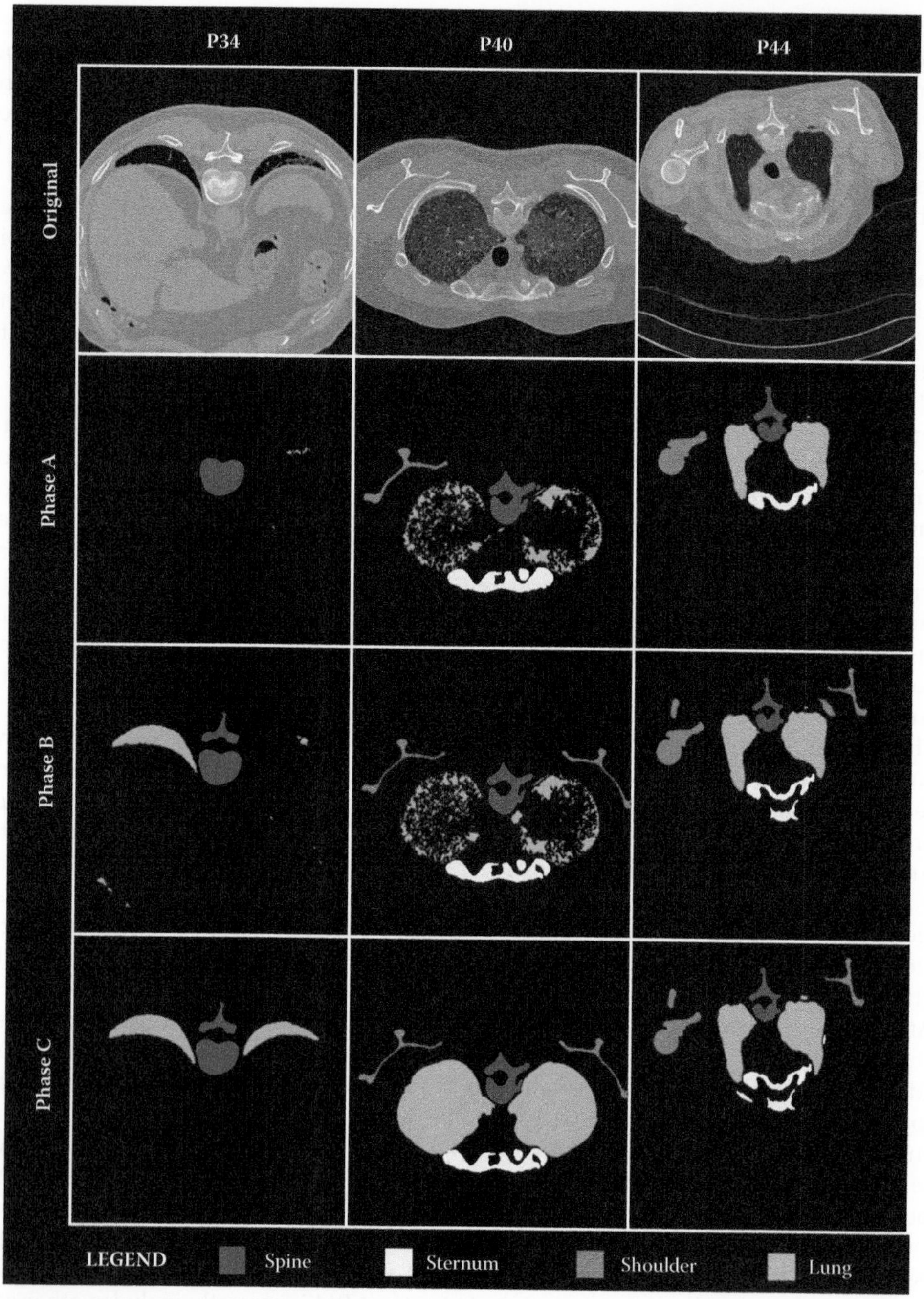

FIGURE 2.10
(See color insert.) Anatomy segmentation results: (left to right) patients P34, P40, and P44; (top to bottom) original HRCT scan, segmentation result after training phases A, B, and C.

ensure that any future changes to the system do not degrade the performance of the processes and system for these cases. Naturally, the strength of such a system lies in the quality of its cornerstone cases. The relatively poor segmentation results for shoulder regions between phases B and C indicate that the current set of cornerstones did not cover the variations present within the test set. Meanwhile, improvements in the segmentation for lung, spine, and sternum regions over the three training phases indicate that the cornerstone cases captured by the relevant processes were indeed representative of the variations in the test set.

Even though the expert is responsible for revising the processes, their efforts were directed and supported by the cornerstone-based validation of ProcessNet. It allows experts the opportunity to identify poorly performing parts of the system and use evidence in the form of cornerstone cases to guide the revisions to improve them. The automatic evaluation of system consistency via the cornerstone cases allows the expert to focus on solving specific vision tasks at each process and make judicious decisions on the quality of any changes. The ProcessNet framework facilitated incremental convergence in the knowledge of the anatomy segmentation system within its source code and rules.

2.4.4 Discussion

The ProcessNet framework helps vision experts in managing the incremental ad hoc revisions that are inevitable because of evolving quasi-expertise and incrementally available data when developing medical image segmentation systems. Experts revise systems, with the intent of addressing the incomplete and incorrect knowledge within the system. However, each revision carries a risk of adversely affecting the system performance for cases that the system handled correctly before the revision.

ProcessNet provides a systematic means to validate the changes at a process and its dependents, allowing the expert to revise each affected process using the cornerstone cases as concrete evidence for the desired handling of data. The management of changes across processes is critical as the complexity of the system grows. In the anatomy segmentation system developed using ProcessNet, the 25 processes were incrementally developed to address their limitations and adapt their content with changes at other processes. The complexity of managing these revisions was significantly reduced for the expert by the identification of specific issues via the cornerstone cases and allowing the expert to focus their effort on addressing each process in turn. The development effort required to engineer a network of processes was found to be manageable despite an increasing number of processes because the expert revises and validates a single process at a time. In addition, the acyclic nature of the dependencies means that the expert considers each process only once.

There are two limitations of the ProcessNet framework. The first is that the framework relies heavily on the expert in incrementally developing a vision system. This makes vision systems likely to be influenced by the level of the expertise at hand. A poor expert is likely to add incorrect knowledge or make imprecise revisions to the system which, in turn, may lead to further changes down the track. This is unavoidable as all expert-based systems, including RDR, fundamentally depend on a sufficient level of expertise (Cao et al. 2004). The role that cornerstone cases play within ProcessNet, however, helps to mitigate the influence of quasi-expertise. Any revisions proposed by the expert must satisfy the consistent handling of the cornerstone cases. Over time with an increasing number of cornerstone cases, the expert can use pattern recognition and machine learning methods that require sufficiently labeled data.

The second limitation is that the quality of the knowledge within the system is also dependent on the nature of cases that the system encountered during development. These cases, which prompted revisions by experts and formed cornerstone cases of processes, justify the knowledge within the process. Therefore, the resulting system is only as good as the quality of its cornerstone cases. This is a challenge faced by all data-driven systems. Over time with sufficient cases, one would expect that the accumulated cornerstone cases would provide better cover over the instance space of the domain. However, no guarantee can be provided on the uniform coverage of the domain by the training data available to a system.

2.5 Conclusions

Incremental and ad hoc development of medical image segmentation systems is an inevitable consequence of engineering systems, as the available data, expertise, and techniques evolve. The risk of a change degrading the system's performance restricts the expert's ability to build complex systems and confidently assimilate new data and techniques. In this chapter, an incremental validated change strategy called ProcessNet that mitigates these risks has been presented. Although ProcessNet may not eliminate all risks of degradation, the experiments support the idea that the accumulated set of cornerstone cases offers a data-driven means to assess the quality of a change to the system. This is the same argument and experience that underlies standard RDR.

ProcessNet captures and validates knowledge represented explicitly (such as in the form of rules) or implicitly in the libraries and algorithms defined in the source code of a process. The use of cornerstones at each process means that the knowledge behind heuristically defined algorithms can be supported by evidence grounded in data. The system developed using ProcessNet demonstrates that despite a large number of ad hoc revisions, a good solution can be discovered and improved on over time in a systematic manner. Although the ProcessNet framework has been applied specifically for the task of segmenting lungs and other anatomical structures in HRCT images, the framework is generic enough to address similar incremental ad hoc engineering for other types of medical image segmentation systems or computer vision systems in general.

References

Agnew, N.M., K.M. Ford, and P.J. Hayes. 1997. Expertise in context: Personally constructed, socially situated, and reality-relevant? In *Expertise in Context: Human and Machine*, Feltovich, P.J., Ford, K.M., and Hoffman, R.R. (eds.), 219–244. AAAI Press/MIT Press.

Amin, A., M. Bamford, A. Hoffmann, A. Mahidadia, and P. Compton. 1996. Recognition of hand-printed Chinese characters using ripple down rules. *Advances in Structural and Syntactical Pattern Recognition*, 371–380.

Archip, N., P.J. Erard, M. Egmont-Petersen, J.M. Haefliger, and J.F. Germond. 2002. A knowledge-based approach to automatic detection of the spinal cord in CT images. *IEEE Transactions on Medical Imaging*, 21:1504–16.

Archip, N., A. Fedorov, B. Lloyd, N. Chrisochoides, A.J. Golby, P.M. Black, and S.K. Warfield. 2006. Integration of patient specific modeling and advanced image processing techniques for image guided neurosurgery. *Proceedings of SPIE on Medical Imaging*.

Armato, S.G., M.L. Giger, and H. MacMahon. 1998. Automated lung segmentation in digitized posteroanterior chest radiographs. *Academic Radiology*, 5:245–255.

Aziz, Z., A. Wells, D. Hansell, G. Bain, S. Copley et al. 2004. HRCT diagnosis of diffuse parenchymal lung disease: Inter-observer variation. *Thorax*, 59(6):506–511.

Ballard, D.H., and J. Sklansky. 1976. A ladder-structured decision tree for recognizing tumors in chest radiographs. *IEEE Transactions on Computers*, C-25(5):503–513.

Ballard, D.H., and C.M. Brown. 1982. *Computer Vision*, Englewood Cliffs, NJ: Prentice-Hall.

Bankman, I.N. 2008. *Handbook of Medical Image Processing and Analysis*. 2nd ed. Elsevier Inc., Maryland Heights, MO, USA, ISBN: 978-0-12-373904-9 2008.

Bekmann, J., and A. Hoffmann. 2005. Improved knowledge acquisition for high-performance heuristic search. *International Joint Conference on Artificial Intelligence*, 19:41–47.

Bovenkamp E.G.P., J. Dijkstra, J.G. Bosch, and J.H.C. Reiber. 2009. User–agent cooperation in multiagent IVUS image segmentation. *IEEE Transactions on Medical Imaging*, 28(1):94–105.

Boykov, Y., and M.P. Jolly. 2001. Interactive graph cuts for optimal boundary and region segmentation of objects in N–D images. *Proceedings of the International Conference on Computer Vision*, 1:105–112.

Boykov, Y., and V. Kolmogorov. 2004. An experimental comparison of min-cut/max-flow algorithms for energy minimization in vision. *IEEE Transactions on Pattern Analysis and Machine Intelligence*, 26(9):1124–1137.

Brown, M.S., L.S. Wilson, B.D. Doust, R.W. Gill, and C. Sun. 1998. Knowledge-based method for segmentation and analysis of lung boundaries in chest X-ray images. *Computerized Medical Imaging and Graphics*, 22(6):463–477.

Cao, T.M., E. Martin, and P. Compton. 2004. On the convergence of incremental knowledge base construction. *Discovery Science*, 207–218.

Clancey, W.J. 1997. *Situated Cognition: On Human Knowledge and Computer Representation*. Cambridge University Press.

Clouard, R., A. Elmoataz, C. Porquet, and M. Revenu. 1999. Borg: A knowledge-based system for automatic generation of image processing programs. *IEEE Transactions on Pattern Analysis and Machine Intelligence*, 21(2):128–144.

Compton, P., and R. Jansen. 1988. Knowledge in context: A strategy for expert system maintenance. *Proceedings of the Australian Joint Artificial Intelligence Conference (AI'88) Adelaide*, 283–297.

Compton, P., and R. Jansen. 1989. A philosophical basis for knowledge acquisition. *European Knowledge Acquisition Workshop*.

Compton, P., L. Peters, G. Edwards, and T. Lavers. 2006. Experience with ripple-down rules. *Knowledge Based Systems*, 19(5):356–362.

Cootes T., C. Taylor, D. Cooper, and J. Graham. 1995. Active shape models—Their training and application. *Computer Vision and Image Understanding*, 38–59.

Cootes, T.F., G.J. Edwards, and C.J. Taylor. 2001. Active appearance models. *IEEE Transactions on Pattern Analysis and Machine Intelligence*, 23(6):681–685.

Cremers D., M. Rousson, and R. Deriche. 2007. A review of statistical approaches to level set segmentation: Integrating color, texture, motion and shape. *International Journal of Computer Vision*, 72(2):195–215.

Crevier, D., and R. Lepage. 1997. Knowledge-based image understanding systems: A survey. *Computer Vision and Image Understanding*, 67(2):161–185.

Cuadra, M.B., C. Pollo, A. Bardera, O. Cuisenaire, J.G. Villemure, and J.P. Thiran. 2004. Atlas-based segmentation of pathological MR brain images using a model of lesion growth. *IEEE Transactions on Medical Imaging*, 23(10):1301–1314.

Declaere, D., C. Smets, P. Suetens, and G. Marchal. 1991. Knowledge-based system for the three-dimensional reconstruction of blood vessels from two angiographic projections. *MBEC North Sea Special Feature*.

Deklerck, R., J. Cornelis, and M. Bister. 1993. Segmentation of medical images. *Image and Vision Computing*, 11(8):486–503.

Doi, K. 2005. Current status and future potential of computer-aided diagnosis in medical imaging. *British Journal of Radiology*, 78(1):S3–S19.

Draper, B., J. Brolio, R. Collins, A. Hanson, and E. Riseman. 1989. The schema system. *International Journal of Computer Vision*, 2(3):209–250.

Draper, B., A. Hanson, and E. Riseman. 1996. Knowledge-directed vision: Control, learning, and integration. *Proceedings of the IEEE*, 84(11):1625–1637.

Draper, B. 2003. From knowledge bases to Markov models to PCA. *Proceedings of Workshop on Computer Vision System Control.*

Drucker, H., C.J.C. Burges, L. Kaufman, A. Smola, and V. Vapnik. 1996. Support vector regression machines. *Advances in Neural Information Processing Systems*, 155–161, MIT Press.

Duda, R.O., P.E. Hart, and D.G. Stork. 2000. *Pattern Classification and Scene Analysis.* 2nd ed., New York: John Wiley & Sons.

Duncan, J.S., and N. Ayache. 2000. Medical image analysis: Progress over two decades and the challenges ahead. *IEEE Transactions on Pattern Analysis and Machine Intelligence*, 22(1):85–106.

Duryea, J., and J.M. Boone. 1995. A fully automated algorithm for the segmentation of lung fields on digital chest radiographics images. *Medical Physics*, 22(2):183–191.

Frangi, A.F., W.J. Niessen, and M.A. Viergever. 2001. Three-dimensional modeling for functional analysis of cardiac images: A review. *IEEE Transactions on Medical Imaging*, 20(1):2–5.

Freuder, E.C. 1977. A Computer System for Visual Recognition Using Active Knowledge Sources. In *International Joint Conference on Artificial Intelligence*, 2:671–677. San Francisco, CA: Morgan Kaufmann Publisher.

Gaines, B.R., and P. Compton. 1995. Induction of ripple-down rules applied to modeling large databases. In *Journal of Intelligent Information Systems*, 5(3):211–228.

Ghosh, P., and M. Mitchell. 2006. Segmentation of medical images using a genetic algorithm. *Genetic and Evolutionary Computation Conference*, 1171–1178.

Giger, M.L., K. Doi, H. MacMahon, C.E. Metz, and F.F. Yin. 1990. Pulmonary nodules: Computer-aided detection in digital chest images. *Radiographics*, 10(1):41–51.

Ginneken, B., H. Romeny, and M.A. Viergever. 2001. Computer-aided diagnosis in chest radiography: A survey. *IEEE Transactions on Medical Imaging*. 1228–1241.

Gong, L., and C. Kulikowski. 1994. VISIPLAN: A hierarchical planning framework for composing biomedical image analysis processes. *Computer Vision and Pattern Recognition*, 718–723.

Grimson, W.E.L. 1990. *Object Recognition by Computer: The Role of Geometric Constraints.* MIT Press.

He, L., Z. Peng, B. Everding, X. Wang, C. Han, K. Weiss, and W.G. Wee. 2008. A comparative study of deformable contour methods on medical image segmentation. *Image and Vision Computing*, 26:141–163.

Heimann, T., and H.P. Meinzer. 2009. Statistical shape models for 3D medical image segmentation: A review. *Medical Image Analysis*, 13(4):543–563.

Hu, S., E.A. Hoffman, and J.M. Reinhardt. 2001. Automatic lung segmentation for accurate quantitation of volumetric X-ray CT images. *IEEE Transactions on Medical Imaging*, 20(6):490–498.

Jain, A.K., M.N. Murty, and P.J. Flynn. 1999. Data clustering: A review. *ACM Computing Surveys (CSUR)*, 31(3):264–323.

Jain, A., R. Duin, and J. Mao. 2000. Statistical pattern recognition: A review. *IEEE Transactions on Pattern Analysis and Machine Intelligence*, 22(1):4–37.

Kaner, C., and W.P. Bond. 2004. Software engineering metrics: What do they measure and how do we know? *International Software Metrics Symposium*, 8:6.

Kass, M., A. Witkin, and D. Terzopoulos. 1988. Snakes: Active contour models. *International Journal of Computer Vision*, 321–331.

Kerr, J. and P. Compton. 2003. Toward generic model-based object recognition by knowledge acquisition and machine learning. In *Proceedings of the IJCAI-2003 Workshop on Mixed-Initiative Intelligent Systems, Acapulco*, 80–86.

Kikinis, R., M.E. Shenton, D.V. Iosifescu, R.W. McCarley, P. Saiviroonporn, H.H. Hokama, A. Robatino, D. Metcalf, C.G. Wible, C.M. Portas, R.M. Donnino, and F.A. Jolesz. 1996. A digital brain atlas for surgical planning, model-driven segmentation, and teaching. *IEEE Transactions on Visualization and Computer Graphics*, 2(3):232–241.

Kolata, G. 2009. Good or Useless, Medical Scans Cost the Same. *New York Times*, March 1.

Kuhnigk, J.M., H.K. Hahn, M. Hindennach, V. Dicken, S. Krass and H.-O. Peitgen. 2003. Lung lobe segmentation by anatomy guided 3D watershed transform, *Proceedings of SPIE on Medical Imaging*, 5032:1482–1490.

Levine, M., and A. Nazif. 1985. Rule-based image segmentation: A dynamic control strategy approach. *Computer Vision, Graphics and Image Processing*, 32(1):104–126.

Li, B., G. Christensen, J. Dill, E. Hoffman, and J. Reinhardt. 2002. 3-D inter-subject warping and registration of pulmonary CT images for a human lung model. *Proceedings of the SPIE Conference on Medical Imaging, San Diego, CA*, 4683:324–335.

Lin, P., C. Zheng, Y. Yang, and J. Gu. 2004. Medical image segmentation by level set method incorporating region and boundary statistical information. In *Computer Science*, 654–660.

Lorenzo-Valdes, M., G. I. Sanchez-Ortiz, R. Mohiaddin, and D. Rueckert. 2002. Atlas-based segmentation and tracking of 3D cardiac MR images using nonrigid registration. In *Lecture Notes in Computer Science*. 2488, Proc. Med. Image Comput. Comput.-Assisted Intervention, 642–650. Berlin: Springer-Verlag.

MacKay, D.J.C. 2003. *Information theory, inference, and learning algorithms*. Cambridge University Press.

Maillot, N., M. Thonnat, and A. Boucher. 2004. Towards ontology-based cognitive vision. *Machine Vision and Applications*, 16:33–40.

Maintz, J., and M. Viergever. 1998. A survey of medical image registration, *Medical Image Analysis*, 2:1–36.

Malik, A., and T. Choi. 2006. A novel algorithm for segmentation of lung images. *Lecture Notes in Computer Science*, 346–357.

Massoptier, L., A. Misra, and A. Sowmya. 2009. Automatic lung segmentation in HRCT images with diffuse parenchymal lung disease using graph-cut. *International Conference Image and Vision Computing New Zealand*, 266–270.

Matsuyama, T. 1988. Expert systems for image processing-knowledge-based composition of image analysis processes. *International Conference on Pattern Recognition*, 125–133.

McInerney, T., and D. Terzopoulos. 1996. Deformable models in medical image analysis. *Proceedings of the Workshop on Mathematical Methods in Biomedical Image Analysis*, 171–180.

McInerney, T., and D. Terzopoulos. 2000. T-snakes: Topology adaptive snakes. *Medical Image Analysis*, 4(2):73–91.

McInerney, T., and D. Terzopoulos. 2009. Deformable models. In *Handbook of Medical Image Processing and Analysis*, 145–166.

McKeown, D.M. Jr., W.A. Harvey, Jr., and J. McDermott. 1985. Rule-based interpretation of aerial imagery. *IEEE Transactions on Pattern Analysis and Machine Intelligence*, 7(5):570–585.

McNitt-Gray, M.F., H.K. Huang, and J.W. Sayre. 1995. Feature selection in the pattern classification problem of digital chest radiograph segmentation. *IEEE Transactions on Medical Imaging*, 14(3):537–547.

Misra, A., A. Sowmya, and P. Compton. 2004. Incremental learning of control knowledge for lung boundary extraction. *Pacific Knowledge Acquisition Workshop as part of Pacific Rim International Conference on Artificial Intelligence (PRICAI)* 2004, 1–15.

Misra, A., A. Sowmya, and P. Compton. 2006. Incremental learning for segmentation in medical images. Biomedical Imaging: nano to macro, *3rd IEEE International Symposium*, 1360–1363.

Mitchell, T. 1997. *Machine Learning*. New York: WCB/McGraw-Hill.

Murthy, S.K. 1998. Automatic construction of decision trees from data: A multi-disciplinary survey. *Data Mining and Knowledge Discovery*, 2:345–389.

Noble, J.A., and D. Boukerroui. 2006. Ultrasound image segmentation: A survey. *IEEE Transactions on Medical Imaging*, 25(8):1–24.

Osher, S.J., and J.A. Sethian. 1988. Fronts propagation with curvature dependent speed: Algorithms based on Hamilton–Jacobi formulations. *Journal of Computer Physics*, 79:12–49.

Ozertem, U., and D. Erdogmus. 2007. A nonparametric approach for active contours. *International Joint Conference on Neural Networks*, 1–4.

Park, M., L.S. Wilson, and J.S. Jin. 2000. Automatic extraction of lung boundaries by a knowledge-based method. Selected papers from the Pan-Sydney workshop on Visualisation, 2:11–16.

Park, M., B. Kang, S. Jin, and S. Luo. 2008. Computer aided diagnosis system of medical images using incremental learning method. *Expert Systems With Applications*, 36:7242–7251.

Paulus, S., U. Ahlrichs, B. Heigl, J. Denzler, J. Hornegger, M. Zobel, and H. Niemann. 2000. Active knowledge-based scene analysis. *Videre: Journal of Computer Vision Research*, 1(4):25.

Pien, H.H., A.J. Fischman, J.H. Thrall, and A.G. Sorensen. 2005. Using imaging biomarkers to accelerate drug development and clinical trials. *Drug Discovery Today*, 10(4):259–266.

Popper, K.R. 1963. *Conjectures and Refutations*. London: Routledge and Kegan Paul.

Prayote, A. 2007. Knowledge based anomaly detection. PhD thesis. University of New South Wales.

Rasband, W.S., 1997. ImageJ, U. S. National Institutes for Health, Bethesda, Maryland, USA (1997–2009), http://rsb.info.nih.gov/ij.

Reinhardt, J.M., R. Uppaluri, W.E. Higgins, and E.A. Hoffman. 2000. Pulmonary imaging and analysis. In *Medical Image Processing and Analysis*, J.M. Fitzpatrick and M. Sonka (eds.), 1005–1060.

Richards, D. 2009. Two decades of ripple down rules research. *The Knowledge Engineering Review*, 24(2):1–26.

Rogowska, J. 2008. Overview and fundamentals of medical image segmentation. In *Handbook of Medical Image Processing and Analysis*, I. Bankman (ed.), 73–90.

Sahba, F.T., H.R. Salama, M.M.A. 2007. A reinforcement agent for object segmentation in ultrasound images. *Expert Systems with Applications*, 1–9.

Singh, P.K., and P. Compton. 2005. Combining machine learned and heuristic rules using GRDR for detection of honeycombing in HRCT lung images. *Knowledge-Based Intelligent Information and Engineering Systems*, 131–137.

Sluimer, I.C., M. Niemeijer, M., and B. van Ginneken. 2004. Lung field segmentation from thin-slice CT scans in presence of severe pathology. *Proceedings of SPIE Medical Imaging*, 5370:1447–1455.

Sluimer, I., A. Schilham, M. Prokop, B.van Ginneken. 2006. Computer analysis of computed tomography scans of the lung: A survey. *IEEE Transactions on Medical Imaging*, 25(4):385–405.

Sommerville, I. 1996. *Software Engineering*. 5th ed. Readwood City, CA: Addison-Wesley.

Stansfield, S.A. 1986. ANGY: A rule-based expert system for automatic segmentation of coronary vessels from digital subtracted angiograms. *IEEE Transactions on Pattern Analysis and Machine Intelligence*, 8(2):188–199.

Sutton, M.A. 2010. Image segmentation by fuzzy clustering: Methods and issues. *Handbook of Medical Image Processing and Analysis*, 91–111.

Ukil, S. and J. Reinhardt. 2004. Smoothing lung segmentation surfaces in 3D X-ray CT images using anatomic guidance. *Proceedings of SPIE*, 1066–1075.

Vernazza, G.L., S.B. Serpico, and S.G. Dellepiane. 1987. A knowledge-based system for biomedical image processing and recognition. *IEEE Transactions on Circuits and Systems*, 1399–1416.

Wangehheim, A.V., H. Wagner, W. Comuello, D. Krechel, M.M. Richter, and P. Conrad. 2000. Cyclops—Expert System Shell for Development of Applications in Area of Medical Image Analysis Workshop 2000 of The German–Brazilian Cooperation Programme on Information Technology, 1:129–134.

Webb, S. 1990. *The Physics of Medical Imaging*. Bristol, PA: Adam Hilger.

Wei, J. 2002. Image segmentation based on situational DCT descriptors, *Pattern Recognition Letters*, 23:295–302.

Wismueller, A. 2009. Segmentation with neural networks. *Handbook of Medical Image Processing and Analysis*:113–143.

Zhang, L., and J. Reinhardt. 2000. 3D pulmonary CT image registration with a standard lung atlas. In *Proceedings of SPIE on Medical Imaging*, 4322:67–77.

Zhang, D., and D.J. Valentino. 2001. Segmentation of anatomical structures in X-ray computed tomography images using artifical neural networks, *Proceedings of SPIE*, 4684:1640–1652.

Zhang, L., E.A. Hoffman, and J.M. Reinhardt. 2003. Atlas-driven lung lobe segmentation in volumetric X-ray CT images. *Proceedings of SPIE*, 5031:306–315.

Zheng, B., J.K. Leader, G.S. Maitz, B.E. Chapman, C.R. Fuhrman, R.M. Rogers, F.C. Sciurba, A. Perez, P. Thompson, W.F. Good, and D. Gur. 2003. A simple method for automated lung segmentation in X-ray CT images. *Proceedings of SPIE on Medical Imaging*, 5032:1455–1463.

Zhou, X., T. Hayashi, T. Hara, H. Fujita, R. Yokoyama, T. Kiryu, and H. Hoshi. 2006. Automatic segmentation and recognition of anatomical lung structures from high-resolution chest CT images. *Computerized Medical Imaging and Graphics*, 30(5):299–313.

3

3D MGRF-Based Appearance Modeling for Robust Segmentation of Pulmonary Nodules in 3D LDCT Chest Images

Ayman El-Baz, Georgy Gimel'farb, Robert Falk, and Mohamed Abo El-Ghar

CONTENTS

3.1 Introduction

Because lung cancer is the most common cause of cancer deaths [1], fast and accurate analysis of pulmonary nodules is of major importance for medical computer-aided diagnostic (CAD) systems. Generally, such a system detects the nodules, quantifies and monitors volumetric changes for a follow-up examination, and classifies their malignancy or benignity. The CAD-based screening is aimed at improving the quality of cancer care management.

In ref. [2] we introduced a fully automatic nodule detection algorithm showing an accuracy of up to 93.3% on the experimental database containing 200 real low-dose computed tomography (LDCT) chest data sets with 36,000 two-dimensional (2D) slices. In the following sections, we focus on the next CAD stage, namely, on accurate segmentation of the detected nodules for subsequent volumetric measurements to monitor how the nodules change in time.

We use a two-step procedure to separate the nodules from their background: (i) an initial LDCT slice is segmented with algorithms introduced in ref. [3] to isolate lung tissues from surrounding structures in the chest cavity as shown in Figure 3.1, and (ii) the nodules in the isolated lung regions are segmented by evolving deformable boundaries under forces

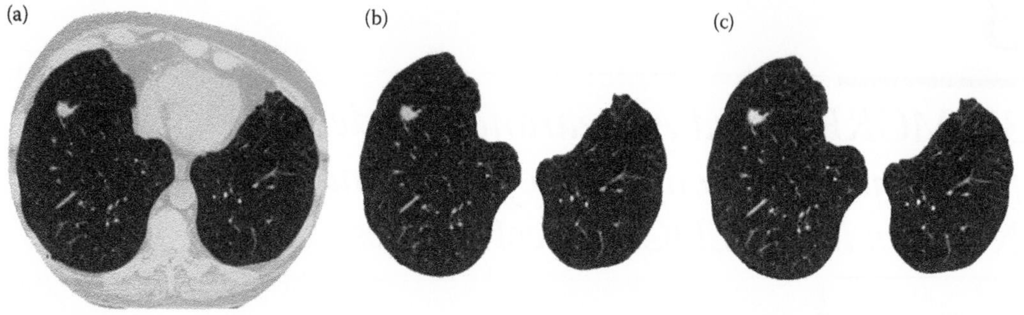

FIGURE 3.1
Step 1 of our segmentation: an LDCT slice (a) with isolated lungs (b), and the normalized segmented lung (c) image.

that depend on the learned current and prior appearance models. At step 1, each LDCT slice is modeled as a bimodal sample from a simple Markov–Gibbs random field (MGRF) of interdependent region labels and conditionally independent voxel intensities (gray levels). This step is necessary for more accurate separation of nodules from the lung tissues at step 2 because voxels of both the nodules and other chest structures around the lungs are of quite similar intensity.

3.1.1 Previous Work

Nowadays, segmentation of pulmonary nodules is being extensively studied. Typical conventional techniques are based on fitting a Gaussian model to empirical data [4], but this approach becomes a challenge when initial measurements are corrupted with outliers and margin truncation because of neighboring structures. For example, the minimum-volume ellipsoid covariance estimator in ref. [5] is robust to outliers but has very limited effectiveness under truncation. Bhalerao and Wilson [6] fit a conventional mixture of Gaussians to a marginal gray level distribution to visualize three-dimensional (3D) vascular structures in magnetic resonance images. Model parameters are estimated by an expectation–maximization algorithm.

Okada et al. [7] proposed an anisotropic intensity model fitting with analytical parameter estimation. However, their model is suitable only for segmenting nodules without cavities. Zhao et al. [8] and Kostis et al. [9] proposed to segment 2D and 3D nodules by thresholding the voxel intensity. Their algorithms accurately segment well-defined solid nodules with similar average intensities but become unreliable on the cavity or nonsolid nodules. Our segmentation overcomes these drawbacks by using deformable boundary models at step 2, such that their evolution is controlled by both a learned prior probability model of the visual nodule appearance and an adaptive appearance model of the nodules in a current image to be segmented.

3.1.2 Basic Notation

Let (x, y, z) denote Cartesian coordinates of points in a finite arithmetic lattice $R = \{(x, y, z): x = 0,\ldots, X-1; y = 0,\ldots, Y-1; z = 1,\ldots, Z-1\}$. It supports a given 3D grayscale image $g = [g_{x,y,z}: (x,y,z) \in R; g_{x,y,z} \in Q]$ with gray levels from a finite set $Q = \{0,\ldots, Q-1\}$ and its region map $m = [m_{x,y,z}: (x,y,z) \in R; m_{x,y,z} \in L]$ with region labels from a finite set $L = \{\text{nd},\text{bg}\}$. Each label

$m_{x,y,z}$ indicates whether the pixel (x,y,z) in the corresponding data set g belongs to the goal object (pulmonary nodule), $m_{x,y,z}$ = nd, or to the background, $m_{x,y,z}$ = bg. Let $b = [P_k: k = 1,\ldots,K]$ be a deformable piecewise-linear boundary with K control points $P_k = (x_k, y_k, z_k)$. The index k can be considered as a real number in the interval K indicating continuous positions around the boundary, e.g., $K = [1,K]$ for the positions from P_1 to P_K.

3.1.3 Our Model versus a Conventional Deformable Model

Conventional deformable models move in the direction that minimizes a boundary energy E such as, e.g., in ref. [10]:

$$E = E_{\text{int}} + E_{\text{ext}} = \int_{k \in K} \left(\zeta_{\text{int}}(b(P_k)) + \zeta_{\text{ext}}(b(P_k)) \right) dk \tag{3.1}$$

where $\zeta_{\text{int}}(b(P_k))$ and $\zeta_{\text{ext}}(b(P_k))$ are internal and external forces, respectively. The internal force $\zeta_{\text{int}}(b(P_k)) = \alpha|b'(P_k)|^2 + \beta|b''(P_k)|^2$ depends on the first, $b'(P_k)$, and second, $b''(P_k)$, derivatives of the contour $b(P_k)$ with respect to the continuous index k (see ref. [10] for details) and weights α and β control the contour tension and rigidity, respectively.

Typical external forces designed in ref. [10] move a deformable contour toward edges in a 2D or 3D grayscale image g: $\zeta_{\text{ext}}(b(P_k)) = -|\nabla g(b(P_k))|^2$, where ∇ denotes the gradient operator. But the deformable contours under this or other traditional external forces, e.g., based on linear edges or gradient vector flow, fail to closely approach intricate boundaries with concavities. Moreover, because of the high computational complexity, segmentation using the deformable models with such external energies is too slow compared with other techniques. To escape these drawbacks, we modify the external energy component in Equation 3.1 by involving two new probability models that roughly describe the visual appearance of the nodules.

The chapter is organized as follows. The prior and current appearance models are described in Sections 3.3 and 3.4, respectively. The prior appearance model considers nodule images as samples of a translation and rotation invariant MGRF with pairwise voxel interaction. The model is identified by analytical estimation of Gibbs potential functions giving quantitative interaction strengths for the nodules from a given training set $S = \{(g_t, m_t): t = 1,\ldots,T\}$ of 3D grayscale images and region maps of the nodules. The visual appearance of the nodules in each current image is also modeled with a linear combination of discrete Gaussians (LCDG) closely approximating the marginal probability distribution of gray levels in the nodules. The model is derived from the mixed empirical distribution of gray levels for the nodules and background using modified expectation–maximization techniques from ref. [3]. Section 3.5 proposes how to control an evolving boundary using the previously mentioned models. Experiments with a number of real LDCT chest slices are discussed in Section 3.6.

3.2 Data Normalization

To account for monotone (order-preserving) changes of signals (e.g., because of different illumination or sensor characteristics), for each segmented data set, we will calculate the occurrence histogram, and then we normalize the segmented data set to make $q_{\max} = 255$ for each segmented data set (e.g., see Figure 3.1c).

3.3 MGRF-Based Prior Appearance Model

To exclude an alignment stage before segmentation, the appearance of both small 2D and large 3D nodules is modeled with a translation and rotation invariant generic MGRF with voxel-wise and central-symmetric pairwise voxel interaction specified by a set N of characteristic central symmetric voxel neighborhoods $\{n_\nu : v \in N\}$ on R and a corresponding set V of Gibbs potentials, one potential per neighborhood.

A central-symmetric voxel neighborhood n_ν embraces all voxel pairs such that (x,y,z)—coordinate offsets between a voxel (x,y,z) and its neighbor (x',y',z') belong to an indexed semiopen interval $[d_{\nu,\min}, d_{\nu,\max})$; $v \in N = \{1,2,3,\ldots\}$ of the intervoxel distances: $d_{\nu,\min} \le \sqrt{(x-x)^2 + (y-y)^2 + (z-z)^2} < d_{\nu,\max}$. Figure 3.2 illustrates the neighborhoods n_ν for the uniform distance ranges $[v - 0.5, v + 0.5)$; $v \in N = \{1,\ldots,8\}$.

The interactions in each neighborhood n_ν have the same Gibbs potential function V_ν of gray level co-occurrences in the neighboring voxel pairs, and the voxel-wise interaction is given with the potential function V_{vox} of gray levels in the voxels:

$$V = V_{\text{vox}} = V_{\text{vox}}(q) : q \in Q \ ; \left\{ V_\nu = V_\nu(q,q) : (q,q) \in Q^2 \ : \nu \in N \right\}$$

3.3.1 Model Identification

Let $R_t = \{(x,y,z): (x,y,z) \in R \wedge m_{t;x,y,z} = \text{nd}\}$ and $C_{\nu,t}$ denote the part of the 3D lattice R supporting the training nodules in the image–map pair $(g_t, m_t) \in S$ and the family of voxel pairs in R_t^2 with the coordinate offsets $(\xi,\eta,\gamma) \in n_\nu$, respectively. Let $F_{\text{vox},t}$ and $F_{\nu,t}$ be a joint empirical probability distribution of gray levels and of gray level co-occurrences in the training nodules from image g_t, respectively:

$$F_{\text{vox},t} = f_{\text{vox},t}(q) = \frac{|R_{t,q}|}{|R_t|} ; \sum_{q \in Q} f_{\text{vox},t}(q) = 1$$

and

$$F_{\nu,t} = f_{\nu,t}(q,q) = \frac{|C_{\nu,t;q,q}|}{|C_{\nu,t}|} ; \sum_{(q,q) \in Q^2} f_{\nu,t}(q,q) = 1$$

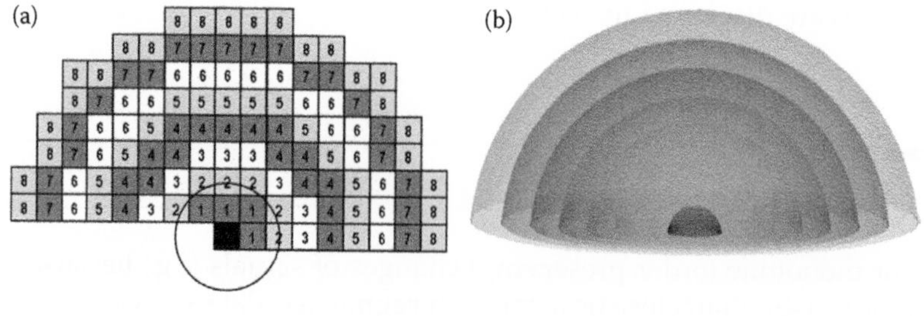

FIGURE 3.2
Central-symmetric 2D (a) and 3D (b) neighborhoods for the eight distance ranges on the lattice R.

where $R_{t,q} = \{(x,y,z): (x,y,z) \in R_t \wedge g_{x,y,z}\}$ is a subset of voxels supporting the gray level q in the training nodules from image g_t and $C_{\nu,t;q,q'}$ is a subfamily of the voxel pairs $c_{\xi,\eta,\gamma}(x,y,z) = ((x,y,z),(x+\xi,y+\eta,z+\gamma)) \in R_t^2$ supporting the gray level co-occurrence (q,q') in the same nodules, respectively.

The MGRF model of the tth object is specified by the joint Gibbs probability distribution on the sublattice R_t:

$$P_t = \frac{1}{Z_t}\exp |R_t| \; V_{\text{vox}}^{\mathrm{T}} F_{\text{vox},t} + \sum_{\nu \in N} \rho_{\nu,t} V_{\nu,t}^{\mathrm{T}} F_{\nu,t} \tag{3.2}$$

where $\rho_{\nu,t} = |C_{\nu,t}|/|R_t|$ is the average cardinality of the neighborhood n with respect to the sublattice R_t.

To simplify the notation, let areas of the training nodules be similar, so that $|R_t| \approx R_{\text{nd}}$ and $|C_{\nu,t}| \approx C_{\nu,\text{nd}}$ for $t = 1,\ldots,T$, where R_{nd} and $C_{\nu,\text{nd}}$ are the average cardinalities over the training set S. Assuming the independent samples, the joint probability distribution of gray values for all the training nodules is as follows:

$$P_S = \frac{1}{Z}\exp \; T R_{\text{nd}} \; V_{\text{vox}}^{\mathrm{T}} F_{\text{vox}} + \sum_{\nu \in N} \rho_\nu V_\nu^{\mathrm{T}} F_\nu$$

where $\rho_\nu = \dfrac{C_{\nu,\text{nd}}}{R_{\text{nd}}}$, and the marginal empirical distributions of gray levels $F_{\text{vox,nd}}$ and gray level co-occurrences $F_{\nu,\text{nd}}$ now describe all the nodules from the training set. Zero empirical probabilities caused by a relatively small volume of the training data available to identify the above model are eliminated if fractions defining the empirical probabilities in terms of cardinalities of the related sublattices or subfamilies are modified as follows: $\dfrac{(\langle \text{nominator} \rangle + \varepsilon)}{(\langle \text{denominator} \rangle + S\varepsilon)}$. With the Bayesian quadratic loss estimate, $\varepsilon = 1$ and $S = Q$ for the first-order or $S = Q^2$ for the second-order interactions. With a more conservative approach in ref. [11], $\varepsilon = \dfrac{1}{S}$.

Using the analytical approach similar to that in ref. [12], the potentials are approximated with the scaled centered empirical probabilities:

$$\begin{aligned} V_{\text{vox,nd}}(q) &= \lambda \; f_{\text{vox,nd}}(q) - \frac{1}{Q} \;;\; q \in Q \\ V_{\text{vox,nd}}(q,q) &= \lambda \; f_{\nu,\text{nd}}(q,q) - \frac{1}{Q^2} \;;\; (q,q) \in Q^2; \nu \in N \end{aligned} \tag{3.3}$$

where the common factor λ is also computed analytically. It can be omitted ($\lambda = 1$) if only relative potential values are used for computing relative energies $E_{\nu,\text{rel}}$ of the central-symmetric pairwise voxel interactions in the training data. The energies that are equal to the variances of the co-occurrence distributions:

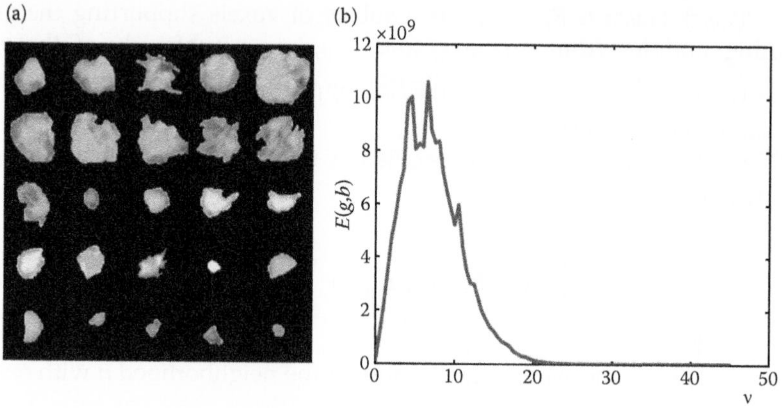

FIGURE 3.3
Training nodule sections (a) and the dependence (b) between the energy of Equation 3.4 and the neighborhood n_v.

$$E_{\mathrm{v,rel}} = \sum_{q,q \in Q^2} f_{\mathrm{v,nd}}(q,q)\; f_{\mathrm{v,nd}}(q,q) - \frac{1}{Q^2}$$

allow for ranking all the central-symmetric neighborhoods n_v and selecting the top-rank, i.e., most characteristic ones $N' \subset N$ to include to the prior appearance model of Equation 3.3. Using this model, any grayscale pattern within a deformable boundary b in an image g is described by its Gibbs energy

$$E(g,b) = V_{\mathrm{vox,nd}}^{\mathrm{T}} F_{\mathrm{vox,nd}}(g,b) + \sum_{\mathrm{v} \in N} V_{\mathrm{v,nd}}^{\mathrm{T}} F_{\mathrm{v,nd}}(g,b) \tag{3.4}$$

where N' is an index subset of the selected top-rank neighborhoods, and the empirical probability distributions are collected within the boundary b in g.

Figure 3.3 shows some samples of typical 2D cross-sections of the 96 training 3D nodules selected from the 350 nodules used for the experiments in Section 3.6, and the dependence of the training Gibbs energies in Equation 3.4 of the neighborhoods similar to those in Figure 3.2.

3.4 LCDG-Based Current Appearance Model

Nonlinear intensity variations in a data acquisition system because of patient weight, radiation dose, scanner type, and scanning parameters affect the visual appearance of nodules in each current data set g presented for segmentation. Thus, in addition to the learned appearance prior, we model the marginal gray level distribution within an evolving boundary b in g with a dynamic mixture of two distributions that characterize the nodules and their background, respectively. The mixture is closely approximated with a bimodal LCDG and then partitioned into the nodule and background LCDGs. The approximation is performed using the modified EM-based approach in ref. [3] adapted to the DGs. The DG $\Psi_\theta = (\Psi(q|\theta): q \in Q)$ is a discrete probability distribution derived from the cumulative Gaussian function $\phi_\theta(q)$ with parameters $\theta = (\mu,\sigma^2)$, where μ and σ^2 are the mean and the variance, respectively: $\Psi(0|\theta) = \phi_\theta(0.5)$, $\Psi(Q-1|\theta) = 1 - \phi_\theta(Q-1.5)$ and $\Psi(q|\theta) = \phi_\theta(q+0.5) - \phi_\theta(q-0.5)$.

Each current appearance model is a bimodal LCDG with two dominant positive DGs approximating the marginal empirical gray level distribution within the evolving boundary and with a number of subordinate sign-alternate DGs approximating deviations of the empirical distribution from the dominant mixture. The mixed nodule–background LCDG model is as follows:

$$p_{\mathbf{w},\mathbf{\Theta}}(q) = \sum_{r=1}^{C_p} w_{p,r}\psi(q\,|\,\theta_{p,r}) - \sum_{l=1}^{C_n} w_{n,l}\psi(q\,|\,\theta_{n,l}) \tag{3.5}$$

where $C_p \geq 2$ and C_n are the total numbers of the positive and negative components, respectively, and $w = (w_{p,.}, w_{n,.})$ are the nonnegative weights. The latter meet the following obvious restriction:

$$\sum_{r=1}^{C_p} w_{p,r} - \sum_{l=1}^{C_n} w_{n,l} = 1$$

To identify the model of Equation 3.5, the numbers C_p, C_n and the parameters w, θ (i.e., the weights, means, and variances) of the positive and negative DGs are first estimated to produce a close initial approximation of the empirical distribution. Under the fixed numbers, C_p and C_n, all other parameters are then refined, and the final LCDG is partitioned into the two LCDGs $p_{\text{vox},l} = [p_{\text{vox},l}(q): q \in Q]$, one per class $l \in L$, such that the misclassification rate is minimal. The LCDG for l = nd describes not only the nodules but also the arteries and veins in the lung regions because of their very similar voxel intensities. The complete process is detailed in ref. [3].

3.5 Boundary Evolution Using Two Appearance Models

The following external energy term in Equation 3.1 combines the learned prior and current appearance models to guide an evolving boundary in such a way that it maximizes the energy within the boundary:

$$\zeta_{\text{ext}}(b(P_k = (x,y,z))) = -p_{\text{vox,nd}}(g_{x,y,z})\pi_P(g_{x,y,z}|S) \tag{3.6}$$

where $p_{\text{vox,nd}}(q)$ is the marginal probability of the gray level q in the LCDG model for the nodules, arteries, and veins (see Section 3.4) and $\pi_P(q|S)$ is the prior conditional probability of the gray level q, given the current gray values in the characteristic central-symmetric neighborhoods of P_k, for the MGRF prior model in Section 3.3:

$$\pi_P\left(g_{x,y,z} \mid S\right) = \frac{\exp\left(E_P(g_{x,y,z} \mid S)\right)}{\sum_{q \in Q} \exp\left(E_P(g_{x,y,z} \mid S)\right)}$$

where $E_P(q|S)$ is the voxel-wise Gibbs energy for a gray level q assigned to P and the current fixed gray levels in all neighbors of P in the characteristic neighborhoods n_v; $v \in N$:

$$E_P\left(g_{x,y,z} \mid S\right) = V_{\text{vox,nd}}(q) + \sum_{v \in N} \sum_{(\xi,\eta,\gamma) \in n_v} \left(V_{v,\text{nd}}(g_{x-\xi,y-\eta,z-\gamma}, q) + V_{v,\text{nd}}(q, g_{x+\xi,y+\eta,z+\gamma})\right)$$

The boundary evolution in each 2D section with the fixed z-coordinate terminates after the total energy E_r of the region $r \subset R$ inside the boundary b does not change:

$$E_r = \sum_{\forall P=(x,y,z) \in r} E_P\left(g_{x,y,z} \mid S\right) \tag{3.7}$$

The deformable boundary b evolves in discrete time, $\tau = 0,1,\ldots,T$, as follows:

ALGORITHM 1: SEGMENTATION ALGORITHM

1. Initialization ($\tau = 0$):
   a. Initialize a boundary inside a nodule (e.g., automatically as in ref. [3]).
   b. Using voxels within and outside the initial boundary, estimate the current "nodule" and "background" LCDGs, $p_{\text{vox,nd}}$ and $p_{\text{vox,bg}}$.
2. Evolution ($\tau \leftarrow \tau + 1$):
   a. Calculate the total energy of Equation 3.7 within the current boundary b_τ.
   b. For each control point, P_k, on the current boundary, indicate the exterior (−) and interior (+) nearest neighbors with respect to the boundary using the method proposed in ref. [13].
   c. For each (+) point, calculate the total energy of Equation 3.1 for each new candidate for the current control point.
   d. Select the new minimum-energy candidate.
   e. Calculate the total energy of Equation 3.7 within the boundary that could have appeared if the current control point has been moved to the selected candidate position.
   f. If the total energy increases, accept this new position of the current control point; otherwise, for each (−) point, calculate the total energy of Equation 3.1 for each new candidate for the current control point.
   g. Select the new minimum-energy candidate.

h. Calculate the total energy of Equation 3.7 within the boundary that could have appeared if the current control point has been moved to the selected candidate position.
i. If the total energy increases, accept this new position of the current control point.
j. Otherwise, do not move the current control point because it is already located on the edge of the desired nodule.
k. Mark each voxel visited by the deformable boundary.
l. If the current control point moves to the voxel visited earlier, then find the edge formed by the previously visited voxels and use the edge points as the new control points of the deformable boundary.
m. If the new control points appear, interpolate the whole boundary using cubic splines and then smooth its control points with a low-pass filter.
n. If the total energy within the boundary does not change, terminate the process; otherwise, return to step 2b.

3.6 Experimental Results

The proposed segmentation algorithm was tested on a database of clinical multislice 3D chest LDCT scans of 29 patients with $0{:}7 \times 0{:}7 \times 2{:}5$ mm^3 voxels that contains 350 nodules, in particular, 150 solid nodules larger than 5 mm in diameter, 40 small solid nodules of less than 5 mm diameter, 10 cavity nodules, 61 nodules attached to the pleural surface, and 89 largely nonspherical nodules. The diameters of the nodules ranged from 3 to 30 mm.

Figure 3.4 illustrates the results of segmenting pleural attached nodules shown by axial, sagittal, and coronal cross-sections. The pixel-wise Gibbs energies in each cross-section

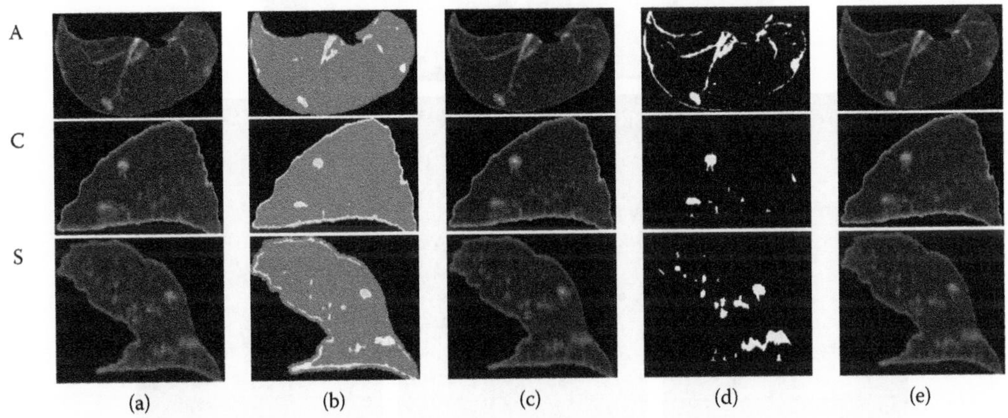

FIGURE 3.4
3D segmentation of pleural attached nodules; results are projected onto 2D axial (A), coronal (C), and saggital (S) planes for visualization: 2D profile of the original nodule (a), pixel-wise Gibbs energies (b) for $\nu = 9$, our segmentation (c), the segmentation with the algorithm in ref. [9] (d), and the radiologist's segmentation (e).

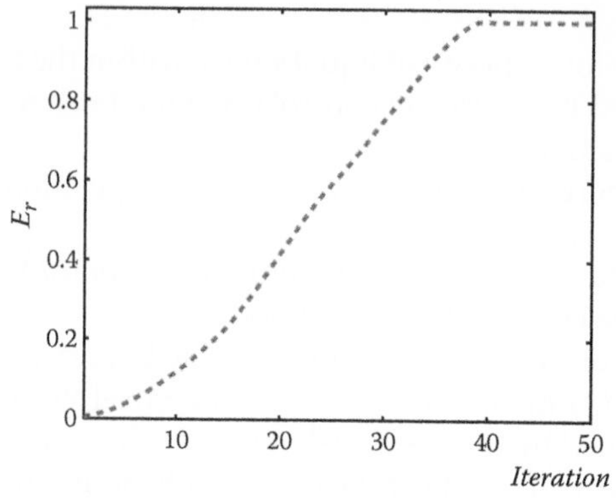

FIGURE 3.5
Convergence of the proposed algorithm for the experiment in Figure 3.4 (the total energy is normalized by dividing each value by the maximum one).

are higher for the nodules than for any other lung voxels including the attached artery. Therefore, our approach accurately separates the pulmonary nodules from any part of the attached artery. Changes in the total nodule energy of Equation 3.7 during the iterations τ of evolving the deformable boundary are shown in Figure 3.5. The evolution terminates after 50 iterations because the changes in the total energy become close to zero. The error of

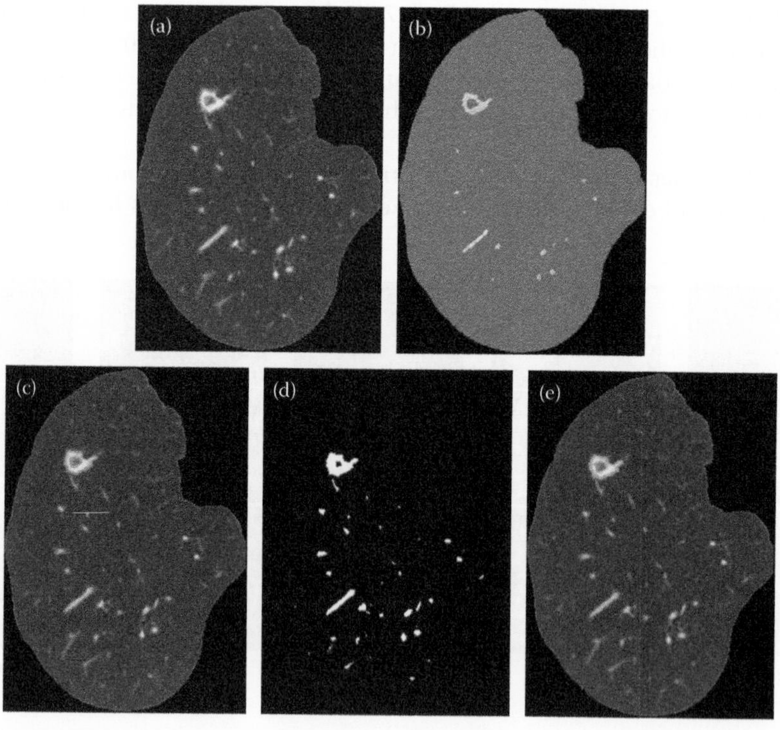

FIGURE 3.6
2D segmentation of cavity nodules: 2D profile of the original nodule (a), pixel-wise Gibbs energies for $\nu = 9$ (b), our segmentation (c), the segmentation using the approach in ref. [9] (d), and the radiologist's segmentation (e).

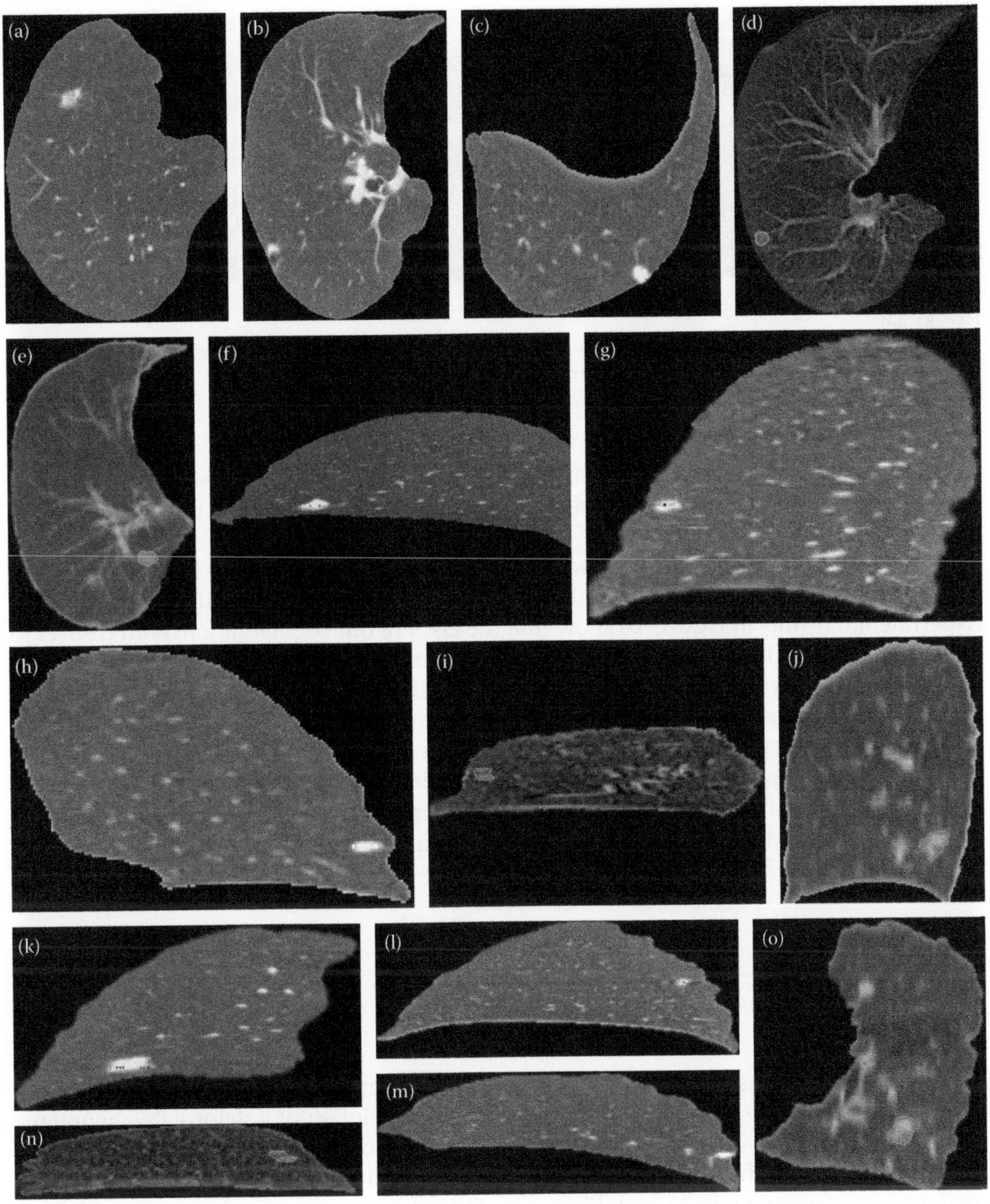

FIGURE 3.7
Our segmentation for five more patients.

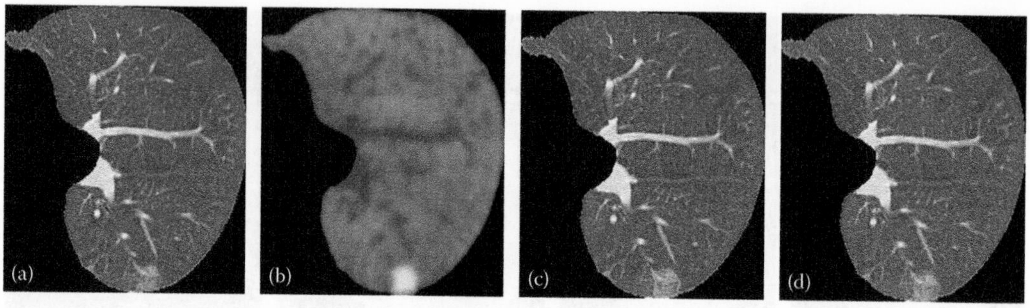

FIGURE 3.8
Segmentation results of a ground-glass nodule: 2D profile of the original nodule (a), pixel-wise Gibbs energies (b), our segmentation (c), and the "gold-standard" radiologist's segmentation (d).

our segmentation with respect to the radiologists' "ground truth" is 2.0%. For comparison, the segmentation error of the FWHM intensity thresholding proposed by Kostis et al. [9] is 46.2%.

The main advantage of our approach over the existing algorithms is in the more accurate segmentation of thin cavity nodules, i.e., the nodules that appear only in a single slice. Experimental results in Figure 3.6 show that the error of our segmentation, with respect to the radiologist, is 2.1%, whereas the segmentation error of the FWHM intensity thresholding [9] is 53.9%. It is noteworthy that the approach of Okada et al. [7] fails to segment this cavity nodule because it is totally inhomogeneous: this approach fails to estimate the nodule's center and thus obtains an inaccurate estimate of the normal density for the nodule. Figures 3.7 and 3.8 present more segmentation results obtained by our algorithm. In total, our segmentation of the 350 data sets has the error range 0.4% to 2.35% with a mean error of 0.96% and a standard error deviation of 1.1% compared with 28.6% to 59.9%, 38.7%, and 21.9%, respectively, for the approach in ref. [9].

3.7 Conclusions

We introduced a new approach to accurately segment small 2D and large 3D pulmonary nodules on LDCT chest images. In our approach, the evolution of a deformable boundary is guided with probability models of visual appearance of pulmonary nodules. The prior MGRF model is identified from a given training set of nodules, and the current appearance model adapts the guidance to each bimodal image of lung regions to be segmented. Both models are learned using simple analytical and numerical techniques. Experiments with real LDCT chest images confirm the high accuracy of our segmentation with respect to the radiologist's ground truth. Our segmentation outperforms other existing approaches for all types of nodules, in particular, for cavity nodules in which other existing approaches fail.

Our experiments show that the proposed accurate identification of the MGRF model demonstrates promising results in segmenting the lung region from LDCT images. Our present implementation on C++ programming language on an Intel quad processor (3.2 GHz each) with 16-GB memory and 2-TB hard drive with RAID technology takes about 17 s to segment a large lung nodule of 30 mm in diameter, and less than 5 s on small lung nodules less than

5 mm in diameter. More experimental results, the algorithm's code, and samples of real data obtained under our own scanning protocol will be provided in our Web page.

References

1. Edwards, B., E. Ward, B. Kohler, C. Eheman, A. Zauber, R. Anderson, A. Jemal, M. Schymura, L. Vogelaar, L. Seeff, M. van Ballegooijen, S. Goede, and L. Ries. 2010. Annual report to the nation on the status of cancer, 1975–2006, featuring colorectal cancer trends and impact of interventions (risk factors, screening, and treatment) to reduce future rates. *Journal of the National Cancer Institute*, 544–573.
2. Farag, A., A. El-Baz, G. Gimelfarb, R. Falk, and S. Hushek. 2004. Automatic detection and recognition of lung abnormalities in helical CT images using deformable templates. *Proceedings of the of International Conference on Medical Image Computing and Computer-Assisted Intervention (MICCAI'04)*, France, Rennes, Saint-Malo, September 26–29, 2004. vol. II, 856–864.
3. Farag, A., A. El-Baz, and G. Gimel'farb. 2006. Precise segmentation of multi-modal images. *IEEE Transactions on Image Processing*, 15(4);952–968.
4. Fukunaga, K. 1990. *Statistical Pattern Recognition*. San Diego: Academic Press.
5. Rousseeuw P.J., and A.M. Leroy. 1987. *Robust Regression and Outlier Detection*. New York: Wiley.
6. Bhalerao A., and R. Wilson. 2001. Estimating local and global structure using a Gaussian intensity model. *Medical Image Understanding and Analysis*, Birmingham, U.K.
7. Okada, K., D. Comaniciu, and A. Krishnan. 2005. Robust anisotropic Gaussian fitting for volumetric characterization of pulmonary nodules in multislice CT. *IEEE Transactions on Medical Imaging*, 24(3):409–423.
8. Zhao, B., D. Yankelevitz, A. Reeves, and C. Henschke. 2003. Two-dimensional multicriterion segmentation of pulmonary nodules on helical CT images. *IEEE Transactions on Medical Imaging*, 22:1259–1274.
9. Kostis, W.J., A.P. Reeves, D.F. Yankelevitz, and C.I. Henschke. 2003. Three-dimensional segmentation and growth-rate estimation of small pulmonary nodules in helical CT images. *IEEE Transactions on Medical Imaging*, 22:1259–1274.
10. Kass, M., A. Witkin, and D. Terzopoulos. 1987. Snakes: Active contour models. *International Journal of Computer Vision*, 1:321–331.
11. Titterington, D.M., G.D. Murray, L.S. Murray, et al. 1981. Comparison of discrimination techniques applied to a complex data set of head injured patients. *Journal of the Royal Statistical Society*, 144:145–175.
12. El-Baz, A., and G. Gimel'farb. 2007. EM based approximation of empirical distributions with linear combinations of discrete Gaussians. *Proceedings of the IEEE International Conference on Image Processing (ICIP'07)*, San Antonio, TX, September 16–19, 2007. vol. IV, 373–376.
13. Kimmel., R. 2004. *Numerical Geometry of Images: Theory, Algorithms, and Applications*. Springer.

4

Ground-Glass Nodule Characterization in High-Resolution Computed Tomography Scans

Kazunori Okada

CONTENTS

4.1 Introduction: Literature Review

Lung cancer is the most common cause of cancer death in the United States for both sexes [1]. Among various types of small cell and non–small cell lung cancers, adenocarcinoma is the most prevalent type, accounting for more than a third of all primary lung tumors, and its incidence has been increasing in the past few decades [2]. X-ray computed tomography (CT) is one of the most sensitive imaging domains for noninvasive diagnostics of adenocarcinomas [3]. The recent advances in three-dimensional (3D) imaging technology, such as high-resolution and multidetector CT, have greatly improved image resolution and scanning time [4], making it possible to detect very small lung tumors. The study of such small tumors is clinically important because they can still be malignant, and early detection of such malignancy could increase the chance of patient survival [5]. This technical advent has also helped us to better understand the intricate pathology of a type of adenocarcinoma known as small peripheral adenocarcinomas [6]. Small peripheral lung adenocarcinomas typically appear radiographically as ground-glass nodules (GGN) [2].

4.1.1 Radiographic Characteristics of GGNs

Radiologically speaking, GGN represents a type of pulmonary nodule (i.e., localized increase of attenuation in the lung parenchyma of an X-ray CT image), which does not completely obscure the underlying normal parenchymal structures, such as airways, vessels, and interlobular septa (i.e., presenting a focal ground-glass opacity or GGO). GGN is also known as a subsolid nodule, whereas those that completely obscure the lung parenchyma are called solid nodules. GGNs cover a spectrum between completely-not-solid and almost-solid opacities, which are clinically categorized into two subtypes: pure and mixed GGNs. For the pure GGNs, the appearance of the entire nodule is subsolid, whereas the mixed GGNs consist of a combination of solid and subsolid components.

4.1.2 Nomenclature of GGNs

There exist varying, sometimes confusing, terms denoting these radiographic classifications. In the literature, GGNs have equivalently been called as GGOs [7], focal GGOs [8], localized GGOs [9], nodular GGOs [10], localized/focal ground-glass attenuations [11], subsolid nodules [2], nonsolid nodules [12], or semisolid nodules [13]. The pure GGNs are also called nonsolid nodules [14], whereas the mixed GGNs are called part-solid nodules [14] or heterogeneous GGOs [15].

4.1.3 Clinical Prevalence: Epidemiology

GGNs are clinically significant because they are the CT appearance of a prevalent and highly malignant class of lung cancers, offering an effective and noninvasive screening and diagnostic means. The spectrum of the small peripheral adenocarcinomas represented by GGNs has been histologically classified by Noguchi et al. [6] and the World Health Organization [16], including special types of the premalignant atypical adenomatous hyperplasia (AAH), the malignant bronchioloalveolar carcinoma (BAC), and more invasive mixed subtype adenocarcinoma. BAC corresponds to Noguchi's type A, B, and C classifications and is the most common form of adenocarcinoma, accounting for 74% of all adenocarcinomas and 2% to 6% of all non–small cell lung cancers. When combining the incidence of BAC with the incidence of the mixed subtype adenocarcinoma with a BAC component, the combined class accounts for 20% of all lung cancers [2].

4.1.4 Malignancy of GGNs

The radiographic findings of the pure and mixed GGNs have been shown to correspond roughly to the AAH, BAC, and other adenocarcinomas [7,9,11,15,17,18]. GGNs are most likely malignant [12], whereas the mixed GGNs are shown to have much higher chance of malignancy than pure GGNs and solid nodules. In a screening study by Henschke et al. [14], the mixed GGNs recorded a malignancy rate of 63%, whereas the pure GGNs and solid nodules were malignant only in 8% and 7% cases, respectively. Several studies have also shown that greater GGO components in the mixed GGN cases correlate with a smaller chance of malignancy [8,10,19] and better prognosis [18,20,21]. Despite these findings, the CT values for differentiating between benign and malignant GGNs have not been confirmed because there are reports with mixed results in the literature [2].

4.1.5 GGNs' Evolution and Histopathological Disease Progression

Studying the subtypes of GGNs is also important for understanding the histopathological evolution of the peripheral adenocarcinomas. The pure GGNs that are less than 5 mm in size nearly always correspond to AAH, whereas the larger pure and mixed GGNs should be treated as malignant BAC or invasive adenocarcinoma [2,8]. It has been observed that at least some cases of benign AAH slowly progress to malignant BAC, and to more invasive adenocarcinoma [22–25]; thus, early detection and treatment of pure GGO can also improve the prognosis of lung cancer [26]. The growth pattern of these GGNs is, however, confusing. Many cases do not show an increase in nodule size and, in some cases, the nodule size can even decrease over time while being malignant [27]. In general, the evolution from AAH to malignant adenocarcinoma is very slow [27] and may not be hypermetabolic at FDG-PET [12], thus requiring a longer interval in a CT follow-up study with more accurate volumetry/change-estimation scheme. This poses a difficult technical challenge because the subsolid opacity of GGNs makes accurate and repeatable 3D lesion segmentation a challenging task, and such accurate segmentation is a prerequisite for an accurate volumetry/change estimation [28–32].

4.1.6 Computer-Aided Detection and Diagnosis of GGNs

Computer-aided detection (CADe) and diagnosis (CADx) for pulmonary nodules is a well-studied field. The improved 3D image resolution helps radiologists detect nodules more accurately [33]; however, it also creates more of a burden by increasing the amount of data they need to interpret. Thus, automation of the analysis with computer-assisted systems is needed to reduce this burden and also to improve the diagnostic accuracy especially for small nodules. Despite the vast existing literature on general lung CAD [3,34–39], studies on applying the CAD approach to GGNs still underrepresent the above clinical interests in the literature. Three different steps, detection [40–47], segmentation [44,47–54], and classification [55–57], of the GGN CAD scheme have been studied by a number of investigators. For GGN detection, most approaches exploit either image processing filters (N-Quoit filter [40,41] and Gabor filter [43]) or machine learning–based classifiers (three-layer artificial neural network [42] and linear discriminant analysis (LDA) [45,47]). Only a few previous studies exist for the classification of GGN subtypes. Suzuki et al. [55] proposed a CAD scheme for classifying the malignancy of pulmonary nodules by using the massive training artificial neural network. Odry et al. [56] proposed an algorithm to automatically estimate the amount of solid components in GGNs. Zheng et al. [57] introduced a voxel-wise GGO index feature that can be used for other applications. For segmentation, various proposals have been made in the literature. The proposed algorithms include robust anisotropic Gaussian fitting (RAGF) [49], shape-based Markov random field [48,50], nonparametric 3D texture likelihood map analysis [44], four-phase level set segmentation [51], six-stage region growing [53], and an LDA-based machine learning approach [47,54]. Most studies focus on maximizing segmentation accuracy rather than robustness/reproducibility. Despite these increasing interests, GGN-CAD remains an open problem with much room for improvement, especially in robustness.

4.1.7 Lung Nodule Volumetry and Its Limitation

Toward realizing a robust volumetry/change estimation of GGNs to diagnose small AAH and BAC more reliably, and to uncover more details of the peripheral adenocarcinomas' disease progression, this study focuses on the segmentation part of the overall GGN-CAD. Segmentation applied in volumetry (i.e., estimation of volume change over time or measuring the doubling time) brings more emphasis to its robustness/reproducibility than its raw accuracy as a domain-specific criterion. Recent studies on CT nodule volumetry have revealed considerable variability in the existing software's estimation results when varying CT reconstruction parameters [58], CT dosage setting [59], software versions [60], algorithm choice [61], and algorithm threshold parameters [58]. These inaccuracies limit the time interval of follow-up studies to some large values, reducing its clinical usability [62]. Note that a fixed-value bias in segmentation error is canceled out when measuring volumetry, so that even an inaccurate segmentation algorithm can be a good choice for volumetry as long as it is reproducible and robust. Thus, a robust algorithm that produces more reproducible/consistent results than existing, more accurate but less robust, solutions can be a better choice in this application context.

4.1.8 GGN Characterization: Our Approach

The RAGF algorithm proposed by our previous work [49,63] is one example of such robust nodule segmentation solution. Instead of finding an accurate nodule boundary estimate, the RAGF algorithm addresses the nodule characterization problem, yielding a robust estimate of ellipsoidally approximated nodule boundary and a set of nodule characterizations in terms of (i) nodule center, (ii) nodule volume, (iii) maximum diameter, (iv) average diameter, and (v) isotropy. The algorithm is designed to be robust against the real CT data with noise that is intrinsic to the measurement process as well as the pathology and anatomy of our interest, including the variability of GGNs,

1. deviation of the signal from a Gaussian intensity model of our choice (i.e., non-Gaussianity: Figure 4.1a,b);
2. uncertainty in the marker location "+" given by system users (i.e., initialization: Figure 4.1a,c); and
3. influences from surrounding structures such as the pleural surface and vessels (i.e., margin truncation: Figure 4.1c,d).

Figure 4.1 illustrates two examples in two-dimensional cross-sectional and one-dimensional profile views of the two lesions for the pure GGN and the juxtapleural cases [29]. The RAGF method succeeds in robustly approximating the nodule boundary (shown by the solid-lined ellipses around the center **x** in the figure) and its volumetric measurements even with the presence of these difficulties. The algorithm is relevant to the GGN characterization because not only is it robust against GGN's variable intensity appearances but it can also handle the cases with pleural surfaces because small peripheral adenocarcinomas have a high likelihood for such wall attachments. An extensive validation study with 1310 cases has demonstrated this method's effectiveness for solitary pulmonary nodules in both primary and secondary lung cancers. However, its effectiveness for GGN cases has not been fully confirmed by our previous studies. In this chapter, we validate the same RAGF algorithm proposed in ref. [49] with a data set of 56 GGN cases. The rest of this chapter presents the summary of the RAGF algorithm, as well as the results of the experimental validation.

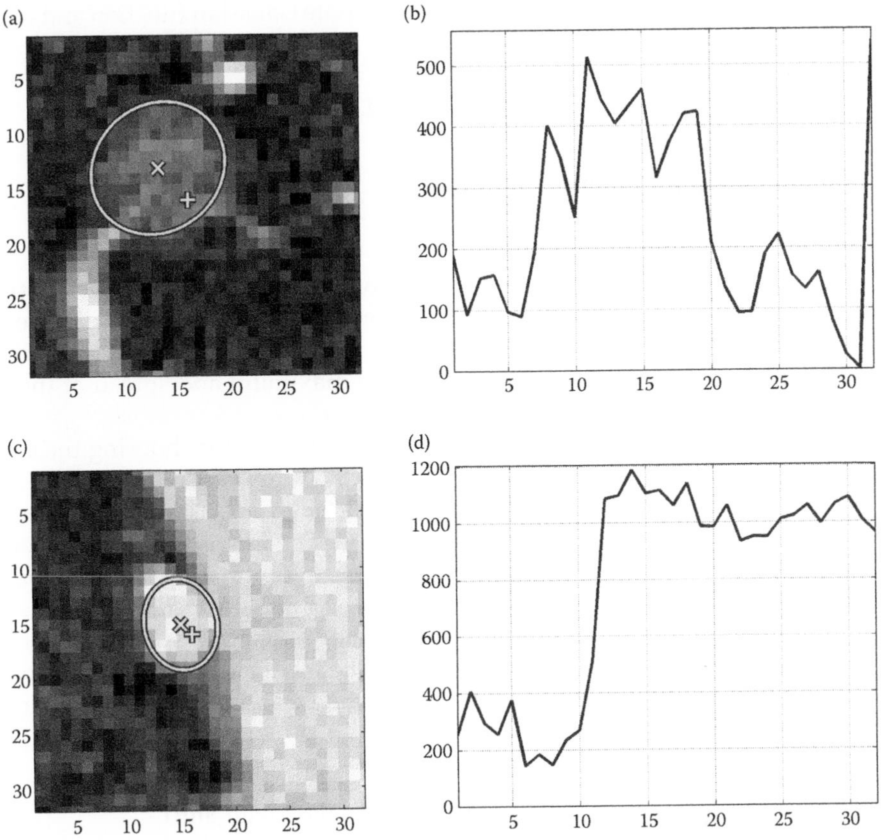

FIGURE 4.1
An illustration of pulmonary nodule examples with typical data noises captured in 3D CT images. (a), Vascularized pure GGN; (b), one-dimensional vertical profile of (a); (c), nodule attached to the pleural surface in two-dimensional dissection; (d), one-dimensional horizontal profile of (c) through the nodule center. The voxel intensities in (b and d) indicate the Hounsfield unit with an offset 1024. "+" denotes markers used as initialization points provided by expert radiologists. The estimated nodule center and anisotropic spread are shown by "×" and 35% confidence ellipses, respectively.

4.2 Methods: RAGF Nodule Characterization

The pulmonary nodule in a chest CT image typically appears as a local concentration of high CT values surrounded by very low CT values of lung parenchyma as background. One of the most common model functions for describing the characteristics of such bounded signals is the Gaussian function [49,64].

The volumetric CT image is treated as the discretization of a d (3)-dimensional continuous nonnegative signal $f(x)$ over a 3D regular lattice. The nonpositiveness is assured by using the offset with 1024 to the CT values in Hounsfield unit. The symbol u is used for describing the location of a spatial local maximum of f. Suppose that the local region of f

around u can be approximated by a product of a d-variate Gaussian function and a positive multiplicative parameter,

$$f(\mathbf{x}) \cong \alpha \times [\Phi(\mathbf{x};\mathbf{u},\Sigma)]_{\mathbf{x}\in S} \tag{4.1}$$

$$\Phi(\mathbf{x};\mathbf{u};\Sigma) = (2\pi)^{-d/2}\left|\Sigma\right|^{-1/2} \exp\left(-\frac{1}{2}(\mathbf{x}-\mathbf{u})^{t}\Sigma^{-1}(\mathbf{x}-\mathbf{u})\right), \tag{4.2}$$

where S is a set of data points in the neighborhood of u, belonging to the basin of attraction of u. The problem of our interest can now be understood as the parametric model fitting and the estimation of the model parameters: mean u, covariance Σ, and amplitude α. The mean and covariance of Φ describe the spatial local maximum and spread of the nodule appearance, respectively.

As discussed in the previous section, the above assumption for choosing the Gaussian intensity model can be largely violated when applied to GGN cases because the intensity distribution of GGNs will most likely not follow that of a Gaussian function (see Figure 4.1b). Two approaches can be pursued in this situation. The first is to choose a model that better fits the data. This is a difficult approach because formulating a functional model that covers all possible GGN appearances is a challenging task. Instead, we take the second approach of devising a robust model-fitting/parameter estimation scheme, which allows the fit of a model to data that do not closely follow the model assumption. The following sections describe one such example by combining the ideas from robust nonparametric density estimation and scale-space data analysis.

4.2.1 Theory: Anisotropic Scale Space and Scale-Space Mean Shift

The scale-space theory [65–67] states that, given any d-dimensional continuous signal f: $\mathbb{R}^d \to \mathbb{R}$, the scale-space representation F: $\mathbb{R}^d \times \mathbb{R}_+ \to \mathbb{R}$ of f is defined to be the solution of the diffusion equation, $\partial_h F = 1/2\nabla^2 F$, or equivalently, the convolution of the signal with Gaussian kernels $\Phi(\mathbf{x};0,\mathbf{H})$ of various bandwidths (or scales) $\mathbf{H} \in \mathbb{R}^{d\times d}$,

$$F(\mathbf{x};\mathbf{H}) = f(\mathbf{x}) * \Phi(\mathbf{x};0,\mathbf{H}). \tag{4.3}$$

When $\mathbf{H} = h\mathbf{I}$ ($h > 0$), F represents the solution of the isotropic diffusion process [67]. When $\mathbf{H}$ is allowed to be a fully parameterized symmetric positive-definite matrix, F represents anisotropic scale space that is the solution to a partial differential equation: $\partial_{\mathbf{H}} F = 1/2\nabla\nabla^t F$.

The gradient vector of the anisotropic scale-space representation $F(\mathbf{x};\mathbf{H})$ can be written as a convolution of f with the Gaussian derivative kernel $\nabla\Phi$ because the gradient operator commutes across the convolution operation. Some algebra reveals that ∇F can be expressed as a function of a vector whose form resembles the fixed-bandwidth density mean shift [68],

$$\begin{aligned} F(\mathbf{x};\mathbf{H}) &= f(\mathbf{x}) * \Phi(\mathbf{x};\mathbf{H}) \\ &= \int f(\mathbf{x})\Phi(\mathbf{x}-\mathbf{x};\mathbf{H})\mathbf{H}^{-1}(\mathbf{x}-\mathbf{x})d\mathbf{x} \\ &= \mathbf{H}^{-1}\int \mathbf{x}\,\Phi(\mathbf{x}-\mathbf{x};\mathbf{H})f(\mathbf{x})d\mathbf{x} - \mathbf{H}^{-1}\mathbf{x}\int\Phi(\mathbf{x}-\mathbf{x};\mathbf{H})f(\mathbf{x})d\mathbf{x} \\ &= \mathbf{H}^{-1}F(\mathbf{x};\mathbf{H})\mathbf{m}(\mathbf{x};\mathbf{H}) \end{aligned} \tag{4.4}$$

$$\mathbf{m}(\mathbf{x};\mathbf{H}) \equiv \frac{\int \mathbf{x}' \Phi(\mathbf{x}-\mathbf{x}';\mathbf{H}) f(\mathbf{x}') d\mathbf{x}'}{\int \Phi(\mathbf{x}-\mathbf{x}';\mathbf{H}) f(\mathbf{x}') d\mathbf{x}'} - \mathbf{x}. \tag{4.5}$$

Equation 4.5 defines scale-space mean shift as the extended fixed-bandwidth mean shift vector for f. Equation 4.5 can be seen as introducing a weight variable $w \equiv f(\mathbf{x}')$ to the kernel $K(\mathbf{x}') \equiv \Phi(\mathbf{x} - \mathbf{x}')$. Therefore, an arithmetic mean of $\mathbf{x}'$ is weighted by the product of the kernel and signal values $K'(\mathbf{x}') \equiv \Phi(\mathbf{x} - \mathbf{x}')f(\mathbf{x}')$. The mean shift procedure [69] is defined as iterative updates of a data point $\mathbf{x}_t$ until its convergence at y_t^m,

$$y_{j+1} = \mathbf{m}(y_j;\mathbf{H}) + y_j \quad y_0 = \mathbf{x}_t. \tag{4.6}$$

Such iteration gives a robust and efficient algorithm of gradient ascent because $\mathbf{m}(\mathbf{x};\mathbf{H})$ can be interpreted as a normalized gradient by rewriting Equation 4.4; $\mathbf{m}(\mathbf{x};\mathbf{H}) = \mathbf{H}\nabla F(\mathbf{x};\mathbf{H})/F(\mathbf{x};\mathbf{H})$. The direction of the mean shift vector aligns with the exact gradient direction when $\mathbf{H}$ is isotropic with a positive scale.

4.2.2 Robust Gaussian Mean Estimation

We assume that the 3D volume is given with information of where the target structure is roughly located, but we do not have explicit knowledge of its spread. The marker point $\mathbf{x}_p$ indicates such location information. We allow $\mathbf{x}_p$ to be placed anywhere within the basin of attraction S of the target structure. In this condition, the Gaussian mean u can be estimated as a local intensity mode of the scale space with a fixed bandwidth $\mathbf{H}$ by using the mean shift procedure in Equation 4.6 with $\mathbf{x}_p$ as its initial point. To increase the robustness of this approach, we run N_1 mean shift procedures initialized by sampling the neighborhood of $\mathbf{x}_p$ uniformly. The majority of the procedure's convergence at the same location (in terms of the Mahalanobis distance with $\mathbf{H}$) indicates the location of the maximum.

4.2.3 Robust Gaussian Covariance Estimation

The Gaussian covariance Σ in Equation 4.1 characterizes the d-dimensional anisotropic spread and orientation of the signal f around the estimated mode u. It can be robustly estimated by using information only sampled within the basin of attraction of the target nodule, ignoring the information that belongs to other structures. This is done by collecting mean shift vectors along convergent scale-space mean shifts from multiple seed points, and then estimating the unknown covariance as a function of the collected mean shifts by solving a constrained least-squares problem.

With the signal model of Equation 4.1, the definition of the mean shift vector of Equation 4.5 can be rewritten as a function of Σ,

$$\begin{aligned}\mathbf{m}(y_j;\mathbf{H}) &= \mathbf{H}\frac{F(y_j;\mathbf{H})}{F(y_j;\mathbf{H})} \\ &\cong \mathbf{H}\frac{\alpha\Phi(y_j;u,\Sigma+\mathbf{H})(\Sigma+\mathbf{H})^{-1}(u-y_j)}{\alpha\Phi(y_j;u,\ \Sigma+\mathbf{H})} \\ &= \mathbf{H}(\Sigma+\mathbf{H})^{-1}(u-y_j).\end{aligned} \tag{4.7}$$

Further rewriting Equation 4.7 results in a linear matrix equation of unknown Σ,

$$\Sigma \mathbf{H}^{-1}\mathbf{m}_j = b_j \tag{4.8}$$

where $\mathbf{m}_j \equiv \mathbf{m}(y_j;\mathbf{H})$ and $b_j \equiv u - y_j - \mathbf{m}_j$. An overcomplete set of the linear equations can be formed by using all the trajectory points $\{y_j | j = 1,\ldots,t_u\}$ that converge to the same u located within the basin of attraction S. For efficiently collecting a sufficient number of samples $\{(y_j,\mathbf{m}_j)\}$, we run N_2 mean shift procedures initialized by sampling the neighborhood of pre-estimated u uniformly. This results in t_u samples ($t_u = \sum_{t=1}^{N_2} t_i$), where t_t denotes the number of points on the convergent trajectory starting from $\mathbf{x}_i$. The system described in Equation 4.8 can be formulated as a constrained least-squares problem,

$$\begin{aligned} &A\Sigma = B \\ &\Sigma \in \text{SPD} \\ &A = (\mathbf{m}_1,..,\mathbf{m}_{tu})^t \mathbf{H}^{-t}, \\ &B = (b_1,..,b_{tu})^t \end{aligned} \tag{4.9}$$

where SPD denotes a set of symmetric positive-definite matrices in $\mathbb{R}^{d\times d}$. The unique closed-form solution Σ^{**} of this system is given by

$$\Sigma^{**} = U_p \Sigma_p^{-1} U_{\tilde{Q}} \Sigma_{\tilde{Q}} U_{\tilde{Q}}^t \Sigma_p^{-1} U_p^t, \tag{4.10}$$

which involves symmetric Schur decompositions [70, p. 393] of the matrices $P \equiv A^t A$ and $\tilde{Q} \equiv \Sigma_p U_p^t Q U_p \Sigma_p$, given $Q \equiv B^t B$, that is,

$$P = U_p \Sigma_p^2 U_p^t$$

$$\tilde{Q} = U_{\tilde{Q}} \Sigma_{\tilde{Q}}^2 U_{\tilde{Q}}^t.$$

The solution Σ^{**} is derived from finding Y^{**} in the Cholesky factorization of $\Sigma = YY^t$. It can be shown that Σ^{**} uniquely minimizes an area criterion $\|AY - BY^{-t}\|_F^2$, where $\|\cdot\|_F$ denotes the Frobenius norm.

4.2.4 Robust Scale Selection

The previous sections explain how the RAGF method estimates the Gaussian center u and spread Σ given an analysis bandwidth **H**. The scale-space–based multiscale analysis treats **H** as a variable parameter. Our procedure repeats the Gaussian fitting for a set of analysis bandwidths $\{\mathbf{H}_k | k = 1,\ldots,K\}$. Then, the bandwidth that provides the optimal K estimate is sought by a certain criterion. The RAGF algorithm exploits the stability test proposed in ref. [68]. Given a set of estimates $\{(u_k,\Sigma_k)\}$ for a series of the successive linear analysis bandwidths $\{h_k | \text{k} = 1,\ldots,K\}$, a form of the Jensen–Shannon divergence is defined by,

$$\mathrm{JS}(k) = \frac{1}{2}\log \frac{\left| \frac{1}{2a+1} \sum_{i=k-a}^{k+a} \Sigma_i \right|}{2a+1\sqrt{\prod_{i=k-a}^{k+a} \left|\Sigma_i\right|}} + \frac{1}{2}\sum_{i=k-a}^{k+a} (u_t - u)^t \left(\sum_{i=k-a}^{k+a} \Sigma_i \right)^{-1} (u_i - u) \tag{4.11}$$

where $u = \frac{1}{2a+1} \sum_{k-a}^{k+a} u_i$ and a defines the neighborhood width of the divergence computation. The most stable estimate across the analysis bandwidths provides a local minimum of the divergence profile. We treat the minimizer as the final estimation of the RAGF method (u^*, Σ^*).

4.2.5 Algorithm Overview

The RAGF algorithm assumes that a marker indicating the rough location of the target nodule is given a priori. Such information can be provided by the user of a graphical user interface-based system. The estimation algorithm is presented below.

Problem: Given the 3D input data, $f(x)$, a marker point, $\mathbf{x}_p$, a set of analysis scales, $\{\mathbf{H}_k | \ k = 1, \ldots K\}$, estimates the 3D anisotropic structure of a nodule (u^*, Σ^*).

Scale-specific estimation: For each k,

1. Perform uniform sampling centered at $\mathbf{x}_p$, resulting in a set of N_1 starting points.
2. Perform the mean shift procedure in Equation 4.6 from each starting point.
3. Take the convergence point of the majority of the points as the location estimate u_k.
4. Perform uniform sampling centered at u_k, resulting in a set of N_2 starting points.
5. Perform the mean shift procedure from each starting point.
6. Construct the system in Equation 4.9 with the mean shift vectors $\{\mathbf{m}(y_j)\}$ along the converging trajectories.
7. Solve the system by Equation 4.10, resulting in the covariance estimate Σ_k.

Scale selection: with K estimates $\{(u_k, \Sigma_k)\}$,

1. Compute the divergence $\{\mathrm{JS}(u_k, \Sigma_k)\}$ using Equation 4.11 for $k = 1 + a, \ldots, K - a$.
2. Find the most stable solution (u^*, Σ^*) by finding a local minimum of $\{\mathrm{JS}_k\}$: argmin_k $\mathrm{JS}(u_k, \Sigma_k)$.

4.2.6 Volumetric Measurements

The multiscale Gaussian-based model fitting, described in the previous sections, results in the mean and covariance estimates (u^*, Σ^*) of a Gaussian function that best fits the given data. Treating the fitted model as a normal probability distribution, $N(\mathbf{x}; u^*, \Sigma^*)$, the tumor boundary segmentation can be approximated by a confidence ellipsoid forming a 3D equal-probability contour. Such a confidence ellipsoid is defined by the solutions to the following generic quadratic equation,

$$(\mathbf{x} - u^*)^t \Sigma^{*-1} (\mathbf{x} - u^*) = \sigma^2 \tag{4.12}$$

where σ^2 is a squared Mahalanobis distance, defining the confidence limit. The volumetry of an ellipsoid can be determined as a function of three radii along its major and two minor orthogonal axes. The radii are denoted by $r_i > 0$ $(r_1 \geq r_2 \geq r_3)$.

The following derives r_i from the eigen decomposition of the covariance Σ^*. Such eigen decomposition can be expressed in a matrix equation: $\Sigma^* \boldsymbol{V} = \boldsymbol{V}\boldsymbol{L}$. $\boldsymbol{V}$ is a column matrix of the eigenvector $\mathbf{v}_i$, and $\boldsymbol{L}$ is a diagonal matrix of the corresponding eigenvalues λ_t^2 $(\lambda_1 \geq \lambda_2 \geq \lambda_3)$. Right-multiplying the matrix equation with $\boldsymbol{V}^t$ yields the symmetric Schur decomposition of Σ^*: $\Sigma^* = \boldsymbol{V}\boldsymbol{L}\boldsymbol{V}^t$. Because $\Sigma^{*-1} = \boldsymbol{V}\boldsymbol{L}^{-1}\boldsymbol{V}^t$, with a coordinate transform $y \equiv \boldsymbol{V}^t(\mathbf{x} - u^*)$, Equation 4.12 can be simplified to: $y^t\boldsymbol{L}^{-1}y = \sigma^2$. Substituting three points, $y = (r_1,0,0)^t,(0,r_2,0)^t,(0,0,r_3)^t$, which are known to lie on the ellipsoid surface, to the quadratic equation results in

$$r_i = \sigma\lambda_i. \tag{4.13}$$

As a result, the following volumetric measurement formula can immediately be derived for the volume $V = \frac{4}{3}\pi\sigma^3 \prod_i \lambda_i$, the maximum diameter $L = 2\sigma\lambda_1$, the average diameter $A = \frac{2}{3}\sigma \sum_i \lambda_i$, and the isotropy $R = \frac{\lambda_2 + \lambda_s}{2\lambda_1}$, where V, L, and A are in the voxel unit and the isotropy R is in the range [0,1], taking the value 1 when it becomes a sphere. The bias of these volumetric measurements is caused solely by the segmentation error. Therefore, these formula are exact and thus free from the partial volume effect when the tumor boundary is well characterized by the ellipsoidal segmentation.

Given a voxel dimension in a physical unit, the volumetric measurement formula shown previously can be revised to produce the measurements in the unit. This is a crucial step for any comparative and differential study because the voxel dimension can vary across different scans. Suppose that a voxel dimension is given as $(\Delta x, \Delta y, \Delta z)$, in millimeters, or in any other unit. After a coordinate transform, eigenvalues in millimeters, λ_i, can be expressed as a function of the voxel dimensions and eigenvectors,

$$\lambda_i = \beta_i \lambda_i \tag{4.14}$$

$$\beta_i = \sqrt{(v_{xi}\Delta x)^2 + (v_{yi}\Delta y)^2 + (v_{zi}\Delta z)^2} \tag{4.15}$$

where the eigenvector is denoted by $\mathbf{v}_i = (v_{xi}, v_{yi}, v_{zi})^t$. This leads us to the following formula which take the voxel dimension into account,

$$V = \frac{4}{3}\pi\sigma^3 \prod_i \beta_i \lambda_i \tag{4.16}$$

$$L = 2\sigma\lambda_{1,} = 2\sigma \max_i \beta_i \lambda_i \tag{4.17}$$

$$A = \frac{2}{3}\sigma \sum_i \beta_i \lambda_i \tag{4.18}$$

$$R = \frac{\lambda_2 + \lambda_3}{2\lambda_1} \tag{4.19}$$

where $\lambda_{1'} \geq \lambda_{2'} \geq \lambda_3$. Note that $\lambda_{1'}$ must be re-sorted from the original order given by the eigen decomposition because the coordinate transform may change such an order.

4.3 Experiments

4.3.1 Data

A data set of 56 clinical GGN cases was used in this study. Thin-section chest high-resolution CT (HRCT) images of 34 patients were recorded by multiple multislice CT scanners (Somatom Volume Zoom and Somatom Sensation 16; Siemens) and anonymitized. Each volumetric image consists of 12-bit positive values over an array of 512 × 512 lattices. The number of slices in a CT volume and the dimensions of a voxel vary across volumes in our data set. The number of slices ranged between 217 and 616. The voxel dimensions ranged within [0.4609–0.8281, 0.4609–08281, 0.5–1] in millimeter. Fifty-six GGN lesions were identified by trained radiologists among the set of volumes. For each GGN lesion, the radiologists provided the initialization marker $\mathbf{x}_p$, indicating its rough location, and a 43-voxel cubic volume-of-interest centered at the marker is extracted as a preprocess. All cases were small (<15 mm) and 44 of them were extremely small (<5 mm). Thirty-nine cases were peripherally located near or attached to the lung wall. Figure 4.2 shows 12 illustrative examples of this data set with circular (a and b), hazy (c–f), small (g–j), and attached (k and l) cases.

4.3.2 Results

A 3D implementation of the RAGF algorithm is evaluated with the above GGN data set. The implementation is straightforward without any 3D specific adaptation. The analysis bandwidths are set to 18 scales with 0.25 interval, $h = (0.50^2, 0.75^2,\ldots, 4.75^2)$. Uniform sampling in the three-voxel neighborhood of the marker (i.e., $N_1 = 7$) was used for estimating the local maximum. The three-voxel size was determined empirically. The same strategy was used for initializing the mean shift trajectories around the local maximum (i.e., $N_2 = 7$). The neighborhood width of the divergence computation is set to $a = 1$ (considering only three adjacent scales).

Figure 4.3 displays the results of the RAGF method for one GGN example case (Figure 4.2a). The second row shows the intensity images generated from the Gaussian model fitted to the data in the first row. The third row shows the result of an approximated nodule boundary shown as two-dimensional intersections of the 35% confidence ellipsoid of the fitted Gaussian. Figure 4.4 shows the RAGF characterization results for the examples in Figure 4.2. Our visual inspection revealed that the marker locations provided by trained radiologists were noticeably off-center in many cases, deviating from the true/estimated nodule centers to a certain degree. The correct estimations for these GGN cases demonstrate the feasibility and effectiveness of the RAGF method for GGN characterization.

Next, the quantitative performance of the RAGF with the above data set was studied. Because of the lack of ground truth for 3D nodule segmentation, the classification of the correct or failure estimation is given manually by visual appraisal of experts using a 3D render view and its corresponding multiplanar reconstruction (MPR) view. Statistical verification using the χ^2 test [49] is also performed for each RAGF result to determine whether to accept or reject it.

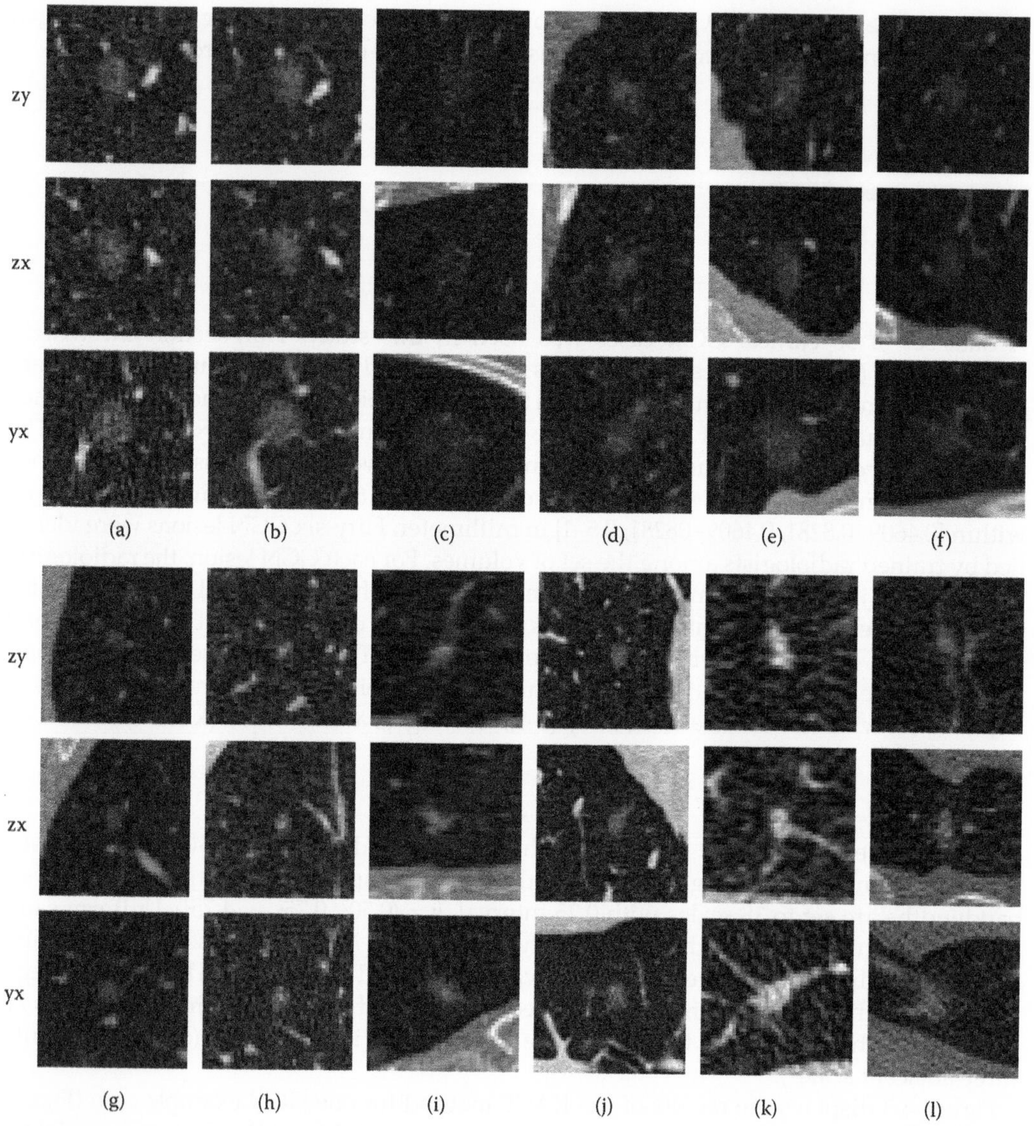

FIGURE 4.2
Twelve GGN examples in 3D HRCT. Each case is shown in the three-plane MPR view of a 43-voxel cubic volume-of-interest. (a) and (b), Circular cases; (c–f), cases with hazy opacity; (g–j), small cases (<5 mm); k and l, cases attached to the pleural surface.

Table 4.1 summarizes the resulting performance statistics. Forty-nine cases (87.5%) resulted in successful nodule characterization confirmed by visual appraisal. For verification, a small percentage of cases resulted in false acceptance (three false positives, 5.4%) and false rejection (five false negatives, 8.9%). The few failures were caused by (a) undersegmentation caused by nearby vessels (two false positives and one true negative), (b) misdetection caused by wall attachment (two true negatives), (c) oversegmentation caused by very hazy opacity (one true negative), and (d) undersegmentation caused by necrosis

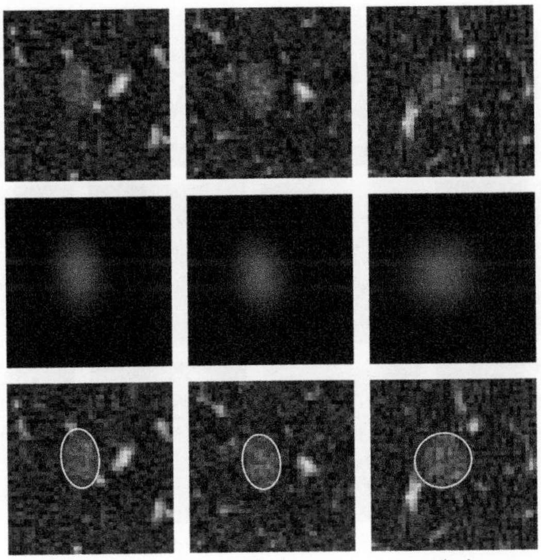

FIGURE 4.3
An example of nodule characterization by the RAGF algorithm. A circular GGN example in Figure 4.2a is shown in the first row. The second row shows the estimated intensity image of the Gaussian model fitted to the above data by the RAGF. The third row shows the final nodule boundary approximation by the 35% confidence ellipsoid of the fitted Gaussian. The marker locations are indicated by "+". The estimated nodule centers are indicated by "×".

(one false positive). Figure 4.5 shows examples for these four causes of failures. Figure 4.5a illustrates failure caused by nearby vessels. The RAGF, in this case, captures a small high-intensity vessel region rather than the GGN attached to the vessel. This case corresponds to a failure of the scale selection process, which mistakenly chose the analysis scale that corresponds to the vessel to be most stable. Figure 4.5b illustrates a case in which a GGN attached to the lung wall is missed. This failure was mainly caused by ill-placed markers. With such markers, nonpathological structures near the markers could be characterized instead of the target nodule and are accidentally well-approximated by the Gaussian distribution (e.g., rib bones). Thirty-seven other peripheral cases were correctly characterized. Figure 4.5c shows failure in which the opacity of GGN was so low that the RAGF's covariance estimation failed. Finally, Figure 4.5d shows a case with necrosis inside of a GGN. In this case, the nodule center was hollow, causing the RAGF to capture a subregion of the target GGN. Overall, the majority of the GGN cases were correctly characterized, except for these special cases, and the results were successfully verified for acceptance or rejection.

4.4 Conclusions

This chapter presents a comprehensive literature review of GGNs across the fields of radiology, pathology, and medical image analysis, and an experimental evaluation of the RAGF nodule characterization method with a clinical data set with 56 pure GGN cases.

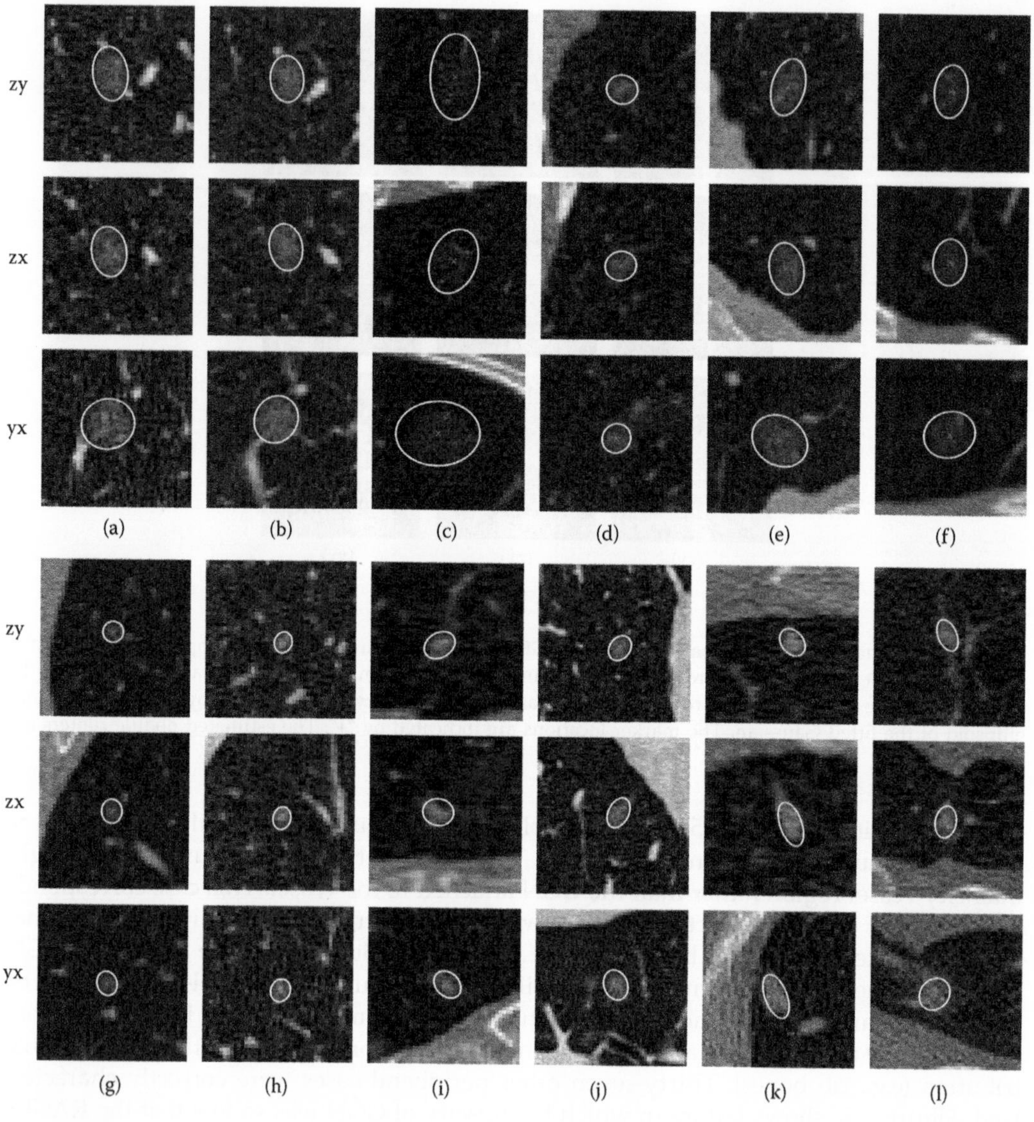

FIGURE 4.4
Nodule characterization results by the RAGF algorithm for the 12 GGN examples shown in Figure 4.2. See captions of Figure 4.2 and Figure 4.3 for details.

GGN is a fairly new subject in all these interdisciplinary fields because we have come to some understanding of them only after the recent advent of high-resolution CT technologies. Although there exist a number of clinical and technical reviews of this subject in the literature, to the best of our knowledge, this is the first to offer a comprehensive review of this subject under these related disciplines together.

The RAGF algorithm was originally proposed as a robust nodule characterization solution for arbitrary types of nodules. Although the original report addressed a potential advantage of the method in some GGN cases, no systematic evaluation of the method's effectiveness toward GGN has been performed to date. This chapter presents the first

TABLE 4.1

Quantitative Performance Evaluation of the RAGF Method

Estimation	No. of Cases (%)	Verification	No. of Cases (%)
Correct	49 (87.5)	TP	44 (78.6)
		FN	5 (8.9)
Failure	7 (12.5)	TN	4 (7.1)
		FP	3 (5.4)

Note: The data set consists of 56 pure GGNs from 34 patients. Multiple scanners were used for data collection.
TP, true positive, accepted correct estimates; FN, false negative, rejected correct estimates; TN, true negative, rejected false estimates; FP, false positive, accepted false estimates.

experimental validation of the RAGF with the clinical data set, demonstrating the feasibility of the method in the GGN application. Note that the RAGF's original performance, with a large clinical data set of 1310 nodules, resulted in an 81.2% success rate. With our GGN data set, the same RAGF algorithm resulted in an 87.5% success rate. The voxel intensity distribution of the GGNs is much more irregular than the typical solid nodules. The favorable performance of the RAGF with GGNs indicates that it is indeed capable of robustly characterizing a wide range of nodule types, including these pure GGNs.

In future work, we plan to improve the performance of the RAGF method for the cases attached to lung walls and vessels (Figure 4.5a and b) to improve the performance further. To derive more clinically conclusive results, we plan to evaluate more GGN cases, especially the mixed cases, as well as to evaluate actual volumetry from follow-up CT data.

Overall, the RAGF method presented is generic and does not depend on semantics of the absolute CT values in the Hounsfield unit. The robustness, flexibility, and efficiency of the proposed framework, therefore, facilitate not only the pulmonary nodule applications in CT sought in this chapter but also various other applications in different imaging domains (e.g., PET scans) and different pathological and anatomical structures (e.g., polyps) involved with the analysis of blob-like geometrical structures. We plan to explore these other applications of our method in the future.

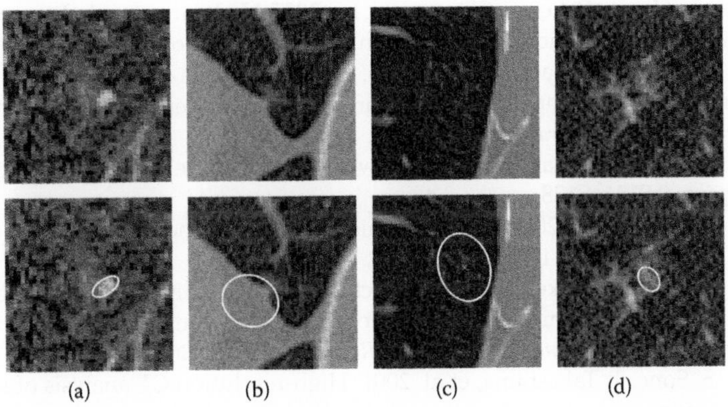

FIGURE 4.5
Examples of failures by the RAGF algorithm. (a), Undersegmentation caused by nearby vessels; (b), misdetection caused by wall attachment; (c), oversegmentation caused by very hazy opacity; (d), undersegmentation caused by necrosis.

Acknowledgments

The author thanks Dorin Comaniciu, Arun Krishnan, Senthil Periaswamy, Toshiro Kubota, Marcos Salganicoff, Visvanathan Ramesh, and Alok Gupta for their support and stimulating discussions.

References

[1] Weir, H.K., et al. 2003. Annual report to the nation on the status of cancer, 1975–2000. *Journal of the National Cancer Institute*, 95(17):1276–1299.

[2] Godoy, M.C.B., and D.P. Naidich. 2009. Subsolid pulmonary nodules and the spectrum of peripheral adenocarcinomas of the lung: Recommended interim guidelines for assessment and management. *Radiology*, 253:606–622.

[3] Ko, J.P., and D.P. Naidich. 2003. Lung nodule detection and characterization with multislice CT. *Radiologic Clinics of North America*, 41:575–597.

[4] Cardinale, L., F. Ardissone, S. Novello, M. Busso, F. Solitro, M. Longo, D. Sardo, M. Giors, and C. Fava. 2009. The pulmonary nodule: Clinical and radiological characteristics affecting diagnosis of malignancy. *La Radiologia Medica*, 114:871–889.

[5] Ohtsuka, T., H. Nomori, H. Horio, T. Naruke, and K. Suemasu. 2003. Radiological examination for peripheral lung cancers and benign nodules less than 10 mm. *Lung Cancer*, 42:291–296.

[6] Noguchi, M., A. Morikawa, M. Kawasaki, et al. 1995. Small adenocarcinoma of the lung: Histologic characteristics and prognosis. *Cancer*, 75:2844–2852.

[7] Kuriyama, K., M. Seto, T. Kasugai, M. Higashiyama, S. Kido, Y. Sawai, K. Kodama, and D. Kuroda. 1999. Ground-glass opacity on thinsection CT: Value in differentiating subtypes of adenocarcinoma of the lung. *AJR. American Journal of Roentgenology*, 173:465–469.

[8] Nakata, M., H. Saeki, I. Takata, Y. Segawa, H. Mogami, K. Mandai, and K. Eguchi. 2002. Focal ground-glass opacity detected by low-dose helical CT. *Chest*, 121(5):1464–1467.

[9] Nakajima, R., T. Yokose, R. Kakinuma, K. Nagai, Y. Nishiwaki, and A. Ochiai. 2002. Localized pure ground-glass opacity on high-resolution CT: Histologic characteristics. *Journal of Computer Assisted Tomography*, 26:323–329.

[10] Park, C., J. Goo, H. Lee, C. Lee, E. Chun, and J. Im. 2007. Nodular ground-glass opacity at thin-section CT: Histologic correlation and evaluation of change at follow-up. *Radiographics*, 27:391–408.

[11] Gaeta, M., R. Caruso, M. Barone, S. Volta, G. Casablanca, and F. La Spada. 1998. Ground-glass attenuation in nodular bronchioloalveolar carcinoma: CT patterns and prognostic value. *Journal of Computer Assisted Tomography*, 22:215–219.

[12] Diederich, S. 2009. Pulmonary nodules: Do we need a separate algorithm for non-solid lesions? *Cancer Imaging*, 9:S126–S128.

[13] Ko, J.P., and D.P. Naidich. 2004. Computer-aided diagnosis and the evaluation of lung disease. *Journal of Thoracic Imaging*, 19:136–155.

[14] Henschke, C.I., D.F. Yankelevitz, R. Mirtcheva, G. McGuinness, D. McCauley, and O.S. Miettinen. 2002. CT screening for lung cancer: Frequency and significance of part-solid and non-solid nodules. *AJR. American Journal of Roentgenology*, 178(5):1053–1057.

[15] Yang, Z.G., S. Sone, T. Takashima, et al. 2001. High-resolution CT analysis of small peripheral lung adenocarcinomas revealed on screening helical CT. *AJR. American Journal of Roentgenology*, 176:1399–1407.

[16] Travis, W.D., K. Garg, W.A. Franklin, et al. 2005. Evolving concepts in the pathology and computed tomography imaging of lung adenocarcinoma and bronchioloalveolar carcinoma. *Journal of Clinical Oncology*, 23:3270–3287.

[17] Suzuki, K., H. Asamura, K. Kusumoto, H. Kondo, and R. Tsuchiya. 2002. Thin-section computed-tomographic scan. *Annals of Thoracic Surgery*, 74:1635–1639.
[18] Kim, E.A., T. Johkoh, K.S. Lee, K. Fujimoto, J. Sadohara, P.S. Yang, T. Kozuka, O. Honda, and S.N. Kim. 2001. Quantification of ground-glass opacity on high-resolution CT of small peripheral adenocarcinoma of the lung: pathologic and prognostic implications. *AJR. American Journal of Roentgenology*, 177:1417–1422.
[19] Li, F., S. Sone, H. Abe, H. MacMahon, and K. Doi. 2004. Malignant versus benign nodules at CT screening for lung cancer: Comparison of thin-section CT findings. *Radiology*, 233:793–798.
[20] Aoki, T., Y. Tomoda, H. Watanabe, H. Nakata, T. Kasai, H. Hashimoto, M. Kodate, T. Osaki, and K. Yasumoto. 2001. Peripheral lung adenocarcinoma: Correlation of thin-section CT findings with histologic prognostic factors and survival. *Radiology*, 220:803–809.
[21] Lee, K.S., Y.J. Jeong, J. Han, B.T. Kim, H. Kim, and O.J. Kwon. 2004. T1 non-small cell lung cancer: Imaging and histopathologic findings and their prognostic implications. *Radiographics*, 24:1617–1636.
[22] Jang, H., K. Lee, O. Kwon, Y.S. Rhee, and J. Han. 1996. Bronchioloalveolar carcinoma: Focal area of ground-glass attenuation at thin-section CT as an early sign. *Radiology*, 199:485–488.
[23] Aoki, T., H. Nakata, H. Watanabe, K. Nakamura, T. Kasai, H. Hashimoto, et al. 2000. Evolution of peripheral lung adenocarcinomas: CT findings correlated with histology and tumor doubling time. *AJR. American Journal of Roentgenology*, 174:763–768.
[24] Takashima, S., Y. Maruyama, M. Hasegawa, T. Yamanda, T. Honda, M. Kadoya, et al. 2003. CT findings and progression of small peripheral lung neoplasms having a replacement growth pattern. *AJR. American Journal of Roentgenology*, 180:817–826.
[25] Kakinuma, R., H. Ohmatsu, M. Kaneko, M. Kusumoto, J. Yoshida, K. Nagai, et al. 2004. Progression of focal pure ground-glass opacity detected by low-dose helical computed tomography screening for lung cancer. *Journal of Computer Assisted Tomography*, 28:17–23.
[26] Watanabe, S., T. Watanabe, K. Arai, T. Kasai, J. Haratake, and H. Urayama. 2002. Results of wedge resection for focal bronchioloalveolar carcinoma showing pure ground-glass attenuation on computed tomography. *Annals of Thoracic Surgery*, 73:1071–1075.
[27] Min, J.H., H.Y. Lee, K.S. Lee, J. Han, K. Park, M. Ahn, and S.J. Lee. 2010. Stepwise evolution from a focal pure pulmonary ground-glass opacity nodule into an invasive lung adenocarcinoma: An observation for more than 10 years. *Lung Cancer*, 69(1):123–126.
[28] Yankelevitz, D.F., A.P. Reeves, W.J. Kostis, B. Zhao, and C.I. Henschke. 2000. Small pulmonary nodules: Volumetrically determined growth rates based on CT evaluation. *Radiology*, 217:251–256.
[29] Kostis, W.J., A.P. Reeves, D.F. Yankelevitz, and C.I. Henschke. 2003. Three-dimensional segmentation and growth-rate estimation of small pulmonary nodules in helical CT images. *IEEE Transactions on Medical Imaging*, 22(10):1259–1274.
[30] Reeves, A.P., A.B. Chan, D.F. Yankelevitz, C.I. Henschke, B. Kressler, and W.J. Kostis. 2006. On measuring the change in size of pulmonary nodules. *IEEE Transactions on Medical Imaging*, 25:435–450.
[31] Jaffe, C.C. 2006. Measures of response: RECIST, WHO, and new alternatives. *Journal of Clinical Oncology*, 24:3245–3251.
[32] Gavrielides, M.A., L.M. Kinnard, K.J. Myers, and N. Petrick. 2004. Noncalcified lung nodules: Volumetric assessment with thoracic CT. *Radiology*, 251:26–39.
[33] Fischback, F., F. Knollmann, V. Griesshaber, T. Freund, E. Akkol, and R. Felix. 2003. Detection of pulmonary nodules by multislice computed tomography: Improved detection rate with reduced slice thickness. *European Radiology*, 13:2378–2383.
[34] Reeves, A.P., and W.J. Kostis. 2000. Computer-aided diagnosis of small pulmonary nodules. *Seminars in Ultrasound, CT, and MR*, 21(2):116–128.
[35] Reeves, A.P., and B.M. Kressler. 2004. Computer-aided diagnostics. *Thoracic Surgery Clinics*, 14:125–133.
[36] Li, Q., F. Li, K. Suzuki, J. Shiraishi, H. Abe, R. Engelmann, Y. Nie, H. MacMahon, and K. Doi. 2005. Computer-aided diagnosis in thoracic CT. *Seminars in Ultrasound, CT, and MR*, 26:357–363.

[37] Sluimer, I., A. Schilham, M. Prokop, and B. van Ginneken. 2006. Computer analysis of computed tomography scans of the lung: A survey. *IEEE Transactions on Medical Imaging*, 25:385–405.
[38] Li, Q. 2007. Recent progress in computer-aided diagnosis of lung nodules on thin-section CT. *Computerized Medical Imaging and Graphics*, 31:248–257.
[39] Goldin, J.G., M.S. Brown, and I. Petkovska. 2008. Computer-aided diagnosis in lung nodule assessment. *Journal of Thoracic Imaging*, 23:97–104.
[40] Ezoe, T., H. Takizawa, S. Yamamoto, A. Shimizu, T. Matsumoto, Y. Tateno, T. Iimura, and M. Matsumoto. 2002. Automatic detection method of lung cancers including ground-glass opacities from chest x-ray CT images. *Proceedings of SPIE*, 1672–1680.
[41] Tanino, M., H. Takizawa, S. Yamamoto, T. Matsumoto, Y. Tateno, and T.A. Iimura. 2003. Detection method of ground glass opacities in chest x-ray CT images using automatic clustering techniques. *Proceedings of SPIE*, 1728–1737.
[42] Kim, K.G., J.M. Goo, J.H. Kim, H.J. Lee, B.G. Min, K.T. Bae, and J.G. Im. 2005. Computer-aided diagnosis of localized ground-glass opacity in the lung at CT: Initial experience. *Radiology*, 237:657–661.
[43] Bastawrous, H.A., N. Nitta, and M. Tsudagawa. 2006. A new CAD system for detecting localized ground glass opacity nodules in lung CT images using cross and coronary section images. *IEEE International Workshop on Medical Measurement and Applications*, Benevento, Italy, 20–21 April 2006, 54–57.
[44] Zhou, J., S. Chang, D.N. Metaxas, B. Zhao, MS. Ginsberg, and L.H. Schwartz. 2006. An automatic method for ground-glass opacity nodule detection and segmentation from CT studies. *International Conference on EMBS, New York*, August 30–September 3 2006, 3062–3065.
[45] Katsumata, Y., Y. Itai, S. Maeda, H. Kim, J.K. Tan, and S. Ishikawa. 2007. Automatic detection of GGO candidate regions employing four statistical features on thoracic MDCT images. *International Conference on Control, Automation and Systems*, Seoul, Korea, 17–20 October 2007, 1278–1281.
[46] Ye, X., X. Lin, J. Dehmeshki, G. Slabaugh, and G. Beddoe. 2009. Shape based computer-aided detection of lung nodules in thoracic CT images. *IEEE Transactions on Bio-Medical Engineering*, 56:1810–1820.
[47] Tao, Y., L. Lu, M. Dewan, A.Y. Chen, J. Corso, J. Xuan, M. Salganicoff, and A. Krishnan. 2009. Multi-level ground glass nodule detection and segmentation in CT lung images. *International Conference on Medical Image Computing and Computer-Assisted Intervention*, London, UK, 20–24 September 2009, Volume 5762, 715–723.
[48] Zhang, L., M. Fang, D.P. Naidich, and C.L. Novak. 2004. Consistent interactive segmentation of pulmonary ground glass nodules identified in CT studies. *Proceedings of SPIE*, 1709–1719.
[49] Okada, K., D. Comaniciu, and A. Krishnan. 2005. Robust anisotropic Gaussian fitting for volumetric characterization of pulmonary nodules in multislice CT. *IEEE Transactions on Medical Imaging*, (24):409–423.
[50] Zhang, L., T. Zhang, C.L. Novak, D.P. Naidich, and D.A. Moses. 2005. A computer-based method of segmenting ground glass nodules in pulmonary CT images: Comparison to expert radiologists' interpretations. *Proceedings of SPIE*, 113–123.
[51] Yoo, Y., H. Shim, I.D. Yun, K.W. Lee, and S.U. Lee. 2006. Segmentation of ground glass opacities by asymmetric multi-phase deformable model. *Proceedings of SPIE*, 6144, 614440.
[52] Browder, W.A., A.P. Reeves, T.V. Apananosovich, M.D. Cham, D.F. Yankelevitz, and C.I. Henschke. 2007. Automated volumetric segmentation method for growth consistency of non-solid pulmonary nodules in high-resolution CT. *Proceedings of SPIE*, 6514, 65140Y.
[53] Kubota, T., A. Jerebko, M. Salganicoff, M. Dewan, and A. Krishnan. 2008. Robust segmentation of pulmonary nodules of various densities: From ground-glass opacities to solid nodules. *International Workshop on Pulmonary Image Analysis*, New York, 6 September 2008, 253–262.
[54] Staring, M., J.P.W. Pluim, B. de Hoop, S. Klein, B. van Ginneken, H. Gietema, G. Nossent, C. Schaefer-Prokop, S. van de Vorst, and M. Prokop. 2009. Image subtraction facilitates assessment of volume and density change in ground-glass opacities in chest CT. *Investigative Radiology*, 44:61–66.

[55] Suzuki, K., F. Li, S. Sone, and K. Doi. 2005. Computer-aided diagnostic scheme for distinction between benign and malignant nodules in thoracic low-dose CT by use of massive training artificial neural network. *IEEE Transactions on Medical Imaging*, (24):1138–1150.
[56] Odry, B.L., J. Huo, L. Zhang, C.L. Novak, and D.P. Naidich. 2007. Solid component evaluation in mixed ground glass nodules. *Proceedings of SPIE*, 6512, 65120R.
[57] Zheng, Y., C. Kambhamettu, T. Bauer, and K. Steiner. 2008. Estimation of ground-glass opacity measurement in CT lung images. *International Conference on Medical Image Computing and Computer-Assisted Intervention*, New York, 6–10 September 2008, Volume 5242, 238–245.
[58] Goo, J.M., T. Tongdee, R. Tongdee, K. Yeo, C.F. Hildebolt, and K.T. Bae. 2005. Volumetric measurement of synthetic lung nodules with multidetector row CT: Effect of various image reconstruction parameters and segmentation thresholds on measurement accuracy. *Radiology*, 235:850–856.
[59] Hein, P.A., V.C. Romano, P. Rogalla, C. Klessen, A. Lembcke, L. Bornemann, V. Dicken, B. Hamm, and H.C. Bauknecht. 2010. Variability of semiautomated lung nodule volumetry on ultralow-dose CT: Comparison with nodule volumetry on standard-dose CT. *Journal of Digital Imaging*, 23:8–17.
[60] Rinaldi, M.F., T. Bartalena, L. Braccaioli, N. Sverzellati, S. Mattioli, E. Rimondi, G. Rossi, M. Zompatori, G. Battista, and R. Canini. 2010. Three-dimensional analysis of pulmonary nodules: Variability of semiautomated volume measurements between different versions of the same software. *La Radiologia Medica*, 115:403–412.
[61] Ashraf, H., B. de Hoop, S.B. Shaker, A. Dirksen, K.S. Bach, H. Hansen, M. Prokop, and J.H. Pedersen. 2010. Lung nodule volumetry: Segmentation algorithms within the same software package cannot be used interchangeably. *European Radiology*, 20(8):1878–1885.
[62] Kostis, W.J., D.F. Yankelevitz, A.P. Reeves, S.C. Fluture, and C.I. Henschke. 2004. Small pulmonary nodules: Reproducibility of three-dimensional volumetric measurement and estimation of time to follow-up CT. *Radiology*, 231:446–452.
[63] Okada, K., D. Comaniciu, N. Dalal, and A. Krishnan. 2004. A robust algorithm for characterizing anisotropic local structures. *European Conference on Computer Vision*, Prague, Czech Republic, 11–14 May 2004, 549–561.
[64] Lee, Y., T. Hara, H. Fujita, S. Itoh, and T. Ishigaki. 2001. Automated detection of pulmonary nodules in helical CT images based on an improved template-matching technique. *IEEE Transactions on Medical Imaging*, 20(7):595–604.
[65] Witkin, A. 1983. Scale-space filtering. *International Joint Conference on Artificial Intelligence*, Karlsruhe, Germany, August 1983, 1019–1021.
[66] Koenderink, J.J. 1984. The structure of images. *Biological Cybernetics*, 50:363–370.
[67] Lindeberg, T. 1998. Feature detection with automatic scale selection. *International Journal of Computer Vision*, 30(2):79–116.
[68] Comaniciu, D. 2003. An algorithm for data-driven bandwidth selection. *IEEE Transactions on Pattern Analysis and Machine Intelligence*, 25(2):281–288.
[69] Comaniciu, D., and P. Meer. 2002. Mean shift: A robust approach toward feature space analysis. *IEEE Transactions on Pattern Analysis and Machine Intelligence.*, 24(5):603–619.
[70] Golub, G.H., and C.F. van Loan. 1996. *Matrix Computations*. Baltimore, MD: Johns Hopkins University Press.

5

Four-Dimensional Computed Tomography Lung Registration Methods

Anand P. Santhanam, Yugang Min, Jannick P. Rolland, Celina Imielinska, and Patrick A. Kupelian

CONTENTS

5.1 Introduction

Lungs are essential respiratory organs that supply the human body with oxygen and remove carbon dioxide. Lungs expand and contract during the respiration process, enabling the air to flow inside it. Knowing the lungs' normal form and how they deform while breathing is an important factor for several different applications. First, a change in the lungs' normal deformation during breathing is a key indicator of a disease state that the human subject may have. Depending on the type of pathophysical condition, the lung's shape may change to minimize the work and stress of breathing that may be associated with breathing when representing the condition. For example, it is known that patients with chronic obstructive pulmonary disease tend to have difficulty breathing and so they alter their breathing pattern to short, shallow breaths that lower the physical stress the subject experiences. Furthermore, patients with disease states such as non–small cell lung cancer tend to develop breathing changes that reflect the presence of tumors. Additional complications arise when the patient has multiple disease states, for instance, the presence of non–small cell lung cancer as well as chronic obstructive pulmonary disease. Based on the type of treatment or therapy the patient is undergoing, the knowledge of the lung's change in shape becomes essential. Second, knowledge of lung motion is essential for understanding the preoperative and postoperative changes in lung functionality. For instance, when patients undergo procedures such as thorectomy or lung transplant, it becomes necessary to monitor the lung's changes in pulmonary function before and after the procedure to understand the functionality of the new anatomy. Third, when patients experience a lung injury, it is vital to the patient's course of treatment to know the changes in the lung's breathing functionality. A vast amount of research has been undertaken to better understand the changes in the respiration process when military service personnel receive shrapnel and bullet wounds. A common injury faced by the subject is open and closed (tension) pneumothorax [1]. In the case of open pneumothorax, the subject has an open wound that fills the pleural cavity with air, disrupting the body's normal system for maintaining a dynamic air volume–pressure relation that enables respiration. The lungs will shrink, unable to respond to the additional air pressure from the open wound and thus disabling them from expanding and contracting after a few breaths. In the case of closed pneumothorax, the subject has a closed wound that fills the pleural cavity with a constant amount of air. The presence of air in the pleural cavity causes constant pain and discomfort to the patient during breathing. The common treatment method involves placing a needle in the chest and removing the air from the pleural cavity. It is important to assess the efficacy and success of the treatment using preoperative (initial or base level lung functionality) and postoperative breathing comparison.

The rest of the chapter is subdivided as follows: we will start by briefly explaining the three-dimensional (3D) computed tomography (CT) and the 3D/four-dimensional (4D) CT imaging processes, which are used clinically for understanding lung motion. We then review the different methods of registration, which forms the main topic of this chapter. They are divided into rigid-body registration, spline-based registration, physics-based registration, inverse consistent registration, and finally, optical flow–based registration. The first two methods can be observed as rigid and nonrigid registration because they determine the type of registration paradigm. The physics-based registration and the inverse consistent registration present additional constraints that can be applied to both rigid and nonrigid registration. The first four methods share the common feature of being based on landmarks, whereas the last method is landmark-independent, nonrigid registration. The next section presents a discussion of validation techniques used for verifying the accuracy of the 4DCT lung registration. Finally, we conclude the chapter by providing an application of 4DCT lung registration: the development of physics-based 3D lung dynamics models and its use in lung radiotherapy.

5.2 CT Imaging Technology

In this section, we discuss the clinical imaging process of CT. Specifically, the 3D and the 4D imaging methodologies are briefly introduced. It is to be noted that peers have extensively investigated these imaging methods and so we outline some of the key efforts.

5.2.1 3DCT Imaging Technology

3DCT is one of modern medicine's most used diagnostic tools. It is an evolution of the simple 2D x-ray. A clinical setup for 3DCT imaging is as follows: the patient lies on a sliding table that passes through the x-ray machine, which is built on a circular gantry. The x-ray circles the patient, obtaining a single transverse slice from multiple angles to provide better resolution to the point of being able to distinguish between different tissue types. The imaging process is schematically represented in Figure 5.1a and b. A series of contiguous slices are taken in this manner and then processed by a computer for tomographic reconstruction. This postprocessing creates the 3D nature that is far more informational than the 2D image. In the field of imaging, when discussing only two dimensions, an imaging primitive is referred to as a pixel. For 3DCT, the basic unit of measurement is a voxel, which also accounts for the thickness of the CT slice. In the case of lung imaging, two different approaches are commonly used. The first approach is referred to as free-breathing

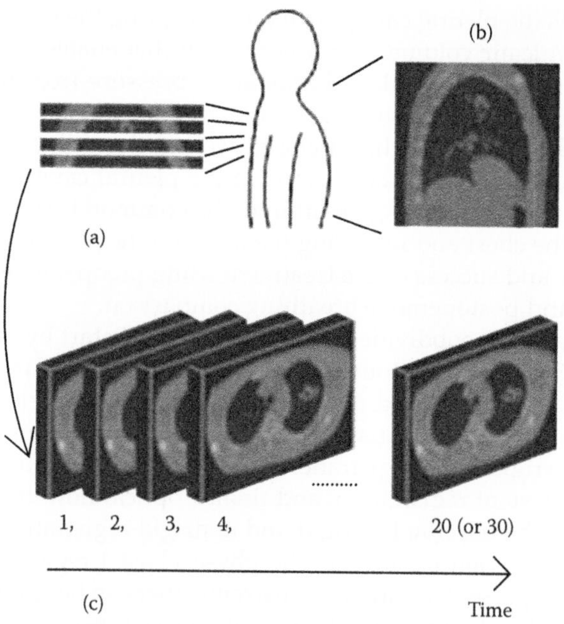

FIGURE 5.1
A schematic representation of the 3DCT acquisition is shown in (a) and (b). 4DCT image acquisition is shown in (c). (Courtesy of McClelland, J.R., et al. *Med. Phys.*, 33(9): 3348, 2006.)

CT (FBCT), in which the patient is allowed to breathe freely while the imaging is done. Such an imaging includes the patient's breathing artifacts. The second approach is referred to as breath-hold, in which the patient is made to hold his/her breath either at the end of inhalation or exhalation. This approach is applied frequently for 4D imaging and is explained further in the following section.

5.2.2 4DCT Imaging Technology

4DCT lung imaging facilitates the estimation of lung motion during the breathing process. As illustrated in Figure 5.1c, 4DCT of the respiratory thorax includes the lungs at different air volumes and the surrounding anatomy (e.g., esophagus, rib cage, trachea, and heart). The uniqueness of this imaging system stems from the fact that it represents a set of 3DCT volumes with the anatomy of interest being the patient's lungs at different volumes through time, as illustrated in Figure 5.1c, during breathing.

In the case of registering human lungs and building a functional model, it is vital to consider their changing shape and volume or the model's usefulness as a diagnostic tool will be highly limited. To create a model that depicts a patient's complete respiratory process, most methods use a 4DCT set that consists of a series of 3DCTs taken at different time steps in the breathing cycle (i.e., each CT depicts a different lung volume). There are two ways to achieve 4DCT imaging. The first method is breath-hold, in which the patient is asked to hold his/her breath for a few seconds while the imaging is acquired. The method is based on the assumption that when patients hold their breath, the lung and its subanatomy do not move. The breath-hold imaging enables the acquisition of lungs only at the end-expiration and end-inspiration. The second method is gated imaging, in which an additional patient-tracking surrogate is used to obtain the patient breathing information. Such a tracking surrogate could be a strain-gauge belt, spirometry flow-volume measurement, or infrared markers. In this case, the 4DCT equipment first images the patient for a few minutes and then re-bins the entire data set at different lung volumes by synchronizing the volume information given by the tracking surrogate.

The type of 4DCT imaging equipment is differentiated according to whether multiple slices or a single slice is acquired at a given time instant. One experiment testing single-slice 4DCT used a commercially available respiratory motion-monitoring system that provided an external tracking signal of the patient's breathing. The monitoring system facilitated time stamping of the CT images by recording the "through the lens x-ray ON" signal from the CT scanner. The CT scan, in this case, was an oversampled spiral scan acquired using a pitch of 0.5 and a scanner rotation time of 1.5 seconds. The images from the scan were sorted by respiratory phase into image bins, the complete set of which made a complete 4DCT data set. This process was used on both a mechanical oscillator phantom and a patient undergoing lung radiotherapy. Results in both cases showed motion artifacts to be significantly reduced as compared with the 3D images in which respiratory motion was not accounted for. It has been found that there are some temporal and spatial limitations to using single-slice 4DCT to track respiratory motion [2,3].

Multislice 4DCT and 4D cone-beam CT scans are being investigated as alternatives to single-slice 4DCT. The number of scans per couch position may vary from 16 to 64. As an example, a multislice 4DCT was acquired in cine mode, gathering 15 scans/couch position [4]. During the process, a patient was hooked up to a digital spirometry monitor surrogate that retrospectively sorted the CT scans by tidal lung volume after scanning was completed. The accuracy of this method was tested by generating a 4DCT set using both free-breathing multislice CT equipment and user-defined tidal volume bins for a set of eight patients. The actual tidal lung volumes agreed with the specified bin volumes within standard deviations ranging between 22 and 33 cm^3. An analysis of sagittal and coronal images demonstrated a relatively small (1 cm) motion artifact along the diaphragm, even for tidal volumes in which breathing motion was greatest.

Helical CTs enable faster image acquisition by spinning the gantry. As a more recent approach, helical CT scanners have been used to perform 4DCT imaging. In one of the experiments detailed by peers, the scanner used for the CT data acquisition was a 16-slice helical CT scanner (MX8000 IDT, version 2.5 scanner; Philips Medical Systems, Cleveland, OH) with a standard physical aperture 70 cm in diameter [5]. The respiration signal was acquired by monitoring the motion of an infrared reflecting marker surrogate placed on the abdomen of the phantom or patient (real-time position management, version 1.5.1 system; Varian Medical Systems, Palo Alto, CA). The CT scanner that initially supported 4DCT of a cardiac signal was shown to be modified to acquire the respiration signal for thoracic 4DCT by reducing the surrogate's frequency from 1 to 0.3 Hz.

5.2.3 How Registration Helps in Knowing the Lung Motion

Registration is about finding a correspondence between a given 3D image primitive (i.e., voxel) in a 3D data set and among a set of voxels in a different 3D data set. The volumetric data sets may be two different volumes of a 4DCT or two different volumes of 3DCT taken at different times, or two different volumes of two different imaging modalities. The correspondences could be based on voxel-specific factors such as the voxel intensity and location, voxel neighborhood factors such as the voxel spatial intensity distribution, or voxel distance factors such as the distance between the given voxel and the voxel in the set being searched. The choice of the method depends mostly on the type of anatomy being investigated and whether voxels belong to the same imaging modality.

It is important to note that there are several methods that have been researched and developed by peers for registering 3D lung models. Also considered is the multimodal registration of lungs, CT, magnetic resonance imaging (MRI), and positron emission tomography (PET), as well as different CT variations that have been extensively used on an everyday basis for improving patient treatment. In this chapter, some of the state-of-the-art algorithms investigated for 4DCT lung registration by peers are discussed. Although no particular approach is championed in this chapter, the need for concrete validation studies for each of the methods is put forth.

5.3 Rigid-Body Transformations

Rigid-body transformations facilitate an automatic way of registering lungs from one air volume to another. The components of the rigid-body transformations include rotation, translation, scaling, and skewing. A simple way to mathematically explain the rigid-body transformation is as follows. Let vector u represent a 3D location that needs to be transformed into a new location given by vector v. The rotational transformation is a matrix vector multiplication that transforms the voxel u. The translation is represented as a vector that is added to the vector u. The scaling factor is represented as a scalar value that is multiplied to the vector u to scale it. The skewing vector is a vector that is a product to the vector u to skew the vector. Registering 3D lung volumes at different breathing volumes using a rigid-body transformation involves solving for the translation, rotation, scaling, and skewing components. The method, being simple, assumes that the lung deformation during breathing is rigid, which is typically not the case when landmarks are tracked visually. Thus, a rigid-body registration of the 3D lungs also aims at numerically minimizing the error involved in the registration of the lung volumes using optimization and convex minimization techniques. The registration error, in this case, is the difference between the 3D target image and the 3D deformed source image. The literature on the minimization and optimization problem has been extensively investigated by peers and lies beyond the scope of this chapter [7].

5.3.1 Automatic 3D Registration of Lung Surfaces in CT Scans

An iterative rigid-body transformation–based approach for registering the lung surface models has been investigated. The steps involved in this approach are as follows: first a set of landmarks with known correspondences was considered [8]. The points were then used to compute the rigid-body transformation components. The method was then repeated until the sum of the squared distances between the target image and the registration image is minimal. This method did not take into account the local continuity in displacement. Additionally, only the surface of the lung was registered. The method, however, accounted for changes in patient orientation.

5.3.2 Deformable 4DCT Lung Registration with Vessel Bifurcations

Another approach to performing 4DCT lung registration is based on max inhale and max exhale CT images [9]. The airway bifurcations were picked from vessel trees as landmarks.

The corresponding feature points were tracked in the airways of two different volumes by using 3D shape context search. To keep the landmark correspondence search automatic, a unique 3D algorithm was developed in which, for each voxel in the vessel bifurcation, an additional value representing the local shape histogram was also considered. The correspondences were computed as a combination of both the voxel intensity as well as the histogram value. The rigid-body transformation was based on this landmark correspondence. This method was also iterative where the affine transformation is optimized using a least squares method.

5.3.3 Landmark Detection in the Chest and Registration of Lung Surfaces with an Application to Nodule Registration

The intensity attenuation technique automatically chooses landmarks and performs landmark correspondences [10]. Figure 5.2 describes the schematic representation of the method. In this case, the choice of the landmarks were in the sternum and vertebra area where the Hounsfield units are much larger than what was observed inside the lung and were significantly different from the soft tissue. As compared with ref. [9], the landmarks in this case were outside the lungs. The center of the entire anatomical component on each 2DCT slice of a 3DCT scan set was taken as a landmark. Additionally, the trachea, in which the Hounsfield (CT attenuation) numbers are much lower than –900, was also considered. The centers of each anatomy in each 2D slice were tracked from one volume to another. Now, the rigid-body transformation parameters were estimated for a given pair of source and target images. For known transformation parameters, the 3D lung volumes were then registered using the iterative closest-point method and Elias's nearest neighbor algorithm. In these steps, the translation vector and the rotation matrix of the rigid-body transformation were iteratively optimized until the sum of the squared distance between the correspondence obtained using the nearest neighbor algorithm and the iterative closest point is minimized.

5.3.4 Modeling Respiratory Motion for Optimization of Lung Cancer Radiotherapy Using Fast MR Imaging and Intensity-Based Image Registration

The rigid-body registration method is not limited to the CT imaging domain. We now discuss, as an example, a method that combines the breath-hold fast MRI with free-breathing MRI [11]. Breath-hold MRI presents an improved shape representation for the 3D lungs. They are, however, in low resolution and contrast as compared with the free-breathing

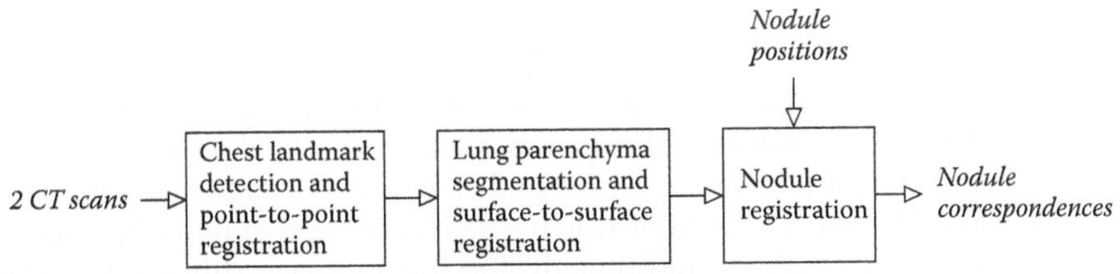

FIGURE 5.2
The schematic diagram of the steps involved in the rigid-body transformation and nodule registration. (Courtesy of Betke, M., et al. *Med. Image Anal.*, 7(3): 265–281, 2003.)

MRI because of increased acquisition time. A registration of the breath-hold MRI with free-breathing MRI enables a prediction of the closest lung air volume that represents free-breathing. Two groups of fast MRI, a breath-hold multiposition MRI and a sequence of dynamic free-breathing MRI, have been registered using rigid-body transformations. Landmarks in this case were picked from the exhalation breath-hold MRI. Voxel similarity, which represents the voxel intensity difference as well as the local shape description, was used for finding the initial correspondences, and the rigid-body transformation parameters were then solved.

5.4 B-Splines and Thin-Plate Splines

4DCT lung registration can be accommodated with the application of splines. Mathematically, splines are higher order polynomials whose coefficients or control points determine the shape of the curve. Splines are fundamentally one-dimensional in nature. They can, however, be extended into 2D and 3D by using a combination of more than one spline for each additional dimension. Since its inception, splines have been used for 2D registration extensively. It is beyond the scope of this chapter to explain in detail how a spline works and its 2D application. However, 4DCT lung registration has benefited significantly from two particular types of splines, B-splines and thin-plate splines (TPS).

5.4.1 B-Splines

B-splines are third-order polynomials in which the control points determine the shape of the 3D object being represented. It is now simpler to walk through how a B-spline model of the lung is generated. For any given 3D segmented lung, the B-splines naturally represent the contours of the lung shape and can be scaled to include the entire lung anatomy. Thus, for a given lung, the B-spline is generated by solving for the control points using simultaneous linear equation-solving techniques. From a registration perspective, for any two given lung CT data sets, their corresponding B-spline models can be generated by solving for the control points of each of the models. Once the control points are known, a registration of the control points from one lung volume to another will register the lung contours of one volume to another. Optionally, the correspondence between the control points of one volume to another can also be done semiautomatically by a clinical expert for better accuracy. The method is also computationally fast because for any given lung, the number of control points is of the order of quarter of the set of voxels that define the lung [12].

5.4.1.1 Quantitative Assessment of Registration in Thoracic CT

Of particular importance was the use of multiresolution B-splines. Specifically, the distribution of the landmarks inside the lungs was divided into four regions for each lung. Multiresolution data for each lung are created and an expert tracked the landmark motion on each resolution. The rest of the lung was registered using B-splines. The accuracy of the landmarks was then studied. Additionally, the interobserver difference is shown to be at least 2 mm. Variations in the accuracy were shown as a function of the number of resolutions used and the number of steps involved in the stochastic gradient descent method [13].

5.4.1.2 A Continuous 4D Motion Model from Multiple Respiratory Cycles for Use in Lung Radiotherapy

In this approach, several CT slabs were scanned during patient FBCT, each slab consisting of 20 to 30 volumes. FBCT has a fast scanning rate; however, it yields relatively low-quality volume data. A higher quality, breath-holding CT scan was then performed as a reference volume. The high-quality scan has thinner slices and a higher resolution, resulting in less noise and more detail in the volume [6]. For gating purposes, the breathing level was determined by two methods: by assessing the volume that was computed from extracted surfaces or by locating the markers attached on the patient chest that are located by stereo camera. Each slab of volume data was then registered to the reference volume by 3D cubic B-spline nonrigid fitting. Two levels of resolution were applied on grid control points. The motion model for each slab was built by temporal fitting of all the registrations. The motion model for the whole lung was constructed by merging the models of all the slabs together. Some discontinuities were observed near the slab boundaries and were validated by visually checking the difference between the predicted volume and the actual volume. The results were evaluated for tumor region, ipsilateral lung, and other tissues. Validation was also applied by point tracking—one landmark was picked in each slab and reference volume by a clinical oncologist who compared the difference between the manually picked ones and the ones in the motion model.

5.4.2 TPS

TPS are second-order polynomials in which the control points lie on the curve generated and also determine the shape of the 3D lung being represented. The advantage of the control points being part of the contour is that the landmarks, manually or automatically, generated and registered can be used for the registration. A simple walkthrough of TPS-based lung registration follows: for a given lung, the TPS control points are first solved as previously discussed for B-splines. Once the TPS model is generated for a given pair of lungs, the control points can then be manually or automatically registered. Mathematically, this step is easier compared with B-splines since the control points do not lie on the contour. Once the correspondences of the control points are known, the lungs are then subsequently registered using the spline function.

5.4.2.1 4DCT Image-Based Lung Motion Field Extraction and Analysis

An effort to register the breath-hold CT, which is a precursor to the 4DCT imaging [14], with FBCT is now discussed. The imaging process involved the patient holding his/her breath at the start of breathing and at the end of breathing. Figure 5.3 shows both the 3D lung images and the surface contours as well as the 3D surface model generated. The end-expiration and end-inspiration CT of the lungs were used for estimating the 3D lung motion. 3DCT volume data are captured as inhale–exhale breath-holding thorax CT images. The lung surface was extracted from the model and then covered with a topologically identical surface mesh for both surfaces. A sparse motion field was constructed by tracking corresponding points on the mesh. A dense motion field was computed from such a sparse motion field by TPS interpolation. TPS, in a 2D case, was similar to the bending force of a thin metal surface. To apply TPS in 2D coordinate transformation, the bending force between the x-axis and the y-axis is the displacement of that node along these axes. A lung surface mesh was generated by performing a connected-component algorithm on

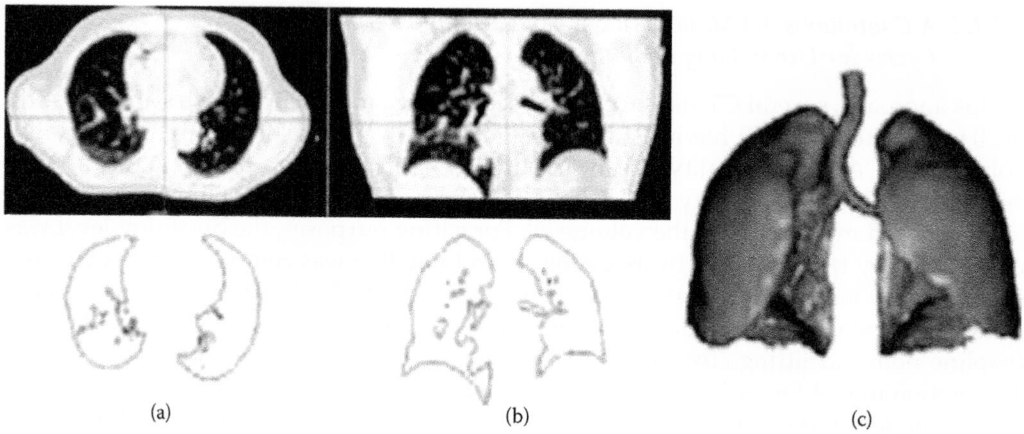

FIGURE 5.3
(See color insert.) The 3DCT is shown along with segmented surface contours for supine (a) and upright orientation (b). (c) The 3D lung models generated from the contours are shown. (Courtesy of Klinder, T., et al. *Proc. SPIE*, 6914(3): 69141L.1–69141.L.11, 2008.)

selected threshold images from reference inhale–exhale volumes. Mesh adaptation was performed iteratively.

5.5 Physics-Based 3D Warping and Registration from Lung Images

One of the earliest approaches for performing 4DCT lung registration was using physics-based 3D lung warping techniques [15]. In this approach, a few landmarks, namely, the airway bifurcations, were tracked from one volume to another. The surrounding anatomy was registered from one volume to another using a continuum mechanics approach. A continuum mechanics model was applied to CT images for nonlinear interpolation with the assumption that the CT image intensity was equivalent to mass density. Three main constraints were used: noncompressibility, divergent free, and continuity preserving. The combination of these three constraints makes the registration math similar to computational fluid dynamics. An anisotropic smoothness filter was applied to maintain the local continuity of the displacement.

5.5.1 Noncompressibility

Noncompressibility is mathematically explained by the following relation. Let f represent the spatial description of the 3D lung volume indexed by t. The noncompressibility relation states that the spatial description f is equal to the negative product of the spatial description of the estimated velocity and the gradient of the spatial description itself. As such, the lung anatomy consists of a combination of solid and liquid substances whose densities vary. To assume noncompressibility, the spatial density was assumed to be a constant.

5.5.2 Divergent Free

The divergent-free constraint states that the divergence of the velocity, which represents the local expansion or contraction of the air, must be zero for regions where the spatial descriptor f is nonzero. Such divergent-free constraints are more commonly used in solving fluid flow problems using computational fluid dynamic techniques. It is to be noted that from a lung biology perspective, the air temperature changes when it flows through the lungs.

5.5.3 Continuity Preserving

Continuity preserving is typically accounting by considering isotropic smoothness constraint. This constraint aims at minimizing the summation of the square of displacements along each direction. However, in this study, the authors have used an anisotropic smoothness constraint by using a weighted value for each direction. Such an approach facilitated motion continuity when the local gray scale differences were large. Of particular importance in the case of lungs is the case where we encounter breathing air coupled with liquid and solid anatomical substances, which causes the lung to move differently from each other. As an alternative, Lame's constants were used for continuity preserving [16]. In the case of lungs, the imaging data typically had a higher slice thickness (resolution along the *z*-axis) than the anatomical landmarks involved. For instance, a given landmark can appear on one slice of a 3D volume and not appear on the other slice of another 3D volume of the same lung. Thus, considering physics-based constraints for registration will compensate for the accuracy of the registration. In conclusion, the continuity-preserving aspect of the registration is the only applicable aspect of the registration. Nevertheless, physics-based registration methods offer a mathematical compact registration system that enforces the continuity of the registration. However, care needs to be given on the applicability of the physics not only from a biology perspective but also from the perspective of imaging limitations.

5.6 Inverse Consistent Registration

The consistency of an image registration approach is a mutual information–based approach [17], in which the registration algorithm is able to obtain the same result when a source image is registered to the target image and when the target image is registered to the source image. When the registration algorithm is unable to uniquely describe the correspondences between two images, the algorithm is deemed inconsistent. The inverse consistent registration aims at maximizing the consistency of a registration by minimizing the registration differences between the source-to-target and target-to-source correspondences. Figure 5.4 represents a schematic diagram of the method. To further explain the method, let us consider the rigid-body transformation. Let S and T be the source and target lung volume, respectively. The rotation, translation, scaling, and skewing components of the rigid-body transformation are required to be inverted when T is registered to S instead of S to T. The key point to observe is that the underlying math in the rigid-body transformation does not guarantee consistency. Adding consistency to the registration method

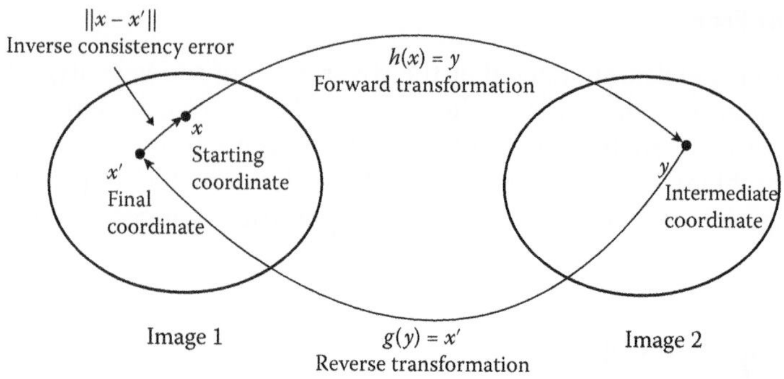

FIGURE 5.4
A schematic representation of the inverse consistent lung representation. (Courtesy of Christensen, G.E., et al. *Med. Phys.*, 34(6): 2155–2163, 2007.)

requires minimizing the differences between the transformations between the S to T and T to S registrations. It is now straightforward to include this constraint to the already iterative methods of solving for rigid-body transformations.

5.6.1 Consistent Landmark and Intensity-Based Image Registration

We now discuss the approach combining TPS with the inverse consistency constraint [18]. Specifically, for TPS to be used for registration, the landmark correspondences are first computed either manually or automatically. Once computed, the TPS function uses the landmark correspondences to compute the correspondences for all the voxels in the 3D volume. A simpler way to achieve consistency is to first formulate a cost function that aims at minimizing the bending energy to avoid large displacements and minimizing the displacement differences between the forward and reverse transforms. From a cost function minimization perspective, whenever there is a function with two independent terms to minimize, a third perturbation term that updates the other two terms in a heuristic manner is introduced. By applying this logic, a third TPS-based perturbation term was used to update both the forward and the reverse TPS transformation functions to minimize the difference between the displacements.

5.6.2 Estimation of Regional Lung Expansion via 3D Image Registration

The inverse consistency can be used in combination with physics-based constraints [19]. Instead of a semiautomatic approach to compute landmark correspondence, a manual way to register landmarks from one airway tree to another was used. It was followed by a cost minimization function that, when used, will give the registration of all the other points. The cost minimization included both linear elasticity constraints and reverse displacement constraints. The latter can be explained as follows. First, the displacement of source a to target b was computed. Then the displacement from source b to target a was computed. Now two different aspects are taken into account: first, the difference between the voxel distribution of the source and the target; second, the difference between the displacement of each voxel when computed using the forward and the reverse manner. The strength

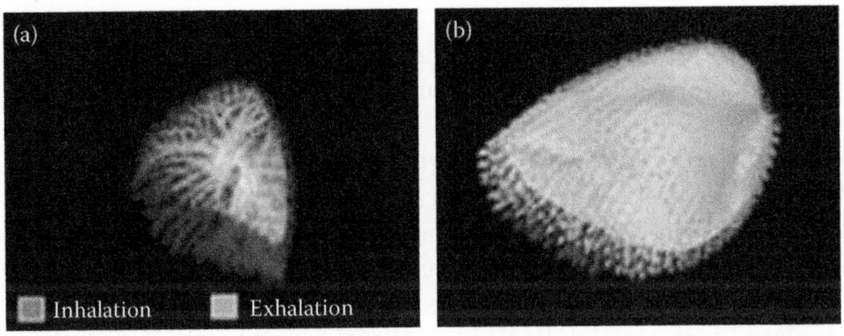

FIGURE 5.5
(See color insert.) (a) The 3D capillary tree of a human lung is shown in end-inhalation and end-exhalation. (b) The 3D surface lung deformation is shown for each surface point. (Courtesy of Christensen, G.E., et al. *Med. Phys.*, 34(6): 2155–2163, 2007.)

of this approach lies in the stability of the algorithm provided by the inverse consistency itself. The method, however, assumed a constant elastic parameter during registration, which is typically not the case.

5.6.3 Tracking Lung Tissue Motion and Expansion Compression with Inverse Consistent Image Registration and Spirometry

In another approach, the small lung deformation is included as a constraint during registration [20]. Tidal breathing (free breathing) volume CT data are collected, followed by the application of a small deformation inverse that is consistent with the linear elastic (SICLE) registration to construct the motion field. The cost function of SICLE was presented as a weighted sum of imaging modality, bending energy, and inverse consistency.

The application of such a registration has been used for the estimation of the lung tissue expansion and tissue mechanics. Figure 5.5a and b show the overlapping regions of lung bifurcations during inhalation and exhalation, along with the direction of the 3D lung surface displacement. The key parameter observed from the 4DCT registration was computed as a Jacobian value, which is the second-order curl of the local gradient. Although the tissue expansion can be obtained from xenon CT imaging, the inverse consistency also helped in obtaining a stable registration while registering multimodal image registration. Additionally, the Jacobian parameter helped in quantifying the lung tissue expansion and contraction.

5.7 Optical Flow–Based Methods

The optical flow method has been previously investigated and published, extensively, by peers. In this section, the application of 4DCT lung registration using optical flow is presented. The 2D and 3D optical flow methods are based on considering both the intensity of the voxel as well as the local gradient of the intensity. Fundamentally, the method aims at minimizing the voxel intensity differences between the target image and the deformed source image. When exact matches are not available, the gradient of the voxel intensity is minimized. The method stands out against other methods because the optical flow is computed using an iterative solution that computes the displacement only using the local voxel gradient and shape description.

The accuracy of the method deteriorates when the displacement is more than one voxel. To alleviate this issue, a multiresolution optical flow–based registration is under investigation. The method starts with a source and a target 3D volume. A multiresolution data set is generated for both the source and target 3D volumes. The initial displacement is assumed to be zero. The source and 3D target data are registered using the optical flow. The results are then extrapolated as the initial displacement of the next level of resolution. The method continues until the source and target 3D volumes are registered at the highest resolution. It can now be observed that no automatic or manual landmark correspondences are initially made for the optical flow, which enables the overall registration to be fully automatic. Guerrero et al. [21] investigated the use of 3D multiresolution optical flow using breath-hold CT for the estimation of regional lung motion.

One of the key limitations of applying optical flow to the registration of 4DCT lungs is that the intensity of landmarks remains the same from one lung volume to another. Based on the patient's breathing and the gating system used, the landmark intensity can significantly vary from one volume to another. Guerrero et al. [21] account for variations in the intensity of landmarks from one volume to another by introducing an error function that is assumed to be small. Min et al. [22] account for the variations in the intensity of landmarks by using a multilevel multiresolution optical flow approach. In this approach, the lung volume is semiautomatically segmented before registration into sublevels. Once segmented, each level of the anatomy is registered with its corresponding level of anatomy at a higher volume using a multilevel optical flow. The intensity of each voxel in the anatomical representation is set to 255. Thus, the local shape description is used to register the 3D lung volumes of an anatomical level.

5.7.1 Nonrigid Registration Method to Assess the Reproducibility of Breath-Holding with Active Breathing Control in Lung Cancer

Another approach to minimize the landmark intensity variation was to use breath-holding CT data with active breath control. During this procedure, airflow halts when the lung reaches a predefined volume. It uses a modified optical flow method for lung motion tracking, which involves a 3D Gaussian recursive filter similar to the viscous fluid regularization method [23].

5.7.2 Evaluation of Deformable Registration of Patient Lung 4DCT with Subanatomical Region Segmentations

In this study, the authors compared two different lung registration methods. In the first method, B-splines were used to register the lung volume from one region to another. In the second approach, which is referred to as demons, subregions inside the lung volume were segmented from 4DCT and are registered using optical flow. Validations were performed to further detail the efficacy of both methods. It was shown that the optical flow–based subanatomical registration yielded an improved result as compared with the 4DCT registration using B-splines. This was because of the optical flow's capability to also account for the local intensity variations for a given landmark [24].

5.8 Validation, the Much Needed Emphasis

The discussion on different methods of 4DCT lung registration clearly depicts the applicability of having a variety of methods. The stability of the 4DCT registration method has been addressed using the inverse consistency approach. However, the accuracy that can be obtained using different methods for a given 4DCT depends on different parameters, including the 3D resolution and contrast of the 4DCT data set, specific patient anatomy (e.g., presence of tumors), and the choice of the landmarks. This section concludes with a discussion of the fact that the metric chosen for quantifying the accuracy of the 4DCT registration also sheds light on the applicability of the registration algorithm for clinical applications.

5.8.1 Deformable 4DCT Lung with Vessel Bifurcations

For additional analyses, the TPS were used for approximating the displacement of other points instead of the rigid-body transformations [9]. To check the validity, clinical experts picked landmarks from both volumes and then compared the locations with those predicted from using the rigid-body transformation as well as the TPS. The other validation method computed volume differences between the target volume and the transformed volume. The key observation made was that when registered with TPS, the overall error in the correspondences in the voxels between the two volumes was lower than when registered by the rigid-body transformation. This result was expected because lung deformation itself is not a rigid-body transformation by nature. The second key observation was with the choice of the landmarks. By considering the 3D shape histogram of each landmark for semiautomatically registering them, the overall registration results were much improved.

5.8.2 Validation Using 3D Lung Phantom

As a first step toward validation, a 4D lung phantom undergoing rigid-body deformation was considered. A physical 3D phantom was created and was CT scanned while the phantom was manually displaced. A 3D optical flow algorithm was then used to track the simulated displacement. For a simulated rigid-body motion, the 3D optical flow registration results showed an accuracy of approximately 2 mm, while a rigid-body registration showed perfect registration [8].

5.8.3 Validation Using Root Mean Square Error

Calculation of root mean square (RMS) error is the standard approach used by peers for measuring accuracy. Although the methods strongly depend on the choice of the data set, Table 5.1 shows the accuracy published for each of the methods. It can be seen that each of the methods reports an accuracy of less than 4 mm for all the registration methods. We have to remember that the results are computed using 4DCT with variations in the imaging modality. Thus, the results may not be directly comparable. The advantage of using RMS as a measure of registration error is that the implication of the error can be directly perceived. For instance, it will be immediately possible to perceive that, for any voxel, the computed displacement may have an error range dictated by the RMS value.

TABLE 5.1

Registration Validation Results Reported from the Literature

Method	Results
[6]	Mean target registration error, 1.26 mm
	Max target registration error, 6.24 mm
[8]	SSD minimum, 7%
	maximum, 86%
[9]	Target registration error (rigid-body transformation), 3.40 ± 2.38 mm
	Target registration error (TPS), 2.85 ± 2. 11 mm
[10]	Target registration error, 4.7 mm for nodules and 4.3 mm for other landmarks
[11]	RMS error
	Inhale/exhale free breathing, 2.93 mm
	Inhale/exhale breath-hold, 6.81 mm
[13]	Target registration error, 0.5–2 mm
[14]	Mean motion error, 4.2 mm
[15]	Warping difference, 10%
[18]	500 times accuracy improvement as compared with TPS
[20]	Correlation of Jacobian value with lung spirometry, $R^2 = 0.538$
[21]	Linear regression correlation, 0.985
[23]	B-splines versus demons comparison (percentage mismatch boundary)
	B-splines, 0.3
	Demons, 1.15
[16]	Mean consistency error
	Point-based methods, 1.33 mm
	Surface tracking methods, 1.25 mm
	Parametric methods, 0.54 mm
	Nonparametric methods, 0.24 mm

5.8.4 Validation Using Regression

The Jacobian value of a given set of 3D voxel displacements represents an increase or decrease in the volume. In the case of lungs, the Jacobian of the group of voxels or the entire lung can be used to characterize the lung deformation. Johnson and Christensen [19] compared the Jacobian computed using inverse consistent registration with the spirometry measurements using a linear regression analysis. As shown in Table 5.1, the results showed a correlation of 0.538. Additionally, Guerrero et al. [21] performed a linear regression analysis for the voxel displacement with the spirometry measurement and, as shown in Table 5.1, the results showed a correlation of 0.985. The implications of the correlation need to be perceived from an application standpoint. For instance, the sensitivity of the regression analysis for a given voxel may not be straightforward, as in the case of RMS-based calculations, for them to be used for clinical setup.

5.8.5 Validation and Comparison Methods for Free-Breathing 4D Lung CT

In this report, a study of comparisons was performed between four different classes of registration methods: point-based tracking, surface-based tracking, parametric volume–based registration, and nonparametric volume–based registration [16]. From the perspective of lung volume change represented by the Jacobian metric, the study showed that the surface-based registration was slightly more accurate than the other registration methods. From a validation perspective, it was shown that the registration error–based estimation of the dose validation was not sufficient because all the methods showed comparative accuracy. When tested for consistency, it was found that the point-based matching method showed the worst performance, followed by the surface, parametric, and physics-based models.

A thorough quantification of the accuracy obtained by different methods is required. Such quantification will enable a better understanding of the registration and how it can be expanded for variations in CT acquisition. To better understand this, let us consider "needle insertion for pneumothorax" and "external beam lung radiotherapy" as two different clinical procedures of concern. In the former, a 2-mm registration error may result in the wrong placement of the needle, thereby further damaging the lung surface tissue. However, the procedure is rather instantaneous as compared with lung radiotherapy in which the external beams target the lung tumor for an average treatment time of 20 to 25 minutes. Additionally, the former procedure has tactile feedback for the clinician, which may help in further reducing the effect of registration errors in the clinical procedure. The latter procedure is fully automatic and the current state-of-the-art clinical follow-up takes days to predict procedural errors. This comparative analysis shows the importance of appreciating the registration accuracy from the standpoint of application itself.

To conclude this section, the validation study has shown that 4DCT lung registration can be obtained using the proposed set of methods within 2 to 8 mm error. However, the accuracy has not been assessed for all methods using the same data set. Additionally, the choice of the parameter used for the validation also varied from one experiment to another. In addition, a better understanding is required about the changes in the accuracy of the proposed method when the CT acquisition is changed from 64-slice CT to 6-slice CT and the slice thickness is decreased to the submillimeter range, providing improved anatomical detail. Such an analysis presents not only the accuracy of the method but also the scalability of the accuracy for CT acquisition improvements.

5.9 Lung Radiotherapy

4DCT lung registration may provide major improvements in lung radiotherapy. Most dose calculations and evaluations of a planned course of treatment are performed on 3D images of the patient taken before treatment. These images are usually high-quality 3DCT and 4DCT scans so that the physician, physicists, and dosimetrists can identify normal structures that need to be spared from radiation and the tumor and other involved tissue that must be targeted. Such dose calculations and evaluations are, however, limited by the variations in the patient position from day-to-day caused by the setup uncertainties, the internal changes from day-to-day (interfraction motion), and the internal changes during a single radiation treatment (intrafraction motion). To alleviate this limitation, a margin is added to the clinical target volume that is visualized on the 4DCT images to ensure adequate coverage of the clinical target volume [26].

In the case of lung tumors, 4DCT facilitates the availability of a description of the patient-specific tumor motion. A detailed discussion on the usage of 4DCT for predicting tumor motion is given in the report of the American Association of Physicists in Medicine Task Group 76 [27]. Dose calculations on 3DCT scans can use many different models. With 3DCT scans, the ability to accurately represent the physics of the radiation beam becomes possible and dose calculations have evolved to use convolution pencil beam algorithms

[25] and Monte–Carlo dose calculations [28]. In the case of lungs, the subject-specific tumor motion and the motion of the surrounding tissues are of particular concern when high radiation doses are delivered with the intent of ablating tumors and gaining local regional control of tumor growth in an environment that includes radiation-sensitive structures such as normal lung tissue, stomach, and the esophagus. As described earlier in this chapter, 4DCT lung data sets provide the tumor motion that inherently occurred during the imaging process and have been used in calculating the dose accumulated on the lung tumor and its surrounding tissues. However, the lung radiotherapy planning methods previously investigated do not take into account the breathing variations that a patient undergoes during a course of treatment.

5.9.1 Simulation and Visualization Requirements for Lung Radiotherapy

From a simulation perspective, the simulation and visualization of subject-specific 3D lung conformal dosimetry are enabled by the use of the following four clinical aspects: (i) use of patient-specific anatomy, (ii) use of patient-specific dose delivery, (iii) use of patient-specific tumor motion, and (iv) real-time dose calculations.

5.9.2 Development of Physics-Based Deformable Lung Models from 4DCT Lung Registration

In this section, the lung surface model and its validation are addressed first, followed by discussion of the volumetric lung deformation model and its use for real-time lung radiotherapy modeling.

5.9.2.1 Physics-Based 3D Deformable Lung Surface Model

A method investigated to obtain changes in 3D lung surface in a physically and physiologically accurate manner was discussed in ref. [29]. The method takes high-resolution 3D lung surface models as input. Such a large number of nodes facilitate effective modeling of both normal and pathophysical lung deformations.

Within the context of physics-based deformation, a Green function (GF)–based deformation was chosen because it has been observed that lung deformations do not undergo vibration motions. Each node is referred to as a mass node. Each link between any two mass nodes forms an elastic connection between the nodes. For computational purposes, a "spring" node between every connected mass node is added. The regional alveolar expandability, which has a linear gradient from the apex of the lung to its base in an upright position, is taken as an indicator of the tissue property. A normalized value of the alveolar expandability was associated to each node based on the node's normalized position. Using the normalized alveolar expandability, an initial estimate of the transfer function was made. Additionally, the airflow inside the lungs was observed to have a linear gradient toward gravity.

A second approach is an inverse deformation analysis of the forward dynamics [30]. In this approach, the deformation operator is represented as a linear combination of the alveolar expandability difference and the geodesic distance between lung surface nodes. The inverse deformation approach aims at computing three unknown constants (A_i, B_i, and C_i) for each node i, which mathematically represent a row of the GF. Additionally, A_i and B_i were shown to be represented in a simultaneous linear equation form. First A_i and B_i were solved by taking a 4DCT data set of a human subject as input. Individual 3D lung surface models are extracted from the 4DCT and registered using the iterative algorithm discussed in ref. [29]. This 3D registration procedure provided us the displacement value associated with each surface node of the lung. Additionally, the geodesic distance between the nodes of the 3D model was precomputed using a level set–based distance vector algorithm. Now, using the forward dynamics algorithm, two estimates of the transfer function, with one of the estimates computed with all its internodal geodesic distances doubled, were computed. Using these two estimates of the transfer function, A_i and B_i were solved for the linear combination for the transfer function. Finally, C_i was computed using the values of A_i and B_i. The GF transfer function matrix in this case was computed by first computing the elastostatic force applied on each node using the estimated transfer function and then solving for the GF transfer function. The elastostatic force (force at equilibrium) applied on each node was computed using an iterative approach.

5.9.2.2 3D Lung Surface Deformations for PET/CT Image Registration

As an application of the deformable surface lung models, a method to nonlinearly register the 3DCT at two lung volumes (end-expiratory and end-inspiratory) with a 3D PET of the thoracic regions using the 3D deformable lung surface models is now described [31]. The 3D deformable lung model was incorporated in the PET/CT registration process to guarantee physiologically plausible deformations. The 3D deformable lung model is generated by using the physical inverse deformation approach with two 3DCT lungs taken as input. Once developed, the 3D lung model that closely represents the 3D PET was generated for different breathing conditions (e.g., rib cage diaphragm compensation). The registration method was based on an automatic selection of anatomical landmark points based on the curvature of the lung surface that closely matches the PET. Additionally, two different landmark selection approaches were investigated. In the first approach, the landmarks were uniformly distributed. In the second approach, the landmarks were nonuniformly distributed. The specific movements of potential tumors were preserved during the registration while guaranteeing a continuous deformation. The results obtained for the PET/CT registration using the deformable lung surface models are shown in Figure 5.6. The usage of 3D deformable surface lung models computed using the physics-based inverse deformation approach is clearly shown for both the landmark selection approaches.

5.9.2.3 Physics-Based Volumetric 3D Lung Model

In this section, a method is presented to estimate the 3D volumetric lung deformation operator for modeling the volumetric lung deformations. The method is inspired by the usage of spherical harmonic transformations for inverse rendering problems in the computer graphics domain [32]. From a computational perspective, a hyperspherical harmonics–based spectral domain method was employed for estimating the 3D volumetric lung tissue elasticity. A frequency domain formulation of the volumetric lung deformation operator was formulated using the hyper spherical harmonics (HSH) coefficients which, in turn, are estimated from known values of an applied force and a displacement. In our formulation, a mixed representation of HSH and the Wigner-d rotation transformations associated with the special orthogonal group 3 (SO(3)) was employed. Specifically, our proposed formulation uses HSH transformations for smooth data and Wigner-d rotation transformations for coarse data, which, in our case, are the airflow distribution inside the lungs and the volumetric lung displacement, respectively. Such a combination helped reduce the amount of data transformation error with a finite number of HSH and Wigner-d coefficients.

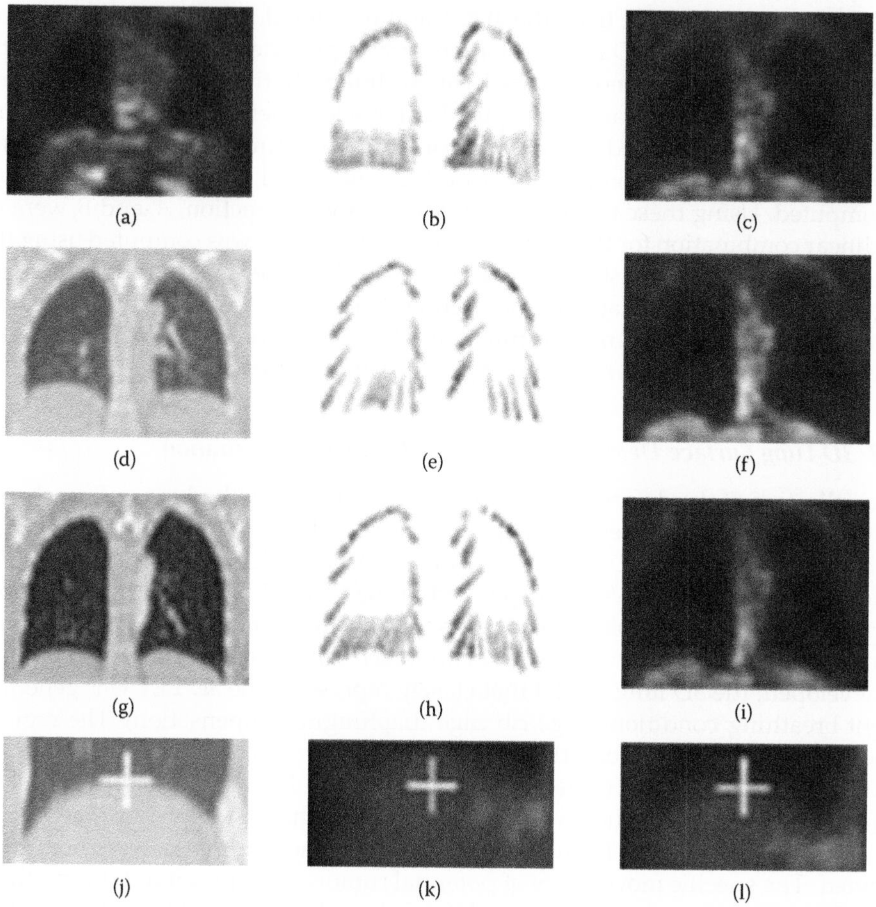

FIGURE 5.6
(See color insert.) Original PET (a) and CT images (d, g) in a normal case. The correspondences between the selected points in the PET image (b) and in the end-inspiration CT image (g) are shown for the direct method. (e) Registration with the breathing model and a nonuniform landmark detection. (h) Registration with the breathing model and a pseudouniform landmark selection (corresponding points are linked). (c) Registered PET is shown for the direct method in (f) for the method with the breathing model with a nonuniform landmark distribution, and in (i) for the method with the breathing model and landmarks pseudouniformly distributed. The fourth row shows the details of registration on the bottom part of the right lung, in a normal case: CT (j), PET registered without breathing model (k), and with a breathing model (l). The white crosses correspond to the same coordinates. The method using the breathing model furnishes a better registration of the surfaces of the lungs. (From Chambon, S., et al. *J. Comput. Assist. Radiol. Surg.*, 13(5): 281–298, 2008. With permission.)

5.9.2.4 *Application of Lung Deformation Estimated from 4DCT for Lung Radiotherapy Applications*

In this section, the lung radiotherapy monitoring using surface lung dynamics and volumetric lung dynamics is discussed. A framework has been implemented that integrates a real-time simulation of lung tumor motion with a 3D display system. The real-time simulation of lung tumor motion takes into account the patient-specific lung tumor motion extracted from 4DCT images and the radiation plan prescribed for the patient [33]. The output of the simulation framework predicted the amount and location of radiation doses deposited in both moving lung tumors and surrounding normal lung tissues during the delivery of radiation. Figure 5.7 shows the radiation dose deposited on the upper and lower lung of two patients considering the 4D lung motion obtained from the model. Radiation dose is represented by blue (85–90%), violet (90–95%), and white (95–100%).

A graphics processing unit–based simulation framework is considered to calculate the delivered dose to 3D lung tumor and its surrounding normal tissues, which are undergoing subject-specific lung deformations [22]. The graphics processing unit–based simulation framework modeled a 3D volumetric lung tumor and its surrounding tissues, simulated subject-specific 4D lung motion during a simulated dose delivery using the dose extracted from a treatment plan, and predicted the amount and location of radiation doses deposited inside the lung. Such a framework enables the development of real-time radiotherapy monitoring and retrospective analyses of the radiation dose delivered during the treatment. A radiation treatment plan of a small lung tumor (1–3 cm diameter) was developed in a commercial planning system (Pinnacle Treatment Planning System, Phillips, Andover, MA) using one of the 3DCTs of the 4DCT data set to simulate the radiation dose delivered. The dose for each radiation field was then extracted from the software. The 4DCT lung data sets were registered with each other using a modified optical flow algorithm. The tumor motion and the motion of the surrounding tissues were simulated by measuring the changes in lung volume during the radiotherapy treatment using spirometry. During the simulation of dose delivery, the 3D lung volume was deformed using the lung volume changes obtained from the spirometry measurements coupled with the displacement obtained using the modified optical flow. The real-time dose delivered to the tumor for each beam is generated by summing the dose delivered to the target volume at each increase in lung volume during the beam delivery time period. The simulation results showed that the dose accumulated on the lung volume varies for variations in breathing. The results also showed the real-time capability of the framework at 20 discrete tumor motion steps per breath, which is higher than the number of 4DCT steps (approximately 12) reconstructed during multiple breathing cycles.

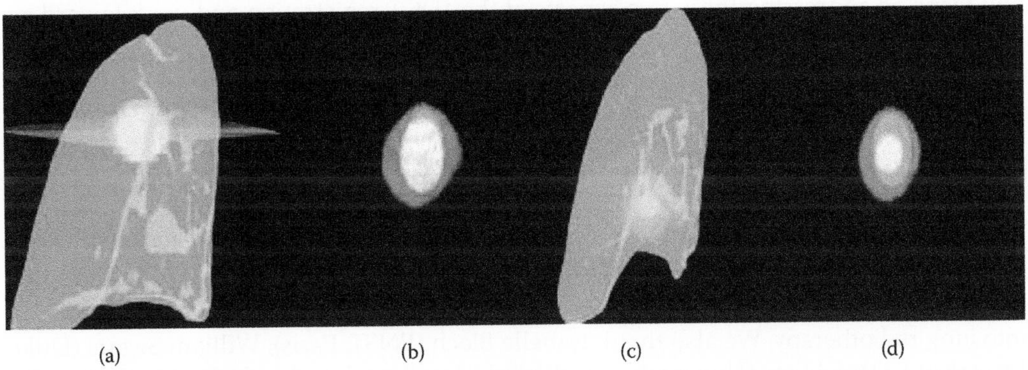

FIGURE 5.7
(See color insert.) (a) The tumor is in the upper lung. The tumor dose delivery is shown in (b). (c) The tumor is in the lower lung. The tumor dose delivery is shown in (d). (Courtesy of Santhanam, A.P., et al. In *Medical Image Computing and Computer Aided Intervention: Lecture Notes on Computer Science*, 2008.)

5.10 Conclusions

An overview of the methods investigated by peers for the 4DCT lung registration problem was discussed. The solutions provided are based on both rigid transformation and nonrigid transformation. Additional physics-based constraints and polynomial continuity constraints have been used for obtaining smooth solutions of the registration. Validations reported by peers have shown that the methods were able to achieve lung registration to within 2 to 3 mm error. However, independent estimations of the consistency obtained by the registration have shown that the results significantly vary for different methods.

Two different facts should be emphasized at this stage. First, the application domain that uses the 4DCT lung registration will dictate the effectiveness of the accuracy obtained by the registration. Toward a comparative study of the registration methods, a study will always be required that sheds more light on the importance of accuracy obtained by the registration. However, it will also be important to know the effectiveness of a 2-mm registration error rate on calculating the treatment delivery and response for a patient. Second, technical advances in the field of imaging equipment developments significantly contribute toward improving the registration errors. Within the last decade, 4DCT imaging has transformed from a single-slice CT imaging to a multiple-slices helical CT system in which the motion artifact is well captured and the CT radiation–induced damage is well minimized. Additionally, multimodal imaging, such as MRI and PET, in combination with 4DCT may enable registration optimizations that further improve the applicability of the registration method. However, registration methods have been under development for several decades, and there is a need to benchmark the accuracy of the methods for the current state of 4DCT imaging. More importantly, it must be noted that the registration accuracy may not be comparable when the imaging systems used for testing the methods differ. In addition, the surrogates used in performing gated imaging need to be carefully taken into account. Patient results may significantly vary for minor changes in the surrogate placement and thus introduce motion artifacts that are not accounted for by the registration algorithm. For instance, although physics-based registration methods are mathematically elaborate, motion artifacts may lead to errors in the 4DCT data that may completely render the governing equations of the registration inapplicable. Future work will focus on addressing these two aspects of the 4DCT registration and work toward an improved benchmarking of the registration accuracy.

Acknowledgments

We thank the James and Esther King Grant Foundation and the Florida I4 Corridor for supporting this research focused on incorporating 3D lung registration and dynamics into lung radiotherapy. We also thank Isabelle Bloch (ENST, Paris), William Segars (Duke University), Daniel Low (University of California, Los Angeles), Bari H. Ruddy (University of Central Florida), Paul Davenport (University of Florida), Olusegun Ilegbusi (University of Central Florida), and Alain Kassab (University of Central Florida) for their close collaboration on various aspects of this project.

References

1. Santhanam, A.P., C. Fidopiastis, J. Anton, and J.P. Rolland. 2006. Pneumothorax influenced 3D lung deformations. *Studies in Health Technology and Informatics*, 119/2005: IOS Press. 480–485.
2. Ford, E.C., G.S. Mageras, E. Yorke, and C.C. Ling. 2003. Respiration-correlated spiral CT: A method of measuring respiratory-induced anatomic motion for radiation treatment planning. *Medical Physics*, 30: 88–97.
3. Vedam, S.S., P.J. Keall, V.R. Kini, H. Mostafavi, H.P. Shukla, and R. Mohan. 2003. Acquiring a four dimensional computed tomography dataset using an external respiratory signal. *Physics in Medicine and Biology*, 48: 45–62.
4. Low, D.A., M. Nystrom, E. Kalinin, P. Parikh, J.F. Dempsey, J.D. Bradley, S. Mutic, S.H. Wahab, T. Islam, G. Christensen, D.G. Politte, and B.R. Whiting. 2003. A method for the reconstruction of four-dimensional synchronized CT scans acquired during free breathing. *Medical Physics*, 30: 1254–1263.
5. Keall, P.J., G. Starkschall, H.P. Shukla, K.M. Forster, V. Ortiz, C.W. Stevens, S.S. Vedam, R. George, T. Guerrero, and R. Mohan. 2004. Acquiring 4D thoracic CT scans using a multislice helical method. *Physics in Medicine and Biology*, 49: 2053–2067.
6. McClelland, J.R., J.M. Blackall, S. Tarte, and D.J. Hawkes. 2006. A continuous 4D motion model from multiple respiratory cycles for use in lung radiotherapy. *Medical Physics*, 33(9): 3348.
7. Tai, X.-C., K.-A. Lie, T.F. Chan, and S. Osher. 2006. Image procesing based on partial differential equations. *Mathematics and Visualization*. Springer.
8. Betke, M., H. Hong, and J.P. Ko. 2001. Automatic 3D registration lung surfaces in computed tomography scans. In *Medical Image Computing and Computer-Assisted Intervention—MICCAI 2001*, 725–733. Berlin-Heidelberg: Springer.
9. Hilsmann, A., T. Vik, M. Kaus, K. Franks, J.P. Bissonette, T. Purdie, A. Beziak, and T. Aach. 2007. Deformable 4DCT lung registration with vessel bifurcations. In *Proceeding of Internatinal Conference of Computer Assisted Radiology and Surgery*. Berlin, Germany.
10. Betke, M., H. Hong, D. Thomas, C. Prince, and J. Ko. 2003. Landmark detection in the chest and registration of lung surface with an application to nodule registration. *Medical Image Analysis*, 7(3): 265–281.
11. Blackall, J., S. Ahmad, M. Miquel, D. Landau, and D. Hawkes. 2004. Modeling respiratory motion for optimization of lung cancer radiotherapy using fast MR imaging and intensity-based image reigstration. *Proceedings of the International Society for Magnetic Resonance in Medicine*, 11: 2610.
12. Farin, G.E. 1987. Geometric modeling: Algorithms and new trends. *SIAM Review. Society for Industrial and Applied Mathematics*.
13. Murphy, K., B. van Ginneken, J.P.W. Pluim, S. Klein, and M. Staring. 2008. Quantitative assessment of registration in thoracic CT. In *The First International Workshop on Pulmonary Image Analysis: MICCAI Workshop*.
14. Klinder, T., C. Lorenz, J. von Berg, S. Renisch, T. Blaffert, and J. Ostermann. 2008. 4DCT image-based lung motion field extraction and analysis. *Proceedings of SPIE*, 6914(3): 69141L.1–69141.L.11.
15. Fan, L. and C.W. Chen. 1999. 3D warping and registration from lung images. *Proceedings of SPIE*, 3660: 459–470.
16. Vik, T., S. Kabus, J. von Berg, K. Ens, S. Dries, T. Klinder, and C. Lorenz. 2008. Validation and comparison methods for free-breathign 4D lung CT. In *Medical Imaging 2008: Image Processing, Proceedings of SPIE*.
17. Rangarajan, A., H. Chui, and J.S. Duncan. 1999. Rigid point feature registration using mutual information. *Medical Image Analysis*, 3(4): 425–440.
18. Johnson, H.J. and G.E. Christensen. 2001. Consistent landmark and intensity based image registration. *IEEE Transactions on Medical Imaging*, 21(5): 450–461.

19. Johnson, H.J. and G.E. Chritensen. 2001. Landmark and intensity-based, consistent thin-plate spline image registration. In *Information Processing in Medical Imaging*, 329–343. Berlin-Heidelberg: Springer.
20. Christensen, G.E., J.H. Song, W. Lu, I. el Naqa, and D.A. Low. 2007. Tracking lung tissue motion and expansion/compression with inverse consistent image registration and spirometry. *Medical Physics*, 34(6): 2155–2163.
21. Guerrero, T., K. Sanders, E. Castillo, Y. Zhang, L. Bidaut, T. Pan, and R. Komaki. 2006. Dynamic ventilation imaging from four-dimensional computed tomography. *Physics in Medicine and Biology*, 51(4): 777–791.
22. Min, Y., A.P. Santhanam, H. Neelakkantan, B.H. Ruddy, S. Meeks, and P. Kupelian. 2010. A GPU-based framework for modeling 3D lung tumor conformal dosimetry with subject-specific lung tumor motion. *Physics in Medicine and Biology*, 55(17):5137–5150.
23. Sarrut, D., V. Boldea, M. Ayadi, J.N. Badel, C. Ginestet, S. Clippe, and C. Carrie. 2005. Nonrigid registration method to assess reproducibility of breath-holding with ABC in lung cancer. *International Journal of Radiation Oncology, Biology, Physics*, 61(2): 594–607.
24. Wu, Z., E. Rietzel, V. Boldea, D. Sarrut, and G. Sharp. 2008. Evaluation of deformable registration of patient lung 4DCT with subanatomical region segmentations. *Medical Physics*, 35(2): 775–781.
25. Chetty, I.J., M. Rosu, D.L. McShan, B.A. Fraass, and R.K. Ten Haken. 2005. The influence of beam model differences in the comparison of dose calculation algorithms for lung cancer treatment planning. *Physics in Medicine and Biology*, 50(5): 801–815.
26. Van-Herk, M. 2004. Errors and margins in radiotherapy. *Seminars in Radiation Oncology*, 14(1): 52–64.
27. Keall, P.J., G.S. Mageras, J.M. Balter, R.S. Emery, K.M. Forster, S.B. Jiang, J.M. Kapatoes, D.A. Low, K. Murphy, B.R. Murray, C.R. Ramsey, M.B. Van Herk, S.S. Vedam, J.W. Wong, and E. Yorke. 2006. The management of respiratory motion in radiation oncology—report of the AAPM Task Group 76. *Medical Physics*, 33(10): 3874–900.
28. Chetty, I.J., M. Rosu, D.L. McShan, B.A. Fraass, J.M. Balter, and R.K. Ten Haken. 2004. Accounting for center-of-mass target motion using convolution methods in Monte-Carlo based dose calculations of the lung. *Medical Physics*, 31(4): 925–932.
29. Santhanam, A.P., C. Imielinska, P. Davenport, P. Kupelian, and J.P. Rolland. 2008. Modeling and simulation of real-time 3D lung dynamics. *IEEE Transactions on Information Technology*, 12(2): 257–270.
30. Santhanam, A.P., S. Mudur, and J.P. Rolland. 2006. An inverse 3D lung deformation analysis for medical visualization. In *Computer Assisted Social Agents*. Switzerland: Computer Graphics Society.
31. Chambon, S., A. Moreno, A.P. Santhanam, J.P. Rolland, E. Angelini, and I. Block. 2008. Using a breathing model for the CT-PET thoracic images with tumors. *Journal of Computer Assisted Radiology and Surgery*, 13(5): 281–298.
32. Santhanam, A.P., Y. Min, S. Mudur, E. Divo, A. Kassab, B.H. Ruddy, J.P. Rolland, and P. Kupelian. 2010. A hyper-spherical harmonic formulation for reconstructing volumetric 3D lung deformations. *Comptes Rendus Mecanique*, 338: 461–473.
33. Santhanam, A.P., T. Willoughby, A. Shah, S. Meeks, J.P. Rolland, and P. Kupelian. 2008. Real-time simulation of 4D lung tumor radiotherapy using a breathing model. In *Medical Image Computing and Computer Aided Intervention: Lecture Notes on Computer Science*, 710–717. Berlin, Heidelberg: Springer-Verlag.

6

Pulmonary Kinematics via Registration of Serial Lung Images

Tessa Cook, Gang Song, Nicholas J. Tustison, Drew Torigian, Warren B. Gefter, and James Gee

CONTENTS

6.1 Introduction

The lung can be described as an elastic body: an elaborate network of fibers connecting the vasculature, airways, and pulmonary interstitium. The functional unit of gas exchange is the alveolus, a tiny sac with thin, capillary-containing walls that form the gas exchange barrier. Specialized alveolar epithelial cells digest foreign matter and produce surfactant, a detergent-like substance that keeps the alveolus patent [1]. Each distinct structure and substance within the lung contributes unique material properties to this composite organ and confers a unique mechanical behavior on the lung.

Numerous pulmonary diseases affect normal lung mechanics by disrupting the healthy material composition of the lung. Lung disease has risen from being the fourth leading cause of chronic morbidity and mortality in the United States in 2007 [2] to the third leading cause today. According to the American Lung Association, one in six deaths in the United States is attributed to lung disease, and more than 35 million Americans live with chronic lung disease [3].

Pulmonary pathologies affect the lung parenchyma in many different ways. Emphysema, an obstructive lung disease, is caused by the proteolytic destruction of the intricate alveolar architecture by elastases, with permanent enlargement of the airspaces and a dramatic increase in lung compliance [4]. Patients with emphysema are unable to effectively expel air from their lungs, a phenomenon known as air trapping. By contrast, pulmonary fibrosis is a restrictive lung disease that can be idiopathic or the final stage of various pathological processes. Fibrosis results in marked thickening of the normally thin alveolar walls and of the pulmonary interstitium—the scaffolding of the lung—because of the increased deposition of collagen in the lung [5,6]. Patients with fibrosis have a very difficult time inflating their lungs and typically require ventilatory assistance as the disease progresses. Vascular pathologies, such as sickle cell disease (SCD), can also affect normal lung function. During periods of hypoxia, the spherical red blood cells of individuals with SCD assume a crescentic shape that makes it difficult for them to pass through the capillaries. Large quantities of oxygen-free radicals are also produced, making these patients highly susceptible to oxidative lung injury. These changes produce pulmonary vascular congestion which leads to hypoventilation, resembling a restrictive etiology [7]. The clinical presentation is described as either acute chest syndrome or chronic sickle cell lung disease, depending on the temporal pattern of the illness.

Physiologically, each of these diseases affects the integrity of the alveolar infrastructure and the lungs' ability to effectively oxygenate the blood. Morphologically, these changes translate to a gross perturbation of respiratory motion. Pulmonary function tests enable clinicians to evaluate an individual's respiratory status via parameters such as forced vital capacity, the largest possible volume of air exhaled after a maximal inhalation [8]. However, the normal range of values for these parameters is dependent on age, gender, race, body habitus, and other factors. In addition, these tests cannot be used to correlate observed aggregate functional performance with regional changes in lung architecture. Furthermore, small, regional changes in pulmonary architecture can be visualized on high-resolution lung imaging before they become clinically significant and produce abnormal pulmonary function tests.

A variety of efforts have been made to study regional lung mechanics and tissue properties *in vitro* by inflating isolated lungs or applying forces to tissue strips [9–19]. However, magnetic resonance (MR) imaging of the lung can be used to study regional motion *in vivo*. Attempts have been made to quantify pulmonary deformation indirectly by tracking the chest wall and diaphragm [20–22]. Other researchers have sought to create synthetic models of parenchymal behavior, especially at the alveolar level [23,24]. Grid tagging, which has been applied extensively to assess cardiac dynamics [25], has also been used to evaluate lung mechanics [26–28]. However, the efficacy of the technique is limited in the lung by the low spatial resolution of currently feasible grids, rapid fading of the grid secondary to the short T_1 relaxation time of lung tissue, and the challenge of applying tags in three-dimensional (3D) imaging [26]. Some work has been done toward the creation of static atlases of the healthy lung by registering computed tomography (CT) volumes [29–31]. Efforts have also been invested in multimodality registration of structural and functional lung images [32].

Variational nonrigid registration has been used to evaluate many types of physiologic motion, including myocardial contraction, abdominal deformation caused by respiration, and tissue changes secondary to tumor growth [33–36]. Hence, a variety of approaches exist to the fundamental problem of motion quantitation. Rueckert et al. [33,36] have modeled both breast deformation and cardiac motion using multilevel free-form deformations to optimize the normalized mutual information (MI) between two images. Rougon and colleagues [34] have also performed registration-based modeling of cardiac motion using specialized image metrics derived from the Ali–Silvey class of measures within a generic optimization framework. This work is an extension of their development of exclusive *f*-information similarity functionals for the matching of facial expressions [37]. Rohlfing et al. have adapted the approaches in refs [33] and [38] to characterize liver deformation during the respiratory cycle and to investigate suspicious breast lesions, respectively [35,39]. Linear elastic models also have been used extensively as reported in the literature [40,41]

In addition to the aforementioned methods, symmetric/consistent registration concerns have been a topic of considerable research effort. Christensen and Johnson proposed consistent image registration in ref. [42] by constraining the forward and inverse transformations to be mutual inverses such that their composition was equal to identity. This implies a constraining criterion that produces improved results over calculating forward and reverse transformations independently. This constraint was applied to lung registration in refs. [41,43,44]. Proximal in motivation for image registration consistency is the diffeomorphic registration framework of Avants et al. [45], who formulate the image registration problem in an inherently symmetric fashion using diffeomorphisms—differentiable maps with differentiable inverses. Diffeomorphism preserves topology, which is essential for physiologically realistic quantitation of pulmonary kinematics. This algorithm has performed quite well in a recent public evaluation [46] of different pulmonary image registration algorithms, as well as in a recent comparison of available brain normalization tools [47].

In this chapter, we present the elastic and diffeomorphic image registration approaches toward motion quantitation and biomechanical modeling in the lung from serial pulmonary imaging data. The registration of pairs of sequential images of the lung produces a dense motion field with displacement information at every image point. This field is acquired using the pulmonary vasculature as a natural source of spatial markers, without requiring knowledge of explicit *a priori* correspondences. The method is validated by tracking the motion of a set of expert-defined anatomic landmarks, and is used to illustrate both normal as well as pathological lung motions. The application of the finite-element method in the variational solution is also highlighted, as it can be solved at physiologically meaningful points within an image and is not restricted to sampling points that lie on or are subsampled from a uniform grid. The sensitivity of pulmonary motion estimation to image resolution, similarity metric, and inflation interval are also discussed and quantitatively evaluated.

6.2 Estimating Pulmonary Motion via Serial Image Registration

The general strategy is to infer the kinematics of lung deformation from observed changes in pulmonary anatomy as revealed on serial scans of the respiratory cycle. Specifically, motion is studied by tracking material points across the configurations of the lung at each imaged instance. The transformation between corresponding material points directly yields the motion between them. The goal of a registration algorithm is to find a transformation that brings the features of one image into correspondence with those of a second image with similar content. Thus, registration algorithms can be used to detect and quantify the change in anatomic configuration in serial studies of moving organs. A variety of nonrigid registration algorithms for medical image data have been developed [48–50], many of which would be appropriate for analyzing lung motion. A long-term aim is to enhance the understanding of lung physiology through the additional study of pulmonary dynamics and the eventual development of models that incorporate this knowledge about lung mechanics. Two mechanics-based registration approaches, elastic matching and diffeomorphic image registration, are presented and evaluated to quantify lung kinematics.

6.2.1 Elastic Matching of the Lung

Elastic matching formulates the registration problem within a continuum mechanical framework [51,52] that is implemented in a natural way using the variational approach. A linear elastic constitutive response is assumed as a first-order approximation to the true material behavior of the lung. Large deformations are accommodated through the application of piecewise constant load increments used to approximate the nonlinear potential energy associated with the image similarity in our variational registration formulation. Specifically, for the sequential pulmonary image pair under consideration, a fixed image, *I*, and a moving image, *J*, we seek the displacement **u** that minimizes the total potential energy.*

$$\Pi = \int \sigma : \varepsilon \, d \quad - \Pi_{\sim}, \tag{6.1}$$

over domain Ω of *I*, in which the stress tensor σ and strain tensor ε are related by Hooke's law, $\sigma_{ij} = C_{ijkl}\varepsilon_{kl}$ (in indicial notation). The elastic coefficients, C_{ijkl}, are components of a tensor describing the material properties of the body. The strain tensor ε is defined as:

$$\varepsilon_{ij} = \frac{1}{2}(\mathbf{u}_{i,j} + \mathbf{u}_{j,i}) \tag{6.2}$$

The work $\Pi_{\sim}$ performed by the loads deforming *I* into register with *J* is maximal when the appropriate correspondence is established between the images. Here, $\Pi_{\sim}$ generalizes any image similarity functions.

Equation 6.1 is easily seen as an instance of the variational energy in variational image registration, and indeed, the preceding development is equivalent to the classic formulation of the elastic matching by Bajcsy and Broit [53], in which the registration process is modeled after the physical task of applying loads to an elastic version of the object depicted in one image so that its deformed configuration resembles the target object in a second image. The appropriate loads are derived from a potential function as described above. The first object is deformed in this way until an equilibrium configuration is reached or,

* The moving image *J* will ultimately be warped into the reference frame provided by *I*. However, the transformation is computed from *I* to *J* and then used to resample *J* to obtain its warped version.

equivalently, until the total potential energy of the system is at a local minimum. The elastostatic configurations therefore represent solutions of the image registration problem as formulated in Equation 6.1.

Using the variational approach, one can show that the Euler–Lagrange equations for the elastostatic potential are of the form

$$\sigma_{ij,j} + f_i = 0 \tag{6.3}$$

where f is the external force applied on the target object and relates to the gradient of the image similarity term, $\Pi_{\sim}$. The first term ($\sigma_{ij,j}$) can be further derived as the Cauchy–Navier operator L:

$$L\mathbf{u} = \mu\nabla^2\mathbf{u} + (\lambda + \mathrm{u})\nabla(\nabla \cdot \mathbf{u}) \tag{6.4}$$

Material properties are determined by the Lamé constants μ and λ for the isotropic material idealization assumed in the current implementation.

6.2.2 Diffeomorphic Image Registration

Compressible and incompressible fluids have the unique property of behavior that corresponds to specific diffeomorphism groups. The theoretical work by Miller et al. [54] focuses on finding geodesic paths across these diffeomorphism manifolds by extending the viscous formulation to also optimize in time. Diffeomorphic transformations are able to preserve the topology, which is fundamental in making comparisons between objects in the natural world because such transformations permit comparisons to be made across time points in an individual's disease process or to study development patterns across a large population. This naturally fits the study of pulmonary kinematics. Some recent work on applying diffeomorphic transformation models on lung image registration is described in refs. [40,55].

We assume that the diffeomorphism, ϕ, is defined on the image domain, Ω. ϕ, over time, parameterizes a family of diffeomorphisms, $\phi(x, t)$: $\Omega \times t \rightarrow \Omega$, which can be generated by integrating a time-dependent, smooth velocity field, $\mathbf{v}$: $\Omega \times t \rightarrow \mathbb{R}^d$, through the ordinary differential equation

$$\frac{\mathrm{d}\phi(\mathbf{x},t)}{\mathrm{d}t} = \mathbf{v}(\phi(\mathbf{x},t),t), \quad \phi(\mathbf{x},0) = \mathrm{x}. \tag{6.5}$$

The deformation field yielded by ϕ is $\mathbf{u}(x) = \phi(x, 1) - x$.

The following minimizing variational form was proposed for optimization in diffeomorphic normalization for inexact image matching in refs. [54,56,57]:

$$\mathbf{v}^* = \underset{\mathbf{v}}{\mathrm{argmin}} \int_0^1 \|L\mathbf{v}\|^2 \,\mathrm{d}t + \lambda \int \|\mathrm{I} \circ \phi(\mathbf{x},1) - J\|^2 \,\mathrm{d} \quad . \tag{6.6}$$

The first term on the right represents a mathematical metric between I and J given an appropriate norm, L, on the velocity field, $\mathbf{v}$. The second term is the image similarity metric of square intensity difference with weight, λ, accounting for the inexact matching.

Similarly as in Equation 6.1, to accommodate a variety of medical image normalization tasks, one typically encounters more complex intensity transfers between one anatomical instance I and another instance J. This leads to the generalization of Equation 6.6:

$$\mathbf{v}^* = \arg\min_{\mathbf{v}} \int_0^1 \|L\mathbf{v}\|^2 \mathrm{d}t - \lambda \int \Pi_{\sim}(I, \phi(\mathbf{x},1), J)\mathrm{d} \tag{6.7}$$

where $\Pi_{\sim}$ is a similarity metric depending on the images and the mapping, and λ controls the degree of exactness in the matching.

6.2.2.1 *Symmetric Normalization*

By exploiting the fact that the diffeomorphism, ϕ, can be decomposed into two components ϕ_1 and ϕ_2 [58], one can construct a symmetric alternative to Equation 6.7. This leads to the symmetric variant of Equation 6.7

$$\left\{\mathbf{v}_1^*, \mathbf{v}_2^*\right\} = \arg\min_{\mathbf{v}_1,\mathbf{v}_2} \int_0^{0.5} \left(\|L\mathbf{v}_1(x,t)\|^2 + \|L\mathbf{v}_2(x,t)\|^2\right)\mathrm{d}t \\ -\lambda \int \Pi_{\sim}(I \circ \phi_1(x,0.5), J \circ \phi_2(x,0.5))\mathrm{d} \Bigg\}. \tag{6.8}$$

The corresponding symmetric Euler–Lagrange equations are similar to ref. [54]. Finding $\mathbf{v}_1^*$ minimizes the variational energy from $t = 0$, whereas $\mathbf{v}_2^*$ minimizes from $t = 1$. Thus, gradient-based iterative convergence deforms I and J along the geodesic diffeomorphism, ϕ, to a fixed point midway between I and J, thus motivating the denotation of the solution strategy as symmetric normalization (SyN).

6.2.3 Image Similarity Functions

The image similarity term $\Pi_{\sim}$ in both Equations 6.1 and 6.7 is essential in driving the deformation of the image warping. Here, we review several widely used image similarity functions.

6.2.3.1 *Optical Flow and Demons Algorithm*

An early contribution was the seminal work of Horn and Schunck [59], who introduced the computation of *optical flow*. The core algorithmic assumption of optical flow is that the intensity representing a particular point is constant between successive image acquisitions regardless of its spatial motion. If we represent the image intensity function as $I(x, t)$, this assumption can be represented formally as

$$I(x,t) = I(x + \delta x, t + \delta t) \tag{6.9}$$

where x denotes spatial location and t denotes acquisition time. Expanding the right side of Equation 6.9 using Taylor's series expansion yields the following relationship:

$$I(x,t) = I(x,t) + \nabla I \cdot \delta x + I_t \cdot \delta t + O^2. \tag{6.10}$$

Ignoring the second and higher-order terms (by assuming small displacements between image acquisitions), Equation 6.10 can be rewritten to yield the traditional optical flow constraint equation, $\varepsilon_{\text{optical flow}}$

$$\nabla I \cdot v + I_t = 0 \tag{6.11}$$

where $v = \frac{\delta x}{\delta t}$ is the sought after displacement. Because this problem is underconstrained, where there is only one equation for determining the multiple components of v, explicit regularization of the velocity field is used as the restriction to the solution space. In the original contribution by Horn and Schunck [59], this involves penalization of deviations from an n-D smooth field measured by

$$\varepsilon_{\text{smooth}} = \| v\|^2 = \sum_{i=1}^{n}\sum_{j=1}^{n} \frac{\partial v_i}{\partial x_j}^2 . \tag{6.12}$$

Minimizing the combined contributions of $\varepsilon_{\text{smooth}}$ and $\varepsilon_{\text{optical flow}}$ using variational calculus, the following iterative solution scheme is obtained:

$$v_{n+1} = v_n - I \frac{v_n \cdot I + I_t}{\lambda^2 + | I|^2} \tag{6.13}$$

where λ is a user-specified weighting term which modulates the solution between contributions of $\varepsilon_{\text{smooth}}$ and $\varepsilon_{\text{optical flow}}$. This technique is used in the recently reported research in refs. [60–62].

Other researchers have used a more recent optical flow variant colloquially known as demons, which was introduced by Thirion [63]. In this proposed variant, the iterative update of the image displacement, v, is given by

$$v = \frac{I_t \; I}{| I|^2 + I_t^2}. \tag{6.14}$$

The iterative update is typically performed in two steps. The first step involves tabulation of the optical flow followed by a regularization step (typically Gaussian convolution characterized by a user-specified σ). We indicate using optical flow as the similarity function with the abbreviation MSQ.

6.2.3.2 Normalized Cross-Correlation

Previous research has used optical flow [62,64] or its variant [65], which implicitly assumes the intensity consistency between two images. However, for pulmonary imaging, the image pairs are usually from two consecutive phases of respiration in which the local density changes are linearly reflected in the intensity changes. In this case, the invariance of cross-correlation to the linear intensity change makes it a suitable similarity function. Furthermore, we compute cross-correlation in a neighborhood around each voxel to accommodate the inhomogeneity of the density changes throughout the whole lung. The local cross-correlation is integrated over the lung volume as the overall similarity in the diffeomorphic transformation. One may write the (squared) cross-correlation for the diffeomorphic image registration as

$$\Pi_{\sim}(I,J) = \mathrm{CC}(x) = \frac{\left(\sum_{i}(I(x_i) - {}_{I(x)})(J(x_i) - {}_{J(x)})\right)^2}{\sum_{i}(I(x_i) - {}_{I(x)})^2 \sum_{i}(J(x_i) - {}_{J(x)})^2}, \tag{6.15}$$

where x is at the center of N^3 square window, μ is the mean value within the window centered at x, and x_i iterates through that window.

6.2.3.3 *MI*

MI was first proposed to register multimodality images [66,67] and is widely used in medical image registration [67,68]. It measures the degree to which information from one image predicts information in another. This information-theoretic criterion does not assume specific intensity relations between two images and can be applied to the registration of different modalities, such as positron emission tomography and CT. Consider images I and J as discrete random variables over intensities. The MI between I and J is defined as:

$$\begin{aligned}\mathrm{MI}(I,J) = &\sum_{i} P_I(i)\log P_I(i) + \sum_{j} P_J(j)\log P_J(j)\\ &-\sum_{i,j} P_{IJ}(i,j)\log P_{IJ}(i,j).\end{aligned} \tag{6.16}$$

$P.$ is the distribution for the random variable (·). P_{AB} is the joint distribution of A and B. Different implementations of MI typically vary the method of Parzen window estimation for the probabilities [32,66,69].

6.2.3.4 *Other Similarity Metrics*

Other researchers have focused more on the similarity between specific anatomic components. For example, Frangi's vesselness measure [70] was adopted in ref. [71] to use the rich information provided by the arborized pulmonary vasculature to match similar vesselness patterns in two images. Registration accuracy was shown to improve when adding the sum of squared vesselness measure difference (noted as SSVMD) to the sum of squared tissue volume difference (noted as SSTVD).

6.2.4 Numerical Implementation

The numerical optimizations of the variational formulation of the registration cost function in Equations 6.1, 6.7, and 6.8 are given in refs. [51,52,57,58].

One practical consequence of the variational formulation of the pulmonary image registration problem is that the finite-element method [72] can be brought to bear on its numerical solution. The details of our finite-element implementation have been reported previously [51,52] and, for the current discussion, it suffices to recall that the method proceeds by restricting the solution to be expressed in terms of a finite number of basis functions, ϕ_i, approximating the true solution

$$u_h(x) = \sum_{i=0}^{n} \alpha_i \phi_i(x). \tag{6.17}$$

The unknowns are the set of scalars, α_i, which are the weights on the basis functions. A special feature of the basis functions is their piecewise definition according to geometric subdivisions of the problem domain (called finite elements). In particular, the subdivision or meshing can be designed to highlight structures of interest in an image. This customization is advantageous for two reasons. First, it allows us to focus on the efficient registration of particular structures (e.g., the pulmonary vasculature) by subdividing more finely over these structures and more coarsely over less relevant regions (e.g., background). Additionally, the deformation of the image can be tailored according to the unique material properties of these structures by assigning different material properties to different elements. Both of these adaptations lay the groundwork for the pulmonary deformation analysis discussed in the sections that follow.

The elastic and the diffeomorphic image registration algorithms are implemented as part of the following open-source libraries: the Insight Toolkit [73] and the Advanced Normalization Tools [74].

6.3 Quantifying Normal Lung Motion in Humans

Images of a healthy young male volunteer acquired with breath-holding on a 1.5-T whole-body Signa Horizon MR scanner (General Electric, Milwaukee, WI) using a two-dimensional TrueFISP sequence (TR, 3.0 ms; TE, 1.5 ms; matrix size, 128 × 128; flip angle, 34 degrees; FOV, 450 mm; slice thickness, 10 mm; acquisition time per image, 0.4 s) were selected for analysis. Five sagittal views of the right lung at phases between full inspiration and full expiration were chosen (Figure 6.1). Three experts, skilled in MR pulmonary

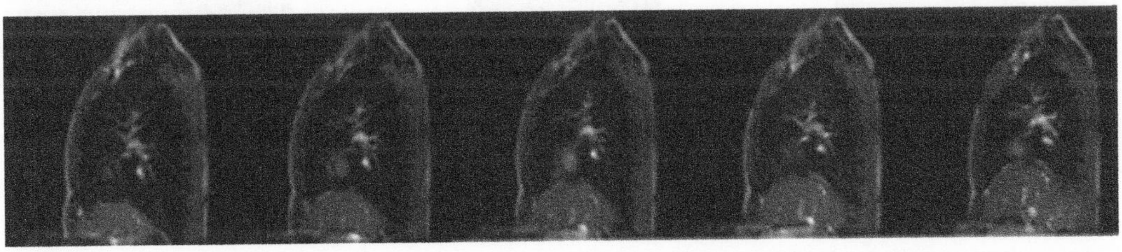

FIGURE 6.1
Serial sagittal MR scans of the right lung of a healthy male during the expiratory cycle. Note the progressive decrease in lung cross-sectional area and the vascular contrast provided by TrueFISP imaging.

anatomy, manually selected 22 landmarks on each image corresponding to a set of pulmonary blood vessels (Figure 6.3a). The three sets of landmarks were then averaged to produce a pseudo–ground truth landmark for each blood vessel.

In the first experiment, sequential pairs of images were registered using the elastic matching approach with cross-correlation as the image similarity term. The image domain was uniformly subdivided into 4 × 4-pixel quadrilateral finite elements, each mesh containing 1024 elements, respectively. Four integration points per element were used with values for Young's modulus (100) and Poisson's ratio (0.2) empirically determined to achieve the reported results. Regions 7 × 7 pixels in size were used to compute the normalized cross-correlation, and each registration ran for 100 iterations at full image resolution. Four displacement fields were generated from the five images. Each displacement field represented the motion of the lung during the interval between the two images. The "ground truth" landmarks were used to evaluate the accuracy of the registration by comparing the displacement of each landmark as computed by the algorithm with the known position of the landmark in the subsequent image.

Registration of the same four image pairs was repeated in a second experiment using anatomy-specific domain discretizations instead of the dense uniform sampling used previously (Figure 6.2). The custom subdivisions were generated by manually segmenting the thorax and the region of vascular prominence within the lung, and feeding the two contours to a quality-constrained triangular mesh generator [75]—see Figures 6.2 and 6.3b for example outputs. The vascular contour was used to ensure that the discretization contained smaller finite elements over the lung and progressively larger elements over other regions. Using smaller elements over a particular region allowed a denser sampling and,

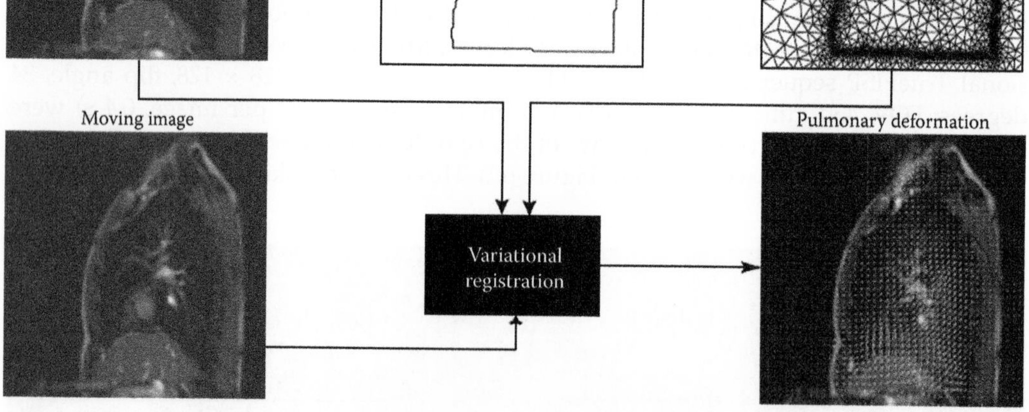

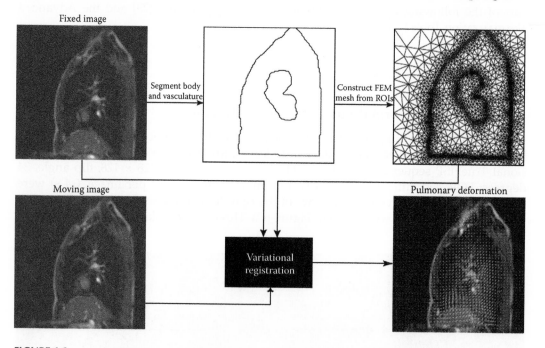

FIGURE 6.2
Use of anatomy-specific meshes for registration-based estimation of pulmonary deformation. Segmentation of the body and vasculature on the fixed image produces contours that are input to a freeware quality-constrained mesh generator. The resulting finite element mesh is then input to the variational registration along with the fixed and moving images, and used to solve the registration at "anatomic" sample points over the domain.

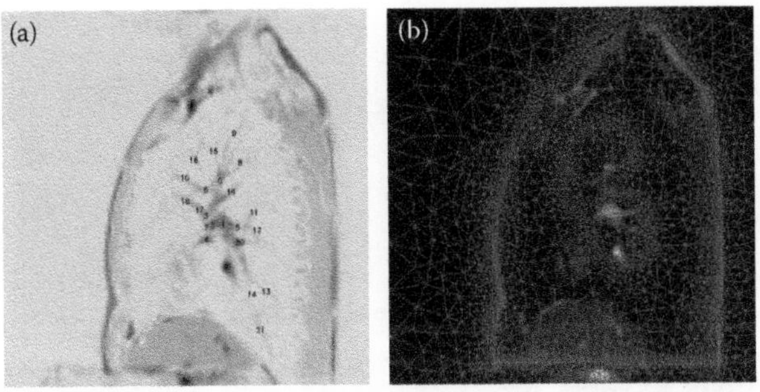

FIGURE 6.3
(a) Twenty-two vascular landmarks defined on a sagittal lung view. Each landmark corresponds to a segmental blood vessel within the right lung. (b) An anatomy-specific domain subdivision used to solve a registration.

in turn, a more precise solution in that region, so anatomy-specific subdivisions were used in anticipation of better motion estimates. In addition to the customized finite-element meshes, more realistic material properties were assumed in different regions of the image. Specifically, the elements over the lung and body were assigned a physiologically elastic behavior, whereas those elements over the image background were made highly compliant in order to mimic the behavior of air. Furthermore, the potential $\Pi_{\sim}$ was nulled over the background to reduce its confounding effect on the registration of structures of interest within the lung. Aforementioned values for the elastic coefficients were used with three integration points per triangle; each mesh contained approximately 5000 triangular elements. The displacement fields obtained using the anatomy-specific finite-element implementation were also evaluated using the known landmark displacements. The elastic registration parameters are listed in Table 6.1.

6.3.1 Quantification of Normal Human Lung Motion

Figure 6.4 shows the motion analysis performed using the homogeneously elastic model of lung deformation with the uniform grids of 4×4 pixel quadrilateral finite elements. The elastic recoil of the diaphragm, the primary driving force during expiration, was partially

TABLE 6.1
Registration Parameters Used for Human and Mouse Experiments

Parameter	Human	Mouse
Element size	4×4 pixels[a]	Variable[b]
Young's modulus (E)	100	100
Poisson's ratio (ν)	0.2	0.2
Integration points	4	3
Metric region	7×7	3×3
Iterations	100	100

[a] Element size is specified for the rectilinear grid experiments; elements of varying sizes were used in the triangular anatomy-specific meshes used in the human data experiments.
[b] Anatomy-specific subdivisions were used exclusively in the mouse experiments.

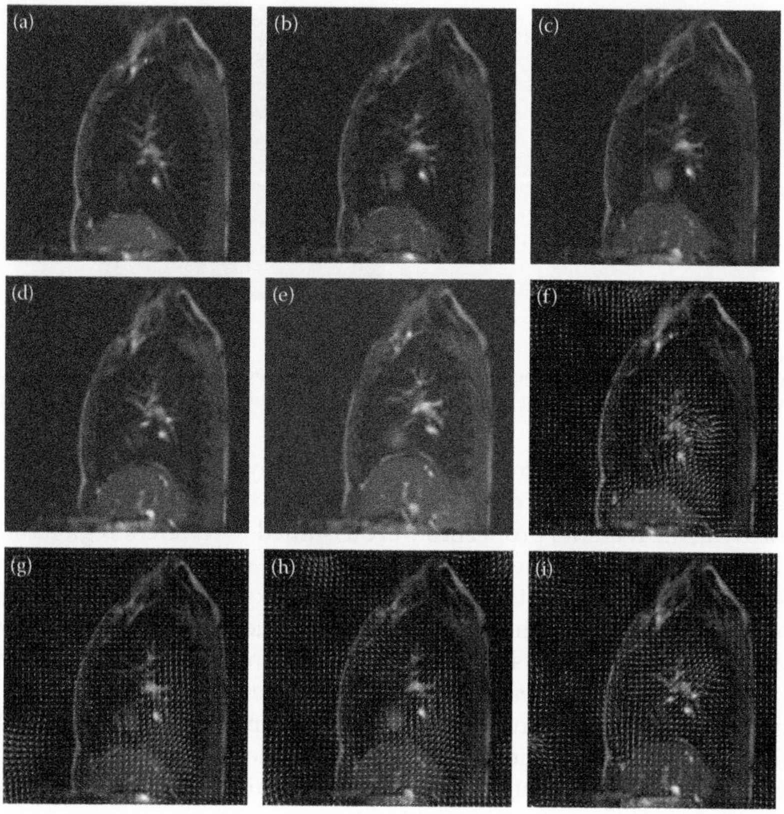

FIGURE 6.4
(a–e) Sequential 2D images of the lung acquired during the expiratory phase of respiration for a healthy adult. (f–i) Resulting motion fields obtained by registration of sequential pairs of images in (a)–(e). For example, (f) is the registration mapping (a) to (b), (g) is the registration mapping (b) to (c), etc.

detected over the posterior portion of the diaphragm in each field. Additional motion was naturally observed over the segmental pulmonary blood vessels, which served as good spatial markers. However, in regions with poor contrast, such as the anterior upper and middle lobes, very little motion information was obtained. The assumption of a homogeneously elastic image body, combined with the inhomogeneity of the background intensities, resulted in the detection of paradoxical motion over the image background. This extraneous motion might confound the pulmonary deformation in the region of interest, but could be reliably removed from the displacement fields computed with the uniform grids.

To improve motion detection in the parenchyma and reduce background motion, the four pairs of images in Figure 6.4 were re-registered, this time using anatomy-specific subdivisions of the image domain. The subdivisions were customized such that the pulmonary and thoracic elements were assigned a physiologic elasticity, whereas the background elements were made highly compliant. Furthermore, loads that were localized to the background elements were nulled to minimize those displacements that could mask true pulmonary motion.

The results acquired by applying the two different problem configurations—rectilinear grid and anatomy-specific mesh—to the first image pair were compared in Figure 6.5. An initial overview revealed that the anatomy-specific model was able to capture the recoil of

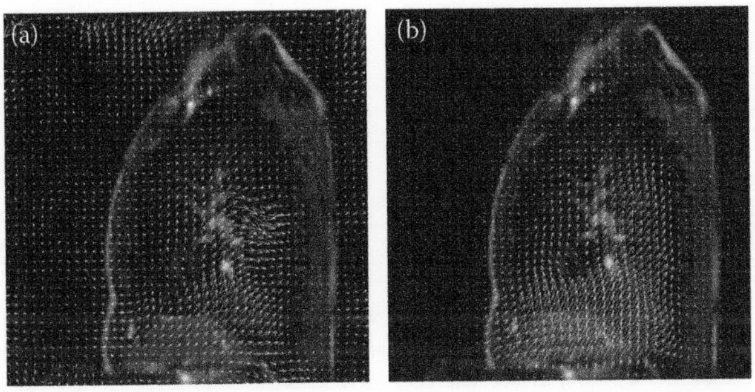

FIGURE 6.5
Comparison of lung motion maps computed using two different registration configurations. (a) A uniform grid of homogeneously elastic elements is used to acquire this displacement field, which reflects some posterior diaphragmatic recoil but also contains background motion. (b) The anatomy-specific mesh used here captures the motion of the entire diaphragm and enables us to focus on the deformation of the pulmonary vasculature and parenchyma. Background motion is also minimized.

the entire diaphragm, whereas the homogeneously elastic model was unable to detect the motion of the anterior diaphragm. The vascular displacements detected by the anatomy-specific model were also much more organized than those detected using the rectilinear grid of elements. In addition, motion in the anterior parenchyma was less obscure in the anatomy-specific result. Furthermore, the unwanted background motion in the customized result was negligible.

The displacements of expert-defined vascular landmarks were used to evaluate the two registration configurations. First, the displacements of the landmarks were calculated using their predefined positions on each image. Then, the displacements computed by the registrations at each landmark location were extracted from each field. These two sets of displacements—landmark-derived and registration-derived—were then compared. For each displacement field, error was computed in terms of the distance between the expected (landmark derived) and achieved (registration derived) vector endpoints. The origins of both vectors were the initial positions of the landmark points, so only the displacement vector endpoints were used to study accuracy. Among all landmarks, the mean endpoint errors for each field were 1.08 ± 0.89, 0.89 ± 0.62, 0.97 ± 0.65, and 1.87 ± 1.57 pixels for the uniform grid results and 1.11 ± 0.91, 0.88 ± 0.54, 1.01 ± 0.71, and 1.78 ± 1.44 pixels for the anatomy-specific meshes. The two methods performed similarly at the landmarks, suggesting that if motion extraction were the only goal, registration with rectilinear grids would suffice. Image contrast at the landmark locations was high, reducing the dependence on the elastic regularization. However, the results indicated that in areas of low parenchymal contrast, the anatomy-specific approach yielded more accurate results. These customized domain discretizations not only produced results with less confounding motion but also set the stage for additional biomechanical modeling that cannot be performed with the uniform grids alone.

6.4 Evaluating Pathologic Lung Motion in Transgenic Mice

Transgenic mouse strains of SCD can be used to evaluate the effects of the disease on lung function using the current methodology [76]. A mouse with SCD was first imaged on a 4.7-T

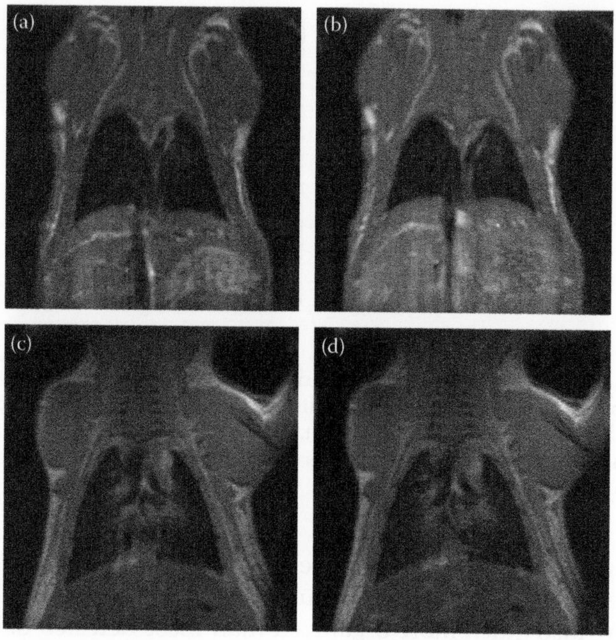

FIGURE 6.6
(a and b) Coronal lung views of a healthy mouse at end-inspiration and end-expiration, respectively. (c and d) Corresponding lung views from a normoxic transgenic mouse depicting a much smaller degree of respiratory excursion.

(Bruker, Karlsruhe, Germany) scanner (TR ≈ 1000 ms; TE, 6.63 ms; FOV, 30 mm; slice thickness, 1 mm) at end-inspiration and end-expiration (Figure 6.6c and d) under normoxic conditions (21% O_2), and then placed in a hypoxic environment (5% O_2) and imaged again at the same points of the respiratory cycle. The inspiratory and expiratory images were registered to extract the expiratory motion of the lungs. The previously discussed values for the elastic coefficients were applied, with three integration points per triangular finite element; both the prehypoxia and posthypoxia results were obtained using slightly more than 3000 triangular elements. Regions 3 × 3 pixels in size were used for the normalized cross-correlation, and the registrations ran for 100 iterations. The resulting displacement fields were compared to demonstrate the effects of hypoxia on an animal with SCD.

This pathologic motion was compared with the lung motion of a healthy mouse (Figure 6.6a and b). The healthy mouse was similarly imaged at end-inspiration and end-expiration (under normoxic conditions only) to generate a displacement field representing normal pulmonary deformation during the expiratory phase. The finite-element discretization used for this registration contained approximately 3100 triangular elements; the same parameter settings were used as in the pathologic case. This resulting displacement field was compared with the displacement field from the SCD mouse to note regional differences in motion associated with acute chest syndrome and ongoing vascular and tissue damage secondary to SCD. The elastic registration parameters are listed in Table 6.1.

6.4.1 Pathologic Lung Motion

One expects to observe decreased respiratory motion in the SCD mouse because of acute chest syndrome. Refined sampling of pulmonary anatomy was achieved by tailoring the

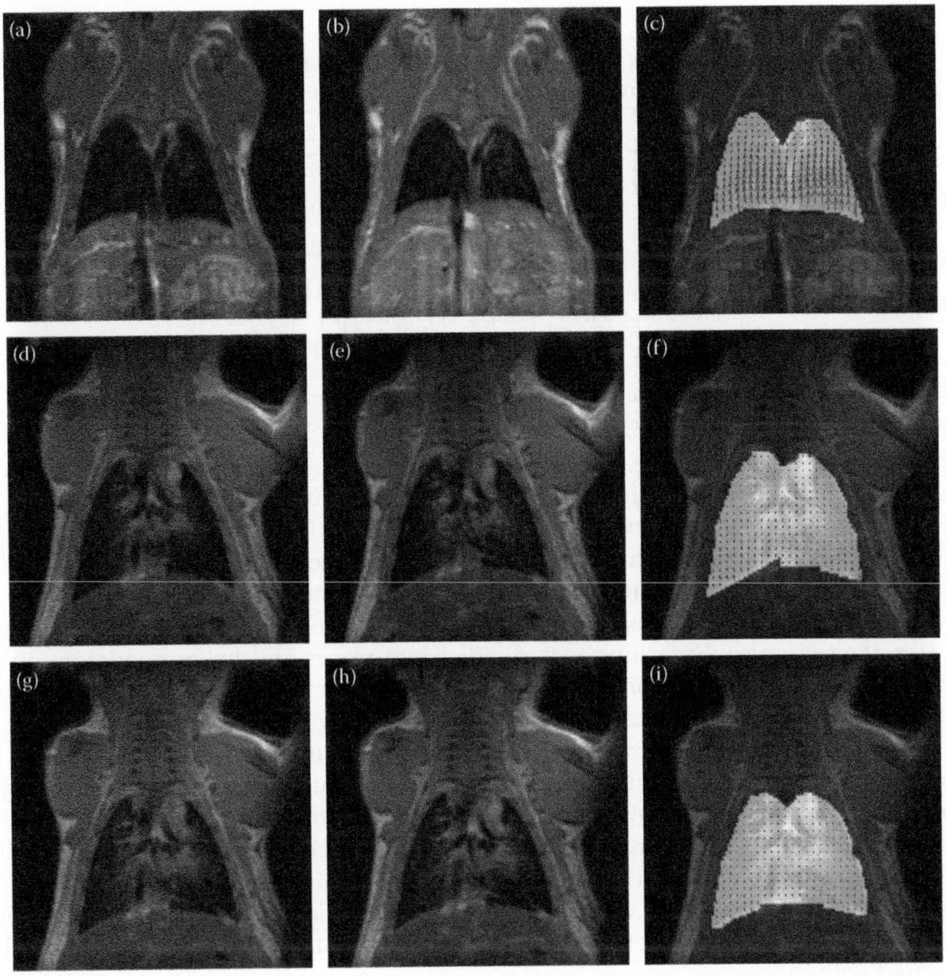

FIGURE 6.7
End-inspiratory images (a,d,g), end-expiratory images (b,e,h), and motion maps (c,f,i) of the expiratory phase of respiration for a healthy mouse (top row), a normoxic SCD mouse (middle row), and the same SCD mouse (bottom row) under hypoxic conditions

finite-element discretizations to lung segmentations produced using the geodesic active contour level set segmentation filter within the Insight Toolkit [73].

First, normal murine lung motion was examined by registering end-inspiratory and end-expiratory images from a healthy mouse. A greater degree of motion in the lower lobes was expected when compared with the upper lobes because of the proximity of the diaphragm; however, continuous motion throughout the lungs was anticipated. The resulting motion field was masked to only show motion over the lungs (Figure 6.7a–c). On these coronal images, observed diaphragmatic recoil, even in the small mouse, could be observed.

Next, this normal motion was compared with the respiratory performance of a transgenic SCD mouse studied under normoxic (Figure 6.7d–f) and hypoxic (Figure 6.7g–i) conditions. Even under normoxic conditions, this mouse displayed less overall respiratory

TABLE 6.2

Comparison of Mean Pulmonary Displacement Magnitudes (in Millimeters) per Quadrant in Mice

Mouse	LL	RL	LU	RU
Normal	1.03	0.73	0.38	0.32
Normoxic SCD	0.16	0.27	0.10	0.09
Hypoxic SCD	0.10	0.16	0.06	0.08

Note: The lungs are divided into four quadrants: left lower (LL), right lower (RL), left upper (LU), and right upper (RU) quadrants. Note that left and right were defined physiologically. A fraction of the respiratory motion in the healthy mouse was observed in the SCD mouse, even when the latter was normoxic.

motion than the healthy mouse, perhaps indicating that the SCD mouse was already experiencing some degree of chronic sickling despite its normoxic environs. Once hypoxia set in, we expected more of the mouse's red blood cells to sickle and clog the smaller arteries and capillaries. The lung was highly susceptible to this process, and the result was a further decrease in observed respiratory motion in the SCD mouse.

A quantitative analysis was performed to localize regional differences in motion between the two mice. Each lung was divided into upper and lower quadrants on the coronal images to define regions for comparison between individuals. The division was determined by drawing a horizontal line across each lung that was equidistant from the highest apical point and the lowest basal point on each lung. Within each quadrant, the mean pulmonary displacement vector length was calculated. This quantitative comparison of the mean displacements in Figure 6.7 emphasized the difference in pulmonary deformation between the normal and SCD mice (Table 6.2). There was a dramatic difference in observed motion between the normal and SCD mice even during normoxia. The decrease in motion coincident with the increase in hypoxia was also evident in the SCD mouse, despite the fact that motion within those murine lungs was already limited when compared with the norm.

This approach could further be adapted for diagnostic purposes. In the previous experiment, we compared the pulmonary effort of a single healthy individual with that of an individual with SCD. The analysis could similarly be applied to serial scans of a patient to determine the progression of disease or the efficacy of a previously applied treatment by quantitatively evaluating the changes in regional lung motion at each clinical visit. Another potential application would be disease screening, whereby a patient's pulmonary motion could be compared with that of previously diagnosed individuals' pulmonary motion to assess the degree of parenchymal involvement.

6.5 Evaluation of SyN in the EMPIRE10 Study

Although many algorithms have been proposed for pulmonary image registration, a systematic evaluation and comparison of different methods remains a problem for the research community. Challenges include the availability of a public database, optimal parameter configurations for different algorithms, and a consistent protocol for evaluating registration quality and the accuracy of results.

The recent Evaluation of Methods for Pulmonary Image Registration 2010 (EMPIRE10) challenge [46,77] provided a public platform for fair and meaningful comparisons of registration algorithms applied to thoracic CT data. The challenge was organized in conjunction with the Grand Challenge workshop at the 13th International Conference on Medical Image Computing and Computer-Assisted Intervention [78]. In the preworkshop session, each participant downloaded a set of 20 thoracic CT image pairs and registered them using individually developed algorithms. The resulting deformation fields were then submitted to the EMPIRE10 organizational team for independent evaluation. On the day of the workshop, each participant registered additional 10 image pairs within 3 hours as part of the live challenge.

By requiring each team to run their own registration algorithm individually, EMPIRE10 avoided the often complex task of configuring and optimizing parameters for unfamiliar registration algorithms. The method of SyN introduced in Section 6.2.2.1 was evaluated [79] in this study and ranked highest among all participants.

6.5.1 Materials and Evaluation Protocol

A total of 30 datasets were provided for the EMPIRE10 study. All datasets were from the same range of sources and had similar properties. The materials used in EMPIRE10 were gathered from a variety of institutions to effectively cover practical clinical scenarios. The subjects included healthy volunteers as well as patients with known pulmonary disease, and were obtained on different CT scanners both with and without contrast administration. Imaging was performed at multiple different breath-holds. In addition to the human data, ovine data with implanted metallic markers and artificially warped image pairs with synthetic deformation fields were also provided. Each image pair was taken from a single subject. The data were cropped using a bounding box around the lungs to reduce unnecessary computation and storage cost.

Unlike other studies in which only the similarity of the image intensities or the displacement of landmarks was evaluated after registration, EMPIRE10 opted for a more comprehensive evaluation protocol. The deformation fields were evaluated in four categories: lung boundaries, fissure alignments, labeled landmarks, and singularities in the deformation. Participating teams were ranked according to their scores in all categories. More details about the study can be found in refs. [46,77].

6.5.2 Results Using SyN

The diffeomorphic model of SyN was applied to the EMPIRE10 database using the open-source Advanced Normalization Tools [74]. The images were first aligned using an affine registration of the binary lung masks. A five-level image resolution pyramid was applied, and the normalized cross-correlation was used as the similarity function with a neighborhood radius of two voxels.

SyN performed the best of the 34 submitted algorithms in the preworkshop session and placed second out of the 20 submitted algorithms in the on-site session. SyN ranked first overall among the 20 algorithms tested in both sessions. Some examples of the registration results are shown in Figure 6.8. The individual score and the ranking for each subject can be found in ref. [77].

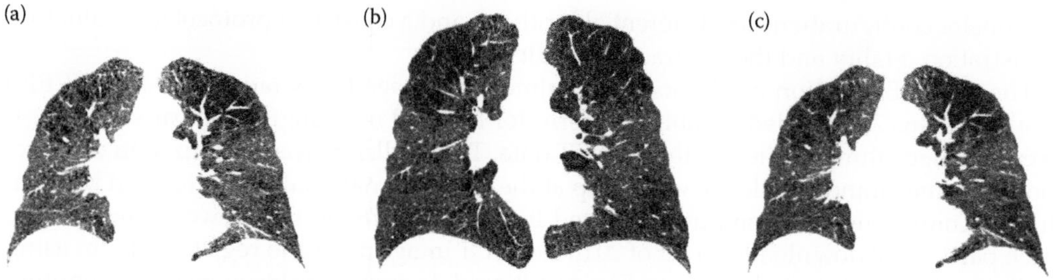

FIGURE 6.8
Sample registration results in the EMPIRE10 challenge obtained using SyN within the Advanced Normalization Tools. Two-dimensional slice from the fixed image (a), the moving image (b), and the moving image (c) after registration.

6.6 Effects of Parameters on Motion Quantitation Accuracy

Validating the accuracy of these motion estimates is a nontrivial problem; ground-truth motion cannot be determined without disruptive methods (such as implantation of tissue fiducials). Less invasive validation approaches for nonrigid registration, in general, include tracking landmarks on images [80], comparison with known synthetic deformations [81], tracking known displacements of a phantom [82], assessment of anatomic overlap [83], and comparison with other modalities [84]. However, these methods are often suboptimal when validating motion quantitation of *in vivo* dynamic organs.

We have previously shown landmark-based validation: identifying and tracking structures that are visible within the lungs, such as airway and vessel bifurcations [85]. The challenges one encountered include the inability to consistently identify points in successive images as well as a limit on the total number of landmarks that can be identified. In this study, ventilated porcine lung explants were imaged using an artificial thorax [86]. Nearly 350 landmarks were identified within the lungs, along the artificial diaphragm, and (as controls) on the hull of the artificial thorax. The "ground-truth" motion of these points was compared with the registration-derived motion estimate to assess the accuracy of the parenchymal dynamics computation with respect to image resolution and similarity metrics. The optimal inflation interval for motion analysis was also quantified.

6.6.1 Data Acquisition

Porcine lung explants from a healthy animal were placed inside a dedicated chest phantom designed by Biederer and colleagues [86]. The phantom was sealed and evacuated to make the lung expand passively. A water-filled elastic diaphragm was used to simulate tidal respiration by cyclic variation of the filling volume at a frequency of 8 cycles/min. Four-dimensional CT images were acquired in dynamic mode with a pitch of 0.1 (Siemens Somatom: slice collimation, 24 × 1.2 mm; rotation time, 1 s; slice thickness, 1.5 mm; increment, 0.8 mm; 120 kV, 400 mAs, lung kernel). Images were reconstructed retrospectively at 0%, 25%, 50%, 75%, and 100% inspiration. The data were acquired with a 512 × 512 matrix. To accommodate technical limitations, image volumes were resampled to dimensions of 256 × 256 × 243 with 1.17-mm isotropic voxels.

A specially trained physician manually selected point landmarks on the 0% inspiration image and then identified them on subsequent images (Figure 6.9). Branching structures

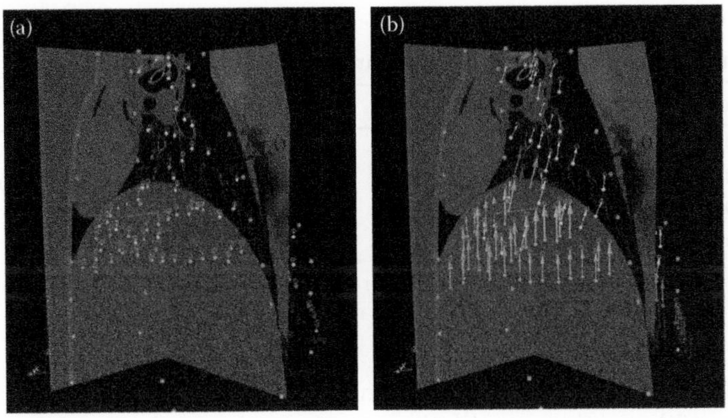

FIGURE 6.9
3D renderings of the landmark displacements between 0% and 25% inflation (a) and 0% and 100% inflation (b). Vectors are rendered in 3D space, whereas orthogonal cross-sections of the image volume are provided for reference. Note that the points on the phantom's hull serve as controls and therefore lack displacement vectors.

(both airway and vascular) were chosen on each image because of their reproducibility and distribution throughout the lungs. In addition, landmarks were placed on the diaphragm—the site of the greatest pulmonary deformation—and on the phantom itself. In total, 125 landmarks were identified as airway and vessel bifurcations, whereas 142 points were selected on the diaphragm and 76 points on the hull of the phantom. Such a distribution of the landmarks throughout the lungs was useful because it allows one to quantify the uncertainty of our registration measurements in different anatomic regions.

The error between the known landmark displacement $\overrightarrow{dx_l}$ and the registration-derived displacement $\overrightarrow{dx_r}$ at each landmark location was computed as the distance between the endpoints of the two displacement vectors $\left(\left\|\overrightarrow{dx_l} - \overrightarrow{dx_r}\right\|\right)$. In the discussion that follows, we report the mean of this endpoint error over the landmarks within the indicated anatomic region (diaphragmatic or parenchymal).

6.6.2 Experiment Setup

The image sequence was processed multiple times with different parameters to study the effect of image resolution and image similarity on the accuracy of motion quantitation over progressively larger inflation intervals. First, we studied the sensitivity of our motion estimates to the number of resolution levels processed. The SyN approach described in Section 6.2.2.1 ran at four increasing levels of resolution (from 1/8 to 1) using MI as the similarity in all cases. Next, the effect of metric choice on motion estimates was examined by running SyN registrations at all four resolution levels with each of the three metrics under investigation (Table 6.3). In both cases, three types of inflation interval were used: sequential, alternating, and phase intervals (see Table 6.3); the latter covers the entire inspiratory phase of respiration. Each level of the multiresolution pyramid was used for no more than 100 iterations.

The performance of the algorithm has previously been evaluated for brain registration [87]. Here, the effectiveness, specifically for lung motion quantitation, was tested. The effect of three different similarity metrics on motion estimates was tested: optical flow (MSQ), a 5 × 5 × 5 neighborhood cross-correlation (CC) based on the implementation in

TABLE 6.3

Summary of 36 Experiments Performed

Iterations		Metric		Intervals
100/1/1/1	×	MI	×	Sequential (0–25%, 25–50%, etc.)
100/100/1/1		MSQ		Alternating (0–50%, 50–100%)
100/100/100/1		CC		Phase (0–100%)
100/100/100/100				

Note: "Iterations" indicates the number of iterations at each of the four levels (from 1/8 of full resolution to full resolution).

ref. [88], and MI. All three were adapted to the symmetric formulation of the registration. The dependence of the motion quantitation process on the resolution of the image was also explored.

6.6.3 Results

Examples of the displacement fields generated via registration of the 0% inflation image to subsequent images in the sequence are shown in Figure 6.10. Figure 6.11 summarizes the errors observed in our experiments.

6.6.3.1 Effect of Image Resolution

When estimating lung motion sequentially, the final result was almost completely achieved at the lowest image resolution, whereas the error within the lung dropped by 0.5–2 mm with processing at higher levels. Errors tended to be 1–2 mm higher at the diaphragm than within the lung, likely because the diaphragm and lung bases moved more than the apical parenchyma. Upon visualization of the registration-derived displacements at the landmarks, it appeared that the error at the diaphragm was angular (vectors were of appropriate magnitude but point in a different direction), whereas within the parenchyma, it was scalar (vectors point in an appropriate direction but were not of the correct magnitude).

Using the alternating inflation intervals, one observed a 1-mm gain in accuracy within the lung by registering at higher levels; errors at the diaphragm remained almost constant.

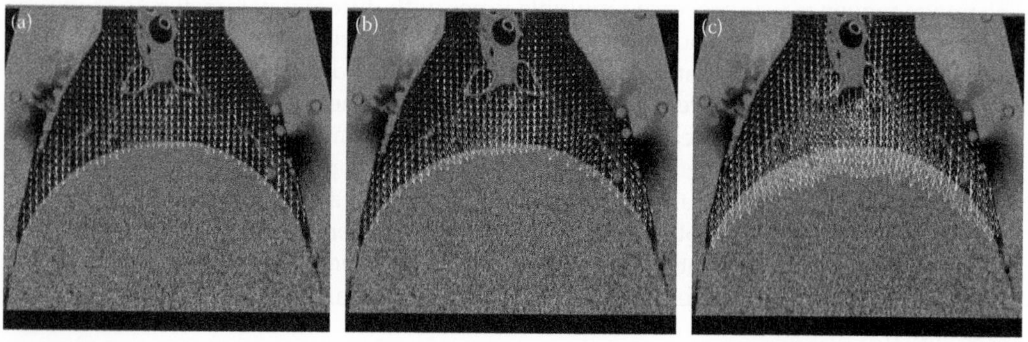

FIGURE 6.10
Sample mid-coronal vector fields (extracted from the 3D displacements) representing expansion from 0% to 25% (a), 0% to 50% (b), and 0% to 100% (c). Vector magnitudes increase nonlinearly as the degree of expansion increases; there is greater motion at the lung bases than the apices.

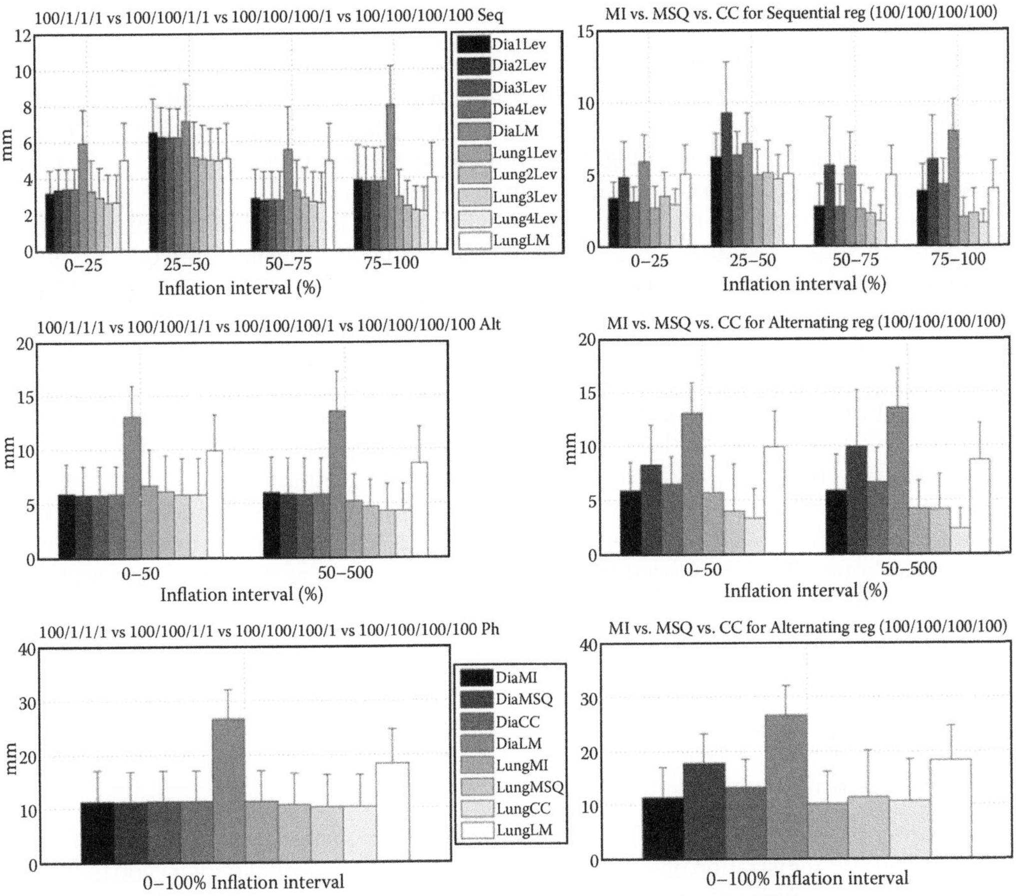

FIGURE 6.11
Mean ± SD endpoint errors for the resolution (left—top legend) and similarity (right—bottom legend) experiments at each of the three intervals (rows). The middle and last bars in each group indicate (for reference) the average motion at each landmark along the diaphragm and within the lung, respectively. #Lev, number of resolution levels used; Dia, diaphragm.

This was likely because the soft tissue–air interface at the diaphragm was not compromised by downsampling and remained a strong contributor to the gradient of the similarity at low image resolutions.

When registering the entire inspiratory phase, one observed an increase in accuracy intraparenchymally with higher levels of processing. However, it was important to note that the mean endpoint error throughout the lung and diaphragm was 11 mm because of the large degree of inflation. By acquiring one additional image (and using alternating intervals), it was able to cut our error in half. Further doubling our sampling frequency increased gains by 25% to 50%.

Overall, errors were at least 1 mm higher along the diaphragm than within the lung parenchyma. In most cases, the magnitude of the resulting endpoint errors was less than 40% of the actual motion in the region. There did not appear to be much improvement between the 128^3 level and the 256^3 level. This suggested that processing at the highest data resolution did not significantly alter the final result, and was encouraging because this level was the most time-consuming.

6.6.3.2 Effect of Image Similarity Metrics

Regardless of the inflation interval, optical flow was consistently the least accurate of the three metrics studied. It resulted in a diaphragmatic error of 0.5–4.5 mm for sequential registrations, 1.9–4 mm for alternating registrations, and 1.8–6.3 mm for the inspiratory phase registrations. Within the lung, however, the MSQ error was within 0.5–1 mm of the MI and CC errors, and occasionally less than the former.

Comparison of the performance of MI and CC yielded some interesting observations. For the sequential registrations, the accuracy of the two metrics was within 0.5 mm of one another. As the inflation interval increased, MI outperformed CC (by an average of 1.8 mm in the phase registrations). However, within the lung, CC was 1.4–1.9 mm better in the alternating registrations (the two metrics were within 0.4 mm of one another in the other experiments). This motivated the anatomic customization of similarity computations. Matching at the diaphragm might be easier because of the clear tissue interface between air and muscle, whereas matching in the parenchyma might require additional regional information (such as that provided the neighborhood integration of CC).

Again, it was important to note that the phase registrations with MI and CC were only accurate to within 11–13 mm at the diaphragm and 10–11 mm within the lung. Adding just one additional image reduced the mean error to 6–7 mm at the diaphragm and only 3–6 mm within the lung.

6.7 Discussion

This chapter presents an approach toward the regional extraction of pulmonary deformation via nonrigid registration of serial lung MR images. Conventional registration methods, as exemplified by a finite-element implementation of the classic elastic matching technique, are shown to perform well over a set of vascular landmarks in the measurement of lung motion. This performance is maintained in an augmented system, incorporating inhomogeneous material properties combined with the use of domain discretizations constructed to reflect the apparent geometry within the image and to reduce background effects. These adaptations represent the first step toward the development of computational models of pulmonary biomechanics.

Registrations performed with anatomy-specific subdivisions of the image thus parsimoniously capture regional deformation within the lung parenchyma, particularly in areas where tissue intensities are somewhat sparse because of the extremely low T_1 of lung tissue. This characteristic of the pulmonary parenchyma poses a number of challenges in the effort to describe respiratory motion. The introduction of manually specified landmarks can circumvent this problem to some degree and is a capability supported by our implementation [89].

Ideally, we would be able to analyze data at the acquired resolution, instead of halving the resolution because of memory limitations. However, it is important to note that the results at the top two resolution levels are very similar. This suggests that slightly augmenting system memory may allow us to register data at the original resolution ($0.5 \times 0.5 \times 0.8$ mm in this case) and result in even better accuracy. Furthermore, we can reduce the number of iterations at the highest level and drastically reduce the runtime required to process an image pair without sacrificing the quality of our motion estimates.

The importance of small inflation intervals is clear through comparing deformation computed from different image pairs. Attempting to quantify lung motion over an entire phase (i.e., end-inspiration to end-expiration), whether we use tidal limits or respiratory extremes, is inaccurate. If a 1-cm error is acceptable, then it is appropriate to acquire only two images, reducing scan time and radiation exposure. However, most clinical applications would not tolerate such a large inaccuracy. Hence, this motivates the need for finer sampling of the respiratory cycle.

One major challenge in quantifying pulmonary deformation is the difficulty associated with *in vivo* validation of motion. Ideally, we would be able to implant a set of parenchymal markers in an animal model, image the respiratory motion of these markers, and compare this to the registration-derived estimates of deformation. However, surgical insertion of markers into the lung introduces the possibility of additionally altering normal alveolar mechanics in the neighborhood of the markers. Surface markers would be helpful in tracking thoracic excursion during breathing, but would not provide insight into regional parenchymal deformation. As a result, we use the empirical validation discussed earlier. The noninvasive tracking of vascular landmarks evident on sagittal sections yields useful information about pulmonary deformation without interfering with normal pulmonary kinematics. However, model-based validation of our algorithm is an ongoing area of investigation.

The results presented here provide an introduction toward biomechanical modeling of pulmonary deformation. In these experiments, we are required to specify the mechanical behavior of the lung and body to compute pulmonary deformation. Despite using the same prescribed material properties, we are still able to quantify differences in lung motion between health and disease states. These differences indirectly represent changes in the material character of the tissue, which cannot directly be estimated using structural imaging modalities. For now, we pursue this image-based approach and note that the image forces used to drive the registration are inferred from the actual mechanical forces (e.g., diaphragmatic recoil, contraction of accessory muscles of respiration) that deform the lung during respiration. Future extensions of this work include the construction of a universal model of pulmonary biomechanics that incorporates the various forces applied by the other thoracic and abdominal structures that affect respiration.

Future efforts include developing the ability to make direct regional comparisons between lungs throughout the respiratory cycle. The ultimate goal of this work is to develop a four-dimensional model of the healthy lung that could be used to (1) evaluate pulmonary motion under various pathologies, (2) compare the respiratory motion of one individual to another, (3) track disease development within an individual, or (4) study the efficacy of a particular treatment or intervention with respect to changes in lung motion. Such a model could also be used to correlate observed functional changes with causative structural variations, or ideally, to build a dynamic atlas of the normal human lung.

References

[1] Murray, J.F., and J.A. Nadel, eds. 2000. *Textbook of Respiratory Medicine*. W.B. Saunders Company, 3rd ed.

[2] Xu, J., K.D. Kochanek, S.L. Murphy, and B. Tejada-Vera. 2010. Deaths: Final data for 2007. *National Vital Statistics Reports*, 58(19).

[3] American Lung Association. 2008. Lung Disease Data. http://www.lungusa.org.
[4] Pratt, P.C. 1988. Emphysema and chronic airways disease. In *Pulmonary Pathology*, 654–659. New York: Springer-Verlag.
[5] Fulmer, J.D., W.C. Roberts, E.R. von Gal, and R.G. Crystal. 1979. Morphologic–physiologic correlates of the severity of fibrosis and degree of cellularity in idiopathic pulmonary fibrosis. *Journal of Clinical Investigation*, 63:665–676.
[6] Gay, S.E., E.A. Kazerooni, G.B. Toews, J.P. Lynch Roberts 3rd, B.H. Gross, P.N. Cascade, D.L. Spizarny, A. Flint, M.A. Schork, R.I. Whyte, J. Popovich, R. Hyzy, and F.J. Martinez. 1998. Idiopathic pulmonary fibrosis: Predicting response to therapy and survival. *American Journal of Respiratory and Critical Care Medicine*, 157:1063–1072.
[7] Knight, J., T.M. Murphy, and I. Browning. 1999. The lung in sickle cell disease. *Pediatric Pulmonology*, 28:205–216.
[8] Gold, W. Pulmonary Function Testing. 2000. In *Textbook of Respiratory Medicine*, 3rd ed, J.F. Murray and J.A. Nadel, eds. 783–804. Philadelphia: W.B. Saunders.
[9] Mead, J., and J. Whittenberger. 1953. Physical properties of human lungs measured during spontaneous respiration. *Journal of Applied Physiology*, 5:779–796.
[10] West, J.B. 1971. Distribution of a mechanical stress in the lung, a possible factor in localisation of pulmonary disease. *Lancet*, 839–841.
[11] Carton, R.W., J. Dainauskas, B. Tews, and G.M. Hass. 1960. Isolation and study of the elastic tissue network of the lung in three dimensions. *American Review of Respiratory Disease*, 82:186–194.
[12] D'Angelo, E. 1975. Stress–strain relationships during uniform and non-uniform expansion of isolated lungs. *Respiration Physiology*, 23:87–107.
[13] Lee, G.C., and A. Frankus. 1975. Elasticity properties of lung parenchyma derived from experimental distortion data. *Biophysical Journal*, 15:481–493.
[14] Liu, S., S. Margulies, and T.A. Wilson. 1990. Deformation of the dog lung in the chest wall. *Journal of Applied Physiology*, 68(5):1979–1987.
[15] Mead, J., T. Takishima, and D. Leith. 1970. Stress distribution in lungs: a model of pulmonary elasticity. *Journal of Applied Physiology*, 28(5):596–608.
[16] Lambert, R.K., and T.A. Wilson. 1973. A model for the elastic properties of the lung and their effect on expiratory flow. *Journal of Applied Physiology*, 34(1):34–48.
[17] Wilson. T.A. 1972. A continuum analysis of a two-dimensional mechanical model of the lung parenchyma. *Journal of Applied Physiology*, 33(4):472–478.
[18] De Wilde, R., J. Clement, J.M. Hellemans, M. Decramer, M. Demedts, R. Boving, and K.P. Van de Woestijne. 1981. Model of elasticity of the human lung. *Journal of Applied Physiology*, 51(2):254–261.
[19] Lai-Fook, S.J., and R.E. Hyatt. 2000. Effects of age on the elastic moduli of human lungs. *Journal of Applied Physiology*, 89(1):163–168.
[20] Suga, K., T. Tsukuda, H. Awaya, K. Takano, S. Koike, N. Matsunaga, K. Sugi, and K. Esato. 1999. Impaired respiratory mechanics in pulmonary emphysema: Evaluation with dynamic breathing MRI. *Journal of Magnetic Resonance Imaging*, 10:510–520.
[21] Cluzel, P., T. Similowski, C. Chartrand-Lefebvre, M. Zelter, J.P. Derenne, and P.A. Grenier. 2000. Diaphragm and chest wall: Assessment of the inspiratory pump with MR imaging—preliminary observations. *Radiology*, 215:574–583.
[22] Ganesan, S., K.E. Rouch, and S.J. Lai-Fook. 1995. A finite element analysis of the effects of the abdomen on regional lung expansion. *Respiration Physiology*, 99:341–353.
[23] Gefen, A., D. Elad, and R.J. Shiner. 1999. Analysis of stress distribution in the alveolar septa of normal and simulated emphysematic lungs. *Journal of Biomechanics*, 32(9):891–897.
[24] Ingenito, E.P., L. Mark, J. Morris, F.F. Espinosa, R.D. Kamm, and M. Johnson. 1999. Biophysical characterization and modeling of lung surfactant components. *Journal of Applied Physiology*, 86(5):1702–1714.
[25] Axel, L., and L. Dougherty. 1989. Heart wall motion: Improved method of spatial modulation of magnetization for MR imaging. *Radiology*, 172:349–350.

[26] Chen, Q., V.M. Mai, A.A. Bankier, V.J. Napadow, R.J. Gilbert, and R.R. Edelman. 2001. Ultrafast MR grid-tagging sequence for assessment of local mechanical properties of the lungs. *Magnetic Resonance in Medicine*, 45:24–28.
[27] Napadow, V.J., V. Mai, A. Bankier, R.J. Gilbert, R. Edelman, and Q. Chen. 2001. Determination of regional pulmonary parenchymal strain during normal respiration using spin inversion tagged magnetization MRI. *Journal of Magnetic Resonance Imaging*, 13:467–474.
[28] Dougherty, L., Q. Chen, J. Asmuth, P. Madhav, V.M. Mai, and V.J. Napadow. 2002. Strain analysis of tagged MR lung images. In *Proceedings of the International Society for Magnetic Resonance in Medicine 2002*, p. 1993.
[29] Hu, S., E. Hoffman, and J. Reinhardt. 2001. Automatic lung segmentation for accurate quantitation of volumetric x-ray CT images. *IEEE Transactions on Medical Imaging*, 20(6):490–498.
[30] Dougherty, L., J.C. Asmuth, and W.B. Gefter. 2003. Alignment of CT lung volumes with an optical flow method. *Academic Radiology*, 10(3):249–254.
[31] Li, B., G.E. Christensen, E.A. Hoffman, G. McLennan, and J.M. Reinhardt. 2003. Establishing a normative atlas of the human lung: Intersubject warping and registration of volumetric CT images. *Academic Radiology*, 10:255–265.
[32] Mattes, D., D.R. Haynor, H. Vesselle, T.K. Lewellen, and W. Eubank. 2003. PET-CT image registration in the chest using free-form deformations. *IEEE Transactions on Medical Imaging*, 22(1):120–128.
[33] Rueckert, D., L.I. Sonoda, C. Hayes, D.L.G. Hill, M.O. Leach, and D.J. Hawkes. 1999. Nonrigid registration using free-form deformations: Application to breast MR images. *IEEE Transactions on Medical Imaging*, 18(8):712–721.
[34] Prêteux F., C. Petitjean, N. Rougon. 2004. Building and using a statistical 3D motion atlas for analyzing myocardial contraction in MRI. In *Proceedings SPIE Conference on Image Processing - SPIE International Symposium Medical Imaging '04, San Diego, CA*, volume 5370, 14–19 February 2004.
[35] Rohlfing, T., C.R. Maurer, Jr., W.G. O'Dell, and J. Zhong. 2004. Modeling liver motion and deformation during the respiratory cycle using intensity-based nonrigid registration of gated MR images. *Medical Physics*, 31:427–432.
[36] Perperidis, D., A. Rao, R. Mohiaddin, and D. Rueckert. 2003. Non-rigid spatio-temporal alignment of 4D cardiac MR images. In *Proceedings of the Second International Workshop on Biomedical Image Registration*, Gee, J.C., J.B.A. Maintz, and M.W. Vannier, eds. LNCS 2717, 191–200.
[37] Prêteux, F., N. Rougon, and C. Petitjean. 2003. Variational nonrigid image registration using exclusive *f*-information. In *Proceedings International Conference on Image Processing (ICIP'2003)*, 2:703–706, September 14–17, 2003, Barcelona, Spain.
[38] Studholme, C., D.L.G. Hill, and D.J. Hawkes. 1997. Automated three-dimensional registration of magnetic resonance and positron emission tomography brain images by multiresolution optimization of voxel similarity measures. *Medical Physics*, 24:25–35.
[39] Rohlfing, T., C.R. Maurer Jr., D. Bluemke, and M. Jacobs. 2003. Volume-preserving nonrigid registration of MR breast images using free-form deformation with an incompressibility constraint. *IEEE Transactions on Medical Imaging*, 22(6):730–741.
[40] Gee, J.C., T. Sundaram, I. Hasegawa, H. Uematsu, and H. Hatabu. 2003. Characterization of regional pulmonary mechanics from serial MRI data. *Academic Radiology*, 10:1147–1152.
[41] Reinhardt, J.M., K. Ding, K. Cao, G.E. Christensen, E.A. Hoffman, and S.V. Bodas. 2008. Registration-based estimates of local lung tissue expansion compared to xenon CT measures of specific ventilation. *Medical Image Analysis*, 12(6):752–763.
[42] Christensen, G.E., and H.J. Johnson. 2001. Consistent image registration. *IEEE Transactions on Medical Imaging*, 20(7):568–582.
[43] Christensen, G.E., J.H. Song, W. Lu, I. El Naqa, and D.A. Low. 2007. Tracking lung tissue motion and expansion/compression with inverse consistent image registration and spirometry. *Medical Physics*, 34(6):2155–2163.

[44] Li, B., G.E. Christensen, E.A. Hoffman, G. McLennan, and J.M. Reinhardt. 2008. Pulmonary CT image registration and warping for tracking tissue deformation during the respiratory cycle through 3D consistent image registration. *Medical Physics*, 35(12):5575–5583.
[45] Avants, B.B., C.L. Epstein, M. Grossman, and J.C. Gee. 2008. Symmetric diffeomorphic image registration with cross-correlation: Evaluating automated labeling of elderly and neurodegenerative brain. *Medical Image Analysis*, 12(1):26–41.
[46] Murphy, K., B. van Ginneken, J.M. Reinhardt, S. Kabus, K. Ding, X. Deng, and J.P.W. Pluim. 2010. In *Evaluation of Methods for Pulmonary Image Registration: The EMPIRE10 Study. Medical Image Analysis for the Clinic - A Grand Challenge*. van Ginneken, B. et al., eds., 11–22.
[47] Klein, A., J. Andersson, B.A. Ardekani, J. Ashburner, B. Avants, M.-C. Chiang, G.E. Christensen, L.D. Collins, J. Gee, P. Hellier, J.H. Song, M. Jenkinson, C. Lepage, D. Rueckert, P. Thompson, T. Vercauteren, R.P. Woods, J.J. Mann, and R.V. Parsey. 2009. Evaluation of 14 nonlinear deformation algorithms applied to human brain MRI registration. *NeuroImage*, 46(3):786–802.
[48] Rueckert, D. 2001. Medical Image Registration, chapter 13. *Non-Rigid Registration: Concepts, Algorithms and Applications*. Boca Raton, Florida: CRC Press LLC.
[49] Maintz, J.B., and M.A. Viergever. 1998. A survey of medical image registration. *Medical Image Analysis*, 2(1):1–36.
[50] D.L.G. Hill, P.G. Batchelor, M. Holden, and D.J. Hawkes, 2001. Medical image registration. *Physics in Medicine and Biology*, 46:R1–R45.
[51] Gee, J.C., and R.K. Bajcsy. 1999. Elastic matching: Continuum mechanical and probabilistic analysis. In *Brain Warping*, Toga, A.W., ed., 183–197. San Diego: Academic Press.
[52] Gee, J.C., and D.R. Haynor. 1999. Numerical methods for high-dimensional warps. In *Brain Warping*, Toga, A.W., ed., 101–113. San Diego: Academic Press.
[53] Bajcsy R., and C. Broit. 1982. Matching of deformed images. In *6th International Conference on Pattern Recognition*, 351–353.
[54] Miller, M.I., A. Trouve, and L. Younes. 2002. On the metrics and Euler–Lagrange equations of computational anatomy. *Annual Review of Biomedical Engineering*, 4:375–405.
[55] Sundaram Cook, T., N. Tustison, J. Biederer, R. Tetzlaff, and J. Gee. 2007. How do registration parameters affect quantitation of lung kinematics? *MICCAI'07 Proceedings of the 10th International Conference on Medical Image Computing and Computer-Assisted Intervention*, (Pt 1):817–824.
[56] Dupuis, P., U. Grenander, and M.I. Miller. 1998. Variational problems on flows of diffeomorphisms for image matching. *Quarterly of Applied Mathematics*, 3:587–600.
[57] Faisal Beg, M., M.I. Miller, A. Trouvé, and L. Younes. 2005. Computing large deformation metric mappings via geodesic flows of diffeomorphisms. *International Journal of Computer Vision*, 61(2):139–157.
[58] Avants B., C. Anderson, M. Grossman, and J.C. Gee, 2007. Spatiotemporal normalization for longitudinal analysis of gray matter atrophy in frontotemporal dementia. *MICCAI'07 Proceedings of the 10th International Conference on Medical Image Computing and Computer-Assisted Intervention*, (Pt 2):303–310.
[59] Horn, B., and B. Schunck. 1981. Determining optical flow. *Artificial Intelligence*, 17:185–283.
[60] Guerrero, T., K. Sanders, E. Castillo, Y. Zhang, L. Bidaut, T. Pan, and R. Komaki. 2006. Dynamic ventilation imaging from four-dimensional computed tomography. *Physics in Medicine and Biology*, 51(4):777–791.
[61] Guerrero, T., R. Castillo, K. Sanders, R. Price, R. Komaki, and D. Cody. 2006. Novel method to calculate pulmonary compliance images in rodents from computed tomography acquired at constant pressures. *Physics in Medicine and Biology*, 51(5):1101–1112.
[62] Guerrero, T., R. Castillo, J. Noyola-Martinez, M. Torres, X. Zhou, R. Guerra, D. Cody, R. Komaki, and E. Travis. Reduction of pulmonary compliance found with high-resolution computed tomography in irradiated mice. 2007. *International Journal of Radiation Oncology, Biology, Physics*, 67(3):879–887.
[63] Thirion, J.P. 1998. Image matching as a diffusion process: an analogy with Maxwell's demons. *Medical Image Analysis*, 2(3):243–260.

[64] Dawood, M., F. Buther, X. Jiang, and K.P Schafers. 2008. Respiratory motion correction in 3-D PET data with advanced optical flow algorithms. *IEEE Transactions on Medical Imaging*, 27(8):1164–1175.
[65] Castillo E., R. Castillo, Y. Zhang, and T. Guerrero. 2009. Compressible image registration for thoracic computed tomography images. *Journal of Medical and Biological Engineering*, 29(5):222–233.
[66] Viola, P.A., and W.M. Wells III. 1995. Alignment by maximization of mutual information. In *ICCV'95*, 16–23, Washington, DC.
[67] Maes, F., A. Collignon, D. Vandermeulen, G. Marchal, and P. Suetens. 1997. Multimodality image registration by maximization of mutual information. *IEEE Transactions on Medical Imaging*, 16(2):187–198.
[68] Pluim, J.P.W., J.B.A. Maintz, and M.A. Viergever. 2003. Mutual information based registration of medical images: A survey. *IEEE Transactions on Medical Imaging*, 22(8):986–1004.
[69] Thévenaz, P., and M. Unser. 2000. Optimization of mutual information for multiresolution image registration. *IEEE Transactions on Image Processing*, 9(12):2083–2099.
[70] Frangi, A.F., W.J. Niessen, K.L. Vincken, and M.A. Viergever. 1998. Multiscale vessel enhancement filtering. MICCAI?98 Proceedings of the International Conference on Medical Image Computing and Computer-Assisted Intervention, *Lecture Notes in Computer Science*, 1496/1998:130–137.
[71] Cao, K., K. Ding, G.E. Christensen, and J.M. Reinhardt. 2010. Tissue volume and vesselness measure preserving nonrigid registration of lung CT images. In *Proceedings of the SPIE Conference on Medical Imaging*, Dawant, B.M., and D.R. Haynor, eds., 7623:762309.
[72] Hughes, T.J.R. 1987. *The Finite Element Method: Linear Static and Dynamic Finite Element Analysis*. Saddle River, NJ: Prentice-Hall, Inc.
[73] National Library of Medicine. 2010. ITK, Insight Segmentation and Registration Toolkit. http://www.itk.org.
[74] Avants, B.B., N.J. Tustison, G. Song, and J.C. Gee. 2010. ANTs, Advanced Normalization Tools. http://www.picsl.upenn.edu/ANTS.
[75] Shewchuk, J. 1996. Triangle: Engineering a 2D Quality Mesh Generator and Delaunay Triangulator. In *1st Workshop on Applied Computational Geometry*, 124–133, Philadelphia, PA, May 1996.
[76] Kiryu, S., M. Takahashi, T.A. Sundaram, J.C. Gee, Y. Mori, H. Uematsu, T. Asakura, and H. Hatabu, 2003. Magnetic resonance lung deformation map of normal mice and transgenic mice model of sickle cell disease. In *Proceedings of the International Society for Magnetic Resonance in Medicine 2003*, page 1313. ISMRM.
[77] EMPIRE10. http://empire10.isi.uu.nl, 2010.
[78] Medical Image Analysis for the Clinic—A Grand Challenge. http://www.grand-challenge.org, 2010.
[79] Song, G., N. Tustison, B. Avants, and J.C. Gee. 2010. In *Lung CT Image Registration Using Diffeomorphic Transformation Models. Medical Image Analysis for the Clinic - A Grand Challenge*. van Ginneken, B. et al., 23–32.
[80] Betke, M., H. Hong, D. Thoams, C. Prince, and J. Ko. 2003. Landmark detection in the chest and registration of lung surfaces with an application to nodule registration. *Medical Image Analysis*, 7:265–281.
[81] Schnabel, J.A., C. Tanner, A.D. Castellano-Smith, A. Degenhard, M.O. Leach, D.R. Hose, D.L.G. Hill, and D.J. Hawkes. 2003. Validation of nonrigid image registration using finite-element methods: Application to breast MR images. *IEEE Transactions on Medical Imaging*, 22(2):238–247.
[82] Dougherty, L., J. Asmuth, A. Blom, L. Axel, and R. Kumar. 1999. Validation of an optical flow method for tag displacement estimation. *IEEE Transactions on Medical Imaging*, 18(4):359–363.
[83] Woods, R.P., S.T. Grafton, C.J. Holmes, S.R. Cherry, and J.C. Mazziotta. 1998. Automated image registration: I. General methods and intra-subject intra-modality validation. *Journal of Computer Assisted Tomography*, 22:141–154.
[84] Ledesma-Carbayo, M.J., P. Mahia-Casado, A. Santos, E. Perez-David, M.A. Garcia-Fernandez, and M. Desco. 2006. Cardiac motion analysis from ultrasound sequences using nonrigid registration: Validation against Doppler tissue velocity. *Ultrasound in Medicine & Biology*, 32(4):483–490.

[85] Sundaram T.A., and J.C. Gee. 2007. Quantitative comparison of registration-based lung motion estimates from whole-lung MR images and corresponding two-dimensional slices. In *Proceedings of the International Society for Magnetic Resonance in Medicine 15th Meeting*, 3039.

[86] Biederer, J., C. Plathow, M. Schoebinger, R. Tetzlaff, M. Puderbach, H. Bolte, J. Zaporozhan, H.P. Meinzer, M. Heller, and H.U. Kauczor. 2006. Reproducible simulation of respiratory motion in porcine lung explants. *Rofo*, 178(11):1067–1072.

[87] Avants, B.B., M. Grossman, and J.C. Gee. 2006. Symmetric diffeomorphic image registration: Evaluating automated labeling of elderly and neurodegenerative cortex and frontal lobe. In *Proceedings of the Workshop on Biomedical Image Registration* 2006, 50–57.

[88] Hermosillo, G., C. Chefd'Hotel, and O. Faugeras. 2002. A variational approach to multi-modal image matching. *International Journal of Computer Vision*, 50(3):329–343.

[89] Sundaram, T.A., and J.C. Gee. 2003. Biomechanical analysis of the lung: A feature-based approach using customized finite element meshes. In *Proceedings of the International Society for Magnetic Resonance in Medicine 11th Meeting*, 410.

7

Acquisition and Automated Analysis of Normal and Pathological Lungs in Small Animals Using Microcomputed Tomography

Xabier Artaechevarria, Mario Ceresa, Arrate Muñoz-Barrutia, and Carlos Ortiz-de-Solorzano

CONTENTS

7.1 Introduction

Studies based on animal models are very useful to characterize lung diseases because they represent an essential intermediate step between *in vitro* experiments and clinical studies on human subjects. A number of animal models exist for a wide variety of pulmonary diseases, including emphysema, fibrosis, asthma, and lung cancer [1–4]. Historically, histology and histomorphometry have been the techniques of choice to assess the evolution of a specific disease in a suitable animal model. The advent of noninvasive imaging techniques suitable for small animal imaging, such as positron emission microtomography and x-ray microcomputed tomography (micro-CT), has widened the range of methods available to monitor disease evolution, eliminating the need to sacrifice the animal [5].

In particular, micro-CT is the most convenient technique to image small animal models of lung disease because of the high difference in x-ray absorption between the lung tissue and the air within the lungs [6]. Many studies have shown that micro-CT can be used to monitor a variety of models of lung disease in mice and rats, such as different models of emphysema [7,8], lung cancer [9,10], and fibrosis [11,12]. Although most of these studies were preliminary—leaving ample room for further advances—it can be said that micro-CT is a reasonably mature technique for lung imaging in small animals.

One of the main challenges faced when acquiring micro-CT images of the lungs is how to minimize movement-related artifacts caused by respiratory motion. Multiple strategies have been proposed, with solutions ranging from the limitation of chest movements using nonelastic tape [9] to prospective and retrospective gating [13,14]. The main strategies will be discussed later in this chapter.

There are very few published studies on the automated analysis of micro-CT images of the lungs, probably because of the relatively short history of this technology and the small number of this type of scanners worldwide. Most published studies rely on manual or semiautomatic tools to quantify different aspects of the physiology and pathology of the lung. However, fully automated algorithms are of great interest because they considerably reduce operator time and increase reproducibility. Rather than performing a thorough review of all the works published, in this chapter, we aim at presenting the main challenges for both image acquisition and quantification, showing the different solutions that have been proposed to address them. The chapter begins with a section on image acquisition that briefly reviews the main factors to keep in mind when imaging the lungs, both on sacrificed or on living animals, i.e., *ex vivo* and *in vivo*, respectively. Next, we address the main applications of automated analysis of lungs in micro-CT images, including the quantification of lung parenchyma, airways, and pulmonary vasculature. Finally, we discuss the main achievements and look into future challenges.

7.2 Image Acquisition

7.2.1 Principles of Micro-CT

The basic principles of micro-CT have been explained elsewhere [15,16]. For image acquisition, the object under study is located between an x-ray source and a detector. In systems for small object imaging, the object rotates and radiographs or shadow images are acquired at different angles. In systems designed for living animals, a gantry containing the x-ray source and the detector rotates around the sample. In both cases, a three-dimensional volume is reconstructed by combining information from individual radiographs.

As in human CT scans, many parameters need to be set when defining a micro-CT imaging protocol; namely,

1. Source voltage (kVp). This parameter defines the maximum energy of the photons emitted by the x-ray source, i.e., a tube voltage of 80 kVp will create x-rays with a maximum of 80 keV. Lower energy rays allow for more contrast between different tissue types, but require longer exposure times. Because of the high x-ray absorption contrast between air and tissue, high voltage values can be used when imaging the lungs.
2. Tube current (μA). This parameter relates to the number of emitted x-rays. A high current implies lower noise but also increases the delivered dose.

3. Filtering. Metal filters, normally made of aluminum, are used to filter out low-energy rays, which contribute to beam-hardening artifacts. The parameter to choose is the thickness of the filter used.
4. Number of projections. The number of projections relates to the amount of information used in the tomographic reconstruction. Thus, the quality of the reconstruction improves with the number of projections, at the expense of a linear increase in dose and acquisition time.
5. Exposure time (ms). It is the time interval between the beginning and the end of the acquisition. The optimum value depends on the x-ray power and the detector sensitivity.
6. Magnification or voxel size. By modifying the source-to-object and the object-to-detector distances, different magnification levels can be achieved, which is reflected by the different voxel sizes.

The specific characteristics of the scanner, the desired image resolution and signal-to-noise ratio, the acceptable radiation dose (in *in vivo* studies), and the scan time are the key elements to be set when defining an imaging protocol.

Table 7.1 shows four different protocols that have been used in different laboratories to image mice lungs. Generally, high voltage values are used because the air in the lungs provides good contrast. Scanners equipped with flat panel detectors are considerably faster, at the expense of lower resolution.

7.2.2 *In Vivo* Imaging

One of the main advantages of micro-CT is that it allows longitudinal animal studies. Because the total dose of radiation delivered to animals during the time extent of an experiment can be considerable, control animals must be used to distinguish the effects caused by radiation from the experimental ones.

Another critical issue that has to be taken into account when using micro-CT to image the lungs is the presence of motion artifacts—because x-ray projections are acquired during

TABLE 7.1

A Summary of Protocols Used for *In Vivo* Micro-CT Mouse Chest Image Acquisition with Different Equipment in Different Research Groups

	Postnov et al. [7]	Artaechevarria et al. [17]	Froese et al. [18]	Ford et al. [8]
Scanner	Skyscan 1070	Siemens micro-CAT II	X-SPECt Gamma Medica-Ideas	GE Locus Ultra
Source voltage	80 kVp	80 kVp	80 kVp	80 kVp
Tube current	100 μA	500 μA	220 μA	50 mA
Filtering	25 μm Ti	0.5 mm Al	Not given	Not given
No. of projections	270 (4 frames/projection)	700	512	4160
Exposure time	8 s/frame	450 ms	Not given	Not given
Voxel size	35 μm	46 μm	490 μm	150 μm
Scanning time	20 min	30 min	120 s	50 s
Gating	No gating	Breath hold	No gating	Retrospective gating

different phases of the respiratory cycle—and how those artifacts affect the tomographic reconstruction. To minimize these motion artifacts, multiple strategies can be adopted:

1. Constraining chest movements. By limiting the movements of the chest, for instance, using nonelastic tape, blurring introduced by the respiratory motion can be reduced [9].
2. Prospective gating. This approach requires monitoring the respiratory cycle of the animal and synchronizing the acquisition of projections with a particular phase of the cycle. In this case, the animals can either be breathing freely or intubated, and the acquisition can be done during inspiration or expiration. Alternatively, breath holds at constant pressure can be forced during the acquisition of x-ray projections. In ref. [19], the three different options are compared, concluding that iso-pressure breath holds provide the best image quality at the expense of a longer acquisition time. Figure 7.1 illustrates the three prospective gating methods mentioned.
3. Retrospective gating. In this case, projections are acquired at any time of the respiratory phase, and the phase at which each projection is acquired is recorded during acquisition or inferred from image projections [20,21]. After acquisition, projections are sorted according to their phases, and different tomographic reconstructions are done for each phase. The advantage of this approach is that it provides information on the respiratory dynamics instead of just static (e.g., one phase) information [14].

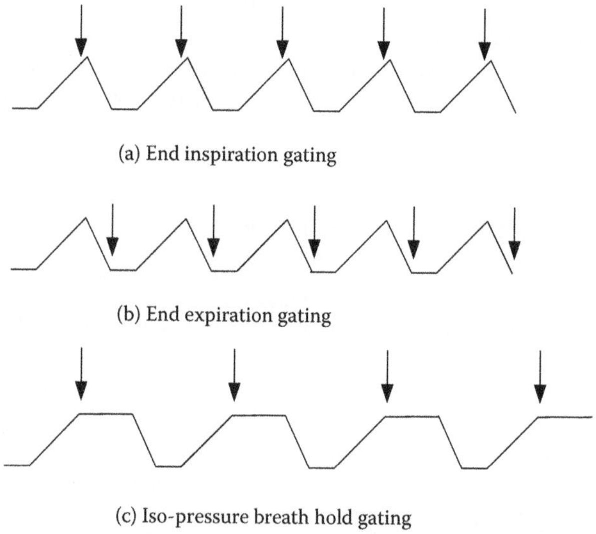

FIGURE 7.1
Existing options in prospective respiratory gating. The black arrows indicate the time point at which each projection acquisition starts. In options (a) and (b), mice can either be breathing freely or intubated. In option (c), intubation is required and the ventilator must be set to induce breath holds regularly. Generally, normal breathings are allowed between breath holds, and special recruitment maneuvers can also be performed.

7.2.3 *Ex Vivo* Imaging

Even when motion correction methods are used, the inherent movements of the animals (reflexes, cardiac-related movement, etc.) still affect the resolution of the images. That is why, if particularly small details of the murine lungs need to be examined, such as the alveoli (approximately 40 μm in diameter) or the alveolar membranes (less than 10 μm), the acquisition of the images must be done *ex vivo* [22]. The obvious drawback is that this cannot be done in longitudinal studies, but there are other advantages besides the increase in resolution associated with the lack of motion artifacts. Namely, the dose limitation problem is avoided, which is of great importance because the dose increases proportionally to the cube of image resolution [22]. Moreover, the pool of candidate contrast agents increase. For instance, blood pool contrast agents are typically used to highlight the pulmonary vasculature on dead animals. This is done by animal exsanguination, perfusion of the circulatory system with a fixative, and injection of an iodine or bromide-derived agent linked to a substance that polymerizes at room temperature inside the blood vessels [23]. This way, the lungs can be excised and imaged at high resolution with the micro-CT. This methodology is applied, for instance, to study the relationship between blood pressure and arterial diameter.

Ex vivo micro-CT imaging is also useful to study the small airways or alveolar microstructure. Because of the small size of the mice, most of the studies to date have used either pigs or rats [24,25]. Staining with radiopaque solutions is generally performed to increase tissue–air contrast. In Figure 7.2a, we can see a micro-CT slice of a murine lung fixed via vascular perfusion [26]. An initial scan of the lungs at a voxel size of 20–28 μm/voxel was used to precisely determine locations inside the lung at which high-resolution (1–2 μm/voxel) volumetric image data sets are acquired nondestructively [27], using a method for optically magnifying projection images from which the reconstructed data

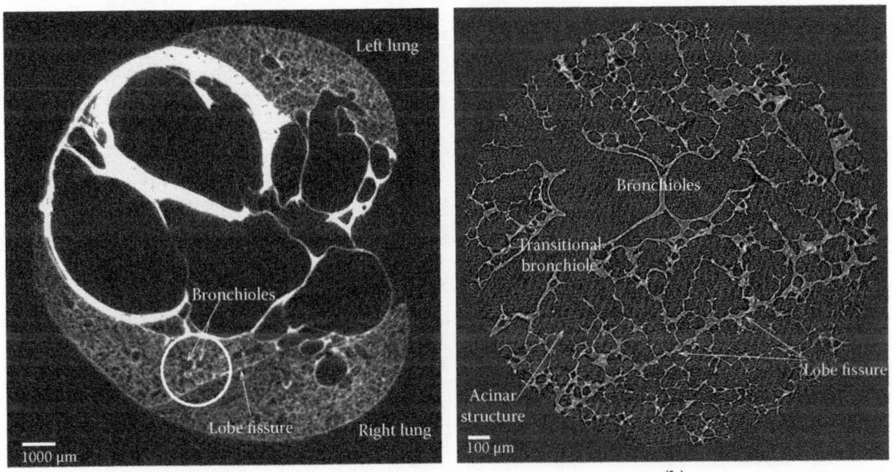

FIGURE 7.2
(a) Micro-CT slice of a murine lung fixed via vascular perfusion at a voxel size of 20–28 μm/voxel. (b) High-resolution (1–2 μm/voxel) image, obtained from local imaging of the intact lung, corresponding to the area encircled in (a). (Courtesy of Dragoş M. Vasilescu and Prof. Eric A. Hoffman, Iowa Comprehensive Lung Imaging Center, University of Iowa, Iowa City, IA.)

are calculated. The resulting volume scan contains multiple acini of high enough quality as to allow a semiautomatic segmentation separating the individual acini from the terminal bronchiole.

7.3 Image Segmentation and Analysis

7.3.1 Lung Parenchyma

7.3.1.1 Normal Lungs and Diseases with Decreased Lung Density

The appearance of the chest in micro-CT images can dramatically change depending on whether the lungs are healthy or pathological, as shown in Figure 7.3. This must be taken into account when approaching the task of automatically segmenting the lungs from the images.

Segmenting healthy mice lungs is a relatively easy task because of the large difference in x-ray absorption that exists between the lungs and the surrounding tissue. Semiautomatic methods are available both in free (e.g., ImageJ) or commercial software (e.g., Amira) [28]. See ref. [29] for other potentially useful programs. Specifically, seeded region-growing algorithms work well for segmenting the lungs in a few seconds. A typical user interface is shown in Figure 7.4. The same method can be applied, for instance, to segment the lungs in mice with emphysema, because the characteristic lung tissue loss of this disease results in even larger contrast.

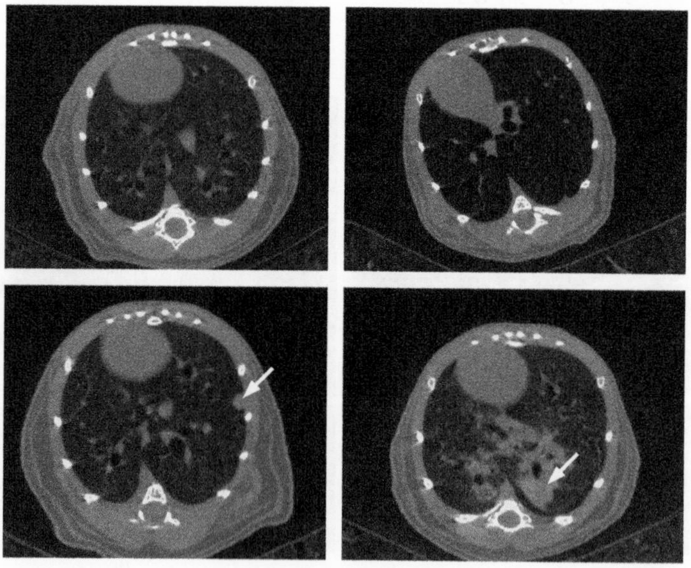

FIGURE 7.3
Sample transversal micro-CT slices of different mouse models of lung disease. A healthy control subject (top left) is displayed for comparison. The elastase-induced emphysema model (top right) results in significant loss of lung tissue; thus the lungs appear darker and more inflated than the healthy lungs. Urethane causes spherical nodules (bottom left, white arrow). Silica aspiration results in heavy inflammation in central areas of the lungs (bottom right, white arrow).

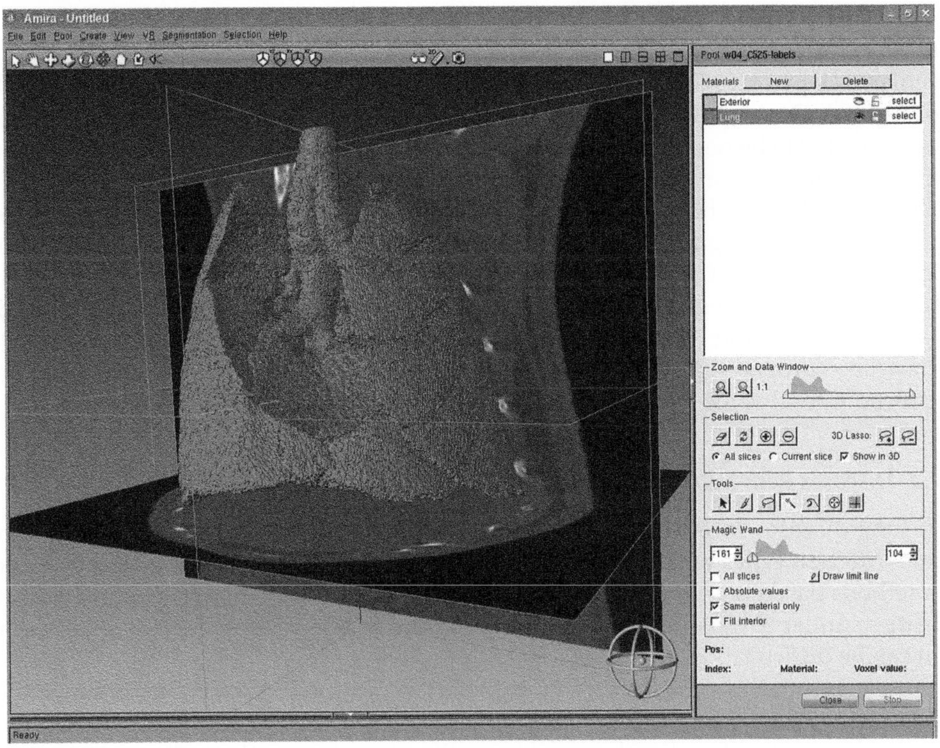

FIGURE 7.4
Screen capture of a seeded region-growing tool in a commercial software used to segment the lungs in a mouse chest micro-CT image. Similar applications can be found, both free and commercial.

Fully automatic segmentation methods can also be used. In particular, popular methods applied to human chest CT images can be translated without major modifications to micro-CT images of mice lungs. The method used regularly in our group is based on the work by Hu et al. [30] and is composed of the following steps:

1. Automatic thresholding. An image threshold is iteratively computed to separate air from tissue parenchyma.
2. Background removal. Air regions connected to the borders are removed by simple connected component analysis.
3. Small volume removal. Small air volumes, which are likely to correspond to air blobs in the digestive tract, are removed. In particular, connected air volumes that represent a volume of less than 4% of the largest volume are rejected.
4. Small vessel inclusion. Possible holes corresponding to vessels within the lung are filled using a reconstruction by erosion filtering.
5. Trachea extraction. The trachea and the main airways are deleted from the volume. To detect the trachea, a circular region is searched in the upper transversal slices of the segmented image. Then, region-growing is applied slice by slice, until a large increase in the grown area is detected, implying that the bronchi have merged with the lungs.

Regardless of the level of interaction required by the chosen segmentation method, the results are similar because of the simplicity of the task. Automatic methods are especially convenient when a large number of images need to be analyzed because user interaction is not needed. Once the lungs have been segmented, morphometric and intensity-based measurements can be performed. Total lung volume (TLV), mean lung intensity (MLI), and emphysema index (EI) are the most widely used measurements. It must be noted that the values obtained using these methods are highly dependent on the gating technique used: images acquired at inspiration will have larger TLV, lower MLI, and larger EI than those acquired at expiration. The optimum threshold used to calculate the EI (i.e., the percentage of lung volume below a given threshold) also depends on the acquisition method used. In humans, values around –920 HU are applied, but in mice and rats, values as high as –600 HU have been proposed [7,18,31]. In our hands, using iso-pressure breath hold gating, –900 HU proved a good value to discriminate healthy versus emphysematous lung volumes.

7.3.1.2 Diseases with Increased Lung Density

Many lung diseases result in increased lung density as seen in micro-CT images. These include different types of fibrosis, infections, or edema. In these cases, simple segmentation methods based on tissue contrast cannot be used because the affected areas display intensities similar to those of the surrounding tissue. In some cases, even manual segmentation can be difficult.

A simple approach to measure the lung volumes affected by bleomycin-induced lung fibrosis was used by Cavanaugh et al. [11]. They imaged the animals before inducing the damage to compute a baseline lung volume following Hu's method. Then, they scanned the animals and computed the air-containing—i.e., healthy—volume of the lungs, once the disease had developed. The disease-affected lung volume was computed by subtracting the healthy lung volume from the baseline volume. This approach does not require long operator times or advanced image segmentation algorithms because it assumes that the TLV is not affected by the disease. However, this assumption may not hold in some cases, especially if artificial ventilation is used, because lungs might get inflated very differently in the presence or absence of disease.

Ask et al. studied a model of fibrosis in rats [32]. They separated larger airways, normal, and fibrotic lung with a semi-automatic region-growing algorithm. We approached a similar segmentation task in a silicosis mouse model using a fully automated algorithm that combined atlas-based segmentation, threshold-based techniques, and level sets, achieving results comparable with manual segmentations [33]. Based on the manual or automatic segmentations, different measurements can be done. Apart from the previously mentioned TLV and MLI, the damaged lung volume or the damaged lung volume fraction can also be measured.

7.3.2 Airways

Multiple groups have looked at rodent airways using micro-CT. Airway remodeling in asthmatic mice was quantified by Lederlin et al. [34]. They intubated the animals, acquired projections at end expiration, and then manually selected 12 bronchi to perform measurements. A representative cross-section from each bronchus was extracted in which they manually delineated the bronchial lumen to measure its area and density. In particular, they defined the peribronchial density as the mean density within a ring-shaped region around the lumen with a radius equal to the lumen's radius.

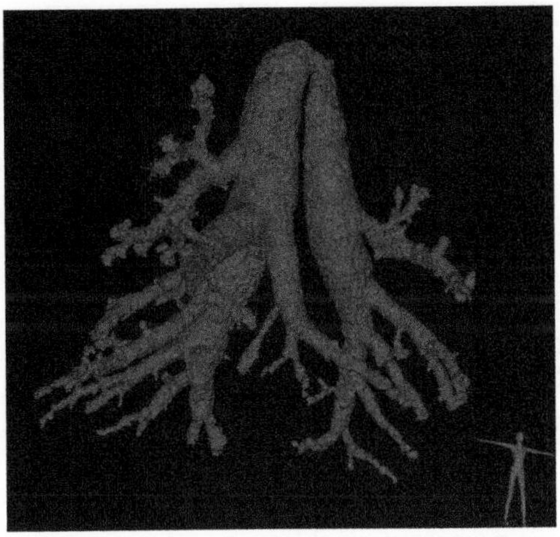

FIGURE 7.5
Image of airway segmentation of an *in vivo* mouse scan. The image was acquired with iso-pressure breath hold gating following the protocol in ref. [19], and segmentation was done with the method detailed in ref. [17]. Pulmonary Workstation (Vida Diagnostics, Iowa City, IA) was used for visualization. (Courtesy of Prof. Joseph M. Reinhardt, Iowa Comprehensive Lung Imaging Center, University of Iowa, Iowa City.)

Ideally, these measurements could be performed fully automatically on the whole bronchial tree. This requires automatic segmentation, labeling, and measurement. Automated segmentation and measurement methods have been reported [17,35], but there is still plenty of room for improvement in this area. Namely, the state-of-the-art methods perform very differently depending on image quality. The currently developed approaches locally adapt to the characteristics of the images to improve the segmentation. Most of the algorithms are based on a propagating front and are not able to segment the bronchi if they are interrupted by noise or disease.

The resolution and noise level of the images is of great importance, especially when smaller bronchi have to be measured. A sample airway segmentation of an *in vivo* specimen can be seen in Figure 7.5.

Ex vivo imaging can provide more insight into airway morphology and airway tree structure. For instance, Chaturvedi and Lee [36] built a silicon cast of mouse airways and developed a method to describe the airway tree geometry. The visualization of finer structures, such as acini, has also been done using synchrotron radiation [37].

7.3.3 Pulmonary Vasculature

Micro-CT is also an interesting tool to visualize the pulmonary arterial tree and study the relationship between pressure and diameter [22,38]. These studies are generally done *ex vivo*. In some initial works, the analysis was performed manually, but more automatic methods have been reported recently [39]. The basic steps are vasculature segmentation, tree generation and labeling, and vessel diameter measurement. Figure 7.6 contains a sample rendering of a mouse airway tree segmentation, along with the skeletonization of the pulmonary vessel tree. To perform these studies *in vivo*, blood contrast agents would be required, as well as very rapid acquisition times to minimize the blurring introduced by cardiac motion. These two methodological developments will open the door to longitudinal studies, which would be of particular interest in anti-hypertension drug testing.

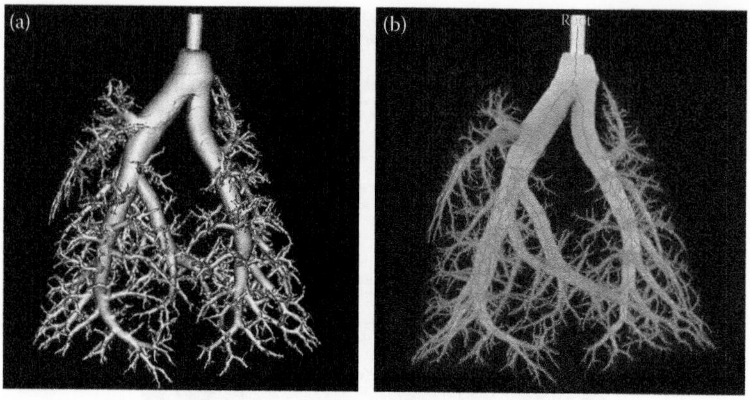

FIGURE 7.6
(a) Shaded surface rendering of a pulmonary vessel tree, imaged *ex vivo* with contrast. (b) Centerlines of the vessel tree, on top of a maximum intensity projection representation of the volume. (Courtesy of Dr. Robert Molthen, Pulmonary Physiology Group, Medical College of Wisconsin, Milwaukee, WI.)

7.3.3.1 Lung Function Imaging

Micro-CT image analysis can also be used to assess lung function by acquiring images at various respiratory phases or inflation levels, thus allowing dynamic respiratory studies. Basic segmentation and registration methods have been used to analyze these images. For instance, Guerrero et al. [40] imaged healthy rat and mouse lungs at different pressures. Then, using nonrigid registration, they were able to compute pulmonary compliance locally, observing significant regional variations. In a different study, Shofer et al. [41] studied mice affected by bleomycin-induced lung injury. They acquired images at both end-inspiration and -expiration and studied lung air recruitment. Another option is to use retrospective gating to separate projections obtained at different respiratory phases [20,21]. The advantage of this method is that animals can be breathing freely and it is likely that, in the near future, more sensitive detectors will allow for faster acquisition and sharper images.

7.4 Discussion

Despite being a very recently developed technology, many studies that report using micro-CT to investigate different aspects of lung pathophysiology in rodents have already been published. Most of these studies used either manual or semiautomatic segmentation and analysis tools, but a trend toward more automated methods has been observed in recent years. Micro-CT–based lung analysis is a rapidly developing area, and numerous advances can be expected in the next few years.

Regarding the scanner hardware and imaging protocols, the advent of new generation scanners is likely to reduce acquisition times, increase image resolution, and reduce radiation dose. Gating techniques will have to be adapted to obtain the maximum benefit from the new possibilities.

Combined single positron emission tomography (SPECT)/micro-CT and fluorescence tomography/micro-CT scanners, applied to study the lung, are also likely to gain importance because of the rich biological information they can provide. We will be able to answer questions relating to the presence and distribution of key molecules—using molecular imaging—while maintaining the morphological information (lung nodule size, emphysema extent, etc.) provided by the micro-CT.

On the image analysis side, several challenges remain for the future. For instance, emphysema analysis to date has been reduced to very simple measurements, such as MLI or EI. More advanced measurements, related to the localization and shape of emphysema lesions, will give valuable insight on dynamic aspects of the disease models.

There have only been preliminary studies using micro-CT for lung nodule assessment in small animal models. Automatic tools for nodule detection and/or volume measurement will be of interest to reduce interoperator variability and operator time. In principle, these algorithms would not need to be very different from those already in use in human CT scans.

To better study lung morphology, higher *in vivo* resolution would be required to allow the study of the temporal evolution of the disease in particular areas of the lung (small airways, alveoli, etc.) as well as the response to treatment. The large size of the data files in these images will probably impose a burden, which will have to be overcome by using more powerful hardware and efficient software. *In vivo* studies of the pulmonary vasculature will benefit from more rapid and higher resolution scanners, together with better contrast agents.

Most of the studies that use synchrotron radiation have not been mentioned in this chapter because of the limited access to this technology. However, it must be noted that very interesting results have been reported both *ex vivo* and *in vivo*, and technical advances in the direction of building compact synchrotron radiation sources might result in the widespread use of this technique [42,43].

Finally, a parallel could be traced between the use of small animals to test therapeutic compounds and the development of image analysis algorithms for micro-CT images. Animal studies are used to assess the potential benefits and side effects of disease treatments. Similarly, micro-CT could be used to develop and test new algorithms for image analysis, the great advantage being that results can be contrasted with histomorphometry. Then, these algorithms could be translated to the clinic with the required modifications. In other words, micro-CT could be used as a test bench for medical image analysis methods.

References

[1] Shapiro, S.D. 2000. Animal models for COPD. *Chest*, 117(5):223S–227S.

[2] Moore, B.B., and C.M. Hogaboam. 2008. Murine models of pulmonary fibrosis. *American Journal of Physiology - Lung Cellular and Molecular Physiology*, 294(2):L152–160.

[3] Meuwissen, R., and A. Berns. 2005. Mouse models for human lung cancer. *Genes & Development*, 19(6):643.

[4] Leong, K. and D. Huston. 2001. Understanding the pathogenesis of allergic asthma using mouse models. *Annals of Allergy, Asthma and Immunology*, 87(2):96–110.

[5] Baker, M. 2010. Whole-animal imaging: The whole picture. *Nature*, 463(7283):977–980.

[6] Johnson, K.A., C. Badea, L. Hedlund, and G.A. Johnson. 2007. Imaging techniques for small animal imaging models of pulmonary disease: Micro-CT. *Toxicologic Pathology*, 35(1):59–64.

[7] Postnov, A., K. Meurrens, H. Weiler, D. Van Dick, H. Xu, P. Terpstra, and N. De Clerck. 2005. *In vivo* assessment of emphysema in mice by high resolution X-ray microtomography. *Journal of Microscopy*, 220(1):70–75.

[8] Ford, N., E. Martin, J. Lewis, R. Veldhuizen, D. Holdsworth, and M. Drangova. 2009. Quantifying lung morphology with respiratory-gated micro-CT in a murine model of emphysema. *Physics in Medicine and Biology*, 54:2121–2130.

[9] De Clerck, N.M., K. Meurrens, H. Weiler, D. Van Dyck, G. Vanhoutte, P. Terpstra, and A.A. Postnov. 2004. High-resolution x-ray microtomography for the detection of lung tumors in living mice. *Neoplasia*, 6(4):374–379.

[10] Cody, D.D., C.L. Nelson, W.M. Bradley, M. Wislez, D. Juroske, R.E. Price, X. Zhou, B.N. Bekele, and J.M. Kurie. 2005. Murine lung tumor measurement using respiratory-gated micro-computed tomography. *Investigative Radiology*, 40(5):263–269.

[11] Cavanaugh, D., E.L. Travis, R.E. Price, G. Gladish, R.A. White, M. Wang, and D.D. Cody. 2006. Quantification of bleomycin-induced murine lung damage in vivo with micro-computed tomography. *Academic Radiology*, 13(12):1505–1512.

[12] Lee, H.J., J.M. Goo, N.R. Kim, M.A. Kim, D.H. Chung, K.-R. Son, H.-C. Kim, C.H. Lee, C.M. Park, E.J. Chun, and J.-G. Im. 2008. Semiquantitative measurement of murine bleomycin-induced lung fibrosis *in vivo* and postmortem conditions using microcomputed tomography: Correlation with pathologic scores—Initial results. *Investigative Radiology*, 43(6):453–460.

[13] Badea, C., L.W. Hedlund, and G.A. Johnson. 2004. Micro-CT with respiratory and cardiac gating. *Medical Physics*, 31(12):3324–3329.

[14] Ford, N.L., A.R. Wheatley, D.W. Holdsworth, and M. Drangova. 2007. Optimization of a retrospective technique for respiratory-gated high speed micro-CT of free-breathing rodents. *Physics in Medicine and Biology*, 52(19):5749–5769.

[15] Kalender, W. 2005. *Computed Tomography: Fundamentals, System Technology, Image Quality, Applications*. Erlangen, Germany: Publicis Corporate Publishing.

[16] Paulus, M., S. Gleason, S. Kennel, P. Hunsicker, and D. Johnson. 2000. High resolution X-ray computed tomography: An emerging tool for small animal cancer research. *Neoplasia*, 1–2:62–70.

[17] Artaechevarria, X., D. Perez-Martin, M. Ceresa, G. de Biurrun, D. Blanco, L.M. Montuenga, B. van Ginneken, C.O. de Solorzano, and A. Munoz-Barrutia. 2009. Airway segmentation and analysis for the study of mouse models of lung disease using micro-CT. *Physics in Medicine and Biology*, 54(22):7009–7024.

[18] Froese, A.R., K. Ask, R. Labiris, T. Farncombe, D. Warburton, M.D. Inman, J. Gauldie, and M. Kolb. 2007. Three-dimensional computed tomography imaging in an animal model of emphysema. *European Respiratory Journal*, 30(6):1082–1089.

[19] Namati, E., D. Chon, J. Thiesse, E.A. Hoffman, J. de Ryk, A. Ross, and G. McLennan. 2006. *In vivo* micro-CT lung imaging via a computer controlled intermittent iso-pressure breath hold (IIBH) technique. *Physics in Medicine and Biology*, 51(23):6061–6075.

[20] Hu, J., S. Haworth, R. Molthen, and C. Dawson. 2004. Dynamic small animal lung imaging via a postacquisition respiratory gating technique using micro-cone beam computed tomography. *Academic Radiology*, 11(9):961–970.

[21] Chavarrias, C., J. Vaquero, A. Sisniega, A. Rodriguez-Ruano, M. Soto- Montenegro, P. Garcia-Barreno, and M. Desco. 2008. Extraction of the respiratory signal from small-animal CT projections. *Physics in Medicine and Biology*, 53:4683–4695.

[22] Ritman, E.L. 2005. Micro-computed tomography of the lungs and pulmonary-vascular system. *Proceedings of the American Thoracic Society*, 2(6):477–480.

[23] Karau, K.L., R.H. Johnson, R.C. Molthen, A.H. Dhyani, S.T. Haworth, C.C. Hanger, D.L. Roerig, and C.A. Dawson. 2001. Microfocal X-ray CT imaging and pulmonary arterial distensibility in excised rat lungs. *American Journal of Physiology - Heart and Circulatory Physiology*, 281(3):H1447–1457.

[24] Litzlbauer, H.D., C. Neuhaeuser, A. Moell, S. Greschus, A. Breithecker, F.E. Franke, W. Kummer, and W.S. Rau. 2006. Three-dimensional imaging and morphometric analysis of alveolar tissue from microfocal X-ray computed tomography. *American Journal of Physiology - Lung Cellular and Molecular Physiology*, 291(3):L535–545.

[25] Sera, T., H. Fujioka, H. Yokota, A. Makinouchi, R. Himeno, R. Schroter, and K. Tanishita. 2003. Three-dimensional visualization and morphometry of small airways from microfocal X-ray computed tomography. *Journal of Biomechanics*, 36(11):1587–1594.
[26] Vasilescu, D.M., R. Ryan, T. Eggleston, M. Ochs, E.R. Weibel, and E.A. Hoffman. 2010. Fixation of murine lung with preservation of *in vivo* morphometry allowing assessment via micro-CT. *American Journal of Respiratory and Critical Care Medicine*, 181,A5513.
[27] Hoffman, E.A., D. Chon, D.M. Vasilescu, M. Cable, H. Chang, T. Fong, O Matthias, and E. Weibel. 2008. Non-destructive unbiased stereological sampling via multi-resolution micro x-ray CT for morphometric assessment of the mouse lung. *American Journal of Respiratory and Critical Care Medicine*, 177: A809.
[28] Jobse, B.N., J.R. Johnson, T.H. Farncombe, R. Labiris, T.D. Walker, S. Goncharova, and M. Jordana. 2009. Evaluation of allergic lung inflammation by computed tomography in a rat model *in vivo*. *European Respiratory Journal*, 33(6):1437–1447.
[29] Walter, T., D. Shattuck, R. Baldock, M. Bastin, A. Carpenter, S. Duce, J. Ellenberg, A. Fraser, N. Hamilton, S. Pieper, M.A. Ragan, J.E. Schneider, P. Tomancak, and J.K. Heriche. 2010. Visualization of image data from cells to organisms. *Nature Methods*, 7:S26–S41.
[30] Hu, S., E. Hoffman, and J. Reinhardt. 2001. Automatic lung segmentation for accurate quantitation of volumetric X-ray CT images. *IEEE Transactions on Medical Imaging*, 20(6):490–498.
[31] Kawakami, M., Y. Matsuo, K. Yoshiura, T. Nagase, and N. Yamashita. 2008. Sequential and quantitative analysis of a murine model of elastase-induced emphysema. *Biological & Pharmaceutical Bulletin*, 31(7):1434–1438.
[32] Ask, K., R. Labiris, L. Farkas, A. Moeller, A. Froese, T. Farncombe, G. McClelland, M. Inman, J. Gauldie, and M. Kolb. 2008. Comparison between conventional and "clinical" assessment of experimental lung fibrosis. *Journal of Translational Medicine*, 6(1):16.
[33] Artaechevarria, X., D. Perez-Martın, J. Reinhardt, A. Munoz-Barrutia, and C. Ortiz-de Solorzano. 2009. Automated quantitative analysis of a mouse model of chronic pulmonary inflammation using micro x-ray computed tomography. *International Conference on Medical Image Computing (MICCAI'09), Second International Workshop on Pulmonary Image Analysis.* September 20th–24th 2009, London, United Kingdom.
[34] Lederlin, M., A. Ozier, M. Montaudon, H. Begueret, O. Ousova, R. Marthan, P. Berger, and F. Laurent. 2010. Airway remodeling in a mouse asthma model assessed by *in vivo* respiratory-gated micro-computed tomography. *European Radiology*, 1:128–137.
[35] Shi, L., J. Thiesse, G. McLennan, E.A. Hoffman, and J.M. Reinhardt. 2007. Three-dimensional murine airway segmentation in micro-CT images. In *SPIE Medical Imaging 2007: Physiology, Function, and Structure from Medical Images*, 6511:651105.
[36] Chaturvedi A., and Z. Lee. 2005. Three-dimensional segmentation and skeletonization to build an airway tree data structure for small animals. *Physics in Medicine and Biology*, 50(7):1405–1419.
[37] Tsuda, A., N. Filipovic, D. Haberthur, R. Dickie, Y. Matsui, M. Stampanoni, and J.C. Schittny. 2008. Finite element 3D reconstruction of the pulmonary acinus imaged by synchrotron X-ray tomography. *Journal of Applied Physiology*, 105(3):964–976. [Online]. Available at: http://jap.physiology.org/cgi/content/abstract/105/3/964.
[38] Karau, K.L., R.C. Molthen, A. Dhyani, S.T. Haworth, C.C. Hanger, D.L. Roerig, R.H. Johnson, and C.A. Dawson. 2001. Pulmonary arterial morphometry from microfocal X-ray computed tomography. *American Journal of Physiology - Heart and Circulatory Physiology*, 281(6):H2747–2756.
[39] Shingrani, R., G. Krenz, and R. Molthen. 2010. Automation process for morphometric analysis of volumetric CT data from pulmonary vasculature in rats. *Computer Methods and Programs in Biomedicine*, 97:562–577.
[40] Guerrero, T., R. Castillo, K. Sanders, R. Price, R. Komaki, and D. Cody. 2006. Novel method to calculate pulmonary compliance images in rodents from computed tomography acquired at constant pressures, *Physics in Medicine and Biology*, 51:1101–1112.
[41] Shofer, S., C. Badea, Y. Qi, E. Potts, W.M. Foster, and G.A. Johnson. 2008. A micro-CT analysis of murine lung recruitment in bleomycin-induced lung injury. *Journal of Applied Physiology*, 105(2):669–677.

[42] Sera, T., K. Uesugi, R. Himeno, and N. Yagi. 2007. Small airway changes in healthy and ovalbumin-treated mice during quasi-static lung inflation. *Respiratory Physiology & Neurobiology*, 156(3):304–311.

[43] Sera, T., H. Yokota, K. Fujisaki, K. Fukasaku, H. Tachibana, K. Uesugi, N. Yagi, and R. Himeno. 2008. Development of high-resolution 4D in vivo-CT. *Physics in Medicine and Biology*, 53:4285–4301.

8

Airway Segmentation and Analysis from Computed Tomography

Benjamin Irving, Andrew Todd-Pokropek, and Paul Taylor

CONTENTS

8.1 Introduction

Airway segmentation from computed tomography (CT) is a useful tool for the detection and visualization of pathology in the chest region. Airway segmentation is generally the first step in the development of a computer-aided detection algorithm for the airways, and can be used to extract features that indicate pathology, such as airway deformation, stenosis, and abnormal wall thickness. Segmentation separates the region belonging to the airways from the surrounding tissue and therefore can also be used to improve visualization, for example, using virtual bronchoscopy, or it can be used to identify related structures, such as the lung lobes, using the position of the airways [1].

This chapter aims to provide an overview of the airway segmentation field and highlight some of the key methods that have been developed. The airway anatomy, imaging of the airways, and airway pathology are briefly discussed in this section. Section 8.2 outlines the general airway segmentation procedure as well as discussing some of the popular algorithms. A recent workshop has attempted to evaluate various airway segmentation methods, and the results are discussed in this chapter. After the airways have been segmented from the CT, there are various steps that can be taken to quantify their shape. Section 8.3 discusses a number of methods that are used to extract the medial line, determine branch points, label the branches anatomically, and analyze the shape of the branches. Shape analysis can take the form of simple measurements or statistical comparisons of a population.

8.1.1 Airway Anatomy

The thoracic cavity is enclosed by the ribs, sternum, and spine, and is divided into two pleural cavities with the mediastinum separating them. The pleural cavities contain the lungs, and the mediastinum includes the heart, trachea, and esophagus. The lungs are divided into separate lobes by fissures; the right lung is divided into three lobes and the left into two lobes. The heart occupies more space on the left side and so the right lung is larger than the left. The left lung does not have a middle lobe but instead has an extra attachment onto the upper lobe, the lingula [2].

The airway tree supplies oxygen to the lungs and forms a branching structure that begins at the trachea and terminates at the alveoli. The trachea bifurcates to form the left (LMB) and right main bronchi (RMB), which enter the lungs. These then divide into the left and right lobar bronchi. The airways continue to divide into smaller and smaller bronchi and bronchioles until they terminate at the alveoli where gaseous exchange takes place. A branch generally divides into two smaller bronchi but can divide into three bronchi. The main divisions of the airway are shown in Figure 8.1, in which the names of the bronchi describe the lung regions that are supplied [2]. The size of the bronchi decreases considerably with bifurcations. Seneterre et al. [3], studying five normal adults, found that the third to sixth generation bronchi decreased in diameter from 8 to 0.8 mm. Another study of 10 healthy adults provides more detailed results of airway diameter and airway wall thickness (see Table 8.1) [4]. The size of the airway affects visualization because of the resolution of CT scanners. This becomes even more problematic for pediatric patients because their bronchi are considerably smaller than in adults. The bronchi are surrounded by dense tissue that makes up the bronchial wall.

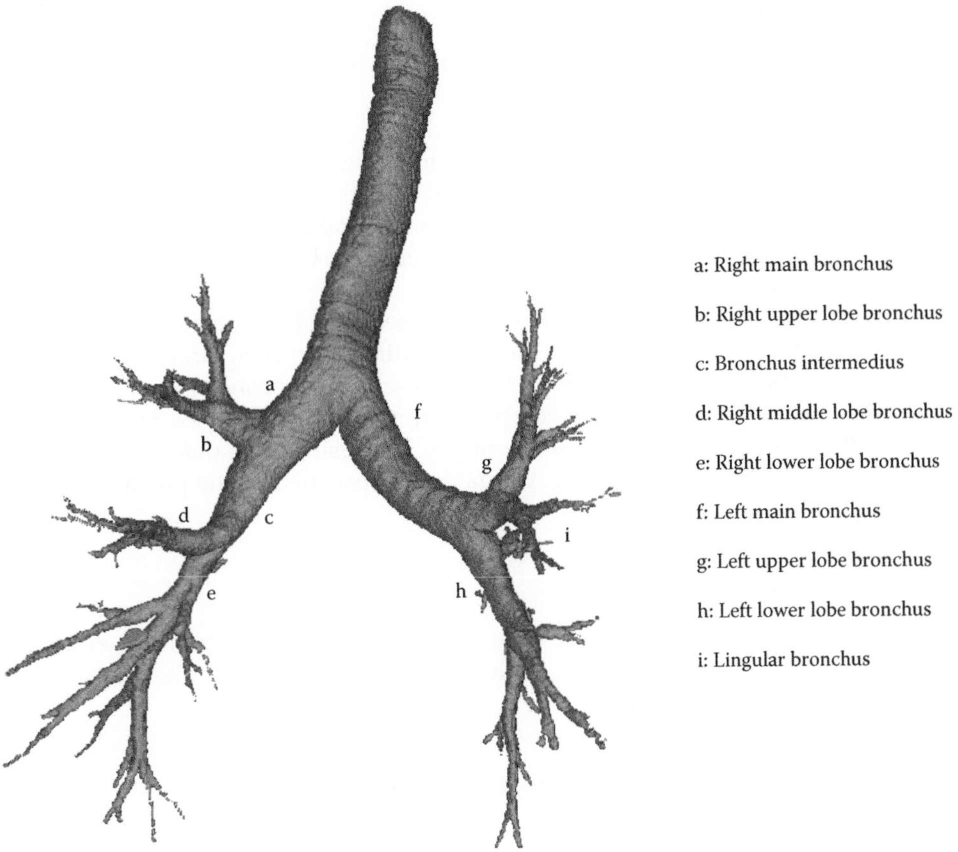

FIGURE 8.1
(See color insert.) An airway segmentation with labeled branches.

TABLE 8.1
Airway Lumen Diameter and Wall Thickness as a Function of Bronchi Generation with Standard Deviation

Generation	Wall Thickness (mm)	SD (mm)	Lumen Diameter (mm)	SD (mm)
0	1.4	0.1	18.5	1.6
1	1.3	0.1	13.9	1.4
2	1.3	0.0	10.4	0.9
3	1.3	0.1	6.8	0.8
4	1.2	0.1	5.0	0.6
5	1.0	0.1	3.6	0.5
6	1.0	0.1	2.8	0.4
7	0.9	0.1	2.5	0.4
8	0.9	0.1	2.4	0.5
9	0.9	0.1	2.4	0.4
10	0.9	0.1	2.4	0.4

Source: Montaudon, M., et al., *J. Anat.*, 211:579–588, 2007.

8.1.2 CT Imaging of the Airways

The larger airways can be separated from the surrounding tissue by a simple threshold [5] because the airways have a low Hounsfield unit (HU) value compared with the brighter airway walls.* However, with the smaller airways, segmentation is more difficult. The walls of the smaller airways can be less than 1 mm and are of a similar order of magnitude to the voxel size. Therefore, partial volume effects could lead to discontinuities in the airway wall and greater HU values for the lumen. Patient movement can also have a considerable effect. Movement artifacts can be limited by a breath hold but this is often not possible in pediatric patients.

CT is considered the "gold standard" for the detection of lymphadenopathy—a cause of airway compression [8]. However, when evaluating narrowing and compression, CT and tracheobronchoscopy are both used. In this case, tracheobronchoscopy is considered the gold standard for evaluating the compression, whereas CT is used to determine the cause [9]. Attempts are being made to use only CT by using edge detection and manual measurements of stenosis on the scan. Virtual bronchoscopy has the potential to replace conventional bronchoscopy [9].

8.1.3 Pathology of the Airways

Pathology can affect the airways directly or through compression from enlarged or deformed external structures, such as the lymph nodes or the heart. The most important examples of pathology of the airways are outlined in this section.

8.1.3.1 Airway Deformation and Pulmonary Tuberculosis

Tuberculosis still has a considerable effect on the quality of life in developing countries—particularly in Africa. The World Health Organization estimates that the annual number of new cases of tuberculosis in Africa is 343/100,000 population/year, higher than in any other region [10]. Tuberculosis is spread from an infected person by *Mycobacterium tuberculosis* in aerosol droplets, for example, by coughing, and a person is infected with tuberculosis by inhaling the bacterium. There are a number of stages in tuberculosis infection, and these stages depend on whether the patient has been previously exposed to tuberculosis [11–13].

Primary tuberculosis is the first infection of tuberculosis and is, therefore, the most common form affecting children. The mycobacterium is inhaled, travels through the airways, and enters the alveoli. Regions of consolidation then develop (a mass that is a combination of bacteria and inflammation from the body's immune response). The consolidation is known as the primary focus (or Ghon focus). At this point, the spread of tuberculosis is generally contained and the patient does not develop symptoms, but the patient will have developed antigens in response to the bacterium and will test positive to an antigen skin test [14].

If the infection is not contained at this point, it will spread via the lymphatic system and infect lymph nodes, typically the hilar, paratracheal, or mediastinal nodes. The combination of the Ghon focus and the infected lymph node is known as the Ghon complex.

* The Hounsfield unit for air is –1000 HU, water is 0 HU, bone is +1000 HU and blood +50 HU [6, 7].

Lymphadenopathy—the pathology of the lymph nodes—causes the lymph nodes to enlarge, which can lead to deformation of the airways [11,14].

Children have more malleable airways than adults and lymphadenopathy is a common feature of pulmonary tuberculosis in children. Therefore, airway compression from the lymph nodes is common, such as displacement of the trachea and bronchi, as well as complete or partial obstruction of the bronchi. Obstruction of the bronchi can, in turn, lead to a hyperinflated or collapsed lobe [11,14,15]. The lymph nodes can also erode through the pleura, causing pleural effusion, or erode into the bronchi [11,14,15]. Airway compression and displacement from lymphadenopathy is most common in young infants. The trachea, LMB, and RMB are generally affected by lymphadenopathy, which can compress the airways externally or erode into the airways [14,15]. This generally results in partial compression of the airways. If the airway is partially obstructed, then a "ball valve" effect may develop in which the vessel becomes blocked only on exhalation, leading to hyperinflation of the lung. If a bronchi is completely obstructed, then lobar collapse could occur. According to Goussard and Gie [15], deviation of the trachea can be an indication of paratracheal lymph gland compression, and if both main bronchi are narrowed, this could indicate enlarged subcarinal lymph nodes.

8.1.3.2 Congenital Cardiac Disease

Congenital cardiac disease can cause airway obstruction by compression from enlarged cardiovascular structures. Lee et al. [16] assessed 52 pediatric patients using bronchoscopy. Each patient had both airway and congenital cardiac disorders. They found that 67% of patients had external compression of the lower airways. Of these cases, 11% had compressions of the trachea, 15% had compressions of the RMB, and 67% had compressions of the LMB. When there was RMB involvement, 75% of these cases also had LMB involvement. The causes of the compression included dilation of the pulmonary arteries or aorta, or aortic arch abnormalities.

8.1.3.3 Lung Cancer

Lung cancer causes the largest number of cancer-related deaths in the world [17]. Tumors can invade a number of lung structures and can result in airway obstruction. Tumors in the trachea are rare but cause increasing airway obstruction and can be inoperable if detected too late. Bronchial tumors are much more common and lead to obstruction of the airways. As the disease progresses, this can lead to lobar collapse and consolidation in the lung lobe. Tumors can also affect the hilar, paratracheal, and mediastinal lymph nodes, causing enlargement and leading to airway obstruction and displacement [17,18].

8.1.3.4 Other Diseases of the Bronchi

Bronchiectasis is a pathological dilation of the bronchi and is caused by a chronic bacterial infection of the epithelium in the lung. The chronic infection causes tissue damage, which leads to bronchial dilation. Tuberculosis or bronchial obstruction (from a bronchial tumor) can lead to bronchiectasis. Chronic obstructive pulmonary disease can cause bronchial obstruction due to inflammation. Smoking is a common cause of chronic obstructive pulmonary disease [17]. This section provides a brief overview on the subject. Further information on respiratory diseases can be found in Brewis et al. [18].

8.2 Segmentation

Airway segmentation is a useful part of airway evaluation and allows automated assessment of the airways. Many algorithms have been used for segmenting the airways from a CT volume. These algorithms tend to have a number of steps in common but often use very different mathematical approaches in each step. An outline of the steps in a typical airway segmentation algorithm is shown in Figure 8.2. The first step defines a seed point. This point is usually at the start of the trachea and is either manually selected or found by identifying a cross-section of the trachea. The second step is often a filter used to enhance the airways. Once possible airways have been identified, then a region-growing method is used to select the connected airway region. Rules are often applied to restrict leakage into non-airway regions or remove leaks, either as part of the region-growing procedure or in the following step.

Algorithms often focus on one of these steps; some algorithms may ignore the airway enhancement stage and focus on rule-based methods to select the correct airways, whereas others may not apply any rule-based restrictions on the region-growing but use sophisticated airway enhancement. For example, Schlathölter et al. [19] apply topological restrictions to the region-growing (see Section 8.2.3), which could be considered a focus on step 4, whereas no step 2 airway enhancement is applied. Other methods, such as the morphology-based methods discussed in Section 8.2.6, could be considered to focus on step 2 by using morphological filtering to enhance the airways.

Algorithms also often distinguish between the main airways and smaller bronchi. The trachea and main bronchi are easier to extract than the smaller bronchi because of a well-defined wall and greater contrast between the lumen and the wall. Therefore, simple thresholding methods are often used to extract the larger airways. This saves processing time and allows the algorithm to be tailored more specifically to the smaller airways. The smaller airways are difficult to segment and this is the focus of airway segmentation algorithms.

Algorithms are often based on a variety of mathematical approaches and often combine or enhance previous methods. This section groups the algorithms according to what is

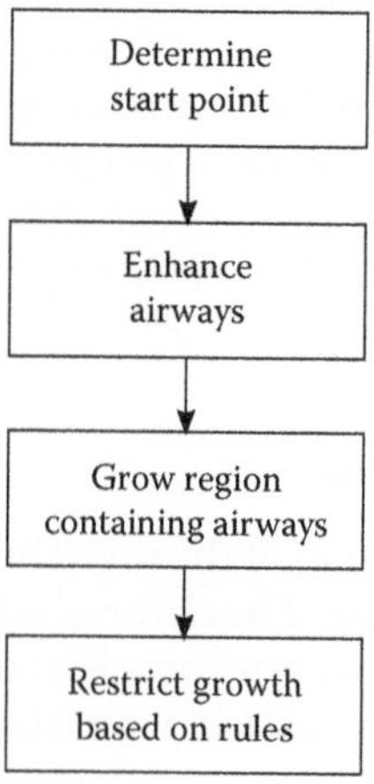

FIGURE 8.2
General stages of a segmentation approach.

perceived to be the main approach used in each. First, the initialization step is described. This is described separately because it is common to most methods. The following six sections describe various segmentation approaches: thresholding, thresholding with topological analysis, rule-based segmentation, fuzzy segmentation, and morphology-based segmentation. Methods are grouped as thresholding where only thresholding and region-growing are used. Methods that build on the basic thresholding methods but include analysis of the airway structure to enhance the airway segmentation are grouped as thresholding with topological analysis. Rule-based segmentation is defined here as the use of rules based on structures beyond the airway tree. Fuzzy segmentation and morphology are methods that apply these techniques. In each of these sections, the key algorithms are presented individually and links between the algorithms are discussed. Evaluation of these methods is difficult because of the varying image quality used in the different data sets. This section discusses a recent airway segmentation challenge, which was organized by Lo et al. [20], as part of the *Second International Workshop on Pulmonary Image Analysis*, in an attempt to evaluate various algorithms.

8.2.1 Initialization

Most methods require seed points to initialize the segmentation of the airways. These seed points are usually a point or points in the airway lumen but can include points in the airway wall [21]. These points are either selected manually by the user [5,7,19,22,23] or found automatically by detecting the cross-section of the trachea in a particular slice.

The trachea is air-filled and, therefore, has a lower HU value than the surrounding tissue. A suitable threshold is chosen that extracts the cross-section of the trachea but not the background. However, the threshold will also extract other objects within the same HU range (see Figure 8.3). Therefore, a number of features are used to select the trachea including the cross-sectional area, location, and circularity [21,24,25].

Mori et al. [25] used a threshold of –900 HU to extract the trachea from the first CT slice. Once potential tracheal cross-sections have been extracted, area and location are used to find the trachea. They use an upper and lower threshold for the area.

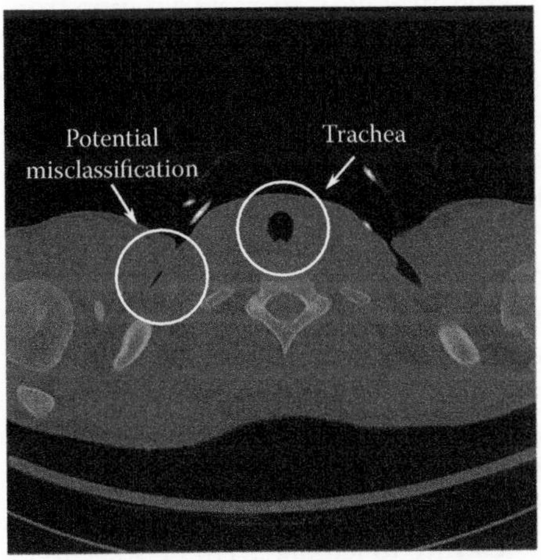

FIGURE 8.3
An axial slice from the CT volume showing the tracheal cross-section and an object of a similar shape that could be misclassified as the trachea.

$$t_{\text{area 1}} < C_{\text{area}} < t_{\text{area 2}} \tag{8.1}$$

where $t_{\text{area 1}}$ and $t_{\text{area 2}}$ are the lower and upper thresholds and were chosen to be 80 and 400 mm^2, respectively. The center of mass (CM) of the trachea candidate is restricted to an allowed region around the CM of the slice.

$$\text{CM} - P_{\text{mar}} < P_{\text{C}} < \text{CM} + P_{\text{mar}} \tag{8.2}$$

where P_{mar} is the allowed distance from the CM. $P_{\text{mar}} = \begin{matrix} 10 \text{ mm} \\ 10 \text{ mm} \end{matrix}$ was chosen [25].

If more than one candidate still exists, then the candidate with the largest area is used [25]. Tschirren et al. [21] used a similar method to that of Mori et al. [25] but also included a circularity measure and a connectivity requirement. A measure of circularity is compactness (C)

$$C = \frac{P^2}{A} \tag{8.3}$$

where P is the perimeter and A is the area of the region of interest (ROI), which is measured in terms of the number of voxels. Smaller compactness means that the region is more circular. Tschirren et al. [21] also found the trachea over a number of slices using these criteria, as well as requiring that the selected regions are connected three-dimensionally (3D).

As additional criteria, Tschirren et al. [21] used two seed points to improve the accuracy of trachea selection, and thus, by searching for a bright voxel near the lumen, a second seed point is found in the airway wall.

8.2.2 Thresholding

A simple way of segmenting the airways is to grow a region from a seed point using a fixed threshold [26]. The air-filled lung region has a very similar HU to the smaller bronchi, and partial volume effects and artifacts lead to discontinuities in the airway wall which, in turn, lead to segmentation leaks into the lungs. A fixed threshold method is often used as the basis of more advanced segmentation methods. Adaptive thresholding improves the performance of a thresholding method.

Mori et al. [27] outlined a method using an adaptive threshold and a region-growing method to segment the airways. The algorithm is automatically initiated in the trachea (see Section 8.2.1). A 3D painting algorithm is then applied to this initial seed point to segment the connected region. Adjacent voxels are connected to the current voxel, provided that the adjacent gray scale values are less than a predefined threshold (the gray scale threshold) and the difference in gray scale intensity between the current voxel and adjacent voxel is less than another threshold (the difference threshold).

The problem with this method is that for a chosen gray scale threshold, the lung region might be extracted as well, leading to leakage. This issue can be overcome by monitoring the volume of the segmented region because the segmented region increases dramatically if the algorithm leaks into the lungs. A minimum and maximum gray scale threshold is defined, in which the lung is never segmented and in which the lung is segmented in all cases. The algorithm is then run for increasingly large gray scale thresholds until the segmented volume exceeds a volume threshold, which means that lung regions have been included. The previous iteration is then used. The problem with algorithms such as these is that although the gray scale threshold is adjusted, it is adjusted globally. This makes the method less accurate for smaller airways [24], particularly those parallel to the slice plane [27].

8.2.3 Thresholding with Topological Analysis

A number of methods use a thresholding and region-growing approach, while including some airway topological analysis to reduce false branches.

8.2.3.1 Branch Validation Region-Growing

Schlathölter et al. [19] used a 3D region-growing method with a fixed threshold to segment the airways. Rules are applied to the bronchi to remove false branches. This method aims to address the problems associated with using a fixed threshold, in which leaks occur before all bronchi of interest have been segmented.

A fast-marching method with a fixed threshold is used as the 3D region-growing technique. The process of fast marching has a similar outcome to that of closed-space dilation (see Section 8.2.6), in which a wave front originating from the trachea moves through the bronchi and divides at branch points, as shown in Figure 8.4. The threshold is chosen to be greater than the gray scale of the lumen of all bronchi of interest. The centroid of the wave front is used to form the centerline, and the connectivity of the wave front is used to find branch points. However, because of the choice of threshold, segmentation leaking will generally occur.

Rules are applied to stop the segmentation from leaking. These rules are based on the shape of the airways and are found from an airway data set. Schlathölter et al. [19] found that children's bronchi tend to be smaller in diameter and length than the parent bronchi,

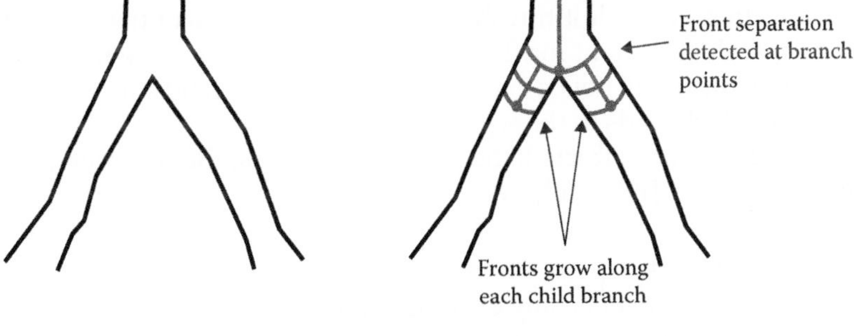

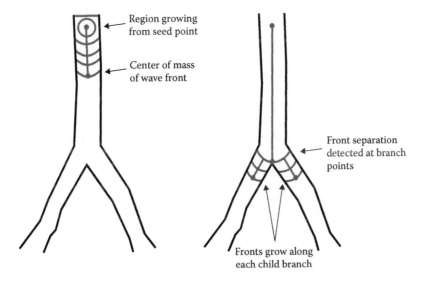

FIGURE 8.4
3D region-growing and centerline extraction using fast marching.

and that leaks tend to consist of a large number of small branches moving in all directions, which means that the density of the branches indicates a leak.

The fast-marching algorithm is manually seeded in the trachea. The algorithm segments the airways using a wave front and is used to segment each branch individually from the trachea (see Figure 8.4). The initial radius of the branch is compared with the radius as the wave front travels through the branch. If the radius increases above a defined threshold, then the connectivity of the wave front is used to determine if branching has taken place.

Once a branch has been segmented (i.e., a new branch point is found), then the branch is validated before the process continues. The radius of the branch is found by calculating the covariance matrix of the positions of the voxels in each wave front of the branch. The first and second eigenvalues are related to the radii of the elliptical wave front.

A branch is valid if

$$r_s < \beta r_{\min} \quad (8.4)$$

where $r_{\min}$ is the smallest radius from all ancestor branches, r_s is the radius of the branch, and β is chosen to be greater than 1 to allow some flexibility in this requirement.

A restriction on the number of branches connected to the branch of interest is also used to remove false branches and, therefore, limit leaking. The neighboring voxels to the surface of the branch are monitored to count the number of connected branches and a threshold is applied to the number of allowed branches.

A variation of the method by Schlathölter et al. [19] is used by Bülow et al. [22] for coronary artery extraction, and a modified version is used by van Ginneken et al. [28] for extraction of the airway. van Ginneken et al. [28] included additional features to the algorithm of Schlathölter et al. [19] to improve accuracy. Branch segments are evaluated instead of entire branches, a multithresholding approach is used instead of a fixed threshold, and additional rules are applied to classify segments correctly. Branch segments are evaluated instead of entire branches. A segment is defined as a region of the airways not having a length of more than five times its radius, and one or more segments make up a branch. This adaptation means that if leaking occurs in a branch, then a number of segments of the branch can still be accepted instead of the whole branch being removed.

van Ginneken et al. [28] applied a similar region-growing approach to that of Schlathölter et al. [19], but instead of a fixed threshold t, a multithresholding approach is used. Initially, $t_0 = -750$ HU is applied to extract each segment. If this threshold leads to a segment being rejected by the validation rules, then a series of thresholds, $t = t_0 + k\Delta t$ (where $k = 1, 2\ldots, 18$ and $\Delta t = -10$), are attempted. Multithresholding is used because of the difficulty in selecting a global gray scale threshold for this algorithm. If the gray scale threshold chosen is too low, then the segment will not be extracted, but if the threshold chosen is too high, then leaking can occur, which leads to the segment being rejected.

Once a segment has been extracted, the rules for accepting the segment also differ from those of Schlathölter et al. [19] as follows:

- $\beta = 1.5$ in Equation 8.4.
- The wave front cannot touch any existing segment.
- The angle between the child and the parent branch must be less than 100°.
- The average ratio of the radius of two consecutive fronts must not exceed 1.1.

The final rule checks for widening, within a segment, that is caused by leaking (in a similar way to that of Irving et al. [29]). Irving et al. [29] used closed-space dilation and compared the radius of the wave front with previous iterations of the wave front instead of previous branches (see Section 8.2.6). However, if this last rule is too restrictive, it can affect the correct segmentation of stenosed branches. Finally, after the completion of segmentation, end segments with lengths and volumes less than 3 mm and 25 mm^3, respectively, are removed in an attempt to remove small false branches that may occur.

8.2.3.2 Centerline-Based Improvement Technique

The algorithm by Swift et al. [5] shares similarities with the previous methods through the use of a region-growing technique with topological restrictions. Although the previous methods [19,22,28] use branch characteristics, Swift et al. [5] used the extracted centerline to improve the segmentation and cross-section evaluation to stop leaking. The focus is to extract a smooth centerline and surface for virtual bronchoscopy.

The algorithm can be divided into two stages: first, a fixed threshold and searching algorithm is used to extract a centerline and, second, this centerline is used along with thresholding and spline fitting to extract the airway surface. Swift et al. [5] defined a few concepts: viewing sites (w_l) are points along the centerline with a position and direction vector, branches (b_m) are defined as a contiguous set of viewing sites that represent one airway branch (i.e., are initiated and terminated by a branch point or end point), and a path (p_n) is defined as a set of connected branches in which the first and last viewing sites of the path are end points. There are 17 viewing sites, 11 branches, and 6 paths illustrated in Figure 8.5.

The algorithm proceeds as follows. In stage 1, start with initialization values w_0, b_0, and p_0, and add w_0 to the queue. Pick $w_l = \{s_l, d_l\}$ from the queue, which includes the 3D coordinates s_l and direction d_l of the centerline at that point. Find the orthogonal plane to d_l and project 16 rays radially outward on this plane from s_l. A gray scale threshold is defined to stop the ray. This threshold is defined so that a stopping point is found at the endoluminal

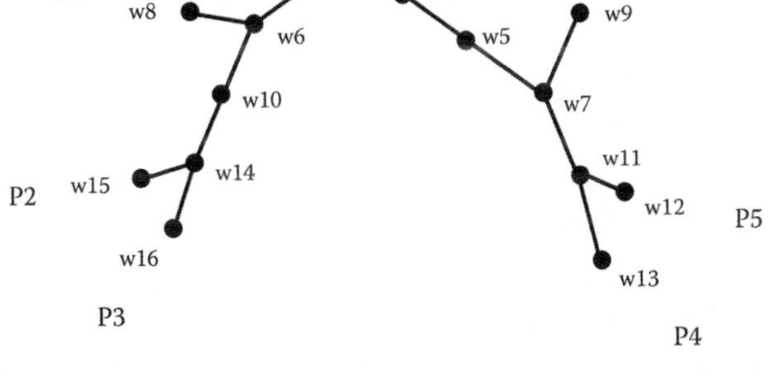

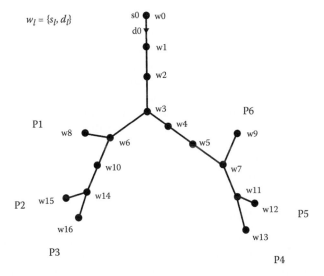

FIGURE 8.5
Extraction of the centerline in terms of w_l, b_m, and p_n.

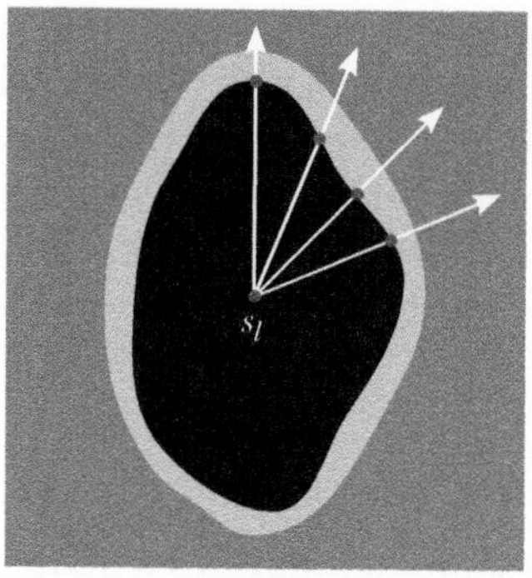

FIGURE 8.6
Intersection of rays projected from s_l with the airway wall.

wall, as shown in Figure 8.6. Once the lumen boundary has been found, the centroid of the boundary points is used to recalculate s_l. This procedure is calculated for every viewing site in the queue.

A new viewing site (w_{l+1}) is determined, as follows, and then added to the queue. A sphere is created with the center at s_l (the position of the current viewing site w_l) and a radius just greater than the airway radius (determined from the boundary points). The intersection of the air-filled lumen with the front sphere surface (represented by vertices) is used to determine s_{l+1}. s_{l+1} is calculated as the centroid of the vertices that intersect the lumen. d_l is calculated as the difference between s_{l+1} and s_l. Two or more separate intersections with the lumen mean that the airway has branched and two new viewing sites are generated. The new viewing sites are added to the queue, and the procedure is repeated until the queue is empty.

Criteria are defined to stop further viewing points from being selected in false branches. A branch is terminated if the radius of the lumen or the circularity is below the defined thresholds. Swift et al. [5] set the radius threshold to half the coarsest spatial resolution, which is generally the resolution in the z direction.

At this point, a segmentation could be created by generating a surface from the boundary points. However, the second stage refines the centerline and boundary points, and fits a generalized cylinder to the surface of each path in the airways. The viewing points (w_l) are used to compute a b-spline centerline and this improved centerline is used—in a similar way to the previous step—to recalculate boundary points. B-splines are used to generate contours from the boundary points and generalized cylinders are fitted to the paths. The generalized cylinders are then merged so that a smooth segmentation of all the branches is produced [5]. Therefore, although the topological structure is used by the previous methods to restrict false branches, Swift et al. [5] used the structure to improve the surface extraction of the branches.

8.2.4 Rule-Based Segmentation

As illustrated in the previous section, segmentation of the airways can be improved by including knowledge about the airway structure. Sonka et al. [7] used rules that apply airway size information and vessel relationships (Figure 8.7). Airways are identified using the rules and a confidence level is assigned to them.

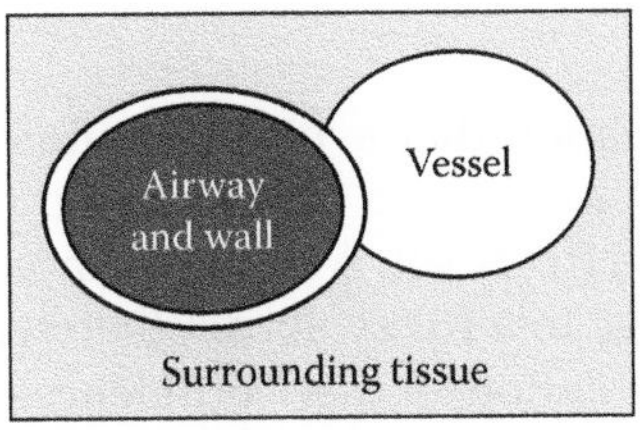

FIGURE 8.7
The relationship and gray scale of the airway, airway wall, and vessel.

The major airways are segmented by first using a gray scale threshold and 3D-seeded region-growing. A conservative threshold is used so that no leaking occurs and only the major airways are segmented. Large vessels are also segmented using a simple threshold [7].

To extract the smaller bronchi and pulmonary vessels, a morphological gray scale filtering method is used to enhance the airways in each slice (morphological filtering–based segmentation methods are discussed in Section 8.2.6). Sonka et al. [7] used a top hat transformation. The top hat transform takes the difference between a gray scale closing and the original image [30]. Top hat filtering is used to enhance the airways and vessels in which the airways are dark and the vessels are bright, and the background tends to have an intermediate gray scale value. The extracted smaller vessels and airways are then combined with the larger segmented airways and vessels.

An edge-based segmentation method is used to divide the image into regions and each region is represented by a single gray scale value.

Rules are used to label the regions as candidate airways, vessels, or background. Additional rules are then used to assign a confidence, of being a vessel or an airway, to each of the candidate regions:

- Rule 1: Labels for background, vessel, big vessel, and airway are assigned to the regions according to the values defining the maximum and minimum sizes of vessels and airways, and gray scale value of the region.

The second pass assigns a confidence to the vessels.

- Rule 2: A vessel confidence of 1 is assigned to the vessel if it is the brightest of all neighbors. A vessel confidence of 0.5 is assigned if it is not the brightest.

The third pass assigns a confidence to the airways.

- Rule 3: Airway confidence is assigned based on the adjacency of a vessel and confidence that the object is a vessel, the darkness of the airway relative to neighbors, and the surrounding airway wall.

A confidence threshold is specified, in which airway regions with a greater confidence are included in the airway tree. Three output regions were produced, the 3D-connected region forming part of the airways, the 3D-connected region and other disconnected regions also classified as airways, and a third region from any shape identified as airways in two-dimensional slices. The results of the first region had low sensitivity compared with the third region. However, the third method identified incorrect airways.

8.2.5 Fuzzy Segmentation

Fuzzy set theory is a representation that avoids definite classification of objects; instead fuzzy rules are used to assign a measure of belonging. Fuzzy rules are used to assign objects to fuzzy subsets within a fuzzy set. A fuzzy membership function is used to assign a measure that an object belongs to a fuzzy subset (between 0 and 1) [23, 30]. The advantage of this method for segmentation is that confidences are assigned to each voxel or region of being part of the airway.

8.2.5.1 Fuzzy Region Classification

Park et al. [23] modified the rule-based method, developed by Sonka et al. [7] (discussed in Section 8.2.4), and included a fuzzy approach to increase the accuracy of airway branch classification. The rule-based approach by Sonka et al. [7] was used to extract candidate airway, candidate vessel, and background regions.

In their rule-based approach, Sonka et al. [7] used rules based on the gray scale of the airways relative to neighboring regions, the confidence of adjacent vessels, and the completeness of the airway wall, to assign a confidence to the airway regions. Park et al. [23] used similar features of the airway except with fuzzy labeling. Fuzzy labeling and then, finally, a defuzzification step are used to assign a confidence to each region. The fuzzy membership functions were designed using a set of labeled CT volumes.

The features used were brightness, the 8-bit gray scale of the airway or vessel; adjacency, the maximum gray scale of the adjacent region; and the degree of wall existence,

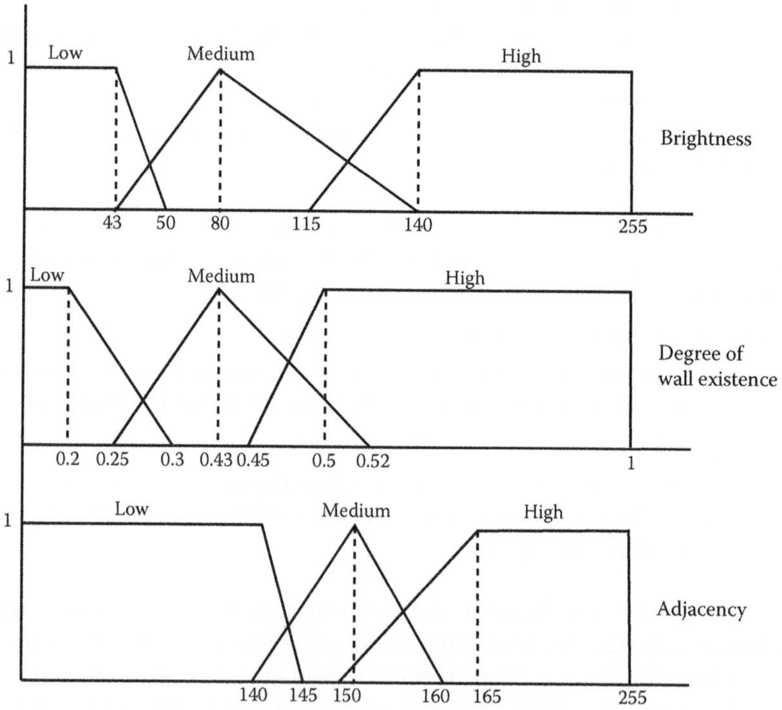

FIGURE 8.8
Fuzzy membership functions for each fuzzy set based on the airway features. (From Park, W., et al., *IEEE Trans. Med. Imaging*, 17:489–497, 1998. Copyright 1999 IEEE. With permission.)

the proportion of the wall that is detected by the bright–dark–bright sequence of a set of rays through the region. These rules were chosen because, first, the airways had low gray scale values; second, the airways were found close to vessels that are bright; and third, the airways have a wall. These features are used to create fuzzy membership functions. Figure 8.8 shows the fuzzy membership functions used by Park et al. [23], where the fuzzy sets of brightness, wall existence, and adjacency are used with subsets of "low," "medium," and "high."

The algorithm proceeds as follows. Using the method by Sonka et al. [7], regions representing possible airway segments are extracted. The region is assigned to fuzzy subsets of "low," "medium," and "high" using the fuzzy membership functions in Figure 8.8 based on its brightness, wall existence, and adjacency features. Next, fuzzy rules (as shown in Figure 8.9) determine the confidence level for each region being an airway, based on the true values obtained using the fuzzy membership functions.

A numerical value is then extracted using defuzzification. The results of this method were compared to that of Sonka et al. [7] on the same data set of 269 airways. The improvement in sensitivity was not statistically significant but the specificity was considerably improved [23].

Adjacency = High

Brightness \ Degree of wall existence	Low	Med	High
Low	Med	High	Very High
Med	Low	Med	High
High	Very Low	Low	Med

Adjacency = Med

Brightness \ Degree of wall existence	Low	Med	High
Low	Low	Med	High
Med	Very Low	Low	Med
High	Very Low	Very Low	Low

Adjacency = Low

Brightness \ Degree of wall existence	Low	Med	High
Low	Very Low	Low	Med
Med	Very Low	Very Low	Low
High	Very Low	Very Low	Very Low

FIGURE 8.9
Fuzzy rules used to assign airway confidence. (From Park, W., et al., *IEEE Trans. Med. Imaging*, 17:489–497, 1998. Copyright 1999 IEEE. With permission.)

8.2.5.2 Fuzzy Connectivity

Tschirren et al. [21] applied fuzzy theory very differently to Park et al. [23]. Tschirren et al. [21] used a fuzzy connectivity approach. Fuzzy connectivity is used in segmentation to assign a fuzzy value based on the similarity between voxels. In this method, fuzzy connectivity analysis is used in the ROI to cluster the voxels in the image into airway lumen (foreground) and the airway wall (background) by calculating the affinity of each voxel to the background and the foreground. The airway tree is then skeletonized and this skeleton is used to guide more accurate wall measurements.

The segmentation is initialized by a seed point in the airway lumen and a seed point in the airway wall for each ROI (see Section 8.2.1). A cylindrical ROI of between 25 and 50 voxels in length is defined as the search area for voxel classification. Affinity functions for the foreground and background are applied to each voxel in the ROI. The affinity is calculated as a function for 18-connected neighbors to the seed voxel. The affinity of nonadjacent voxels is calculated by analyzing each possible path between the seed voxel and the voxel of interest. Each path is represented by the voxel in the path with the weakest affinity. The affinity of a voxel is taken to be the affinity of the strongest path [21].

The affinity function for foreground objects depends only on the gray scale (i) of the voxel:

$$(i) = \exp \; -\frac{(i - {}_0)^2}{2\sigma^2} \tag{8.5}$$

where Tschirren et al. [21] determined the constants $\mu_0 = 0$ and $\sigma = 100$ experimentally. Gray scale values of 0 have the highest foreground affinity and, therefore, the highest probability of being part of the airway. A gray scale value of 0 has the highest probability because Tschirren et al. [21] converted the image to 8 bit where –1000 HU corresponds to 0 on the new scale. This 8-bit resampling is designed to preserve gray scale without loss in the range of the airway gray scale values of between –1000 and –800 HU.

The affinity function for a voxel belonging to the background (i.e., the airway wall) is based on differences between the gray scale of the background seed voxel and the current voxel, instead of just the gray scale of the voxel of interest.

$$(i_1, i_2) = \exp \; -\frac{[(i_1 - i_2)/2 - {}_0]^2}{2\sigma^2} \tag{8.6}$$

This is because partial volume effects could have a considerable effect on the gray scale variation of the wall. A directional restriction is also added to the the affinity to reduce leaks.

Each voxel in the ROI is classified as background or foreground, depending on which affinity is greater. Once the voxels are classified, a queue-based region-growing algorithm is used to segment the surface of the airways. The algorithm grows along foreground voxels that are 6-connected to background voxels and the airway skeleton is extracted from the segmentation. The segmentation and skeleton are used to initialize new ROIs that are, in turn, segmented using fuzzy connectivity. New foreground and background seed points are required for each new ROI. The foreground seed point is chosen as the first centerline point in the new ROI that was generated from the previous ROI and a seed point in the lumen is found by searching for bright gray scale voxels adjacent to the airway lumen. Following this fuzzy logic–based segmentation, additional steps were taken by Tschirren et al. [21] to take more accurate measurements of the airway walls by extracting slices perpendicular to the centerline of the airways.

8.2.6 Morphology

Morphology-based methods are commonly used to enhance smaller airways. The top hat transform used by Sonka et al. [7] (discussed in Section 8.2.4) is an example of a morphological filtering method.

Two variations of morphological filtering, used to extract the airways, are discussed in this chapter. The first method uses gray scale closing and reconstruction with region-growing [24,29,31,32]. The second method uses connection cost between voxels and energy minimization region-growing [33,34].

8.2.6.1 *Morphological Reconstruction*

The first method discussed here uses morphological reconstruction and region-growing, and a number of algorithms share these key elements [24,29,31,32]. The larger airways are generally segmented using thresholding, and the smaller airways are enhanced using gray scale morphological reconstruction. A threshold is then applied to the difference between the original image and the reconstructed image which leaves a binary image of possible airway locations. A seeded region-growing technique is then applied to extract the connected region representing the airways.

The methods used to segment the larger bronchi are similar to those discussed in Section 8.2.2. Aykac et al. [24] segmented the trachea using an automatically detected seed point (see Section 8.2.1). Each slice is then thresholded and segmented using the segmented region from the slice above as seed points. This method is only used to find the first bifurcation of the airways and is repeated until the segmentation spreads into the lungs, which is monitored by the size of the region on the current slice. Kiraly et al. [31] used a similar method with an adaptive region-growing. As shown in Figure 8.10, an initial threshold

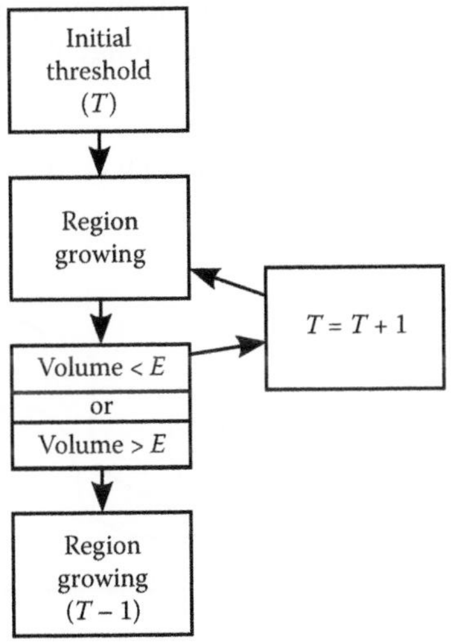

FIGURE 8.10
The adaptive region-growing method used by Kiraly et al. [31] for extraction of the main bronchi, where T is the selected gray scale threshold and E is the explosion parameter.

(T) is chosen and region-growing is applied using that threshold. The volume of the segmented area is used as a measure of leakage. If the volume is lower than an explosion parameter (E), then the threshold is increased until the volume exceeds E. The region segmented using T from the previous step is then used. Gray scale thresholding is only used to segment larger branches because if smaller branches are included in the segmentation, the similar gray scale intensities of the small bronchi and lungs, along with discontinuities caused by artifacts and partial volume effects, will cause leaking into the lungs.

Once the larger airways have been extracted, then gray scale morphological reconstruction is used to enhance the smaller airways. Gray scale reconstruction can be used to enhance gray scale peaks (or valleys) and is applied to each CT slice to enhance the regional minima and, therefore, extract the smaller airways [24,29,31,32].

Gray scale reconstruction is an extension of binary reconstruction and so it is useful to discuss binary reconstruction first. Binary reconstruction is the application of successive dilations within objects of a binary image as shown below:

$$\rho_B(X) = \lim_{n \to +\infty} \delta_B^{(n)}(X) \tag{8.7}$$

where $\delta_B^{(1)}(X) = (X \quad K) \cap B$ and $\delta_B^{(n)}(X) = \delta_B \circ \delta_B \circ \ldots \delta_B(X)$ n times.

The (X) markers are seed points and are a subset of the mask (B). Therefore, X is where the dilation starts in the object [35,36]. K is a structuring element (SE) used in the dilation.

A similar definition is used for gray scale reconstruction [35,36]; a marker and mask image are used in which every voxel in the marker image has a voxel intensity less than or equal to the intensity of the corresponding voxel in the mask image. The marker and mask images are then thresholded over a range of thresholds and binary reconstruction is performed on each threshold. The maximum voxel intensities of the binary reconstructed images form the gray scale reconstructed image [35,36]. With a good choice of a marker image, this method creates an image with the peaks removed (see Figure 8.11). This can then be subtracted from the original image to enhance the peaks.

For the gray scale reconstruction to select the airway regions, a suitable marker image needs to be chosen. A gray scale closing of the image can be used as a suitable marker [24,29,31] as shown below:

$$X = B \bullet D = (B \oplus D) \ominus D \tag{8.8}$$

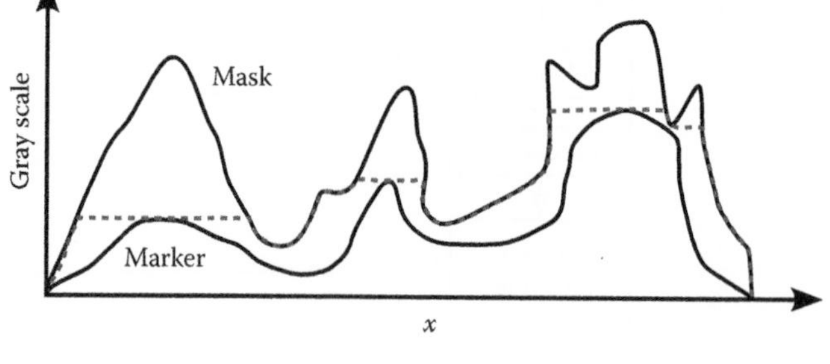

FIGURE 8.11
An illustration of gray scale reconstruction in one dimension, showing the mask and marker gray scale values, in which the dashed line is the gray scale reconstructed image.

where X is the marker image, B is the original image (used in reconstruction as the mask image), and D is the SE. D will control the shape of the marker image and, therefore, what size airways are enhanced in the reconstruction. Note that gray scale closing will create an image that always has a greater or equal gray scale than the original image. Therefore, reconstruction is applied using the inverted original image and the inverted gray scale closed image. Figure 8.12 shows gray scale closing and reconstruction on a CT slice containing the RMB and LMB.

The gray scale morphological reconstruction is applied to each CT slice using a range of marker images created from gray scale closing the original image with a range of SEs. These SEs are chosen to be of similar size to the cross-section of the airways present in the slice in order to enhance them. A difference image between the original image and each reconstructed image is calculated which results in an image of the airways with the background subtracted. A threshold is then applied to extract the airways and the union of the resulting binary images used as airway candidates.

The choice of SE varies among the algorithms discussed. Pisupati et al. [32] fitted ellipses to the segmented airways of the previous slices. The longest short axis of the ellipses is used as the diameter for the largest circular SE, which will be applied to the current slice. Multiple SEs with decreasing diameters are used to enhance airways of various sizes.

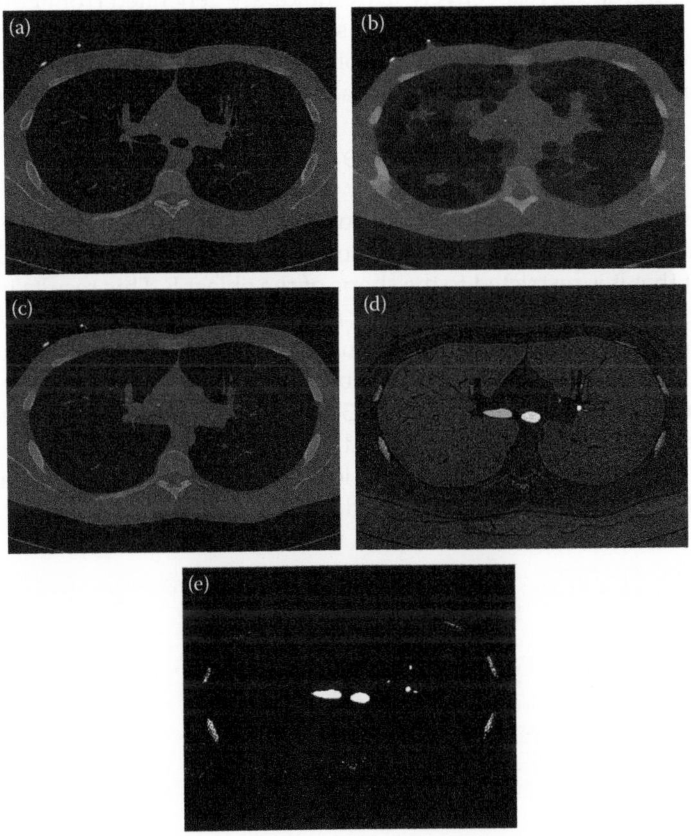

FIGURE 8.12
Gray scale closing and reconstruction. (a) Original image. (b) Gray scale closed image. (c) Reconstructed image. (d) Subtracted image. (e) Threshold.

Aykac et al. [24], Kiraly et al. [31], and Irving et al. [29] used a binary 4-connected SE (B_4) as the smallest SE. B_4 is then dilated using itself to create a range of SEs that will extract different airway sizes (i.e., $nB_4 = B_4 \oplus B_4 \oplus \ldots \oplus B_4$ n times). Aykac et al. [24] used a range of SEs from $n = 1$ to $n = 15$. Kiraly et al. [31] used SEs up to $n = 18$ for large airways and up to $n = 3$ for small airways. A threshold of 0.2 of the difference between the minimum gray scale (g_{min}) and the maximum gray scale value in the current slice is used to threshold the difference image for airways below the carina [24,31].

$$T_{morph} = \beta(g_{max} - g_{min}) + g_{min} \tag{8.9}$$

where $\beta = 0.2$ and T_{morph} is the threshold applied to the difference image.

Aykac et al. [24], Kiraly et al. [31], and Pisupati et al. [32] applied the filtering to each axial slice. Irving et al. [29] extended this method and applied filtering in 3D, i.e., to each slice in the axial, coronal, and sagittal planes. This is because if only one direction is used, the detection of branches parallel to the slice is poor. The axial plane is filtered last to enhance the segmentation of bifurcation areas that can appear large and noncircular from the axial plane if branches are parallel to the slice. Smaller branches parallel to the axial plane are, therefore, segmented first, leaving circular bifurcation areas that are then detected with the axial filter (see Figure 8.13). SEs up to $n = 12$, $n = 6$, and $n = 6$ are used for the axial, coronal, and sagittal slices, respectively. Thresholds are generated from Equation 8.9 using $\beta = 0.3$, $\beta = 0.4$, and $\beta = 0.4$ for these directions.

The images are stacked to create a 3D volume and the airways are segmented using closed-space dilation [24,29,31,32]. Closed-space dilation is described as follows

$$X \oplus_B K = X_N = (X_{N-1} \oplus K) \cap B = (X_{N-2} \oplus K)\ldots \tag{8.10}$$

where $X = X_0$ is the initial seed, B is the region being segmented, K is the opening kernel, and $\oplus$ is the morphological dilation operation [37]. Closed dilation acts like the dilation operator except that it is restricted to the shape of the object B. This results in a binary, connected volume of the segmented airway that can be used for analysis of the airways.

Once possible regions have been detected using morphological filtering and reconstruction, bounded space dilation is applied to the binary volume as a region-growing technique from the initial seed point in the trachea [37]. Some methods used a two-dimensional bounded space dilation with seed points and backward and forward passes [24], whereas other methods used 3D-bounded space dilation [29,31]. 3D dilation allows any complexity of topology to be followed without backward and forward passes.

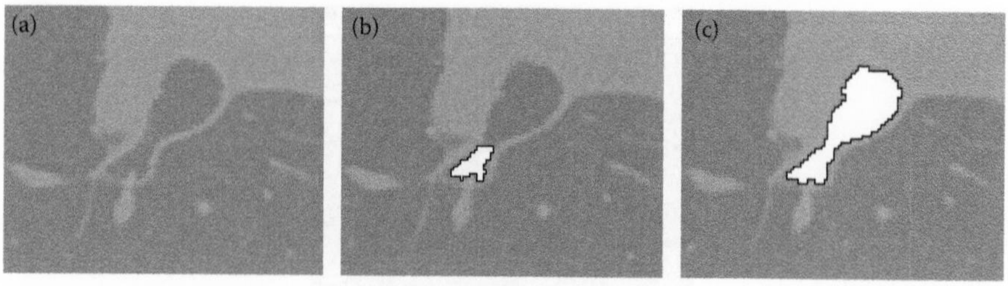

FIGURE 8.13
Part of a CT slice showing a segmentation using 3D filtering to extract airways that are noncircular in the plane. (a) Unsegmented section of the airway tree. (b) Parallel vessels segmented using coronal and sagittal filtering. (c) Axial filtering applied.

In some cases, objects that are of a similar size and shape to that of the airways are enhanced by the morphological reconstruction and remain when thresholded. If the object is 6-connected to the airway region it will be segmented, this causes leaks. These leaks can be minimized by applying a restriction to the dilation. The change in the cross-section of each branch can be monitored by calculating the area of the growth front of each branch and comparing it to previous growth fronts [29,37]. The growth front of each branch is calculated by labeling in 3D each connected object of the growth front and labeling the connected growth front from the previous step. To detect leakage where the volume increases substantially, the volumes of the last three dilations for each branch are compared with the three dilations before that. If the ratio of the volumes is above a specified threshold of double the size, then closed-space dilation along this branch is stopped. This leak removal method is similar to the rules applied by van Ginneken et al. [28] in Section 8.2.3.

8.2.6.2 Connection Cost and Energy Minimization

Fetita et al. [33] used a morphological filtering connection cost approach to select airway candidates and an energy-based region-growing approach for extraction of the distal airways. This is an extension of their earlier work [34].

The key principle behind their airway enhancement approach is that of connection cost between voxels in an image (a related concept is that of fuzzy connectivity in Section 8.2.5). Connection cost is based on gray scale values of the path between voxels and is defined as [33,34]:

$$C_f(x,y) = \Lambda\{\lambda \in \mathbb{R} \mid \delta_f, \lambda(x,y) < +\infty\} \tag{8.11}$$

where Λ is the infinum operator and δ is the geodesic distance between x and y for a threshold λ applied to the gray scale function f. Therefore, $C_f(x, y)$ between two points x and y is the minimum gray scale value λ that when applied as a threshold to f results a connected path between x and y (see Figure 8.14a). $C_f(x, Y)$ can also be represented as a function of a set of chosen reference points and is illustrated in Figure 8.14b. This shows that connection cost can be used as a method to fill valleys and, therefore, enhance the airways. However, there are larger gray scale changes between bone and tissue than the airways. Therefore, Fetita et al. [33] used connection cost operation with a method of marking bronchi to create an operator that fills in only the airway regions.

An operator is introduced: the selective marking and depth-constrained (SMDC) operator using the basis of connection cost along with markers to fill in only potential airways. The markers used to find potential airways are found using the morphological operator (Of).

$$Of = \min(f \quad B, f \quad \breve{B}) \tag{8.12}$$

where f is the gray scale function of the CT volume. This operator is the minimum of the dilation of f with B and the dilation of f with $\breve{B}$. If x is the current voxel, then B is an upstream neighborhood of x and $\breve{B}$ is symmetric to B with respect to x. Figure 8.15a shows the two operators and the gray scale function f. Local minima in Of are used as markers to select airway candidates and the minimum value of the marker in a "trough" is used as the gray scale filling of that trough.

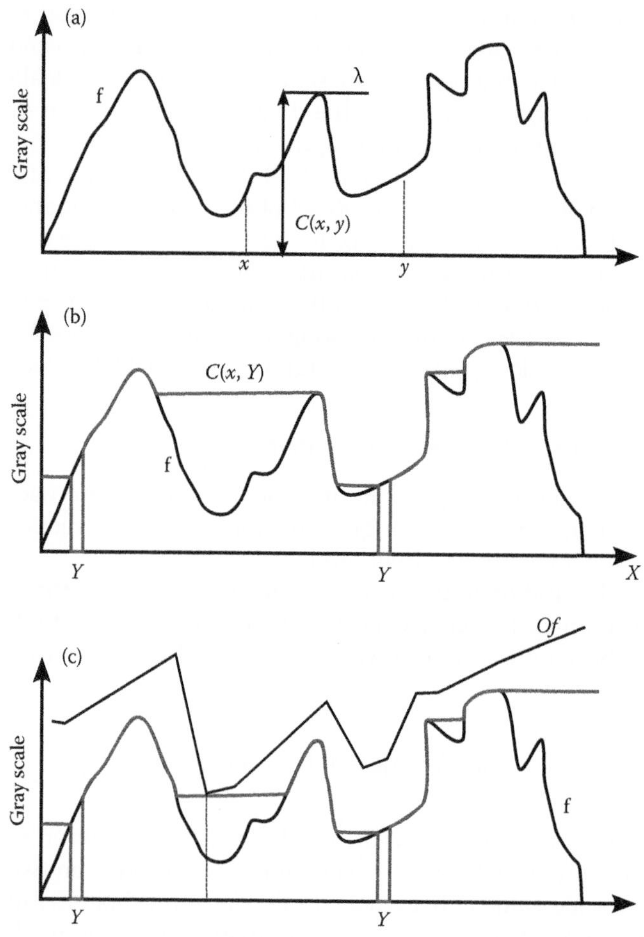

FIGURE 8.14
Connection cost function. (a) Connection cost between two points x and y. (b) Connection cost using a set of reference points (Y). (c) Selecting seed points from *Of*.

Therefore, SMDC creates an output that is identical to f, except that potential airways have been filled. The size of B must be chosen to detect airway regions. This method produces a similar result to using morphological closing and reconstruction as discussed in Section 8.2.6.1.

Airway segmentation is performed using this method as follows. Low order airways are extracted first and then an energy minimization method is used to extract the higher order airways. The trachea is identified in the first axial slice and the diameter is found. This value is used to define x_1 of the structuring element B_{x1} used in *Of* to extract the lower order airways using the SMDC. The algorithm is also applied using B_{x2} of $x_2 = 2$. The second run identifies noise in the image which is then subtracted from the first output. Note that B_x is the 3D SE of size x.

An energy-based 3D region-growing method is used to segment the distal airways. The propagation is controlled by minimizing energy

$$\varepsilon = \exp(-\alpha V_{prop}) \tag{8.13}$$

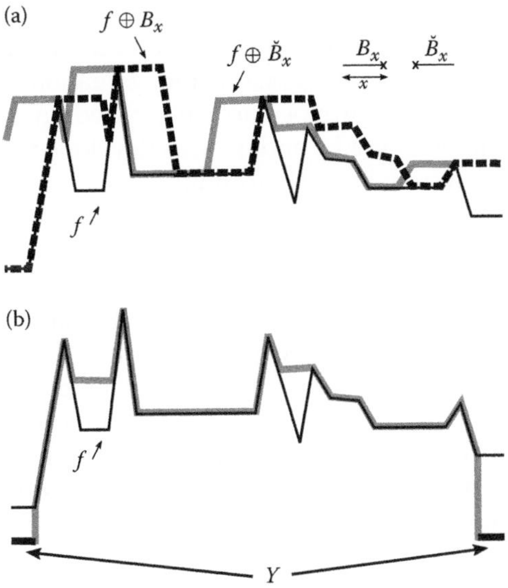

FIGURE 8.15
(a) Two structuring elements B and $\breve{B}$ of Of. (b) Potential airways filled using SMDC. (From Fetita, C.I., et al., *IEEE Trans. Med. Imaging*, 23:1353–1364, 2004. With permission.)

where α is a constant and V_{prop} is the potential of a voxel and is used to guide the region-growing. This potential is in terms of the binary value of the 26-connected neighborhood of voxels. V_{prop} has radial, distal, and control propagation components:

$$V_{\text{prop}} = V_{\text{radial}} + V_{\text{distal}} + V_{\text{control}} \tag{8.14}$$

V_{radial} controls radial propagation and is directed toward the high-density gray scale values of the wall, V_{control} limits the propagation to the bronchial lumen, and V_{distal} directs the region growing along the length of the bronchi.

8.2.7 Other Methods

This section has selected some of the key methods used to segment the airways and a number of algorithms have not been included. Additional methods worth mentioning include the following: Summers et al. [38] used a manual threshold and region-growing approach, Law and Heng [39] used a thresholded region-growing approach and a genetic algorithm for seed point selection, Kitasaka et al. [40] performed a ROI bronchial extraction method, and Reinhardt et al. [41] used a maximum-likelihood approach to identify the airway wall.

8.2.8 Airway Segmentation Evaluation (EXACT'09 Challenge)

Segmentation methods using a variety of techniques have been discussed. However, the evaluation of airway segmentation methods is a difficult task because different CT data sets and varying performance measures are used by each group; the CT data sets often vary considerably in resolution and image quality. The Pulmonary Image Analysis workshop* at MICCAI 2009 held the EXACT'09 airway segmentation challenge in an attempt to evaluate various airway segmentation methods. Twenty-two teams registered for the challenge and 15 teams submitted results for evaluation [20].

Their methods evaluated each team's performance based on the accuracy of segmentations of a set of 20 CT volumes. A gold standard was developed for each volume and compared with the segmentation from each algorithm.

8.2.8.1 Methods

Forty CT scans were selected as the EXACT'09 data set, and divided into 20 training images and 20 testing images. The CT images contained a selection of different acquisition conditions and pathologies. These CTs were provided to the teams and the segmentations from each team were submitted to EXACT'09 for evaluation. A reference segmentation was found for each test CT scan by combining the segmentations from each algorithm and using trained observers to remove false branches. Each segmentation from each team was evaluated by comparing the segmentation to the appropriate reference segmentation.

The segmentations were divided into individual branches for evaluation. Branch points were found using a fast marching algorithm as a region-growing method—in a similar way to Schlathölter et al. [19] in Section 8.2.3. A number of slices from each branch, containing image and segmentation information, were then viewed by trained observers (medical students) and evaluated. More than one observer viewed each branch and labels of "correct," "partly wrong," "wrong," or "unknown" were assigned. The labeled branches from all segmentation algorithms were combined and correct voxels were used to form the reference segmentation for each test CT volume. Each segmentation was then evaluated by comparing each segmented branch to the reference segmentation [20].

8.2.8.2 Results and Discussion

Evaluation measures included *Branch Detected, Tree Length Detected,* and *False Positive Rate. Branch Detected* is the mean proportion of branches detected with respect to the reference segmentations. *Tree Length Detected* is the mean proportion of tree length detected with respect to the reference segmentations. *False Positive Rate* is the proportion of the total segmentation volume that is incorrect [20].

These measures were calculated for each of the 15 teams using the 20 test images. Figures 8.16 and 8.17 show the *Branch Detected* and *Tree Length Detected* plotted in terms of the *False Positive Rate* for the 15 teams. The number in each figure refers to the team number and each team's algorithm is outlined in Table 8.2.

These graphs seem to indicate that, in general, algorithms that detect a greater proportion of the tree tend to have a greater false positive rate. If a method has the ability to adjust the strictness of the segmentation and, therefore, adjust the position on the graph, then comparisons become difficult. Better comparisons could be made by using a receiver operating characteristic (ROC) curve for each method.

It is also worth noting that a considerable proportion of the airway tree was not segmented by the algorithms, which means that there is room to improve the airway segmentation methods.

---

* http://www.lungworkshop.org.

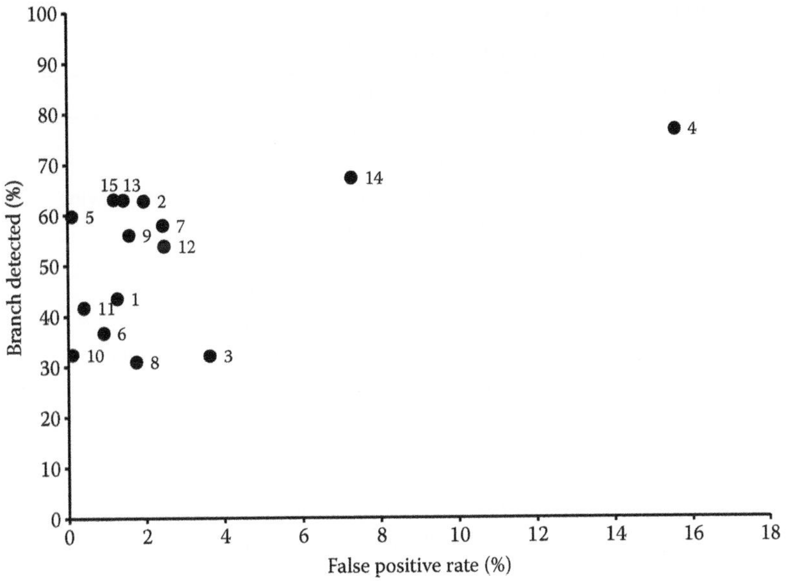

FIGURE 8.16
Branches detected versus false positive rate.

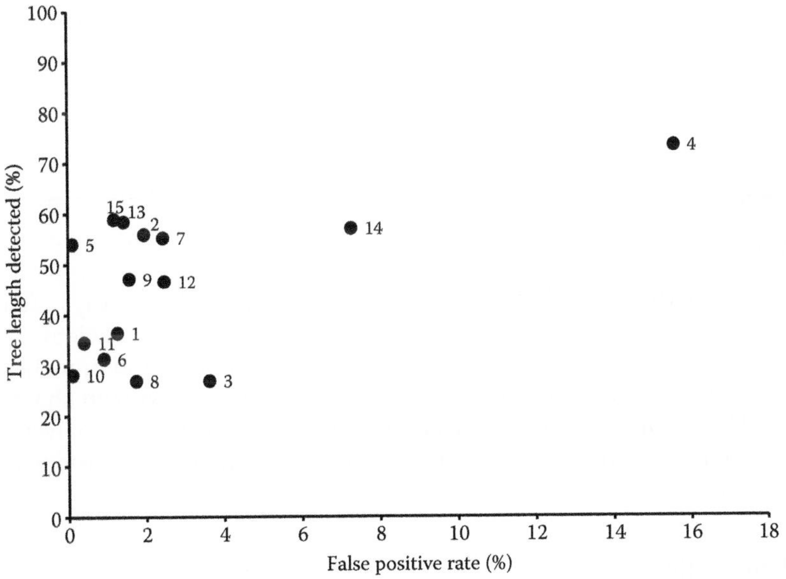

FIGURE 8.17
Tree length detected versus false positive rate.

TABLE 8.2

Segmentation Methods Evaluated in EXACT'09

Method	Summary
1	Morphological filtering and region growing Irving et al. (Section 8.2.6.1)
2	Morphological filtering, connection cost, and region-growing Related to Fetita et al. (Section 8.2.6.2)
3	Restricted region-growing
4	Branch edge detection and region-growing
5	Airway appearance model and airway/vessel guide Method was submitted by EXACT'09 challenge evaluator
6	Region-growing with reevaluation of ROI
7	Tube detection and knowledge-based region-growing
8	Adaptive region-growing
9	Local centricity region-growing
10	Region-growing with leak detection
11	Wave propagation and template matching
12	Adaptive region-growing
13	Gradient vector flow
14	Multithreshold with topological restrictions Method based on van Ginneken et al. (Section 8.2.3)
15	Region-growing User manually corrects branches Based on Mori et al. (Section 8.2.2)

Source: Lo, P., et al., In *Second International Workshop on Pulmonary Image Analysis*, 2009; Irving, B.J., et al., In *Second International Workshop on Pulmonary Image Analysis*, 2009; Fetita, C.I., et al., *IEEE Trans. Med. Imaging*, 23:1353–1364, 2004; van Ginneken, B., et al., *Med. Image Comput. Comput. Assist. Interv.*, 11:219–226, 2008; Mori, K., et al., *Proc. Intl. Conf. Pattern Recognition*, 3:528–532, 1996.

8.3 Analysis

This section briefly discusses further steps in the analysis of the airways after they have been segmented. Steps include extraction of the medial line using skeletonization, finding branch points, and labeling of branches. Once branch points and branches have been found, then branches can be labeled by matching the airway to known characteristics of each branch. The advantage of branch labeling is that branch-specific analysis can be performed. Branch analysis might include measurement of branch dimensions or statistical surface analysis.

8.3.1 Skeletonization

A medial line—a line that travels through each branch and is at the center of a branch cross-section—is generally required to identify the topology of the airways and, therefore, to label branches. Having extracted the medial line, there are a number of other benefits, such as directing virtual bronchoscopy and extracting airway cross-sections. A number of methods can be used to skeletonize the airways. However, many cannot produce a one-voxel-thick medial line, which is required for branch point analysis. Skeletonization of branching structures has been the focus of a number of algorithms (for example, refs. [37,42]); however, this section will focus on examples of algorithms that have been successfully applied to the airway tree segmentations from CT images.

8.3.1.1 Region-Growing Methods

Some methods identify the medial line as part of the airway segmentation step [5,19,22,28] (as discussed in Section 8.2.3). Swift et al. [5] calculated points on the medial line by finding the centroid of boundary points in the cross-section of the airway. Schlathölter et al. [19] grew the skeleton as a product of their branch point detection step in their method.

Extraction of the medial line is performed in a similar way by Wood et al. [26]. The centroid of the wave front is used to form the medial line and corrections are made to the bifurcation points using the medial lines of the three branches of the intersection. A seed point at the base of the trachea, in the segmented airway, is used to initialize the method and is labeled 0. Voxels that are 26-connected to the 0 voxel are labeled 1 and unlabeled voxels that are 26-connected to voxels labeled 1 are labeled 2, etc. This is repeated until all voxels are labeled. To extract the medial line, the centroid is found for each connected set of voxels with the same label, and neighboring centroids are connected with a line, i.e., the centroid with label n is connected with a line to the centroids labeled $n + 1$ and $n - 1$. At bifurcation points, both child branches are given the same label.

However, extracting the medial line from the wave front means that the branches are disconnected in the bifurcation region (see Figure 8.18a). Wood et al. [26] overcame this problem by fitting lines to each of the three branches forming the bifurcation and used a minimization algorithm to find the best intersection of these lines, which is labeled as the bifurcation point (see Figure 8.18b). The middle 70% of each branch is used to fit the line because of noise in the medial line around the bifurcation point.

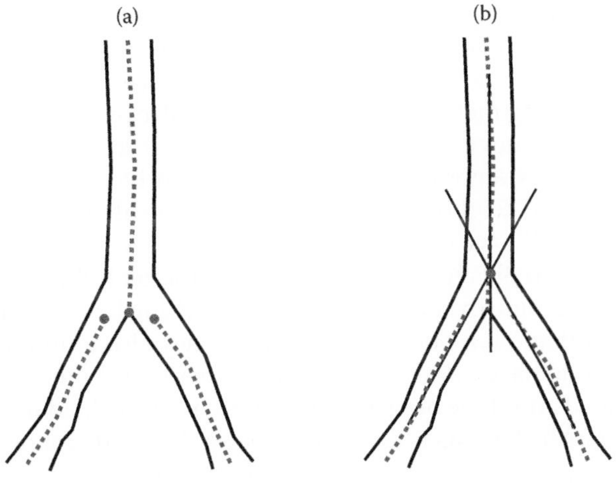

FIGURE 8.18
Bifurcation point detection.

8.3.1.2 Thinning Methods

Region-growing methods are not the only way to extract the medial line from the airway tree; Palágyi et al. [43,44] used a thinning algorithm. Their algorithm can be divided into two steps: topological correction and centerline extraction, and these steps employ a number of techniques to make the skeletonization robust. In the first step, morphological closing removes small holes, bays (surface deformations), and cavities in the segmentation. These small irregularities would cause unwanted changes such as false branches.

Once the segmentation has been corrected, the second step extracts the centerline by iteratively thinning the segmentation. Each surface voxel is analyzed for orientation and connectivity. If the surface voxel is classified as a simple point and is not an end point, it is removed, leaving a one-voxel-thick medial line. This is repeated until no more voxels are removed. This method has also been used successfully by other researchers [45].

The algorithm proceeds as follows. A base point is found as the center of the first slice containing the trachea and this point is preserved. Next, surface voxels of the segmentation are identified as points that are 6-connected to a 0 voxel (a background voxel) in one direction. They are grouped as U (up), N, E, S, W, and D (down) voxels depending on the direction of the 6-connectivity to a background voxel. Simple points are points that can be removed without changing the topology of the skeleton, and line-end points are points that are 26-connected to only one other one voxel (an airway voxel).

Therefore, simple points that are not line-end points are selected and iteratively removed for each directional grouping U, N, E, S, W, and D. For a voxel i in the current directional grouping:

- Check if i is a simple point and line-end point.
- Remove i if a simple point and not a line-end point.
- Also, if the point is a line-end point and a simple point but the number of deleted 6-connected neighbors is greater than or equal to t, then also delete i.

t controls the sensitivity of the algorithm to surface effects and the sensitivity of the algorithm to branching. Simple points and line-end points are checked during the initial selection of points as well as at the point deletion stage because deleting surrounding points will change the point. This algorithm acts to iteratively thin the airways down to a one-voxel-thick skeleton and is repeated until no more changes occur.

Even after morphological closing in the first step, surface irregularities can still cause false branches, so a pruning method is used to remove false branches by cutting circularly connected regions and removing branches based on their length and distance from the airway surface. Using this algorithm, branch points can be identified by the centerline points with more than two neighbors because this thinning algorithm guarantees that end points and line points will have one and two 26-connected neighbors, respectively.

Mori et al. [25] also used 3D region thinning to find the centerline and label the branching structure. They overcame the problem of false branching by observing that, in general, false branches are short and have no child branches. They also found that branches with a large diameter tended to have more false branches. Therefore, branches that have no child branches are examined and if the branch is shorter than a threshold (t_{length}) or if the branch is connected to a branch that has a diameter greater than a threshold (t_{diameter}), then the branch is deleted. t_{length} and t_{diameter} were found experimentally.

Figure 8.19 shows an example of voxels representing the medial line of an airway tree. The connectivity of the medial line has been used to assign three different colors to

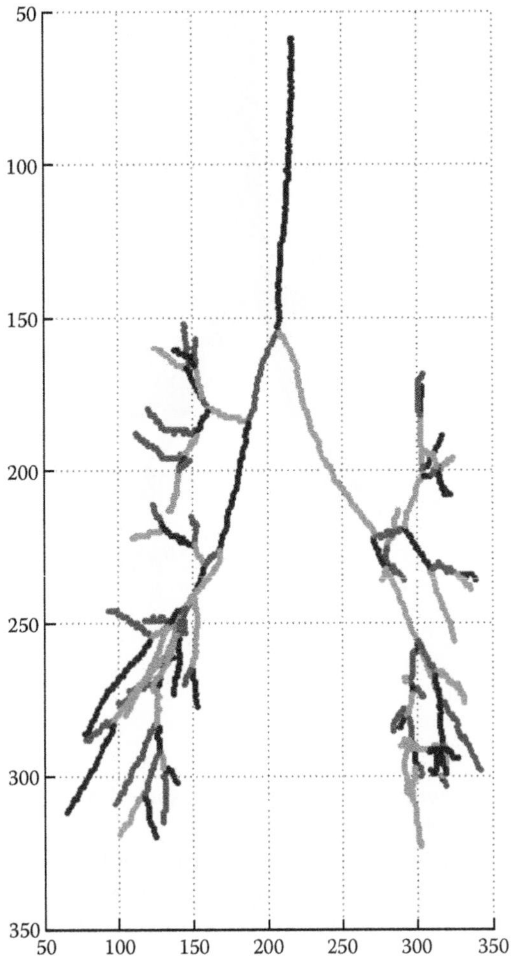

FIGURE 8.19
(See color insert.) An example of a labeled airway skeleton.

branches that connect at a branch point. Figure 8.20 shows the segmentation with branches identified using the skeleton.

8.3.2 Anatomical Branch Labeling

Once the airway has been segmented and branch points found, branches can be matched to their anatomical labels. This is necessary for almost any analysis because it allows branch-specific comparisons to be made. Examples include locating the position of abnormalities in the airway tree and using the branching structure of the airway to identify lung structures.

Tschirren et al. [46] outlined a method for matching airway branches to anatomical labels. They assume that the first three or four generations of the airway can be matched and further generations differ for each individual. Their method uses the medial line to convert each airway tree into a graph where vertices represent branch points. An associative graph

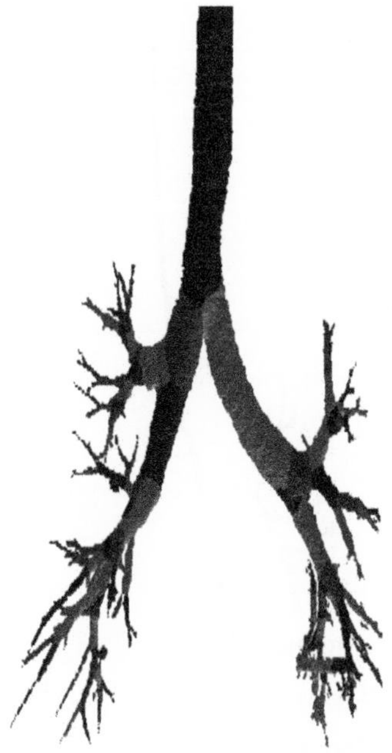

FIGURE 8.20
An example of a labeled segmentation.

is then built between an airway of interest and a labeled anatomical model and used to find the best match between the trees.

The medial line and branch points are used to represent the airways as a directed acyclic graph in which the vertices represent end points and branch points, and the vertices are connected by edges that are representative of the connectivity of the airway tree (as shown in Figure 8.21).

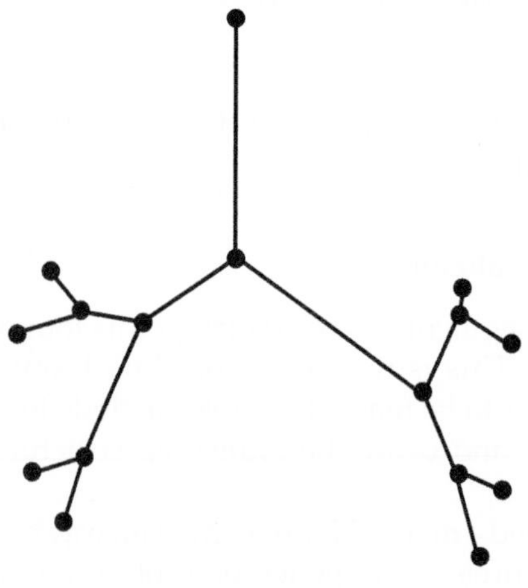

FIGURE 8.21
Graph representation of the airway tree.

The association graph is used to match an airway tree to an anatomically labeled population average. An association graph G_{assoc} is a measure of the similarity between two graphs (G_1 and G_2) and has a vertex for every possible pairing of vertices consisting of vertices from G_1 and G_2. An edge connects two vertices in G_{assoc} if the relationship between the corresponding vertices in G_1 is the same as that between the vertices in G_2. Tschirren et al. [46] used inheritance and topological distance to define this relationship. Therefore, in the association graph, maximum clique (the largest subset of vertices in which every vertex is connected to every other vertex) represents the set of vertices of G_1 and G_2 that have the same relationship. This maximum clique represents the best match between the two trees and forms the basis of the algorithm by Tschirren et al. [46]. However, a number of steps are taken to reduce the computational complexity of the task of finding the maximum clique.

The anatomical model, which is matched to each airway, is a population average, created from a data set of labeled segmentations. A number of measures are used to define the anatomical model, including individual measures of branch length and orientation, as well as measures between branches, of inheritance (e.g., parent and child), angle between segments, spatial relationship, and topological distance.

Every branch is represented in terms of a start vertex, end vertex, and edge. Edges between vertices are only added to the association graph if the inheritance relationship is the same and the topological distance is similar for a branch of the tree and the population average. Vertices and edges in the association graph are then assigned weights according to the measures discussed earlier. Vertices and edges with low weights are removed to reduce the computational complexity of finding the maximum clique. The maximum clique is then found which represents the match of the branches from the airway tree to the anatomical model. Therefore, using a population average, labels can be assigned to each branch of a segmented tree.

An alternative method is discussed by van Ginneken et al. [28]. They use a training set of airway segmentations that are manually labeled using the same labels as Tschirren et al. [46]. Probabilities based on orientation, average radius, and angle are used to label branches. Starting from the trachea, each branch is labeled based on the label of the parent and the probabilities of the child and grandchild branches.

Mori et al. [25] also proposed a template-matching algorithm. Their method is similar to that of Tschirren et al. [46] in that they use branch position and hierarchy to match the branches. However, their labeling is based on minimizing a global fitting function instead of using an associative graph.

Their approach is divided into two levels of detail: (a) labeling of the RMB and LMB, and (b) labeling the smaller bronchi. Candidate RMB branches and LMB branches are found by identifying branches with the trachea as the parent and an end point that is less than k from a template

$$\left\| Q_{b_i} - Q_{\text{template}} \right\| < k \tag{8.15}$$

where Q_{b_i} is the location of the end point of branch B_i and Q_{template} is the location of the template end point. If more than one candidate exists, then an evaluation based on the child branches is performed. Other potential branches exist because the skeletonization method can create false branches [25] and this algorithm is designed to minimize the risk of breaking labeling at the RMB/LMB level.

Smaller branches are labeled by comparing each branch to a template branch using an energy function E, where:

$$E_{B_i K_j} = \frac{d^{B_i} \cdot d^{K_j}}{\left\| d^{B_i} \right\| \left\| d^{K_j} \right\|} \quad (8.16)$$

where B_i is the branch under consideration, K_j is the labeled template branch, and d^{B_i} and d^{K_j} are the directions of B_i and K_j, respectively. Therefore, E is greatest when B_i is in the same direction as K_j, and this is used to label a branch.

Therefore, starting from child branches of the main bronchi, each branch (B_i) is compared to template branches with the same parent branch. B_i is assigned the label which yields the highest E. If that label has already been assigned to another branch, then the branch with the highest E is assigned the label and it is removed from the other branch. This method is applied iteratively until all branches have been labeled. Finally, if more than one candidate LMB or RMB exists, then each candidate is tested and all child branches are matched. The candidate with the largest sum of all energy from the child branches is selected. This method successfully labeled 93% of branches that were successfully segmented and skeletonized.

8.3.3 Branch Analysis

Analysis of the structure of each branch is a useful outcome of the segmentation and branch labeling procedure. The degree of complexity varies considerably depending on the goal of the branch analysis.

Schlathölter et al. [19] calculated the average diameter of each branch as part of their airway segmentation algorithm (Section 8.2.3).

Palágyi et al. [44] performed simple measurements on each branch including length, volume, surface area, and average radius. These measures are calculated from the skeleton length and the number of voxels belonging to a branch. Their analysis is restricted to the part of the branch not considered to be part of the bifurcation area. The volume is taken as the sum of the number of voxels in a branch multiplied by the voxel dimension, the length is calculated from the sum of voxels in the skeleton, and the average branch radius is calculated as:

$$\text{radius} = \sqrt{\frac{\text{volume}}{\pi \text{ length}}} \quad (8.17)$$

These are useful but only consider average measures for the whole branch. Tschirren et al. [21], on the other hand, performed a number of airway measurements along each branch by measuring the diameter of a section of the branch that is perpendicular to the centerline. Wood et al. [26] used the segmentation and skeleton to measure the bronchi length, bifurcation angles, and cross-sectional area at points along a branch. The length of each bronchus is approximated as the linear distance between the branch points that initialize and terminate the branch. The bifurcation angle is measured as the angle between lines fitted to the child branches. The cross-sectional area is the area of the voxels in a plane perpendicular to the skeleton.

8.3.4 Statistical Shape Models of Airway Trees

Beyond simple branch measurements, there is potential to use statistical modeling to detect pathological deformation and stenosis in the airway tree from a data set of segmentations. This is a relatively unexplored approach to airway tree analysis. This section briefly highlights the potential of statistical models for analyzing airway shape variation.

Heimann and Meinzer [47] provided an overview of statistical shape models in 3D. The main representations that are suitable for quasi-tubular objects—that is, objects showing similarities to tubes—include point distribution models (corresponding points placed on the surface) and medial models (objects represented by centerlines and radii). Other methods include Fourier surfaces and spherical harmonics. Examples of applications of these methods are given to demonstrate the potential for modeling the airways.

Point distribution models are a commonly used representation and can be used to determine the main modes of variation within a set of training shapes. Each shape in the training set is described by a set of corresponding landmark points. These shapes are then aligned by rotation, translation, and scaling using generalized Procrustes analysis. Principal component analysis (PCA) can then be applied to the aligned shapes to extract the main modes of variation [48]. The mean shape and the modes of variation can be useful in modeling shape changes in a data set of airways and, thus, identify pathology.

Point distribution models and statistical analyses have been applied successfully to other organs. Hutton et al. [49] and Paulsen et al. [50] both use point distribution models for analyzing shape changes in the face and ear canal, respectively. They used a set of sparse landmarks which are selected manually and then performed thin-plate spline warping of a template to obtain dense surface correspondence between the object surfaces (between 2000 and 20,000 vertices [49,50]). Dense correspondence is made by mapping the vertices of the template shape to the closest points on the surface of the warped objects. Hutton et al. [49] used the mean landmarks as the template, whereas Paulsen et al. [50] used one of the training objects. Generalized Procrustes analysis is used to align the objects before PCA is used to reduce dimensionality, and multivariate analysis is used to extract the variation. Each airway is represented in terms of the extracted eigenvalues in the eigenvector space. Hutton et al. [49] took a standard approach to deciding how many components to retain so that 98% of the variance in the data set is represented. Classifiers are trained using labeled data sets and determine a decision hyperplane that best separates the labeled shapes in the eigenvector space. Hammond et al. [51] and Hutton et al. [49] tested a number of classifiers for differentiating between Noonan syndrome and controls. Noonan syndrome can be identified by a number of facial features. The classifiers were the nearest mean, decision trees, neural networks, logistic regression, and support vector machines. They found support vector machines to be the most effective classifier for this data set with an average sensitivity of 92% and an average specificity of 93%. However, the nearest mean, neural networks, and logistic regression all had sensitivities and specificities greater than 83% and 86%, respectively.

An alternative representation is the medial model. Pizer et al. [52,53] used discrete medial representations of shapes. The basic component of a discrete m-rep model is the atom and a set of atoms represent a shape. An atom consists of a hub, which is the center of the maximal sphere, and two spokes to represent the two radii whose end points are tangent to the surface of the object being modeled (as shown in Figure 8.22). Conditions restrict folding in the surface of this model. PCA cannot be applied to this representation because it is not Euclidean. Therefore, principal geodesic analysis was developed, which applies PCA using geodesic distance on the manifold [54]. Statistics can be applied to m-rep figures on a global level or on an atomic level (analyzing the connectivity between atoms) [55].

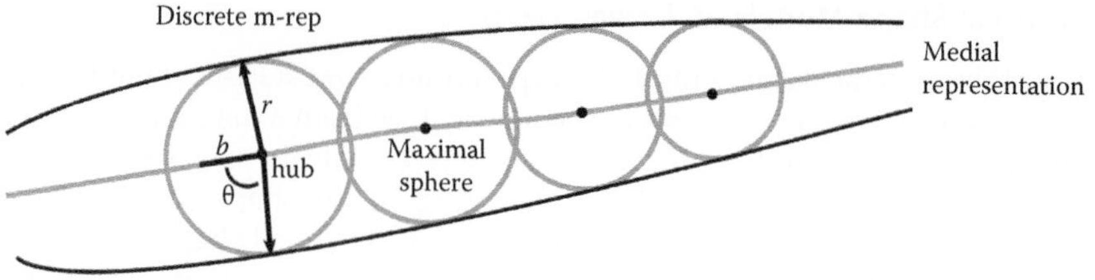

FIGURE 8.22
Medial representation.

As can be seen, a key element of statistical analysis of the airways is developing correspondence between the airways in a data set. Correspondence is usually found in point distribution models by labeling or identifying a set of landmarks on each shape and then aligning these landmarks. The correspondence problem is slightly different for the airways because of the lack of anatomical landmarks on the surface of the airway, and the topological structure must be used instead.

Huysmans et al. [56] developed correspondence using a cylindrical parameterization approach. Initially, an iterative closest point algorithm is used to align the shapes by obtaining a best match of the two shapes. They use cylindrical parameterization to develop correspondence, whereby the mesh representing the object is iteratively collapsed, minimizing the error between the collapsed shape and the original shape, until there are six vertices. These vertices are then transformed to the cylindrical triangulation and the vertices are split to rebuild the mesh. All objects in the data set are parameterized in this way to establish correspondence. Pinho et al. [57] used the method of obtaining correspondence developed by Huysmans et al. [56] to assess tracheal stenosis. They do this by estimating the healthy trachea of a patient with tracheal stenosis. They applied the method to nine shapes and placed 1024 landmarks on each shape. The method was also tested on tubular phantoms, in which local erosion had been applied to produce stenosis. However, considerable modification is required for a branching tubular structure.

Vitanovski et al. [58] developed patient-specific models of shape changes to the pulmonary trunk. Their model is based on a training set and is fitted to individual patient scans. The model consists of landmarks, centerlines, and surface approximations. First, five anatomical landmarks are placed on the pulmonary trunk. These landmarks are then used to guide the centerline extraction of the tube and the surface of the pulmonary artery is modeled using nonuniform rational B-splines. For a specific patient, the landmarks are detected and the centerline is extracted using the landmarks and a trained circle detector. The section that is relevant to airway modeling is Vitanovski et al. [58]'s use of a mean surface and the skeleton to develop correspondence. The centerline is sampled equidistantly and a local coordinate is constructed at each point. Points on the surface of the mean model are related to the local coordinate system by their Euclidean distance. Therefore, mapping the centerline of the mean model to that of a specific model will map the related surface points—developing correspondence.

This section outlines a generic method of analysis variation in a data set of shapes by developing point correspondence and determining the variation. Methods that have been used to create correspondence in tubular structures are also discussed.

8.4 Summary

This chapter introduced airway segmentation and analysis techniques. The airways can be extracted from a CT using various segmentation procedures. Once segmented, further analysis includes finding the medial line and assigning anatomical labels, which can be used to make individual branch measurements and model the variation of airways in a data set.

Segmentation algorithms were grouped according to what was considered to be the defining method used in each algorithm. This included thresholding, thresholding with topological analysis, rule-based, fuzzy logic, and morphology-based segmentation. Comparing these algorithms is difficult because of the differing image qualities used in each of the studies. The EXACT'09 challenge was created as an opportunity to evaluate various airway segmentation algorithms [20]. Some methods performed better than others but, in general, greater branch segmentation sensitivity led to poorer specificity. This challenge provided a useful comparison but there is scope to extend this challenge, especially by including algorithm results at a range of sensitivities and specificities.

Once the airways have been segmented, branch detection and anatomical labeling can be used for more specific airway analysis. The medial line is generally the first step in airway analysis and can also be used as a guide for virtual bronchoscopy and cross-sectional measurements. This chapter discusses region-growing and thinning methods to extract the medial line.

Anatomical branch labels allow intrapatient and interpatient branch measurements to be compared. Each branch is given an anatomical label by using the detected branch points and an anatomical model of the airways. A number of branch measurements can be performed on these labeled branches and include average branch measurements, cross-sectional measurements, and branch curvature.

There is a large scope for further research in this field. The results of EXACT'09 showed that a considerable portion of smaller bronchi were missed by all algorithms and, therefore, there is room to improve airway segmentations with the possibility of combining algorithms that missed different bronchi. A relatively unexplored area of airway research is using segmentation and analysis techniques to quantify normal and pathological variations of the airway, and develop tools to detect disease from airway variation. These tools could also form a component of computer-aided detection for the lungs.

Acknowledgments

We thank Professor Robert Gie and Dr. Pierre Goussard, University of Stellenbosch, for their clinical assistance and providing CT images used to produce certain figures in this chapter. Funding is provided by the Commonwealth Scholarship Commission.

References

[1] Boiselle, P.M., K.F. Reynolds, and A. Ernst. 2002. Multiplanar and three-dimensional imaging of the central airways with multidetector CT. *American Journal of Roentgenology*, 179(2):301–308.

[2] Moses, K., J.C. Banks, P.B. Nava, and D. Petersen 2005. *Atlas of Clinical Gross Anatomy*. Philadelphia, PA: Mosby/Elsevier.

[3] Seneterre, E., F. Paganin, J.M. Bruel, F.B. Michel, and J. Bousquet. 1994. Measurement of the internal size of bronchi using high resolution computed tomography (HRCT). *European Respiratory Journal*, 7:596–600.

[4] Montaudon, M., P. Desbarats, P. Berger, G. De Dietrich, R. Marthan, and F. Laurent. 2007. Assessment of bronchial wall thickness and lumen diameter in human adults using multi-detector computed tomography: Comparison with theoretical models. *Journal of Anatomy*, 211:579–588.

[5] Swift, R.D., A.P. Kiraly, A.J. Sherbondy, A.L. Austin, E.A. Hoffman, G. McLennan, and W.E. Higgins. 2002. Automatic axis generation for virtual bronchoscopic assessment of major airway obstructions. *Computerized Medical Imaging and Graphics*, 26(2):103–118.

[6] Sonka, M., and J.M. Fitzpatrick. 2000. *Handbook of Medical Imaging*, vol. 2. Bellingham, WA: SPIE Press.

[7] Sonka, M., W. Park, and E.A. Hoffman. 1996. Rule-based detection of intrathoracic airway trees. *IEEE Transactions on Medical Imaging*, 15:314–326.

[8] Andronikou, S., E. Joseph, S. Lucas, S. Brachmeyer, G.D. Toit, H. Zar, and G. Swingler. 2004. CT scanning for the detection of tuberculous mediastinal and hilar lymphadenopathy in children. *Pediatric Radiology*, 34:232–236.

[9] du Plessis, J., P. Goussard, S. Andronikou, R. Gie, and R. George. 2009. Comparing three-dimensional volume-rendered CT images with fibreoptic tracheobronchoscopy in the evaluation of airway compression caused by tuberculous lymphadenopathy in children. *Pediatric Radiology*, 39:694–702.

[10] World Health Organization. Summary for TB-HIV estimates for 2005 by WHO regions. http://www.who.int/tb/country/tb_burden/en/index.html (Accessed September 2008).

[11] Grainger R.G., and D.J. Allison. 1986. *Diagnostic Radiology: An Anglo-American Textbook of Imaging*. Edinburgh, New York: Churchill Livingstone.

[12] Collins J., and E.J. Stern. 2007. *Chest Radiology: The Essentials*. Philadelphia, PA: Lippincott Williams & Wilkins.

[13] Marais, B.J. 2007. Childhood tuberculosis—risk assessment and diagnosis. *South African Medical Journal*, 97:978–982.

[14] Gie, R. 2003. *Diagnostic Atlas of Intrathoracic Tuberculosis in Children: A Guide for Low Income Countries*. Paris: International Union against Tuberculosis and Lung Disease.

[15] Goussard, P., and R. Gie. 2007. Airway involvement in pulmonary tuberculosis. *South African Medical Journal*, 97:986–988.

[16] Lee, S.L., Y.F. Cheung, M.P. Leung, Y.K. Ng, and N.S. Tsoi. 2002. Airway obstruction in children with congenital heart disease: Assessment by flexible bronchoscopy. *Pediatric Pulmonology*, 34:304–311.

[17] Bourke, S.J. 2007. *Respiratory Medicine*, 7th ed. Oxford: Blackwell Publishing.

[18] Brewis, R.A.L., B. Corrin, D.M. Geddes, and G.J. Gibson. 1995. *Respiratory Medicine*, 2nd ed. London: W.B. Saunders Company.

[19] Schlathölter, T., C. Lorenz, I.C. Carlsen, S. Renisch, and T. Deschamps. 2002. Simultaneous segmentation and tree reconstruction of the airways for virtual bronchoscopy. *SPIE*, 4684:103–113.

[20] Lo, P., B. van Ginneken, J. Reinhardt, and M. de Bruijne. 2009. Extraction of airways from CT. In *Second International Workshop on Pulmonary Image Analysis*.

[21] Tschirren, J., E.A. Hoffman, G. McLennan, and M. Sonka. 2005. Intrathoracic airway trees: segmentation and airway morphology analysis from low-dose CT scans. *IEEE Transactions on Medical Imaging*, 24:1529–1539.

[22] Bülow, T., C. Lorenz, and S. Renisch. 2004. A general framework for tree segmentation and reconstruction from medical volume data. *Medical Image Computing and Computer-Assisted Intervention*, 3216: 533–540.

[23] Park, W., E.A. Hoffman, and M. Sonka. 1998. Segmentation of intrathoracic airway trees: A fuzzy logic approach. *IEEE Transactions on Medical Imaging*, 17:489–497.
[24] Aykac, D., E.A. Hoffman, G. McLennan, and J.M. Reinhardt. 2003. Segmentation and analysis of the human airway tree from three-dimensional X-ray CT images. *IEEE Transactions on Medical Imaging*, 22:940–950.
[25] Mori, K., J. Hasegawa, Y. Suenaga, and J. Toriwaki. 2000. Automated anatomical labeling of the bronchial branch and its application to the virtual bronchoscopy system. *IEEE Transactions on Medical Imaging*, 19:103–114.
[26] Wood, S.A., E.A. Zerhouni, J.D. Hoford, E.A. Hoffman, and W. Mitzner. 1995. Measurement of three-dimensional lung tree structures by using computed tomography. *Journal of Applied Physiology*, 79:1687–1697.
[27] Mori, K., J. Hasegawa, J. Toriwaki, H. Anno, and K. Katada. 1996. Recognition of bronchus in three-dimensional x-ray CT images with application to virtualized bronchoscopy system. *Proceedings of the International Conference on Pattern Recognition*, 3:528–532.
[28] van Ginneken, B., W. Baggerman, and E.M. van Rikxoort. 2008. Robust segmentation and anatomical labeling of the airway tree from thoracic CT scans. *Medical Image Computing and Computer Assisted Intervention*, 11:219–226.
[29] Irving, B.J., P. Taylor, and A. Todd-Pokropek. 2009. 3D segmentation of the airway tree using a morphology based method. In *Second International Workshop on Pulmonary Image Analysis*.
[30] Sonka, M., V. Hlavac, and R. Boyle. 1999. *Image Processing, Analysis and Machine Vision*. London: International Thomson Publishing.
[31] Kiraly, A.P., W.E. Higgins, G. McLennan, E.A. Hoffman, and J.M. Reinhardt. 2002. Three-dimensional human airway segmentation methods for clinical virtual bronchoscopy. *Academic Radiology*, 9:1153–1168.
[32] Pisupati, C., L. Wolff, W. Mitzner, and E. Zerhouni. 1996. Segmentation of 3D pulmonary trees using mathematical morphology. *Mathematical Morphology and Its Applications to Image and Signal Processing*, 409–416. Norwell, MA: Kluwer Academic Publishers.
[33] Fetita, C.I., F. Preteux, C. Beigelman-Aubry, and P. Grenier. 2004. Pulmonary airways: 3D reconstruction from multislice CT and clinical investigation. *IEEE Transactions on Medical Imaging*, 23:1353–1364.
[34] Prêteux, F., C.I. Fetita, A. Capderou, and P. Grenier. 1999. Modeling, segmentation, and caliber estimation of bronchi in high resolution computerized tomography. *Journal of Electronic Imaging*, 8:36–45.
[35] Vincent, L. 1993. Morphological grayscale reconstruction in image analysis: Applications and efficient algorithms. *IEEE Transactions on Image Processing*, 2:176–201.
[36] Vincent, L. 1992. Morphological grayscale reconstruction: definition, efficient algorithm and applications in image analysis. In *Proceedings of Computer Vision and Pattern Recognition*, 92:633–635.
[37] Masutani, Y., T. Schiemann, and K.H. Hoehne. 1998. Vascular shape segmentation and structure extraction using a shape-based region-growing model. *Lecture Notes in Computer Science*, 1496:1242–1249.
[38] Summers, R.M., D.H. Feng, S.M. Holland, M.C. Sneller, and J.H. Shelhamer. 1996. Virtual bronchoscopy: Segmentation method for real-time display. *Radiology*, 200(3):857.
[39] Law, T., and P. Heng. 2000. Automated extraction of bronchus from 3D CT images of lung based on genetic algorithm and 3D region growing. *SPIE*, 3979:906–916.
[40] Kitasaka, T., K. Mori, J. Hasegawa, Y. Suenaga, and J. Toriwaki. 2003. Extraction of bronchus regions from 3D chest X-ray CT images by using structural features of bronchus. *International Congress Series*, 1256:240–245.
[41] Reinhardt, J.M., N. D'Souza, and E.A. Hoffman. 1997. Accurate measurement of intrathoracic airways. *IEEE Transactions on Medical Imaging*, 16:820–827.
[42] Toriwaki, J., and K. Mori. 2001. Distance transformation and skeletonization of 3D pictures and their applications to medical images. *Lecture Notes in Computer Science*, 2243:189–200.

[43] Palágyi, K., J. Tschirren, and M. Sonka. 2003. Quantitative analysis of intrathoracic airway trees: Methods and validation. *Lecture Notes in Computer Science*, 2732:222–233.
[44] Palágyi, K., J. Tschirren, E.A. Hoffman, and M. Sonka. 2006. Quantitative analysis of pulmonary airway tree structures. *Computers in Biology and Medicine*, 36:974–996.
[45] Tschirren, J., K. Palágyi, J.M. Reinhardt, E.A. Hoffman, and M. Sonka. 2002. Segmentation, skeletonization, and branchpoint matching—a fully automated quantitative evaluation of human intrathoracic airway trees. *Lecture Notes in Computer Science*, 2489:12–19.
[46] Tschirren, J., G. McLennan, K. Palágyi, E.A. Hoffman, and M. Sonka. 2005. Matching and anatomical labeling of human airway tree. *IEEE Transactions on Medical Imaging*, 24:1540–1547.
[47] Heimann, T., and H.P. Meinzer. 2009. Statistical shape models for 3D medical image segmentation: A review. *Medical Image Analysis*, 13:543–563.
[48] de Bruijne, M., B. van Ginneken, M.A. Viergever, and W.J. Niessen. 2003. Adapting active shape models for 3D segmentation of tubular structures in medical images. *Lecture Notes in Computer Science*, 2732:136–147.
[49] Hutton, T.J., B.F. Buxton, P. Hammond, and H.W.W. Potts. 2003. Estimating average growth trajectories in shape-space using kernel smoothing. *IEEE Transactions on Medical Imaging*, 22:747–753.
[50] Paulsen, R., R. Larsen, C. Nielsen, S. Laugesen, and B. Ersboll. 2002. Building and testing a statistical shape model of the human ear canal. *Lecture Notes in Computer Science*, 2489:373–380.
[51] Hammond, P., T.J. Hutton, J.E. Allanson, L.E. Campbell, R.C.M. Hennekam, S. Holden, M.A. Patton, A. Shaw, I.K. Temple, M. Trotter, et al. 2004. 3D analysis of facial morphology. *American Journal of Medical Genetics*, 126A:339–348.
[52] Pizer, S.M., P.T. Fletcher, S. Joshi, A. Thall, J.Z. Chen, Y. Fridman, D.S. Fritsch, A.G. Gash, J.M. Glotzer, M.R. Jiroutek, et al. 2003. Deformable M-reps for 3D medical image segmentation. *International Journal of Computer Vision*, 55:85–106.
[53] Pizer, S.M., P.T. Fletcher, A. Thall, M. Styner, G. Gerig, and S. Joshi. 2003. Object models in multiscale intrinsic coordinates via m-reps. *Image and Vision Computing*, 21:5–15.
[54] Fletcher, P., C. Lu, SM Pizer, and S. Joshi. 2004. Principal geodesic analysis for the study of nonlinear statistics of shape. *IEEE Transactions on Medical Imaging*, 23:995–1005.
[55] Han, Q. 2008. *Proper Shape Representation of Single Figure and Multi-Figure Anatomical Objects*. PhD thesis, Chapel Hill.
[56] Huysmans, T., J. Sijbers, F. Vanpoucke, and B. Verdonk. 2006. Improved shape modeling of tubular objects using cylindrical parameterization. *Lecture Notes in Computer Science*, 4091:84–91.
[57] Pinho, R., J. Sijbers, and T. Huysmans. 2007. Segmentation of the human trachea using deformable statistical models of tubular shapes. *Lecture Notes in Computer Science*, 4678:531–542.
[58] Vitanovski, D., R.I. Ionasec, B. Georgescu, M. Huber, A.M. Taylor, J. Hornegger, and D. Comaniciu. 2009. Personalized pulmonary trunk modeling for intervention planning and valve assessment estimated from CT data. *Lecture Notes in Computer Science*, 5761:17–25.

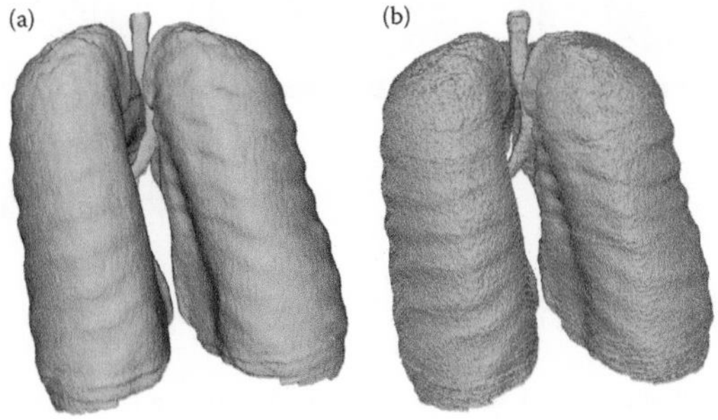

FIGURE 1.10
3D visualization of a healthy lung with no nodules: (a) our results and (b) result with the algorithm in ref. [40] (note that to be included in a software package usable at hospitals, the latter segmentation result based on the 2D algorithm still requires postprocessing for reconstruction of data in 3D space).

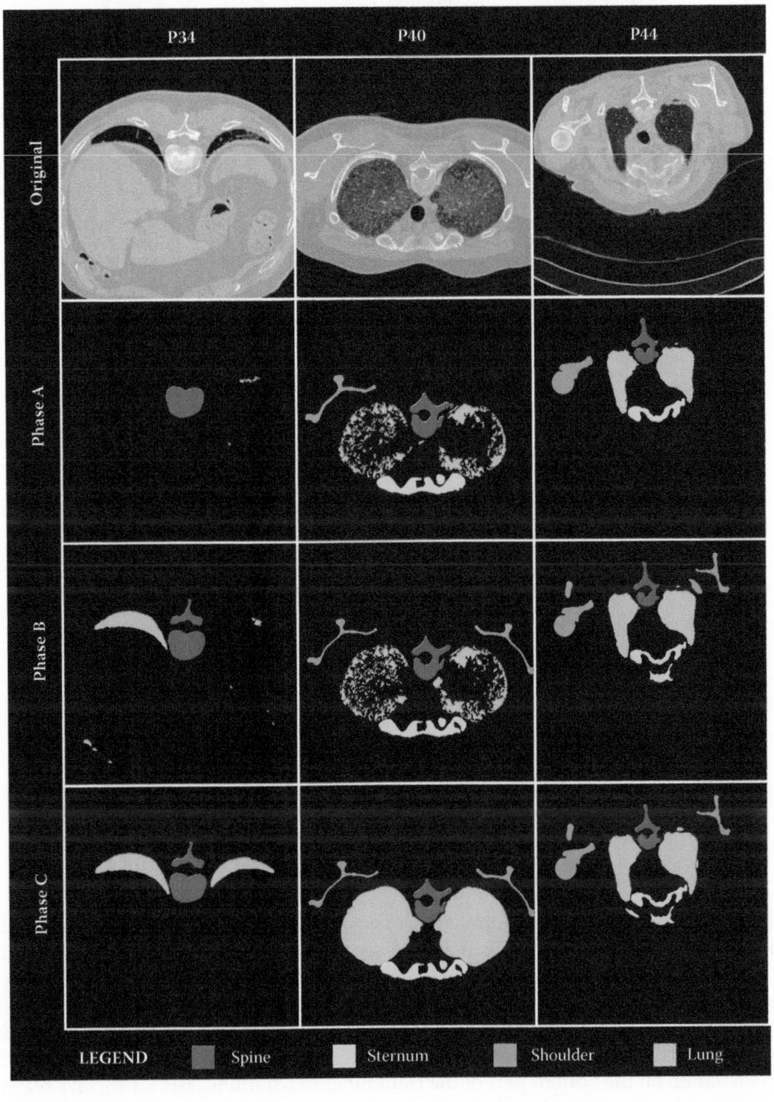

FIGURE 2.10
Anatomy segmentation results: (left to right) patients P34, P40, and P44; (top to bottom) original HRCT scan, segmentation result after training phases A, B, and C.

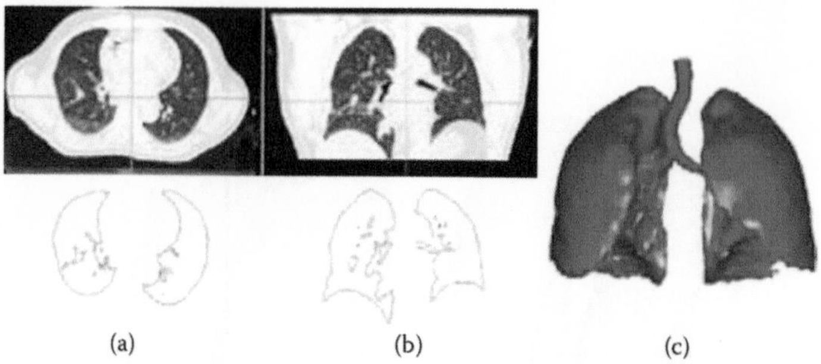

FIGURE 5.3
The 3DCT is shown along with segmented surface contours for supine (a) and upright orientation (b). (c) The 3D lung models generated from the contours are shown. (Courtesy of Klinder, T., et al. *Proc. SPIE*, 6914(3): 69141L.1–69141.L.11, 2008.)

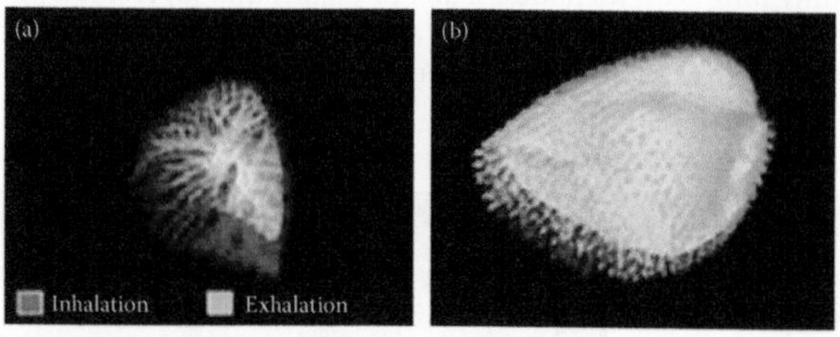

FIGURE 5.5
(a) The 3D capillary tree of a human lung is shown in end-inhalation and end-exhalation. (b) The 3D surface lung deformation is shown for each surface point. (Courtesy of Christensen, G.E., et al. *Med. Phys.*, 34(6): 2155–2163, 2007.)

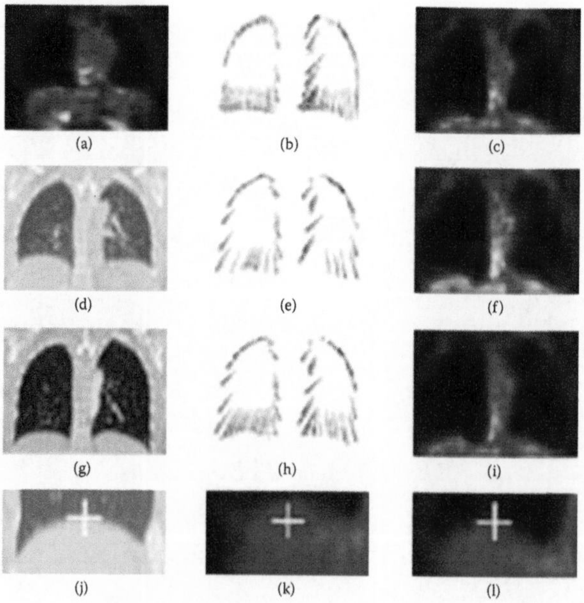

FIGURE 5.6
Original PET (a) and CT images (d, g) in a normal case. The correspondences between the selected points in the PET image (b) and in the end-inspiration CT image (g) are shown for the direct method. (e) Registration with the breathing model and a nonuniform landmark detection. (h) Registration with the breathing model and a pseudouniform landmark selection (corresponding points are linked). (c) Registered PET is shown for the direct method in (f) for the method with the breathing model with a nonuniform landmark distribution, and in (i) for the method with the breathing model and landmarks pseudouniformly distributed. The fourth row shows the details of registration on the bottom part of the right lung, in a normal case: CT (j), PET registered without breathing model (k), and with a breathing model (l). The white crosses correspond to the same coordinates. The method using the breathing model furnishes a better registration of the surfaces of the lungs. (From Chambon, S., et al. *J. Comput. Assist. Radiol. Surg.*, 13(5): 281–298, 2008. With permission.)

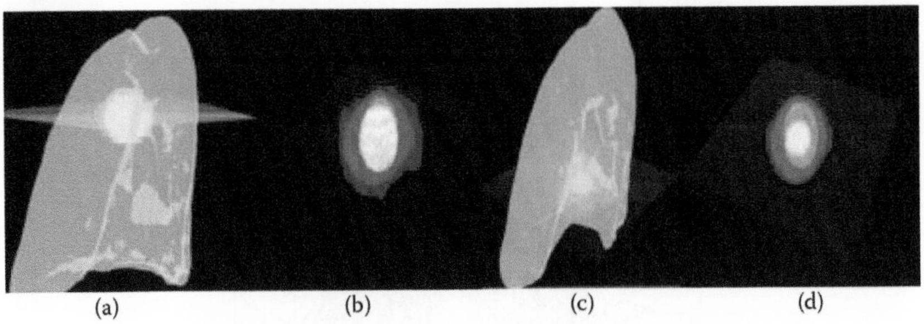

FIGURE 5.7
(a) The tumor is in the upper lung. The tumor dose delivery is shown in (b). (c) The tumor is in the lower lung. The tumor dose delivery is shown in (d). (Courtesy of Santhanam, A.P., et al. *Medical Image Computing and Computer Aided Intervention: Lecture Notes on Computer Science*, 2008.)

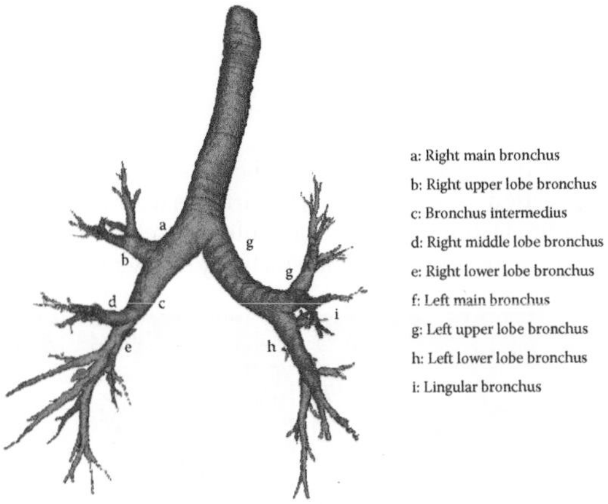

FIGURE 8.1
An airway segmentation with labeled branches.

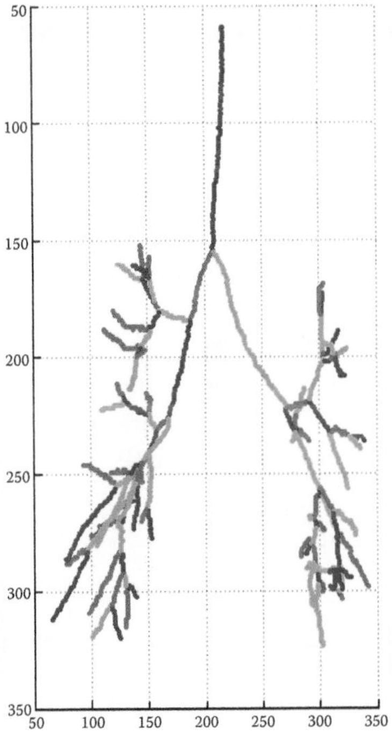

FIGURE 8.19
An example of a labeled airway skeleton.

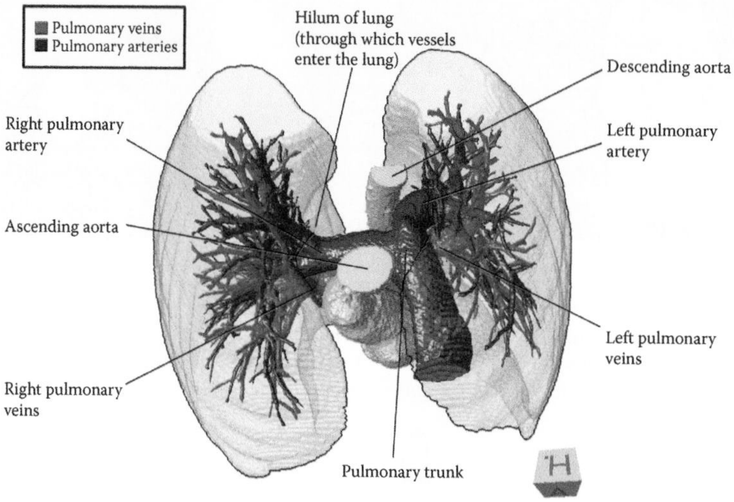

FIGURE 9.1
Anatomy of the pulmonary artery trees. The vessels inside the left and right lung were automatically segmented using the method described in Section 9.2.4. Afterward, the arteries were interactively separated from the veins using the random walker algorithm [3] limited to the segmented vessels. The mediastinum has been cropped to the heart region and the containing structures were interactively segmented using random walker as well.

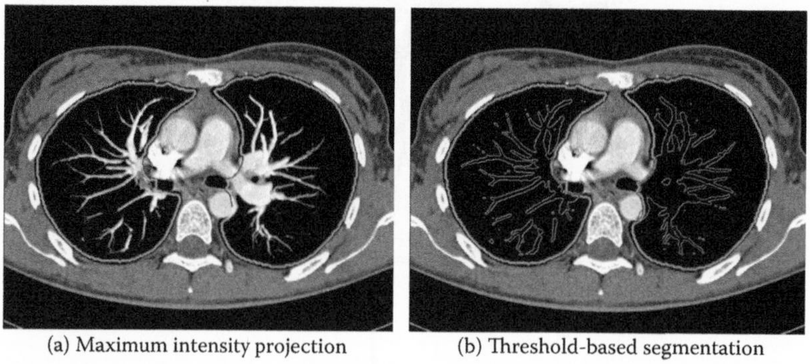

FIGURE 9.5
Segmentation result using a simple threshold operation. (a) A thoracic CT scan using a windowing of C/W = 100/600 HU. The interior of the lung regions (green contour) are shown as thick maximum intensity projection over 25 slices. (b) Segmentation results using a threshold range of $0 < I(\mathbf{x}) < 1476$ HU as contours.

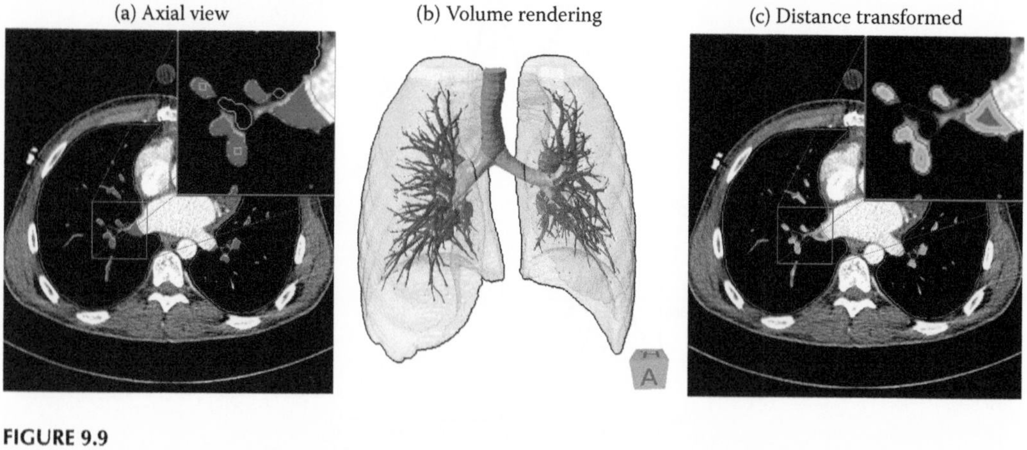

FIGURE 9.9
(a) The core vessel segmentation [2] is shown as an overlay to the axial view. The extracted seed points are shown as small boxes. (b) The corresponding result is shown as volume rendering. For each voxel within the segmentation result, the minimal 3D Euclidean distance to the vessel surface has been calculated and is shown color-coded in (c).

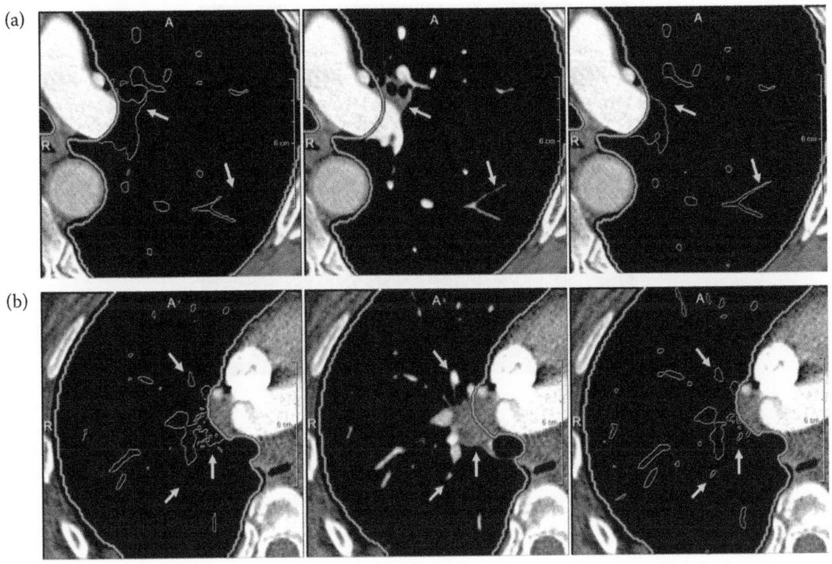

FIGURE 9.11
Segmentation results using the multimodal affinity function [1] (right) in comparison with the intensity-based affinity function [2] (left) shown as contours corresponding to two different patients (original images shown in the center). One can observe that the multimodal segmentation extends further to the periphery than the purely intensity-based one. At the same time, leakage into nonvessel regions is suppressed. In particular, please compare the segmentation outcome at the positions highlighted by arrows, for instance pointing towards branches that have not been delineated (and hence do not appear as contours) in the left image, but are correctly delineated in the right image.

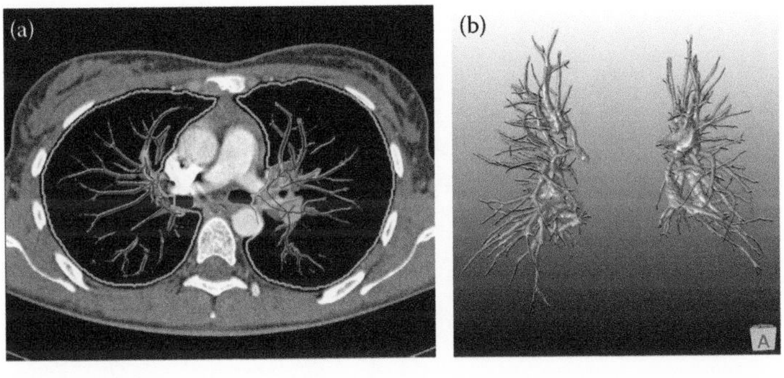

FIGURE 9.12
Segmentation result and corresponding centerlines using the multimodal affinity function with $P_{vessel} > 0.57$ using the same data and visualization settings as shown in Figure 9.5. Note that it features almost no false-positives in the hilum area compared with the threshold-based segmentation, whereas small vessels are not always segmented to their distal end. Decreasing P_{vessel} would add smaller branches to the segmentation at the cost of increasing false-positives.

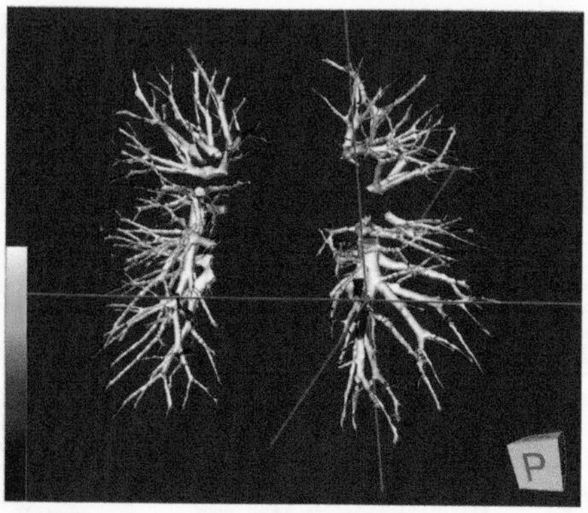

FIGURE 9.13
Vessel segmentation with the outer surface colored by the inner contents [41,42]. Unlike in the original work, potential PE regions are color-coded, with dark colors corresponding to low HU values, to avoid confusions between regular 3D shading and emboli visualization. A marked PE is shown with cross-hairs, which is also shown in 2D in Figure 9.2(b).

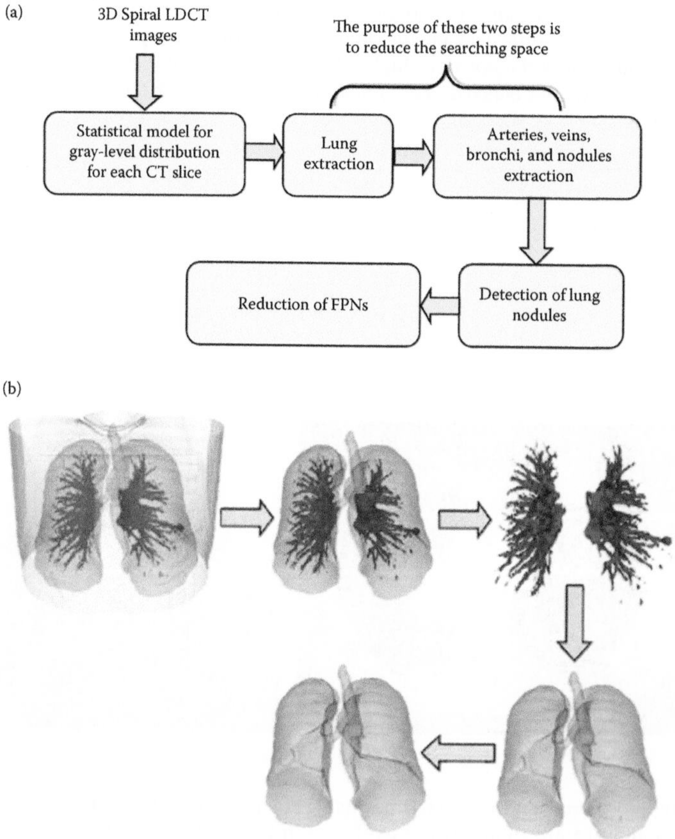

FIGURE 10.1
The lung abnormality detection system: (a) block diagram and (b) illustration example.

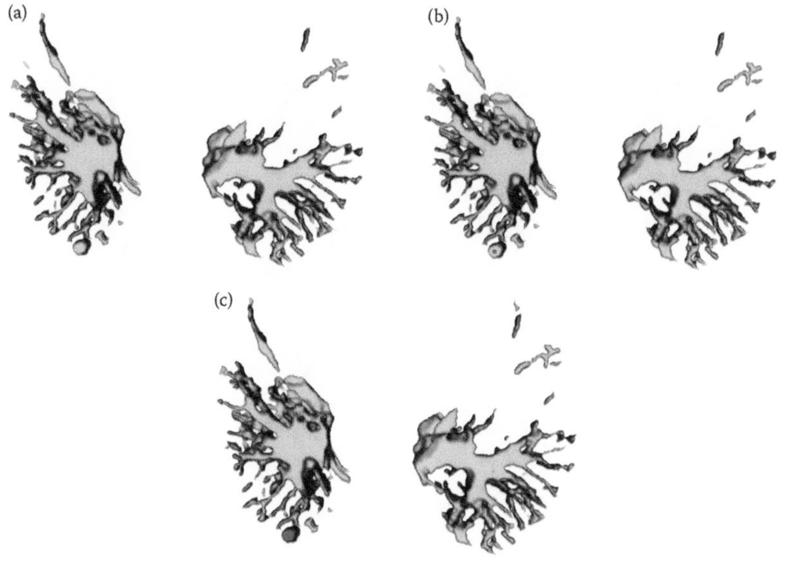

FIGURE 10.3
(a) Part of the separated 3D lung objects, (b) the initialized level set shown in red, and (c) the finally extracted potential nodule candidate.

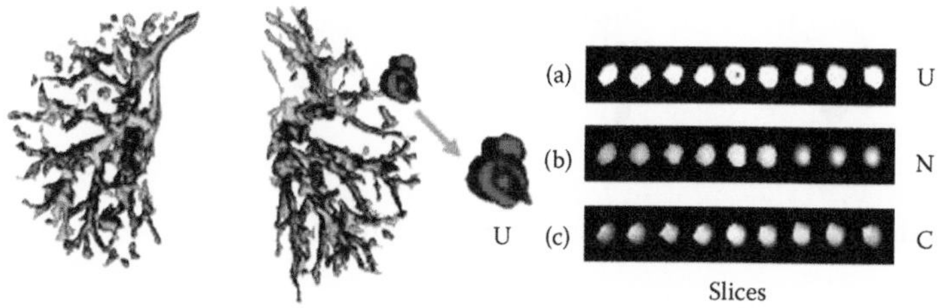

FIGURE 10.5
Detected nodule candidate: (a) slices of the extracted voxel set U, (b) the gray-level prototype N, and (c) the actual gray levels C (the correlation $\text{Corr}_{C,N} = 0.886$).

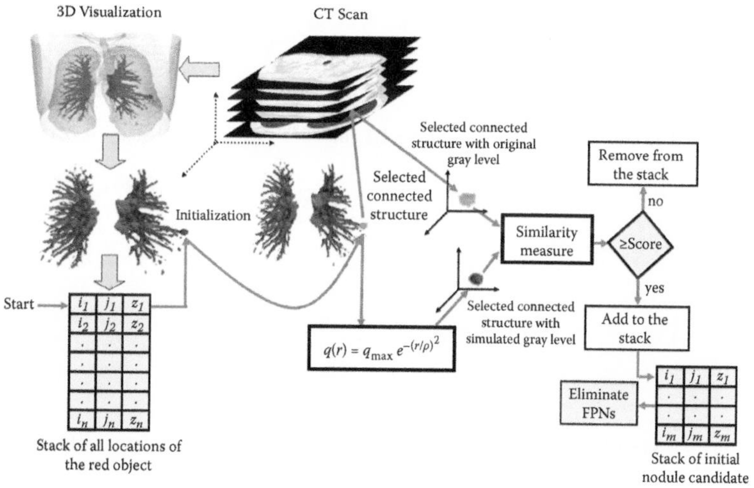

FIGURE 10.6
Step-by-step illustration of the proposed CAD detection system.

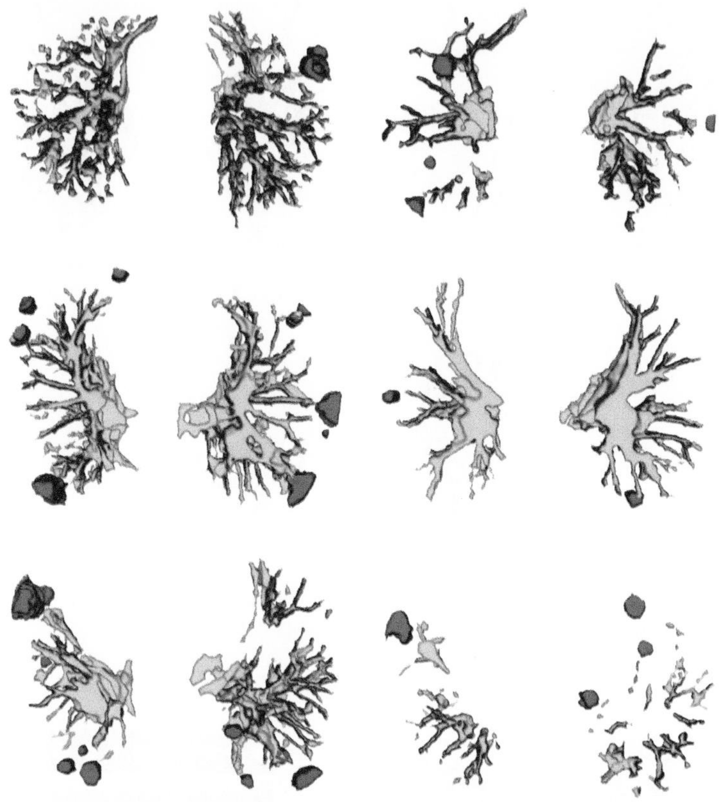

FIGURE 10.8
Large candidate nodules (shown in red) detected with our approach.

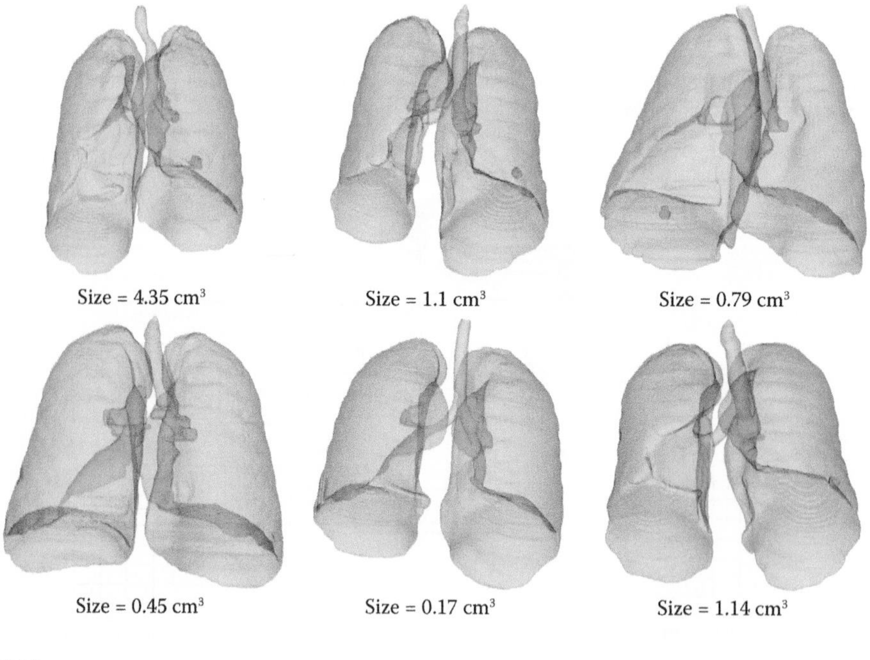

FIGURE 10.9
Large candidate nodules (shown in green) detected with our approach.

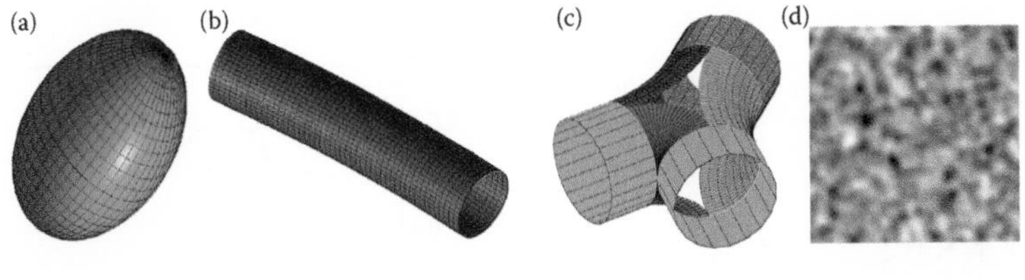

FIGURE 11.6
Graphical representation of the nodule, vessel, junction, and parenchyma models. (a) The nodule model is represented by an ellipsoid with axes $a = b \le c$. The vessel model is represented by a segment of a torus with minor and major radii given by $r \le R$. (c) Three tori with adequate parameters form the junction model, with the cylindrical extensions are included for clarity. (d) In contrast to the previous three models, the parenchyma model is not represented through a geometric shape, but as an isotropic Gaussian random field.

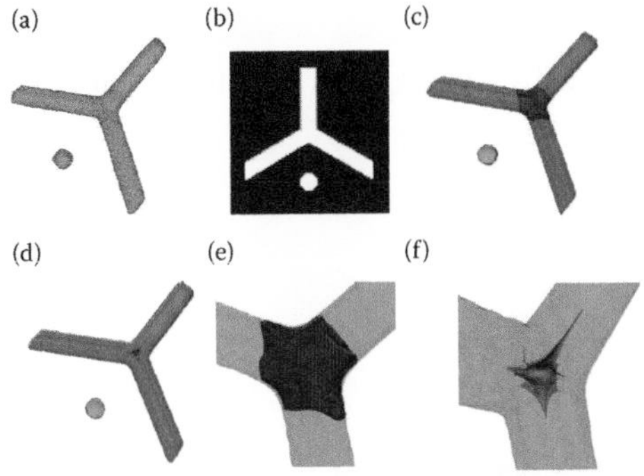

FIGURE 11.9
Experiments on synthetic data. (a) 3D rendering and (b) 2D slice of a phantom vessel bifurcation. Bayesian voxel labeling results (c) with and (d) without including the junction model with zoom-in views shown in (e) and (f), respectively. Each voxel is colored according to the model with the highest probability using red for vessels, green for nodules, and blue for junctions. Note that without the junction model, (d) and (f) show nodule responses at the bifurcation center.

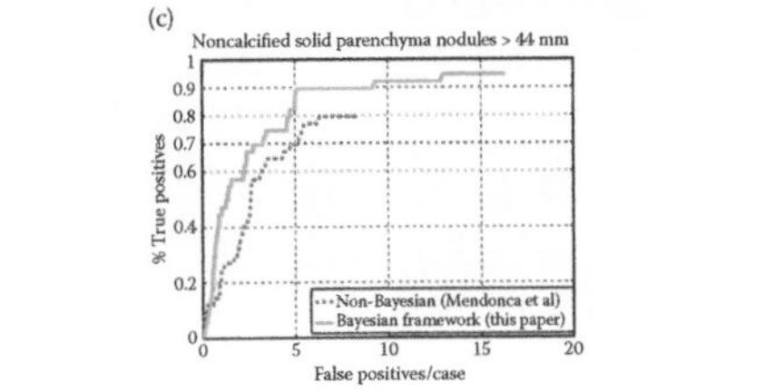

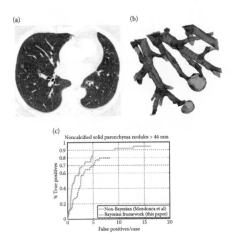

FIGURE 11.10
Experimental validation. (a) A 2D slice of a high-resolution CT scan with nodule labels overlaid in green on the intensity image. (b) A 3D rendering of the voxel labeling for a small region from the same case showing nodules (green), vessels (red), and junctions (blue). (c) FROC curves comparing performance of the Bayesian voxel labeling framework to a curvature-based nonprobabilistic approach given in ref. [32].

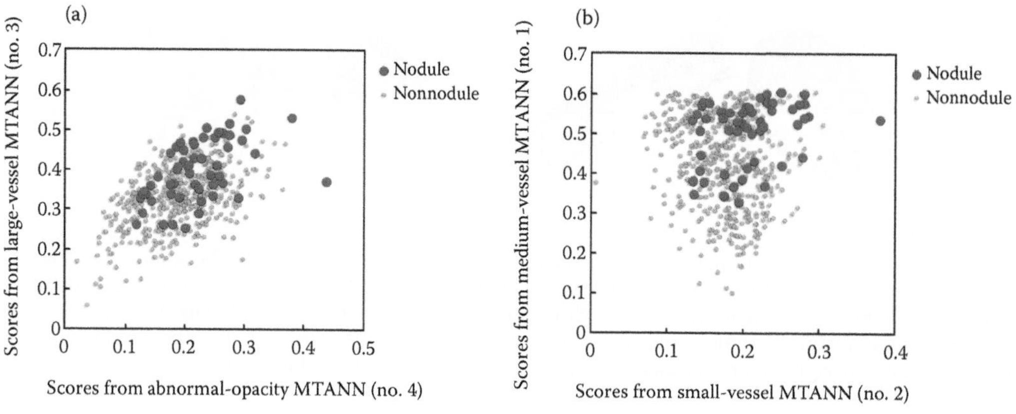

FIGURE 13.10
Distributions of scores from expert MTANN nos. 1–4 for reduction of four different types of FPs.

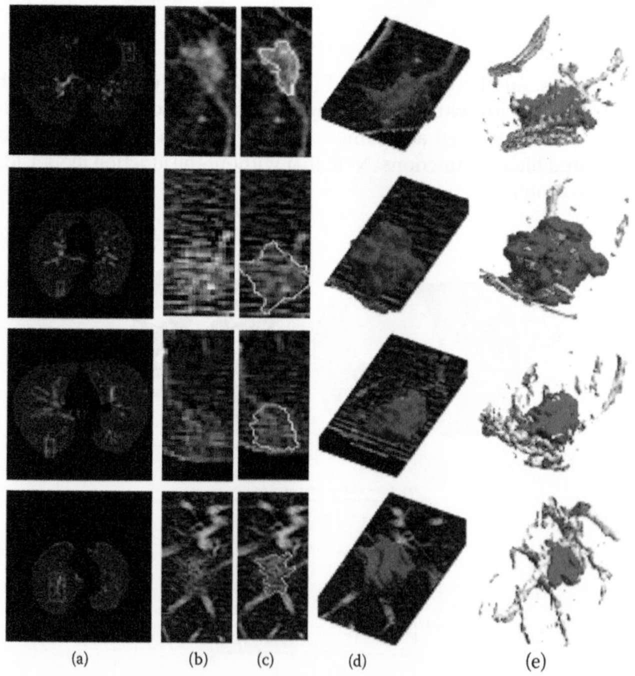

FIGURE 14.8
GGO segmentation—four segmented GGO nodules are shown: (a) original CT images containing GGO nodules, (b) enlarged GGO areas, (c) segmented GGO, (d) 3D reconstruction of segmented GGO overlaid with original CT images in (a), and (e) 3D reconstruction of segmented GGO with other nearby structures.

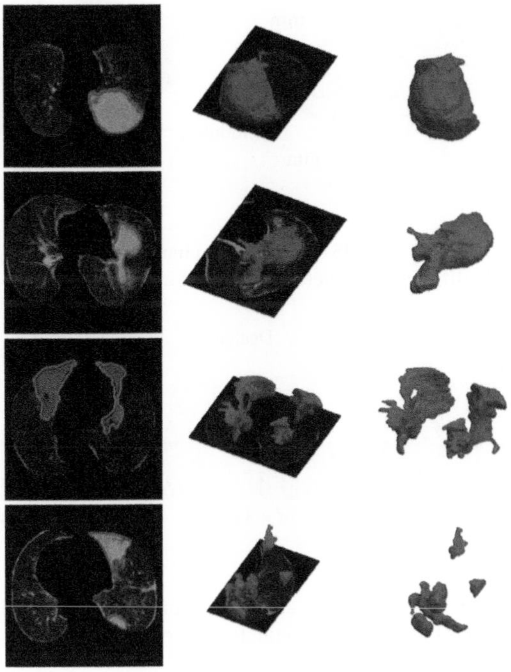

FIGURE 14.12
Results: (left) segmented large lung lesions projected onto a slice and (middle and right) corresponding 3D lesions.

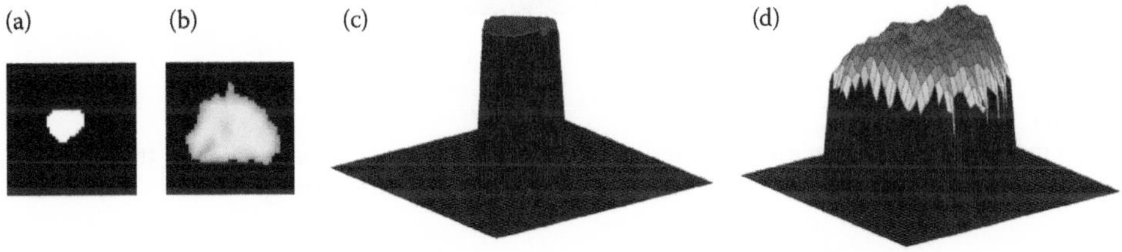

FIGURE 17.2
(a, b) 2D and (c, d) 3D visualization of Hounsfield values over an axial cross section of a (a, c) benign and (b, d) malignant nodule.

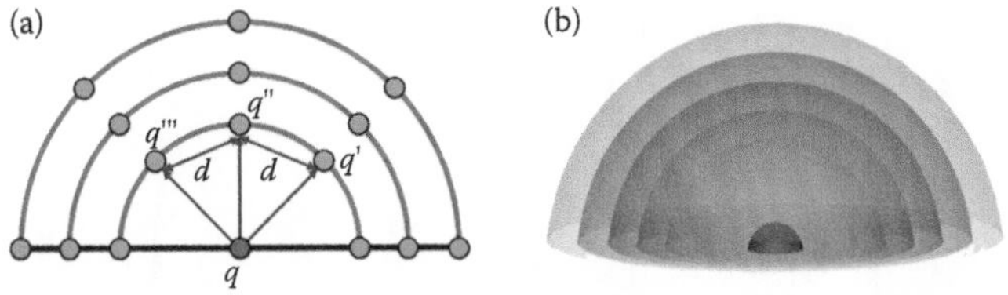

FIGURE 17.3
Central-symmetric second-order (a) 2D and (b) 3D neighborhood system.

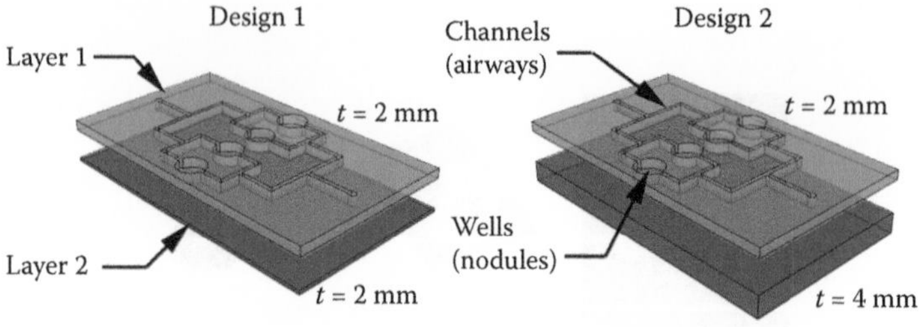

FIGURE 18.1
The first phantom model consists of two PDMS devices, with channels representing the airways and wells representing the nodules. The only difference between the two devices is the thickness of the bottom layer.

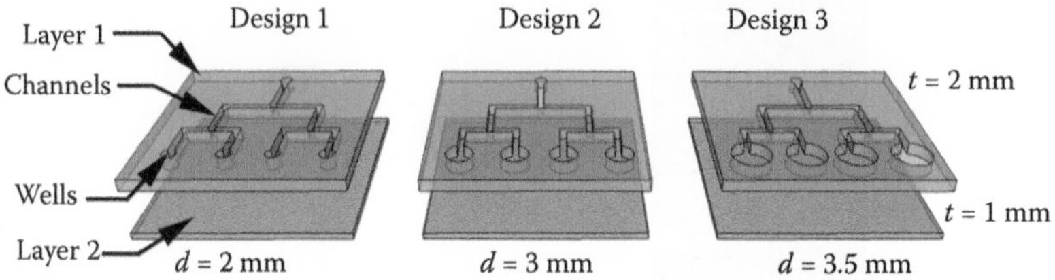

FIGURE 18.2
The second phantom model mimics tumor progression and is similar in construction to model 1. The only difference among the three designs is the increasing diameter of the nodules.

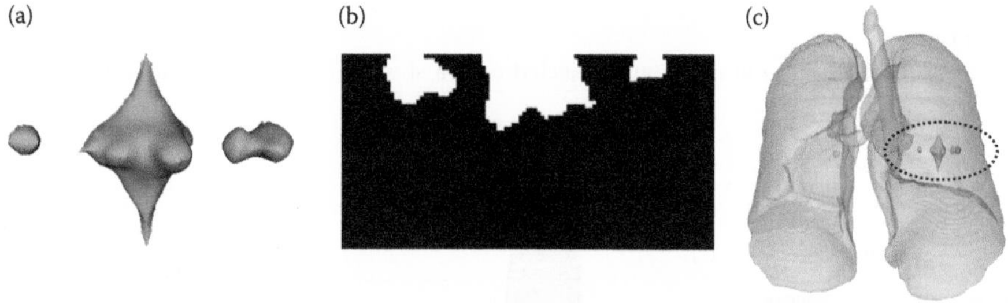

FIGURE 18.3
(a) The 3D neighborhood system estimated for the lung tissues, (b) its 2D cross section in the plane $\zeta = 0$ (in white), and (c) its superposition onto the lungs reconstructed from the LDCT images.

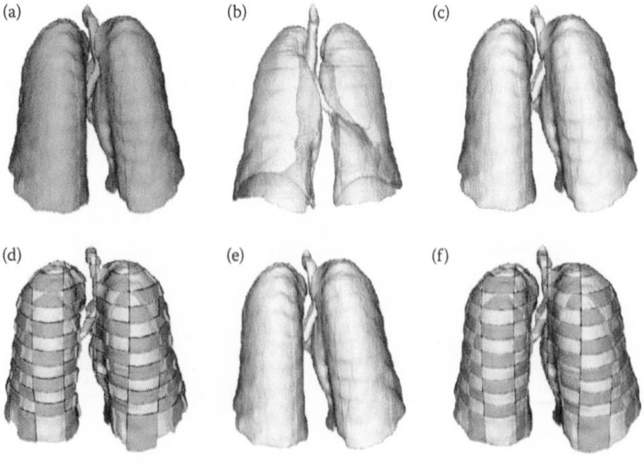

FIGURE 18.4
3D global and local registration: (a) reference data, (b) target data, (c) target data after 3D affine transformation, (d) checkerboard visualization to show the motion of lung tissues, (e) results of our nonrigid registration, and (f) checkerboard visualization to show the quality of the proposed local deformation model.

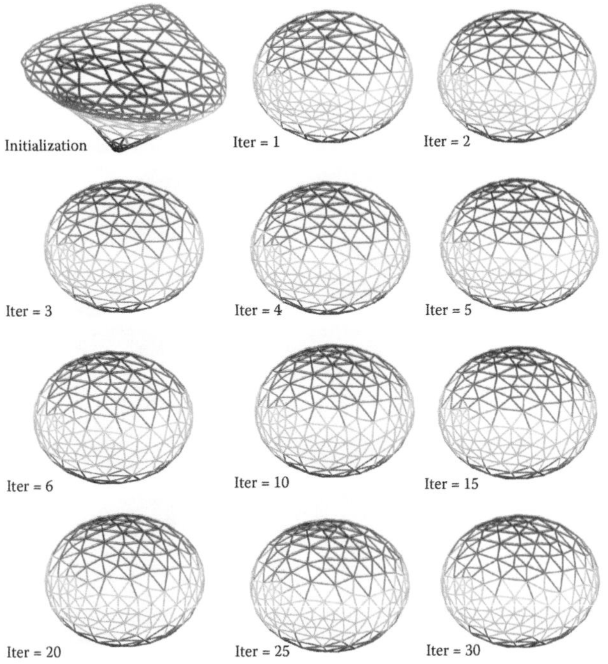

FIGURE 19.7
A step-by-step illustration of the output of attraction–repulsion algorithm at different iterations.

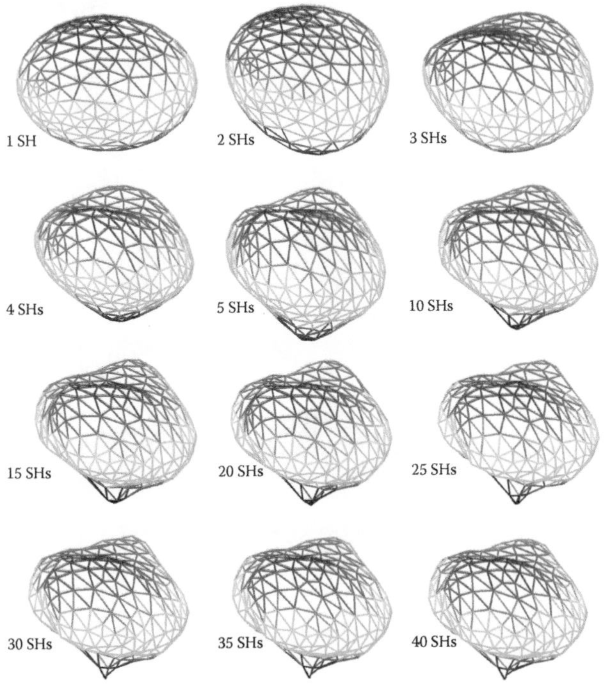

FIGURE 19.9
A step-by-step lung nodule surface reconstruction using SHs.

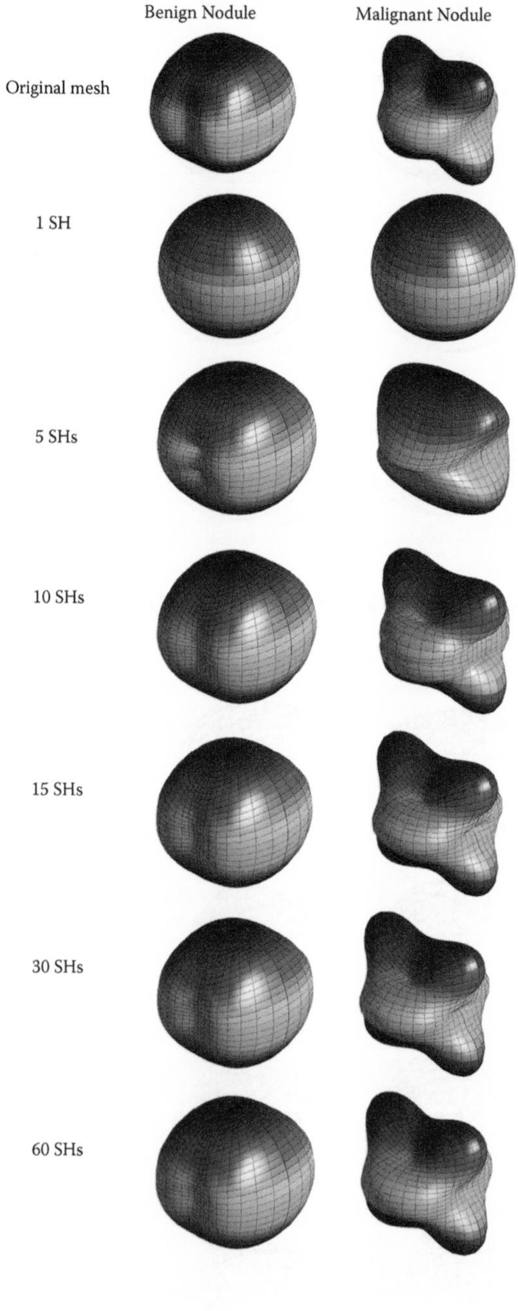

FIGURE 19.10
Approximation of the 3D shape for malignant and benign lung nodules.

TABLE 18.7

3D Visualization of the Detected Lung Nodules in End-Expiration BH and End-Inspiration BH CT Scans

	Benign Cases		Malignant Cases	
	Subject 1	**Subject 2**	**Subject 3**	**Subject 4**
End-expiration BHs	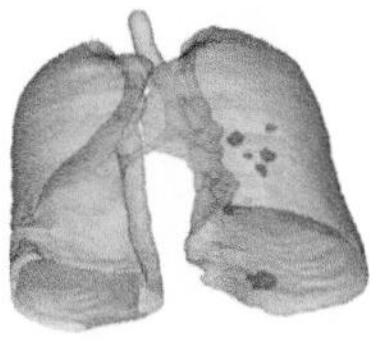	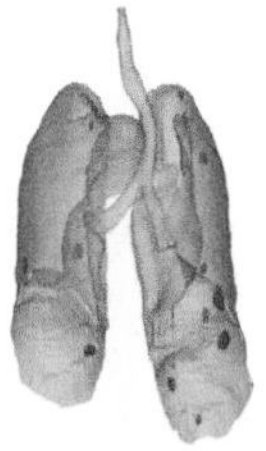	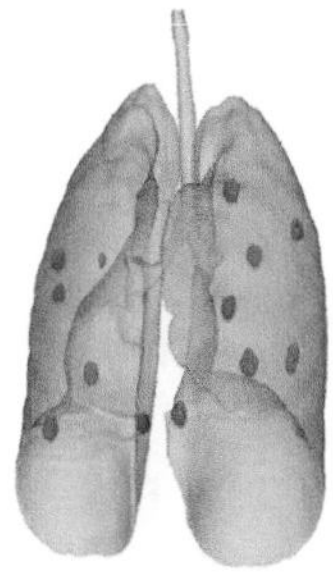	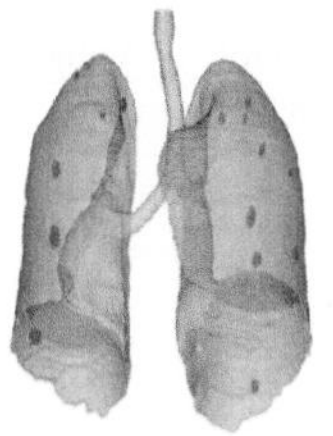
End-inspiration BHs	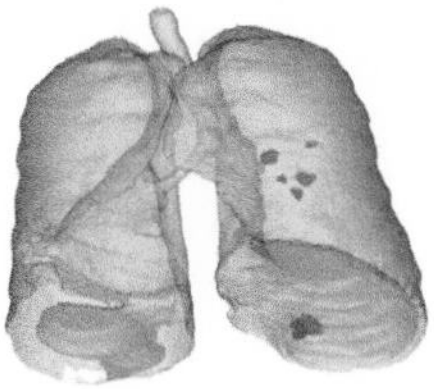	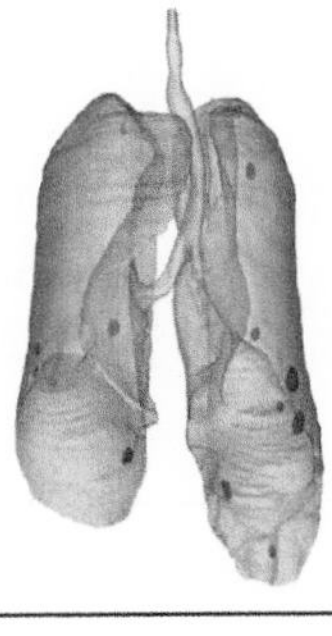	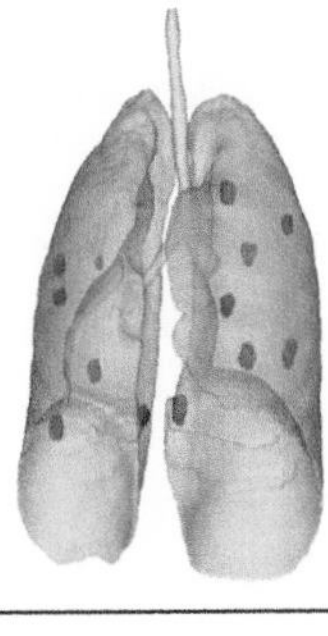	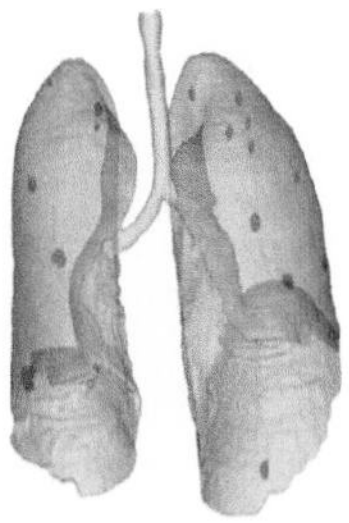

TABLE 18.8

3-D Illustration of the Registration Results

		End-Expiration BH (Reference)	End-Inspiration BH (Target)	Registration Results	Checkerboard Visualization
Benign cases	Subject 1	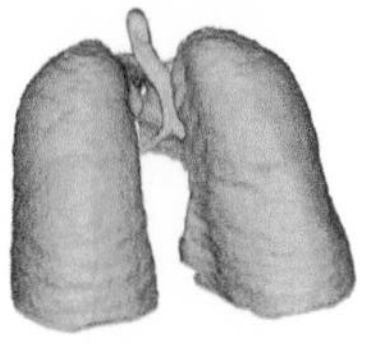	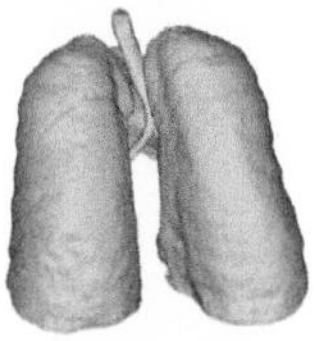	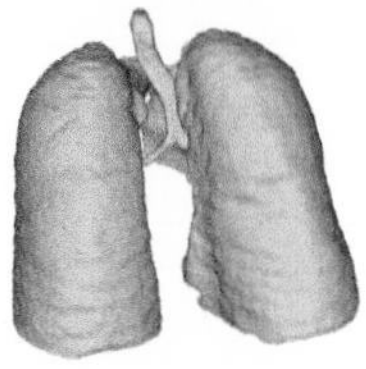	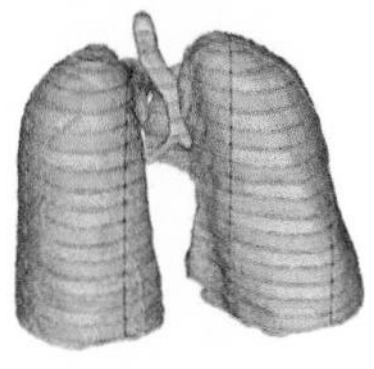
	Subject 2	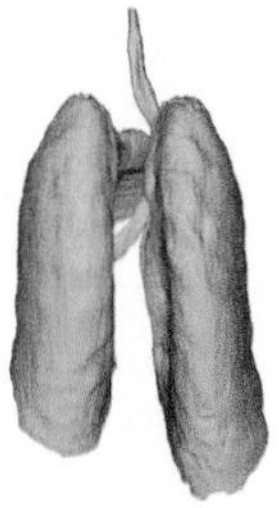	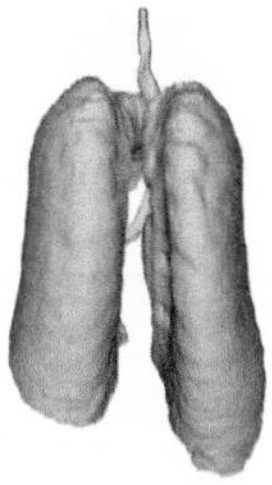	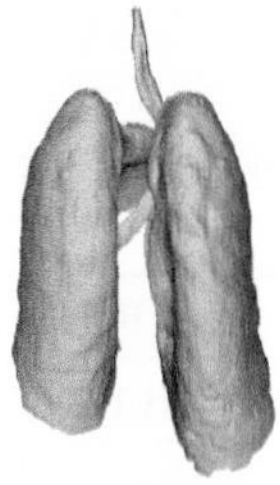	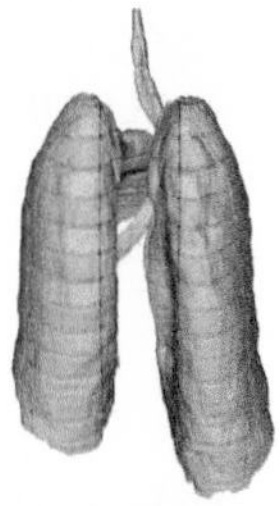
Malignant cases	Subject 3	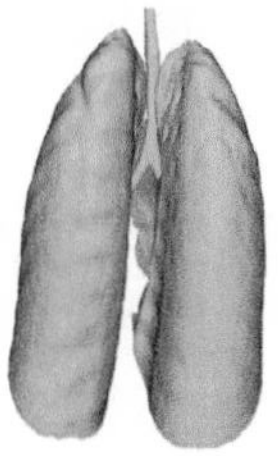	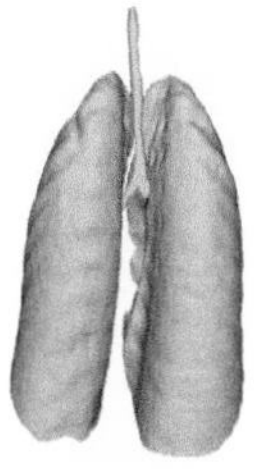	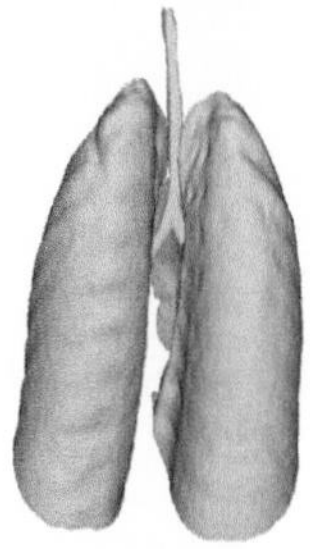	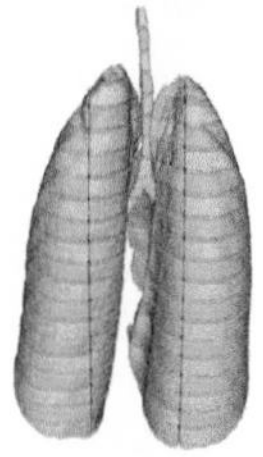
	Subject 4	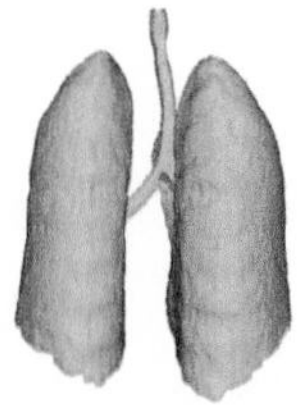	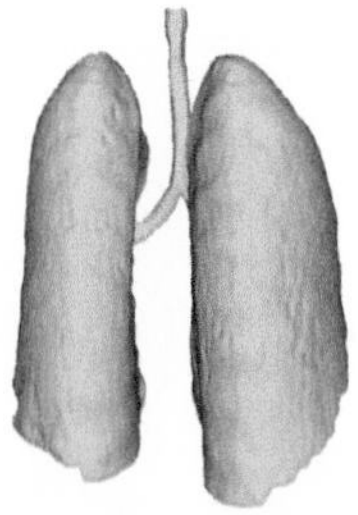	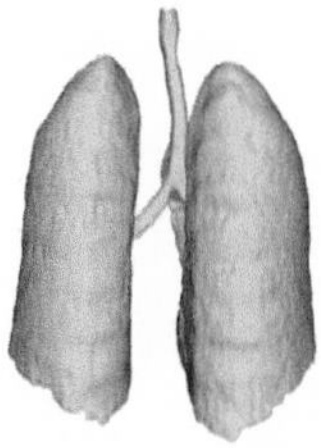	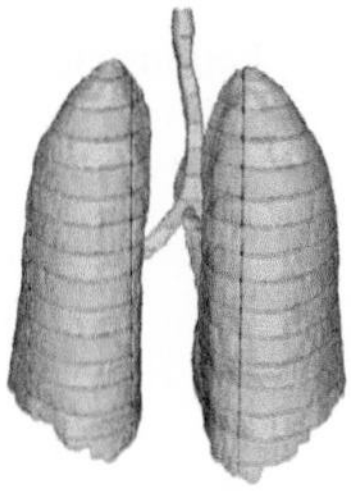

9

Pulmonary Vessel Segmentation for Multislice CT Data: Methods and Applications

Jens N. Kaftan and Til Aach

CONTENTS

9.1 Introduction

The detection and delineation of vascular structures from computed tomography (CT) angiography (CTA) data is often a prerequisite for diagnosis, treatment planning, and follow-up studies in clinical applications. To this end, a (iodine-based) contrast agent is typically injected to give blood a higher attenuation, allowing its better distinction from surrounding tissues. Such examinations using a CT device are then referred to as CTA. With recent advances in image acquisition technologies, the spatial resolution of image data has been significantly increased. Consequently, the number of slices that need to be read by the physician during a typical examination has been constantly increasing, whereas CT images reveal increasingly more details, allowing an improved diagnosis of diseases that had been previously difficult to detect. Considering the limited time a radiologist may typically spend on a case in clinical routine, imaging applications that support the examiner's tasks and optimize the clinical workflow have become more and more important.

The remainder of this chapter is organized as follows. First, the pulmonary anatomy is illustrated and medical applications that directly impact the vasculature are summarized. Subsequently, different methods for segmenting pulmonary arteries and veins from CT data with or without contrast agent are detailed in Section 9.2, with particular focus on a fuzzy segmentation scheme (Section 9.2.4). Besides computer-aided detection (CAD) of diseases directly influencing the appearance of the vascular trees, other algorithms could also benefit from vessel segmentations. In particular, further segmentation algorithms can be improved by using additional knowledge from the vessel tree. These applications, which might already be established procedures or still limited to research, are summarized in Section 9.9.3. Finally, we give a summary and draw conclusions.

9.1.1 Anatomy

The vascular system transports the blood and the substances it carries to and from all parts of the body. It can be divided into two parts, the systemic circulation, which serves the body as a whole (except the lungs), and the pulmonary circulation, which carries the blood to and from the lungs. Vessels that carry blood away from the heart are called arteries, whereas vessels returning to the heart are called veins.

The pulmonary vessels consist of two trees, the pulmonary venous and the pulmonary arterial tree (cf. Figure 9.1). Both tree structures enter the lung area through the hilum. The pulmonary arterial tree, originating in the right ventricle of the heart, pumps oxygen-poor blood into the lungs. The pulmonary veins carry oxygen-rich blood from the capillaries in the lungs into the left atrium. The region that contains, among others, the heart and the major blood vessels close to the heart is called the mediastinum. The third tubular tree structure present in the lungs is the bronchial tree. It supplies the lungs with air and starts from the trachea and then splits into the left and right main bronchus. Generally, every bronchus is accompanied by an artery, with both having similar diameters [4].

9.1.2 Vascular Diseases

Diseases affecting the vascular system are common and can be lethal. Cardiovascular diseases, as an example, are widespread, with an estimated number of 80 million American adults having one or more types of cardiovascular disease. In 2005, approximately 860,000 deaths in the United States were attributed to cardiovascular disease [5]. Vascular diseases include, but are not limited to:

- Blood clots—occurring in a deep vein, are referred to as deep venous thrombosis, whereas those occurring inside the lung are known as pulmonary emboli (PE).
- Stenosis—an abnormal narrowing of the vessel.
- Aneurysm—an abnormal bulge in the wall of a blood vessel, most commonly occurring in the aorta.

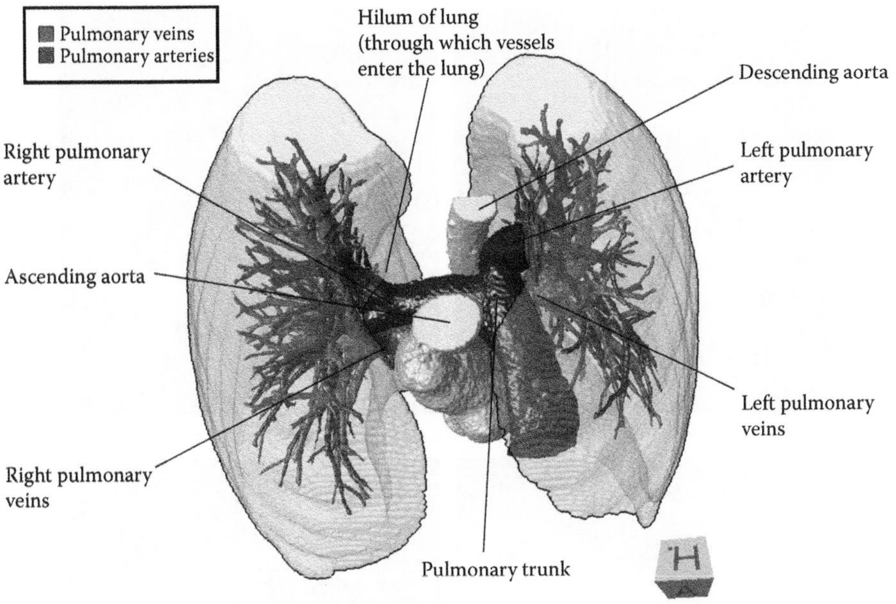

FIGURE 9.1
(See color insert.) Anatomy of the pulmonary artery trees. The vessels inside the left and right lung were automatically segmented using the method described in Section 9.2.4. Afterward, the arteries were interactively separated from the veins using the random walker algorithm [3] limited to the segmented vessels. The mediastinum has been cropped to the heart region and the containing structures were interactively segmented using random walker as well.

The most prominent application considering pulmonary vessels directly is probably the examination for PE. However, imaging the lung may also unveil other pulmonary diseases for which the knowledge of the vessels' location is useful. For instance, it can be used to improve the outcome of airway and lung fissure segmentation algorithms, which, in turn, affect several applications such as virtual bronchoscopy or lobectomy planning. Additionally, vessel bifurcations might serve as potential landmarks for registration purposes for follow-up examinations. At the same time, different diseases that do not affect the vasculature directly but may influence the segmentation performance can be frequently observed in conjunction with vascular diseases including PE. Some examples are shown in Figure 9.2.

9.1.2.1 Pulmonary Embolism

PE is the obstruction of a pulmonary artery by, e.g., a blood clot (cf. Figure 9.3). Such a thrombus typically forms in the deep venous system of the lower extremities (deep venous thrombosis), becomes detached from its origin, and travels through the vasculature to the lung. Large thrombi lodge at the bifurcation of the main pulmonary artery or the lobar branches and cause hemodynamic compromise. Smaller emboli continue traveling distally, occluding smaller vessels in the lung periphery (Figure 9.3).

PE is a common, potentially fatal, disorder occurring in some 600,000 to 630,000 patients per year in the United States [6]. Of these cases, 11% die in the first hour and it has been estimated that PE will remain undiagnosed in approximately 70% of patients who survive the initial thromboembolic event. Overall, 200,000 patients (31.7%) will die from this disease

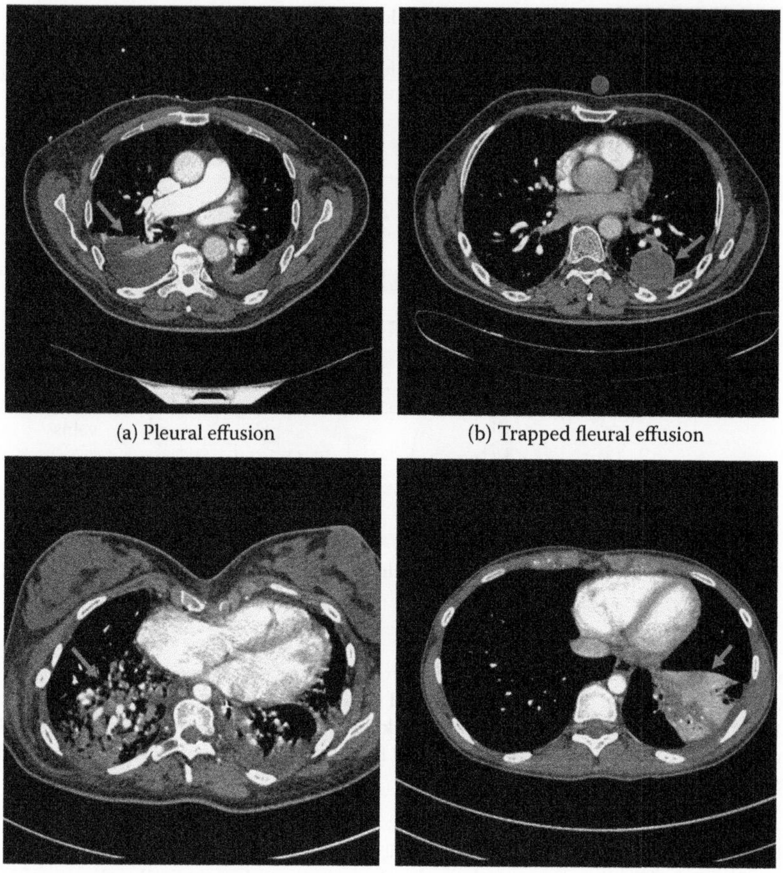

(a) Pleural effusion (b) Trapped fleural effusion

(c) Pulmonary infiltrates (d) Atelectasis

FIGURE 9.2
Examples of nonvessel related diseases.

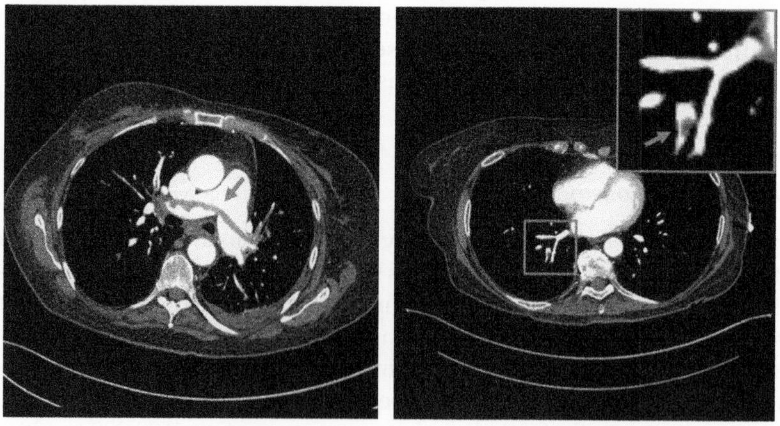

(a) Mediastinal PE (b) Segmental PE

FIGURE 9.3
Examples of PE in contrast-enhanced CT.

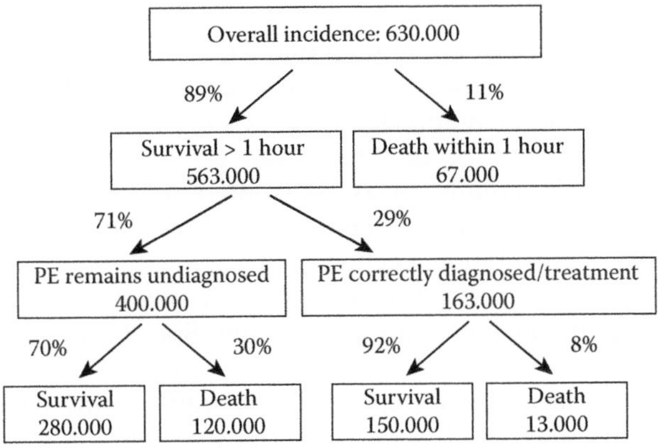

FIGURE 9.4
Incidence of PE in the United States [6].

(Figure 9.4). PE is therefore the second most frequent cause for unexpected death (after sudden cardiac death), and the third most common cause of death in hospitalized patients [7].

Although PE is a frequent cause of death, an early and reliable diagnosis and an appropriate treatment with anticoagulant drugs to dissolve the clot can prevent mortality (the survival rate after PE was correctly diagnosed is approximately 92%). The fast treatment with anticoagulant drugs is therefore essential on the one hand, but on the other hand, it also involves some risks requiring a correct diagnosis before treatment.

9.1.2.2 Pulmonary Hypertension

Pulmonary hypertension (PH) is defined as an increase in blood pressure in the lung vasculature, often caused by a recognizable cardiac or pulmonary disorder. PH can be observed in pulmonary arteries and veins and, in association with disorders of the respiratory system or hypoxemia, caused by thrombotic or embolic diseases, or by disorders directly affecting the pulmonary vasculature. In CTA examinations, PH often appears as enlarged central pulmonary arteries with an abrupt reduction in vascular diameter. In general, it has been shown that patients with pulmonary arterial hypertension have central pulmonary arteries larger than patients with normal arterial pressure. PH should be suspected when the diameter of the main pulmonary artery is larger than 2.8 cm or larger than the aortic diameter. Another finding is an increased diameter of the right and left pulmonary arteries of more than 1.6 cm. An enlargement of more peripheral arteries can be observed when the ratio between the arterial diameter and the diameter of its accompanying bronchus exceeds a normal bronchoarterial diameter ratio between 1.0 and 1.2 on segmental and subsegmental level [4].

9.2 Vessel Segmentation

Pulmonary vessel segmentation from CT data has been intensively studied with a focus on different applications [1–2, 8–25]. Typical pulmonary vessel segmentation approaches vary from threshold operations to front propagation techniques. These algorithms usually limit themselves to the lungs (cf., Chapters 1–2) as the region of interest (ROI). Some approaches, however, extract lung and vessel regions simultaneously. Because the lung exhibits considerable contrast between vessels and their surroundings, many techniques rely solely on intensity information as a segmentation feature (Section 9.2.1). Besides that, Hessian-based vessel enhancement techniques (Section 9.2.2) are a popular choice in pulmonary vessel segmentation (Section 9.2.3). Finally, fuzzy segmentation techniques have been recently proposed that compute, for each voxel, the likelihood of it belonging to the vasculature rather than to a binary segmentation (Section 9.2.4).

In practice, accurate and quick modeling of blood vessels in contrast-enhanced CT images is still a challenging task in many applications. Specifically,

1. Intensity contrast may change depending on scan-specific parameters or even within a single vascular structure/along a single vessel.
2. Nearby bright, high-density structures, such as bones or airway walls, might be confused with vessels.
3. A single vessel tree can have large and small vessels, i.e., the vessel scale changes significantly.
4. Local vessel structures may deviate from a tubular structure because of the presence of pathologies, such as PEs.
5. Vessels in close proximity might cause their segmentation to overlap, resulting in a potential merging of different vascular structures, e.g., arteries and veins.

In clinical applications, a vessel segmentation algorithm must be able to produce robust and accurate results despite the listed difficulties meeting certain time constraints.

9.2.1 Intensity-Based Approaches

The major pulmonary vessels appear brighter than other objects inside the lungs in CT angiography data, with reasonably good contrast relative to their surroundings. In many cases, efficient threshold operations limited to the lungs as ROI provide good results for segmenting those very bright vessels. For instance, Figure 9.5 shows the major pulmonary

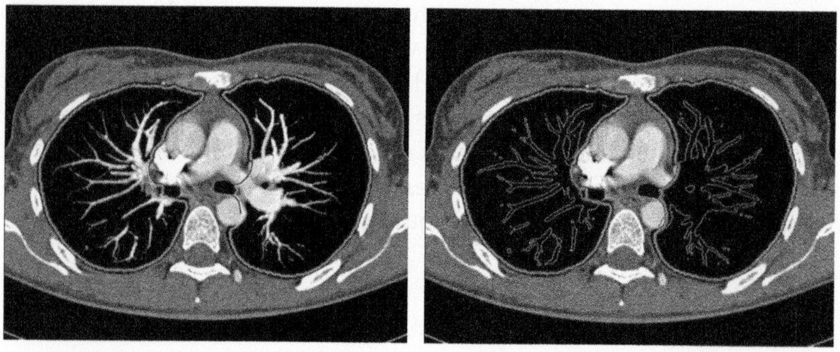

(a) Maximum intensity projection (b) Threshold-based segmentation

FIGURE 9.5
(See color insert.) Segmentation result using a simple threshold operation. (a) A thoracic CT scan using a windowing of C/W = 100/600 HU. The interior of the lung regions (green contour) are shown as thick maximum intensity projection over 25 slices. (b) Segmentation results using a threshold range of $0 < I(\mathbf{x}) < 1476$ HU as contours.

vessels inside the lungs as a maximum intensity projection over 25 slices using a window setting of center/width (C/W) = 100/600 Hounsfield units (HU) and the resulting segmentation using an interval banded by thresholds of $0 < I(\mathbf{x}) < 1476$ HU.

However, there are several reasons why such a simple approach is not sufficient in most applications. In particular, smaller vessels have lower CT values than the main and lobar branches because of, for example, partial volume effects and inhomogeneous contrast agent distribution. More specifically, small vessels might appear darker than connective tissue near the mediastinum or airway walls, preventing the separation of vessels and nonvessels with a single threshold. Additionally, the observed vessel intensities in each data set might vary depending on contrast agent, bolus phase, scan protocol, etc., or even within one data set. As a consequence, most purely intensity-based approaches determine an initial segmentation using a threshold operation, which is refined by further postprocessing steps and/or more sophisticated segmentation algorithms.

The method presented in ref. [8] segments the lung vessels in contrast-enhanced CT data by first applying a fixed threshold to the lung areas. Regions above that threshold are then analyzed by a connected component labeling method, and small, isolated components that do not exceed a minimal volume are disregarded. Such an initial threshold can be further adapted based on the intensity histogram of the data set in consideration. Figure 9.6 shows exemplarily three histograms of the data shown in Figure 9.5. To this end, the histogram is plotted over the entire volume, inside the body volume [9], and inside the lung regions [2], showing several characteristic peaks.

Masutani et al. [9] used an initial lower threshold that corresponds to the identified peak position of the opacified vessels at more than 176 HU (with an upper threshold of 1476 HU to exclude metal artifacts). In contrast, Bouma et al. [10] defined the initial threshold as the average value between 0 HU and the histogram peak above 150 HU. For CT images without any contrast, Zhou et al. [11] proposed to use the local minimum that is closest to 0 HU as lower threshold. What all methods have in common is that the resulting segmentations are only used as input for a subsequent region-growing or front propagation step.

Given one or more seed positions, Bülow et al. [13] proposed to use a fast-marching front propagation process to segment the vascular trees. In their implementation, they define an intensity-based, constant front propagation speed function. That is, front voxels that exceed

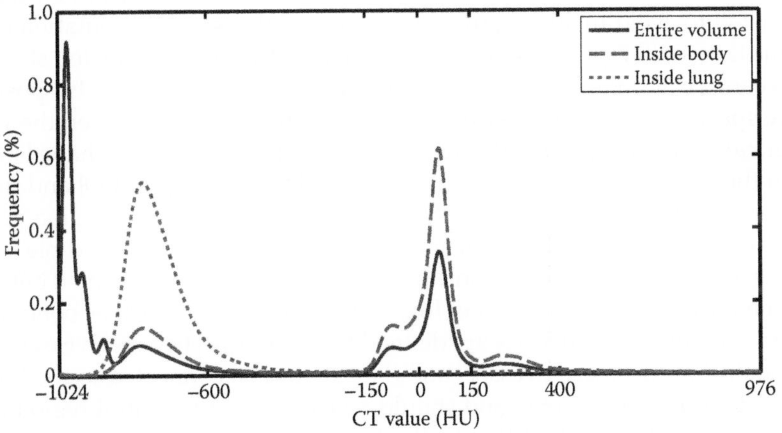

FIGURE 9.6
Histogram of a CTA chest scan (entire volume, inside body volume, inside lung regions). Note that percentages are normalized by the corresponding total volume for each plot.

a lower threshold of −600 HU are included in the object, whereas the front stops at voxels of lower intensities. The front arrival time, however, is only dependent on the distance to the seed point because of the constant speed term. Altogether, such front propagation can be considered as a region-growing process, with the advantage that branching points are simultaneously extracted if the front splits into two or more disconnected components (cf. [26]). Such geometrical clustering into segments or branches allows for locally adapting segmentation parameters or to use higher-level knowledge. In the described framework, a segment is rejected if its radius exceeds twice the radius of the parent segment. In addition, terminal segments less than 5 mm in length are pruned.

This method is also used in ref. [10] to connect isolated vessel regions to the main vasculature. After segmenting the major vessels using a global threshold, peripheral vessels are addressed separately. In particular, a lower threshold of T_{min} = −150 HU is applied for regions with a distance above 15 mm to the mediastinum and only resulting components with radii < 2.4 mm are kept. As a consequence of using threshold operations (particularly when using even different thresholds for different regions) resulting vessels might lack connectivity. To connect isolated vessels to the main vasculature, a front propagation is used to extract the minimal cost paths with respect to intensity and distance. In particular, the front propagation is limited to regions with intensities above −150 HU.

Alternatively, Zhou et al. [11] reported a refinement method similar to methods commonly applied to airway tree segmentation for segmenting vessels from multislice chest CT images without any contrast enhancement. Using the initially detected vessel regions as seed points, an intensity-based region-growing process including branching point detection is started. The intensity threshold is consecutively reduced until leakage into nonvessel regions is detected and the lowest value that does not cause leakage is selected. Moreover, this process is repeated on a branch-by-branch basis. That is, after determining the "optimal" threshold for a vessel tree given its root, each child branch is considered as the root of an independent subtree, which again is refined using the described procedure. Finally, voxels near the surface of airways are considered as bronchial wall and hence removed from the vessel segmentation based on a simple distance threshold. Fetita et al. [12] also paid particular attention to removing airway walls from the vessel segmentation in their intensity-based segmentation approach from noncontrasted data. To this end, the intensities in the airway wall regions defined by an airway lumen segmentation were attenuated to avoid including these into the initial vessel segmentation obtained by a fixed-value threshold (T_{min} = −145 HU). Additionally, they filter extracted skeleton points from the reconstructed vessels using a geometric feature to remove false-positive candidates. More specifically, for each skeleton point, the intersection between the vessel mask and a spherical structuring element is determined and its cylindrical shape is validated.

Although the previous approaches were all limited to the lungs as ROI and the resulting segmentation is optionally extended to the mediastinum using, e.g., region-growing, the hysteresis thresholding approach of Masutani et al. [9] is applied to the whole body region. That is, using an initial threshold, not only pulmonary vessels are segmented but also vessels inside the mediastinum as well as other high-density structures such as bones (spine, ribs, etc.). To this end, different heuristics are defined to distinguish between vessel and nonvessel components. For instance, a vessel candidate should be connected to the lung regions, should exceed a minimal volume, and should be located in the central region of the body to exclude ribs. One drawback of this method is that bones and vessels cannot always be separated using intensity information only. In particular, one connected component might include vascular as well as bone structures. Finally, a region-growing process with constant parameters ($-124 < I(\mathbf{x}) < 1476$ HU) is applied, starting from the initial segmentation.

In his PhD thesis designated to artery–vein separation from thoracic CTA scans, Park [14] used an intensity-based expectation–maximization algorithm to separate each voxel in the volume into one of six classes: air, lungs, muscles, soft tissue, blood vessels, and bones, and high intensity values, represented by a mixture model of eight intensity ranges. Subsequently, the lungs are extracted by identifying the largest connected components of the class "lung" and removing bones in the next step. Subsequently, various morphological operations are applied to classify the remaining voxels into heart region, small radius blood vessels, and so on. Finally, the skeleton of the vasculature is extracted and analyzed (see Section 9.2.5).

A quite different approach was proposed by Bruyninckx et al. [15]. They first track the minimal cost paths from each lung voxel that significantly exceeds the (local) average parenchyma intensity to the closest of the manually defined root points. From these paths, a set of bifurcations is detected. It is self-evident that a bifurcation is formed at any location in which at least two paths join. Finally, in the resulting graph, using the bifurcation as nodes and the segments between the nodes as edges, the optimal tree that reaches the whole organ is determined by minimizing an energy functional that incorporates physiological knowledge about tree-like structures.

9.2.2 Vessel Enhancement

Vessels can also generally be characterized by their tubular shape. That is, the local image signal can be expected to be almost constant along the direction of the vessel whereas exhibiting strong variations perpendicular to it (Figure 9.7). Such properties are reflected in the Hessian matrix **H** that includes the second-order partial derivatives of a function $I(\mathbf{x})$:

$$\mathbf{H}(\mathbf{x}) = \begin{pmatrix} \frac{\partial^2}{\partial x^2} I(\mathbf{x}) & \frac{\partial^2}{\partial x \partial y} I(\mathbf{x}) & \frac{\partial^2}{\partial x \partial z} I(\mathbf{x}) \\ \frac{\partial^2}{\partial y \partial x} I(\mathbf{x}) & \frac{\partial^2}{\partial y^2} I(\mathbf{x}) & \frac{\partial^2}{\partial y \partial z} I(\mathbf{x}) \\ \frac{\partial^2}{\partial z \partial x} I(\mathbf{x}) & \frac{\partial^2}{\partial z \partial y} I(\mathbf{x}) & \frac{\partial^2}{\partial z^2} I(\mathbf{x}) \end{pmatrix}. \tag{9.1}$$

(a) Ideal vessel model

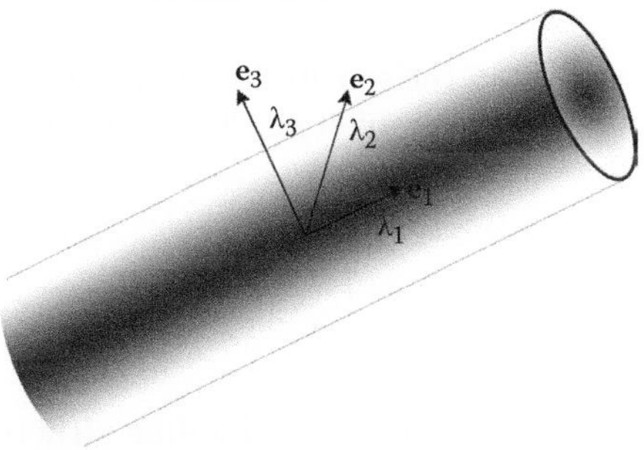

(b) Associated shapes

Eigenvalues	Shape
$\lambda_1 \leq 0, \lambda_2 \leq 0, \lambda_3 \leq 0$	blob
$\lambda_1 \approx 0, \lambda_2 \leq 0, \lambda_3 \leq 0$	tube
$\lambda_1 \approx 0, \lambda_2 \leq 0, \lambda_3 \leq 0$	plane

FIGURE 9.7
Vessel model of cylindrical shape (a). The cross-sectional plane is defined by the eigenvectors $\mathbf{e}_2$ and $\mathbf{e}_3$ with the corresponding eigenvalues λ_2 and λ_3. It is assumed that the intensity profile along the cross-section is Gaussian-like. The resulting shapes from different eigenvalue combinations are listed in (b).

In this framework, differentiation is defined as a convolution with derivatives of Gaussians:

$$\frac{\partial}{\partial x} I(\mathbf{x}, \sigma) = I(\mathbf{x}) * \frac{\partial}{\partial x} G(\mathbf{x}, \sigma), \tag{9.2}$$

where the scale parameter σ corresponds to the standard deviation of the Gaussian kernel G.

The local orientation at $\mathbf{x}$ can then be assessed via eigenvalue analysis of the Hessian matrix. The resulting eigenvalues $\lambda_{1,2,3}$ describe the intensity deviation along the corresponding eigenvectors $\mathbf{e}_{1,2,3}$ and hence allow the formulation of a vesselness measure of which several examples are known in the literature [27–29]. For bright, tubular structures, and eigenvalues that are ordered by their magnitude, $|\lambda_1| \le |\lambda_2| \le |\lambda_3|$, we expect the following criteria to be met according to the vessel model:

1. Elongated structure: $|\lambda_1| \approx 0$
2. Locally bright structure: $\lambda_2 \ll 0$ and $\lambda_3 \ll 0$
3. Symmetric structure: $|\lambda_2| \approx |\lambda_3|$

Lorenz et al. [27] hence define the filter response as

$$\mathfrak{L}(\mathbf{x}) = \sigma^{\gamma} \frac{|\lambda_2| + |\lambda_3|}{2}, \tag{9.3}$$

where γ normalizes responses across scales σ. The filter defined by Sato et al. [28] is given by

$$\mathfrak{S}(\mathbf{x}) = \begin{cases} \sigma^2 |\lambda_3| \left(\frac{\lambda_2}{\lambda_3}\right)^{\gamma_{23}} \left(1 + \frac{\lambda_1}{|\lambda_2|}\right)^{\gamma_{12}} & \lambda_1 \le 0 \\ \sigma^2 |\lambda_3| \left(\frac{\lambda_2}{\lambda_3}\right)^{\gamma_{23}} \left(1 - \alpha\frac{\lambda_1}{|\lambda_2|}\right)^{\gamma_{12}} & 0 < \lambda_1 \le \frac{|\lambda_2|}{\alpha} \\ 0 & \text{otherwise} \end{cases}, \tag{9.4}$$

where $\gamma_{23} \ge 0$ controls cross-section asymmetry, $\gamma_{12} \ge 0$ the sensitivity to blob-like structures, and $0 \le \alpha \le 1.0$ the sensitivity to the vessel curvature. Frangi et al. [29] defined their filter as

$$\mathfrak{F}(\mathbf{x}) = \left(1 - e^{-\frac{\mathfrak{R}_A^2}{2\alpha^2}}\right) e^{-\frac{\mathfrak{R}_B^2}{2\beta^2}} \left(1 - e^{-\frac{S^2}{2c^2}}\right), \tag{9.5}$$

with $\mathfrak{R}_A = \frac{|\lambda_2|}{|\lambda_3|}$ designed for distinguishing between plate- and line-like structures (controlled by α), $\mathfrak{R}_B = \frac{|\lambda_1|}{\sqrt{|\lambda_2 \lambda_3|}}$ discriminates from blob-like structures (controlled by β), and $S = \sqrt{\lambda_1^2 + \lambda_2^2 + \lambda_3^2}$ (controlled by c) eliminates background noise. Opposed to the previous definitions that formulate normalization across scales within the vesselness functions, Frangi et al. accounted for different scales by using scale-normalized derivatives.

In conjunction with pulmonary vessel segmentation, other vesselness functions have been additionally reported, e.g., Zhou et al. developed a new multiscale response function in ref. [20], again, using scale-normalized derivatives:

$$\mathfrak{Z}(\mathbf{x}) = \begin{cases} \frac{|\lambda_2| + |\lambda_3|}{2} e^{-\left|\frac{|\lambda_3|}{s} - c\right|} & \lambda_1, \lambda_2, \lambda_3 \leq 0 \\ 0 & \text{otherwise} \end{cases}, \tag{9.6}$$

with c being a constant, which should be set between 0.57 and 0.71. More recently, a vesselness function that is directly calculated from a predefined vessel model without any further parameters than the scale σ has been published by Erdt et al. [30] in conjunction with hepatic vessel segmentation:

$$\mathfrak{E}(\mathbf{x}) = \kappa \cdot \sigma^{-3/2} \cdot \frac{2}{3}\lambda_1 - \lambda_2 - \lambda_3 , \tag{9.7}$$

with κ being an isotropy factor:

$$\kappa = \begin{cases} 0 & \lambda_2 > 0 \text{ or } \lambda_3 > 0 \\ 1 - \frac{|\lambda_2| - |\lambda_3|}{|\lambda_2| + |\lambda_3|} & \text{otherwise} \end{cases}. \tag{9.8}$$

Shikata et al. [18] argued that criteria (1) and (3) are not always particularly met in real-world data and, hence, define a filter output function that takes only criterion (2) into account:

$$\mathfrak{H}(\mathbf{x}) = -\frac{\sigma^2 \lambda_2}{I(\mathbf{x})}. \tag{9.9}$$

Thus, it may also enhance blob-like structures as well as image noise, whereas image noise is claimed to be less enhanced than vessels and can be consequently eliminated by post-processing steps.

Filter responses at different scales σ_i are typically combined into a final estimate of vesselness using a maximum operator. One general, well-known drawback of Hessian-based enhancement techniques is the implicit assumption that there locally exists only one oriented structure. Consequently, filter responses often lack in areas with multiple orientations such as bifurcations (see also ref. [31]).

9.2.3 Vesselness-Based Approaches

Vessel enhancement filters have been applied in a variety of approaches [16–23, 25]. Segmentation systems designed for CT examinations without contrast agent have especially taken advantage of the shape characteristics of vascular structures. Hence, vesselness-based systems often allow a better distinction between vessel and nonvessel regions, but frequently need multiple scales to capture all vessel details. Coupling this necessity with the multiple computations required for each scale tends to make these methods computationally rather intense and therefore slow.

For instance, Zhu et al. [16] extended the level set framework for pulmonary vessel segmentation by a vesselness-based compensation of the curvature term to allow a faster front propagation along the vessel direction, while still maintaining the smoothness of vessel walls. In particular, they used the speed function

$$F = g(\nu - \varepsilon \cdot \kappa), \tag{9.10}$$

with κ being the local curvature including a weighting factor ε. This weighting factor is regulated based on the vesselness measure $\mathfrak{F}$ (Equation 9.5). It allows the front to propagate faster along the vessels (because of large vesselness response along the centerline), whereas the curvature penalty is larger when the front is near the boundary. The edge-stopping function g is also defined based on $\mathfrak{F}$. Finally, the external propagation force ν is defined as a function of the joint intensity and vesselness statistics.

The method presented in refs. [17, 18] determines an initial segmentation by thresholding the filtered output of CT scans performed without imposition of an X-ray contrast agent. To this end, the vesselness filter (Equation 9.9) is computed with different scales (a subset from a total of five scales) depending on a local vessel radius estimate $\tilde{r}$. The radius information is estimated by first segmenting vessels by using an intensity-based threshold of −600 HU. Afterwards, a distance transformation is applied to determine $\tilde{r}$. To fill the resulting gaps, especially at bifurcations, which usually do not have high responses to line filters, a tracking algorithm is used [32]. To this end, seeds at the center of each segment are identified. During vessel traversal, the eigenvectors and eigenvalues are examined, serving as termination criterion. In particular, branches are detected based on the eigenvalues along the extracted trajectory. Finally, the vessel radius along the trajectory is estimated to reconstruct the vessels and resulting vascular structures with less than 100 bifurcations are disregarded. More recently, Liu et al. [19] used this approach as the initial segmentation for their graph-based segmentation of vascular trees across bifurcations. By using its medial axes to guide a resampling method, they are able to extract sufficient information and construct a graph to identify the optimal surfaces using a min-cut/max-flow algorithm [33] to reconstruct the vessel surfaces.

Zhou et al. [20] developed their own filter response function (Equation 9.6), which was designed to enhance vessels as well as bifurcations and to suppress nonvessel structures. This filter is applied using 12 different scales with $\sigma_i \in [1,\ldots,12]$ mm. Then, vessels inside the lung regions are extracted using an expectation–maximization algorithm at each individual scale, and the resulting segmentation results are combined in a hierarchical manner. The same approach was used in ref. [21] as an initial segmentation. Additionally, to correct possible oversegmentations, a refinement method based on texture classification is proposed. In particular, a support vector machine, in conjunction with co-occurrence texture features, is used to differentiate between vessels and interstitial pneumonia patterns.

A different approach [22] uses the eigenanalysis of the Hessian matrix to trace vessels along the estimated direction of a vessel $\mathbf{e}_1$ in a first step, and subsequently, to extract the cross-sectional planes orthogonal to the vessels (defined by $\mathbf{e}_2$ and $\mathbf{e}_3$; cf. Figure 9.7(a)). These are then the basis to detect bifurcation points using AdaBoost. Finally, the vessels are reconstructed with deformable sphere models at each of the detected center points as well as the detected branching points.

Contrary to Hessian-based enhancement filters that depend on second-order partial derivatives, an enhancement filter based on the structure tensor is proposed in ref. [23], with application to pulmonary vessels. More specifically, the filter employs three sets of eigenvalues of the correlation matrix of image gradients within a local window to distinguish between vessels, junctions, and nodules. First, a set of candidates C are detected using the voxel intensity information $I(\mathbf{x})$, the eigenvalues of the Hessian matrix, and the first-order partial derivatives of $I(\mathbf{x})$. Then, the gradient vector field is computed and regularized in an adaptive local window at each center location $c \in C$. Afterward, three principal directions are iteratively detected based on the eigenvalues of the resulting structure tensor by first determining the most prominent orientation and later removing the gradients supporting this direction. The resulting eigenvalues of each principal direction are used to define filters to enhance vessels, junctions, and nodules. Afterward, vessels are extracted using adaptive thresholds, which are automatically determined based on the local neighborhood [24]. Then, the result is used to build fuzzy spherical objects representing the vessels using regulated morphological operations. Finally, a vessel tree reconstruction algorithm is used to connect the spherical objects into vessel segments and then into trees.

Furthermore, Song et al. [25] proposed an iterative system that optimizes both the segmentation and the orientation estimation of the vessel tree. To initially estimate the orientation, a bank of directional filters is applied. They use elongated second-order derivate filters, such as:

$$F(\alpha,\beta,\gamma) = u(\tilde{x}) \frac{1}{C} \frac{\partial^2}{\partial \tilde{y}^2} e^{\frac{\tilde{x}^2}{\lambda_x \sigma^2} + \frac{\tilde{y}^2}{\sigma^2} + \frac{\tilde{z}^2}{\lambda_z \sigma^2}} \Bigg|_{(\tilde{x},\tilde{y},\tilde{z})^T = \mathbf{R}(\alpha,\beta,\gamma)(x,y,z)^T}, \tag{9.11}$$

with $u(\tilde{x})$ being the unit step function, which is responsible for the filter responding only to the forward direction. The scale of the filter is controlled by σ, whereas λ_x and λ_z control the elongated scale along the x-axis and the filter thickness. $\mathbf{R}$ is the rotation matrix defined by (α,β,γ). By rotating and applying the filter for a distinct set of predefined directions, more than one orientation can be described at each location. In particular, the number of orientations is limited to three (describing bifurcations) using orientation histogram analysis. Then, for each iteration, the estimated orientation is regularized with a fixed segmentation mask and, consecutively, the segmentation mask is updated using the min-cut/max-flow algorithm [34] using the orientation estimates for defining the cost function.

9.2.4 Fuzzy Segmentation

A pulmonary vessel segmentation approach based on a fuzzy segmentation concept was presented in ref. [2]. It combines the strengths of both threshold- and seed-point–based methods by first identifying multiple seed points with a high specificity and then continuously adding neighboring voxels based on a probability-like measure. The result is a fuzzy segmentation, in which sensitivity/specificity can be adapted to the application-specific requirements. The method consists of two principal phases as shown in the flowchart in Figure 9.8. The first phase identifies the core components of the vascular tree within the lung areas with a high specificity. This step performs an initial segmentation using a threshold-based approach as described in Section 9.2.4.1. Subsequently, each resulting region is reduced to one or more seed positions, which are used as input to the second

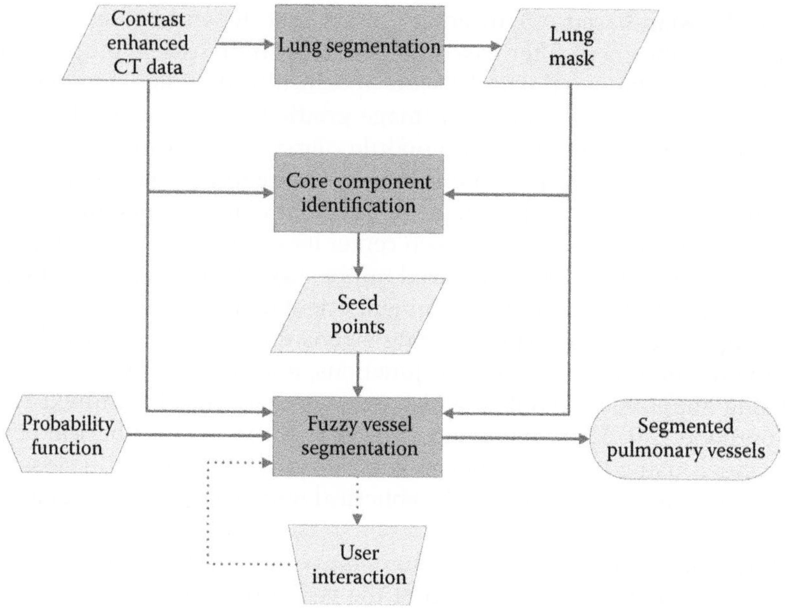

FIGURE 9.8
A high-level diagram of the steps and output of the proposed method [2]. The input consists of the original, contrast-enhanced CT data. A lung segmentation method is applied to identify the left and right lungs as the ROIs. The core component identification step is then used to automatically identify seed points within the core lung vessels. These are used along with a probability function as input to the fuzzy vessel segmentation step. If necessary, this step might be repeated, guided by user interaction. The final output is then the segmentation of the pulmonary vessels within the lung mask.

phase. In this phase, an improved fuzzy segmentation is created, which is described in detail in Section 9.2.4.2. Assuming the seed positions are located inside the pulmonary vessels, the probability that a voxel of interest also belongs to the vascular tree is determined by examining the paths between the voxel and the seed points. It allows the sound integration of multiple features such as intensity information, vesselness response, or higher-level knowledge. The final binary segmentation is obtained by applying a threshold, allowing the sensitivity of the method to be adjusted *a posteriori* in this last step. Additionally, the user can further efficiently influence the outcome of the segmentation system by adding seed points into subtrees that were not previously detected or by deleting wrongly located seed points.

9.2.4.1 Core Component Identification

To identify reliable seed positions within the lung vessels, the core vessel components are first extracted from the masked input data, in a manner similar to the vessel segmentation method described in ref. [8]. A threshold with "conservative" boundaries, e.g., T_{min} = 150 HU and T_{max} = 600 HU, is applied to slightly eroded lung regions to create an initial segmentation with a high specificity. Thus, voxels identified at this early stage most likely belong to the vascular tree. To eliminate further false-positive regions, a connected-component analysis is performed on the segmented structures. Components that do not exceed a minimal volume V_{min} in size, e.g., V_{min} = 400 voxels, are discarded. Based on the chosen thresholds and the parameter V_{min}, this stage will identify n distinct components.

These could be many components or just a few, in which a large value of V_{min} will result in a small number n, and vice versa. Small holes within this segmentation output are closed using morphological operations. Compared with ref. [8], the parameters are chosen to obtain a core segmentation with a very high specificity, rather than a segmentation of a complete tree structure (see Figure 9.9(a) and (b)).

Next, the segmentation mask is partitioned using a tubular component labeling approach. To this end, the segmented components are converted into a structure that reflects the likelihood of centerlines C, based on a three-dimensional (3D) Euclidean distance transform. Voxels within the segmentation output with a higher distance to the closest vessel surface are located further inside the vessels and, hence, are more likely to correspond to the centerline (see Figure 9.9(c)). This means that local maxima within such a structure most likely correspond to the centerline and that the associated distance value corresponds to a radius estimate. Hence, local maxima within a kernel window of size 5 × 5 × 5 voxels for which the radius estimate is within the range of radii of interest, e.g., $r_1, r_2 = \sqrt{2}, \infty \cdot$ voxel size, become seed-point candidates.

Depending on the physical location and the radius estimates, these seed candidates are clustered together. Therefore, starting with the seed candidate with a maximum radius estimate, we assign each further seed candidate within a certain distance to the same group/component. In particular, two seed candidates s_1 and s_2 are grouped together if the Euclidean distance $d(\mathbf{s}_1,\mathbf{s}_2)$ is smaller than twice the maximal radius estimate of both positions, i.e., if

$$d(\mathbf{s}_1,\mathbf{s}_2) \leq 2 \cdot \max(r(\mathbf{s}_1), r(\mathbf{s}_2)). \tag{9.12}$$

This is continued until all seed candidates are assigned to one group, whereas a considered point that is not assigned to another candidate will find a new component. Finally, for each tubular component, the seed candidate with the largest radius estimate is chosen as a cluster representative. This means that the cluster representatives, which are the final seed positions for the subsequent fuzzy segmentation, tend to be located toward the origin of each component because the radius estimates are maximal in that area. The number N of detected seed points, however, depends on the chosen parameters.

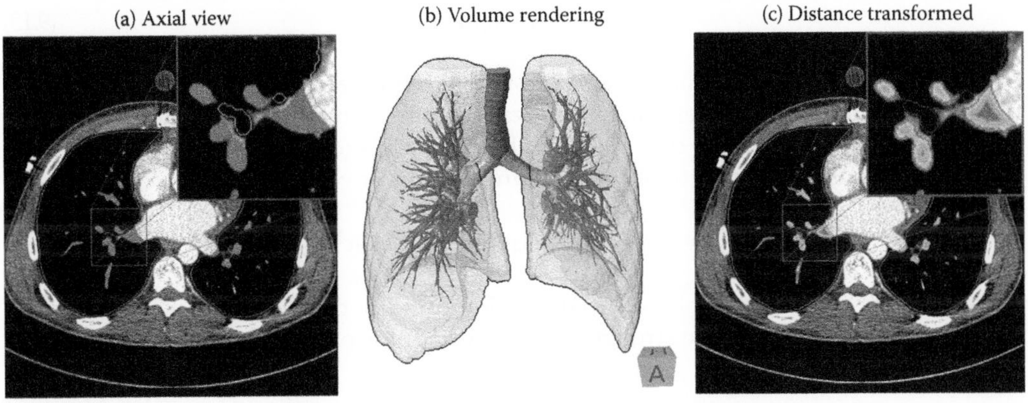

FIGURE 9.9
(See color insert.) (a) The core vessel segmentation [2] is shown as an overlay to the axial view. The extracted seed points are shown as small boxes. (b) The corresponding result is shown as volume rendering. For each voxel within the segmentation result, the minimal 3D Euclidean distance to the vessel surface has been calculated and is shown color-coded in (c).

9.2.4.2 Fuzzy Vessel Segmentation

After identification of multiple seed points throughout the whole lung (Section 9.2.4.1), these seeds are used as input for a seed-point–based segmentation approach. Assuming all seed points are located within the vascular tree, we create a probability map in which the "belongingness" of each voxel to one of the seed points and hence to the class "vessel" is stored using the CT data masked by the lung segmentation. Finally, this probability map is converted into a binary segmentation by applying a threshold, depending on the application-specific requirements.

To calculate such a probability measure, the vessel probability of each seed position is first set to one. Next, starting from the seed positions, neighboring voxels receive a vessel probability based on local image features and the probability measure of their neighbors, whereas those not visited have a vessel probability of zero. This is repeated in an iterative fashion, where voxels with a high probability are processed first, until the probability that a newly visited voxel belongs to one of the seed positions drops below a specified value. Thus, the process can be compared to a front evolution or region-growing process in which neighboring voxels that are more likely to belong to a vessel are added earlier than unlikely ones.

In practice, this is realized using the fuzzy connectedness algorithm [35], which is used to calculate a probability measure that a voxel belongs to one or more seed points modeling the so-called "hanging togetherness" of voxels within the scene. An object O with its seed positions $\mathbf{s}_i \in \mathbb{O}$, $i \in [0, N-1]$ and the background B are separated by dividing the set of voxels present in the scene in such a way that the hanging togetherness or belongingness of each object voxel to $\mathbb{O}$ is larger than the belongingness of each background voxel.

The probability that two neighboring voxels $\mathbf{c},\mathbf{d}$ belong to the same group is therefore defined by a local fuzzy relation called "affinity" $\mu_\kappa(\mathbf{c},\mathbf{d})$. The neighborhood of a voxel in 3D data is typically defined either by its 6- or 26-nearest neighbors. The affinity of non-neighboring voxels equals zero and the affinity of a voxel to itself equals one (reflexive condition): $\mu_\kappa(\mathbf{c},\mathbf{c}) = 1$. For all other pairs of voxels, the affinity is defined by a probability function to be defined. The local affinity is designed to be symmetric, i.e.,

$$\mu_\kappa(\mathbf{c},\mathbf{d}) = \mu_\kappa(\mathbf{d},\mathbf{c}). \tag{9.13}$$

The "strength of connectedness" of two distant voxels $\mathbf{c},\mathbf{d}$ along a certain path $p_{\mathbf{c},\mathbf{d}}$ within the scene is simply the smallest pairwise fuzzy affinity along this path, whereas the path $p_{\mathbf{c},\mathbf{d}}$ from $\mathbf{c}$ to $\mathbf{d}$ is a sequence of $m > 2$ neighboring voxels $\langle \mathbf{c}^{(1)},\mathbf{c}^{(2)},\ldots,\mathbf{c}^{(m)} \rangle$, such that $\mathbf{c}^{(1)} = \mathbf{c}$ and $\mathbf{c}^{(m)} = \mathbf{d}$. Thus, the "strength of connectedness" equals:

$$\mu_N(p_{\mathbf{c},\mathbf{d}}) = \min[\mu_\kappa(\mathbf{c}^{(1)},\mathbf{c}^{(2)}),\mu_\kappa(\mathbf{c}^{(2)},\mathbf{c}^{(3)}),\ldots,\mu_\kappa(\mathbf{c}^{(m-1)},\mathbf{c}^{(m)})]. \tag{9.14}$$

As there are various possible paths connecting $\mathbf{c}$ and $\mathbf{d}$, the global connectivity $\mu_K(\mathbf{c},\mathbf{d})$ is defined as the largest of the strengths of connectedness of all possible paths between $\mathbf{c}$ and $\mathbf{d}$:

$${}_K(\mathbf{c},\mathbf{d}) = \max_{p_j \in \mathbb{P}_{\mathbf{c},\mathbf{d}}} \quad {}_N(p_j) \quad \forall\, j, \tag{9.15}$$

where $\mathbb{P}_{\mathbf{c},\mathbf{d}}$ denotes the set of all possible paths p_j.

Assigning a probability value of $P_{\text{vessel}}(\mathbf{s}_i) = 1$ to all seed points $\mathbf{s}_i$, fuzzy connectedness efficiently computes a probability measure for a voxel x by examining the paths between x and the seed points that are independent of the length of the path, yielding a probability measure

$$P_{\text{vessel}}(\mathbf{x}) = \max_{\mathbf{s}_i \in \mathcal{O}} \mu_{\kappa}(\mathbf{x}, \mathbf{s}_i) \quad \text{with} \quad P_{\text{vessel}}(\mathbf{s}_i) = 1 \; \forall \, i. \tag{9.16}$$

Note that even if P_{vessel} decreases to less than 0.5 for a voxel, this voxel can still most likely belong to the vascular tree. An appropriate threshold has to be chosen for binarization, allowing the sensitivity of the method to be adjusted *a posteriori*. Figure 9.10 shows exemplary segmentation results using different thresholds.

9.2.4.3 Probability Function

The local affinity $\mu_\kappa(\mathbf{c},\mathbf{d})$ in Section 9.2.4.2 describes the likelihood that two neighboring voxels $\mathbf{c},\mathbf{d}$ belong to the same class.

Such a function typically considers the image content using an intensity- or gradient-based probability function, or a combination of both. In the context of pulmonary vessel segmentation, an intensity-based probability-like function has proven to yield good segmentation results [2]:

$$\mu_{\kappa,I}(\mathbf{c},\mathbf{d}) = e^{-\frac{1}{2\sigma_I^2}\left(\frac{I(\mathbf{c})+I(\mathbf{d})}{2} - \mu_I\right)^2}. \tag{9.17}$$

In this expression, μ_I and σ_I^2 represent the expected intensity and variance of the object in consideration. In other words, $\mu_{\kappa,I}$ becomes large if the input value of $\frac{I(\mathbf{c})+I(\mathbf{d})}{2}$ agrees well with the assumed intensity-based vessel model. The parameter σ_I controls how fast the probability function drops toward zero for values distant from the expected ones.

(a) $P_{\text{vessel}} > 0.78$ (b) $P_{\text{vessel}} > 0.39$ (c) $P_{\text{vessel}} > 0.04$

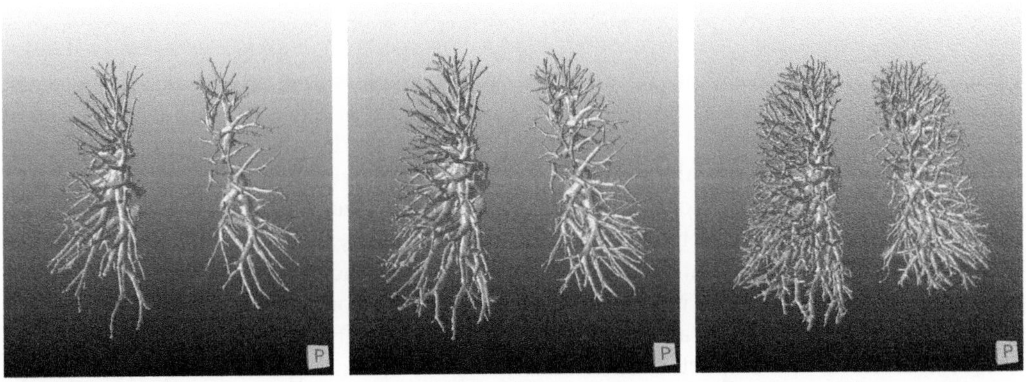

FIGURE 9.10
3D renderings of the segmentation result using the fuzzy connectedness implementation and an intensity-based affinity function [2]. For each figure, only voxels with a probability P_{vessel} larger than a certain threshold are visualized, thus resulting in different segmentation sensitivities/specificities.

For the particular objective of pulmonary vessel segmentation, it is reasonable to slightly modify the local affinity function. As blood vessels are the brightest objects within the lungs, it is reasonable to define a piecewise function that increases Gaussian-like for intensities below μ_I, that is constant for values above μ_I, and zero for values below a minimal intensity value $I_{\min}$ as follows:

$$_{\kappa,I}(\mathbf{c},\mathbf{d}) = \begin{cases} 0 & \frac{I(\mathbf{c})+I(\mathbf{d})}{2} < I_{\min} \\ e^{-\frac{1}{2\sigma_I^2}\left(\frac{I(\mathbf{c})+I(\mathbf{d})}{2} - {}_I\right)^2} & I_{\min} < \frac{I(\mathbf{c})+I(\mathbf{d})}{2} < {}_I \\ 1 & \text{otherwise} \end{cases} . \qquad (9.18)$$

One can observe that using a solely intensity-based affinity function with global parameters tends to assign a larger probability measure P_{vessel} to nonvessel structures in close proximity to vessels with larger diameters than to small vessels itself (Figure 9.11). This is caused by the fact that smaller vessels often appear darker as expected by a constant intensity model. To overcome this shortcoming, the enhancement of particularly smaller vessels using a Hessian-based enhancement filter (Section 9.2.2) has been proposed in ref. [1].

To this end, a vessel enhancement filter has been computed, preferably using only as few scales as possible to preserve the computational efficiency of the system. In particular, a combination of $\sigma_i = [1,2,4]$ mm using Erdt's filter (Equation 9.7), which does not require any further parameters, is used. Having the original intensities $I(\mathbf{x})$ and the filter output $\mathfrak{E}(x)$, one can define a second affinity term $\mu_{\kappa,\mathfrak{E}}$ using the filter response instead of the intensity values in Equation 9.17. The scalar output of μ_κ has been chosen to be the maximum value of $\mu_{\kappa,\{I,\mathfrak{E}\}}$ with the additional parameters $\mu_{\mathfrak{E}}$ and $\sigma_{\mathfrak{E}}$.

The expected values μ_I in Equation 9.18, resp., $\mu_{\mathfrak{E}}$ are estimated from the input data by averaging the intensity values $I(\mathbf{x})$ and $\mathfrak{E}(\mathbf{x})$ of all N seed positions $\mathbf{s}_i$ (Section 9.2.4.1), respectively:

$$_I = \frac{1}{N}\sum_{i=0}^{N-1} I(\mathbf{s}_i), \quad _{\mathfrak{E}} = \frac{1}{N}\sum_{i=0}^{N-1} \mathfrak{E}(\mathbf{s}_i). \qquad (9.19)$$

Using this estimate rather than a predefined value considers intensity variations between different patients caused by, for example, the contrast agent used, bolus phase, and most importantly, the scan protocol. The variance σ_I is set to a predefined value, e.g., $\sigma_I = 200$ HU and the minimal intensity value to $I_{\min} = -400$ HU. However, the choice of σ_I is not crucial in this setting because it can be regarded as a normalization constant with respect to image noise within the object of interest. More particularly, the segmentation algorithm will yield identical segmentations with different σ_I when adapting the threshold to convert the fuzzy segmentation to a binary segmentation accordingly. A more lengthy and formal discussion of redundant parameters in local affinity functions can be found in ref. [36]. However, σ_I is important in relation to $\sigma_{\mathfrak{E}}$ if considering both image features. An experimental study [1] analyzing the vessel segmentation performance independently for regions with predominantly larger, resp., smaller vessels has shown that if using intensity information alone, large vessels are best segmented using a threshold to convert the fuzzy segmentation into a binary segmentation that differs from thresholds optimal for small

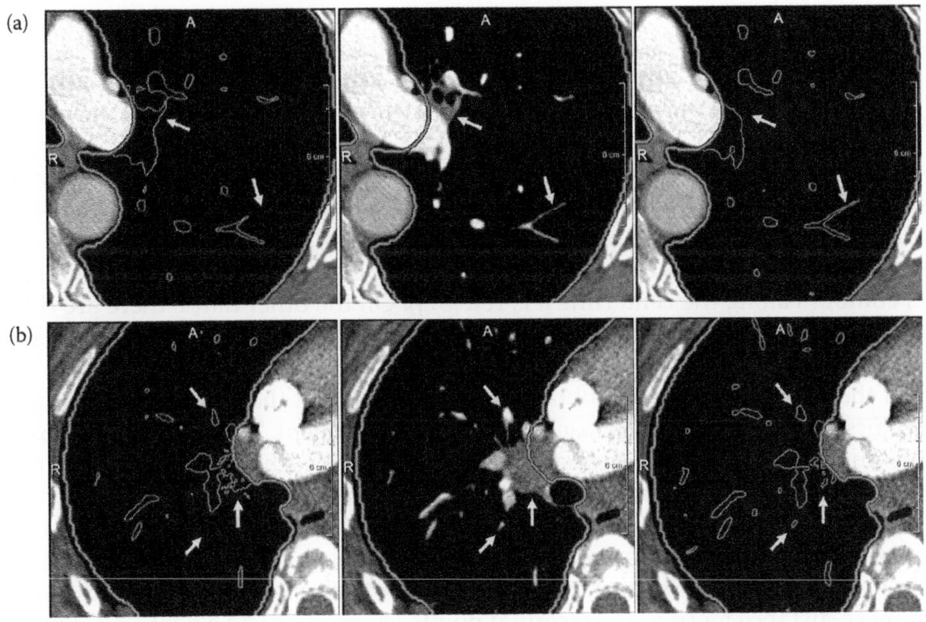

FIGURE 9.11
(See color insert.) Segmentation results using the multimodal affinity function [1] (right) in comparison with the intensity-based affinity function [2] (left) shown as contours corresponding to two different patients (original images shown in the center). One can observe that the multimodal segmentation extends further to the periphery than the purely intensity-based one. At the same time, leakage into nonvessel regions is suppressed. In particular, please compare the segmentation outcome at the positions highlighted by arrows, for instance pointing towards branches that have not been delineated (and hence do not appear as contours) in the left image, but are correctly delineated in the right image.

vessels. One can observe that if additionally using the filter response with, e.g., $\sigma_{\mathfrak{E}} = 3000$, the segmentation accuracy of small vessels is improved using the same threshold for large as well as smaller vessels.

The resulting multimodal affinity function, which considers the intensity information as well as the filter response, allows for accurate vessel segmentation with only a few filter scales. More specifically, the filter response needs to be computed only for a very limited number of smaller scales, whereas the segmentation of larger vessels is not influenced. Using this filter response alone would not be adequate to extract the whole vascular tree except if adding multiple scales, which would make this method significantly more computationally expensive. In addition, the intensity information is capable of steering the fuzzy-connectedness region-growing process in areas such as bifurcations for which the filter output is lacking. The result is a synergy of the benefits of the individual methods compensating their individual drawbacks. The speed of intensity-based methods is preserved as best as possible with the specificity benefits of vessel enhancement filtering. Finally, using only small scales also avoids the localization problem caused by smoothing with larger scales (especially in areas with close-by high-intensity structures).

In addition to the above-described probability functions, higher-level knowledge might also be encoded into this framework. For instance, similar to ref. [11], voxels in close spatial proximity to the airway lumen might be considered as the airway wall and, hence, should receive a low vessel probability. Such *a priori* knowledge can be described as a function based on the distance to the segmented airway lumen (Chapter 8), in particular, when no segmentations of the outer airway walls are available [2].

9.2.4.4 Centerline Extraction

To extract the centerline of vascular structures, there are two fundamentally different strategies. On the one hand, there exist different techniques to extract the vessel centerline directly (without prior vessel segmentation), typically referred to as vessel tracking. Additionally, the extracted centerline can be used to optionally delineate the vessel contours along the centerline (cf., ref. [37]). On the other hand, there are different algorithms known for extracting the centerline from a given segmentation (e.g., refs. [38,39]).

Given the binary vessel mask obtained by thresholding the fuzzy segmentation output, we first locate a root site for each connected component. To this end, the voxel with the maximal distance to the vessel surface is selected for each component. Next, the centerline tree can be determined by computing the 3D skeleton and capturing the data in a tree representation $T = \{S,B\}$ consisting of branches B and sites S [38]. To this end, two distance metrics are computed for all voxels within the mask. These metrics give information on the distance of each voxel from the tree's root site and outer surface, respectively. Using these distance metrics, the terminal points are marked. As a next step, an iterative thinning procedure is applied until a single-voxel-thick skeleton along the ridges of the vessel is obtained without changing the topology. Afterward, this skeleton is captured in a tree structure containing hierarchically ordered branches $B = \{\mathbf{b}_1,\ldots,\mathbf{b}_M\}$ consisting of connected sites $S = \{\mathbf{s}_1,\ldots,\mathbf{s}_L\}$. Each site $\mathbf{s}$ additionally stores the distance to the closest surface as an approximation of the vessel radius $r(\mathbf{s},\mathbf{b})$. Because of imperfect segmentation results and nonsmooth vessel surfaces, the tree will include false-positive branches as well as nonsmooth centerlines. To address these issues, several postprocessing steps that might delete or move centerline points as well as delete false branches are applied [38]. In particular, branches resulting from small irregularities on the vessel surface are eliminated by deleting terminal branches that are shorter than twice the radius at the bifurcation point. Additionally, bifurcation points are re-centered to obtain a smooth transition between each branch and its children. Finally, intermediate sites are eliminated to create smooth branches using cubic Hermite spline interpolation that are equidistantly sampled. Figure 9.12 shows exemplarily the resulting centerline tree for a vessel segmentation.

9.2.5 Artery–Vein Separation

The separation of vascular tree structures (cf. Section 9.1.1) is still one of the major challenges in vascular image processing. Recent techniques still often require massive user interaction for providing reliable separation results. In practice, the separation of different vascular structures such as pulmonary arteries and veins is challenging for several reasons:

1. Different structures appear in the same HU range, except when specialized scan protocols define particular bolus phases for enhancing only parts of the vasculature.
2. Arterial and venous trees might approach or even touch each other at multiple locations involving branches of varying scale, whereas each tree in itself already

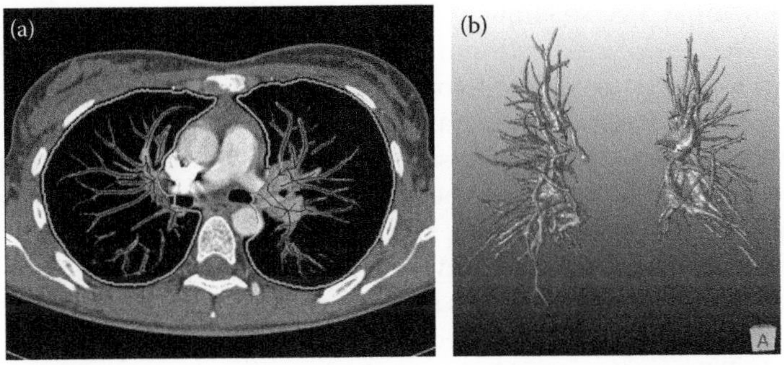

FIGURE 9.12
(See color insert.) Segmentation result and corresponding centerlines using the multimodal affinity function with $P_{vessel} > 0.57$ using the same data and visualization settings as shown in Figure 9.5. Note that it features almost no false-positives in the hilum area compared with the threshold-based segmentation, whereas small vessels are not always segmented to their distal end. Decreasing P_{vessel} would add smaller branches to the segmentation at the cost of increasing false-positives.

consists of branches of varying sizes forming highly variable and complex branching patterns.

3. Often, no trace of intensity gradient is recognizable at locations of fusing vessels.
4. Anatomical variations and pathologies additionally affecting the vessels are not uncommon in routine.
5. Limited resolution, suboptimal signal-to-noise-ratio, and other imaging artifacts may hamper a clear distinction.

In contrast with other applications, the identifiable parallelism between arteries and airways within a certain range of hierarchical generations allows the incorporation of an additional feature into the separation algorithms. This property is used in ref. [13] to define an "arterialness" measure based on the spatial proximity of a bronchus to a given vessel on the one hand, and a co-orientation measure on the other hand. That is, for each sampling point along the vessel centerline, bronchi candidates within a plane normal to the vessel orientation are locally detected within a square of edge length $8 \times r_{ves}$, with r_{ves} being the vessel radius at that point. Candidates include all local intensity minima after smoothing, from which candidates above −800 HU are excluded as well as candidates with the 2D Gaussian curvature being smaller than twice the maximal curvature among all candidates. Ideally, only one candidate having a much larger Gaussian curvature than all other initial candidates is left in the resulting reduced candidate set. If there are too many (>5) left, Bülow et al. argue that the centerline point most likely belongs to a vein, in which case, no such outlier is expected. For the remaining candidates, a co-orientation feature between the vessel and the suspected bronchus is evaluated. Such a feature compares the orientation estimate of the candidate, which is determined by eigenanalysis of the structure tensor at that point, to the orientation of the vessel. Additionally, the orientedness, which is a function of the corresponding eigenvalues, is evaluated at the candidate point. Finally, the arterialness of a centerline point corresponds to the maximal co-orientation value among all candidates and the arterialness of a vessel segment is defined as the top 50% of arterialness values along its centerline.

Other approaches address the artery–vein separation in a more general way without considering pulmonary-specific features. Park [14] labeled arteries and veins based on their origin following a reverse strategy. That is, each distal end of the segmented vasculature is backtracked to the mediastinum and vessels connecting to the pulmonary trunk are labeled as arteries, whereas vessels connecting to other parts of the heart are classified as veins. This method employs radius and orientation information via local spheres to resolve areas with unclear boundaries using a rule-based system. More particularly, local spheres are fitted into the vessels from the terminal ends toward the heart. As soon as two spheres overlap from different branches, spheres are pregenerated along the blood vessel directions. If the shortest connection between the centers of the different spheres is completely inside one branch, both branches shall be merged, forming a Y-junction. If at least one connection between the pregenerated sphere centers intersects with a vessel surface, both branches shall be continued independently, forming an X-junction.

Most recently, Saha et al. [40] proposed an iterative separation scheme using multiscale topological and morphological features to separate two iso-intensity structures without using any gradient- or edge-based features. Given a fuzzy segmentation, the user is asked to manually place seed points on the approximate center of each vascular structure. Based on a fuzzy distance transform (FDT), both objects are separated starting at large scales and processing toward smaller scales. To this end, the FDT values are normalized using local scale information and an FDT-based relative connectivity is used. This process equals fuzzy connectedness (cf. Section 9.2.4.2) using the normalized FDT map as input and each point is assigned to the object to which the connectivity is strongest.

9.3 Applications

Vascular tree segmentation in pulmonary CT images is a core component of a variety of applications. As the computer-aided diagnosis of PE is the most prominent application, it is described in more depth in the following. Additionally, other applications, such as lung nodule-CAD, airway and lung fissure segmentation, and lung registration, are summarized in subsequent subsections.

9.3.1 PE-CAD

Both CAD and visualization of PE (Section 9.1.2) require vessel segmentation [10, 41–44]. Ideally, such vessel segmentation would be separated into arteries and veins because PEs only occur in arteries but not in veins. A robust separation could potentially significantly reduce the false-positive rate by excluding PE candidates located in veins. Additionally, in 3D visualization, the pulmonary venous tree could be hidden such that it is neither blocking the user's view on potential PEs nor attracting the user's attention during evaluation.

One PE visualization system that supports the examiner's task was proposed by Pichon et al. [41]. It uses the density values inside the segmented vessels to color the outside of a shaded surface display of the vessel tree to highlight potential PEs in a 3D view (see Figure 9.13). In a multiple-reader study with 10 cases and 69 validated PEs, the authors have shown that such a 3D visualization of pulmonary arteries allows the reader to detect a significant number of additional emboli not detected during the traditional 2D axial readings. The study showed an increase in sensitivity from 66% using 2D views to 74% using both the 2D and 3D methods. At the same time, the number of false-positives increased from 0.23 (2D only) to 0.4 (combined reading) per case [42].

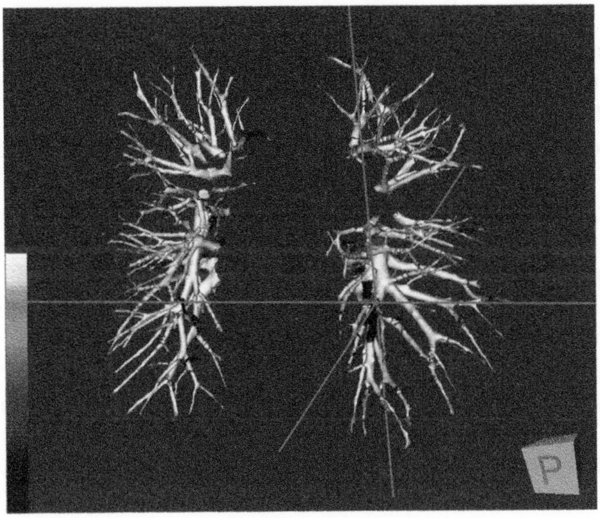

FIGURE 9.13
(See color insert.) Vessel segmentation with the outer surface colored by the inner contents [41,42]. Unlike in the original work, potential PE regions are color-coded, with dark colors corresponding to low HU values, to avoid confusions between regular 3D shading and emboli visualization. A marked PE is shown with cross-hairs, which is also shown in 2D in Figure 9.2(b).

Besides advanced visualization techniques, several CAD systems have been suggested as a second reader. For instance, Masutani et al. [43] proposed a feature-based approach, for which the search space is limited to the segmented vessel volume. That is, on a voxel level, PE candidates are extracted using intensity properties, local contrast, and the degree of curvilinearity, computed via eigenvalue analysis of the Hessian matrix. The resulting connected components are evaluated according to volume, effective length, and mean local contrast. The volume threshold was used to adjust the sensitivity/specificity of the system. As a result, a sensitivity of 100% with 7.7 false-positives per case and 85% sensitivity with 2.6 false-positives is reported based on 19 clinical data sets with 21 overall thrombi.

Very similarly, Bouma et al. [10] proposed a system that also includes a candidate detection step on a voxel level and subsequent classification of resulting PE candidates. In the first step, three features are used to detect candidate voxels inside the vessel segmentation, namely, CT values, eigenvalues of the Hessian matrix, and local contrast. For the second step, a set of features among intensity, shape, location, and size features are selected in conjunction with multiple classifiers. Results indicate that a bagged tree classifier with a stringness criterion (shape of the blood vessel near PE candidates) and the distance to the vessel boundary, as features, performs best. Using this method on an evaluation data set of 19 positive cases (including scans with considerable motion artifacts, suboptimal contrast, a variety of thrombus load, and parenchymal diseases) with a total of 116 PEs resulted in a sensitivity of 63% at 4.9 false-positives per data set.

In contrast, Zhou et al. used an adaptive multiscale expectation–maximization algorithm to screen the segmented vessel volume for potential PEs [44]. Subsequently, they applied a linear discriminant analysis classifier using nine features such as contrast, intensity difference between the detected object and its background, object size, etc., to reduce the number of false-positives. In a study using two databases of 59 and 69 PE cases, respectively, a sensitivity of 80% was reported with 18.9 and 22.6 false-positives per case depending on the choice of training set versus test set. Note, however, that a computer-detected volume of interest was considered true positive when it overlapped with only 10% or more with the manually identified PE.

Several studies evaluating CAD systems for detecting PEs in CT examinations have been published. A review covering the years between 2002 and 2007 is presented in ref. [45]. More recently, in a multireader study, Das et al. [46] found that the additional use of a CAD system increases the radiologists' performance from an average of 82% to 94.3% based on 33 patients with a total of 215 thrombi. Later, Dewailly et al. [47] reported CAD accuracies under the focus of varying scanning conditions and image qualities using 74 data sets, of which 21 scans were positive for PE with a total of 93 peripheral clots. The overall sensitivity of the CAD tool was reported as 86% for detecting peripheral clots with a mean of 5.4 false-positives per patient. No significant difference in sensitivities between scans of varying scanning conditions and image quality was observed. Finally, Wittenberg et al. [48] performed a CAD evaluation in an on-call setting with 210 negative studies and 68 positive studies for PE, including a total number of 377 emboli. The CAD system found PE in seven patients originally reported as negative. On a per-patient basis, 64 scans were found positive (sensitivity of 94%), and in 44 scans without findings, no false-positives were detected by the CAD algorithm (specificity of 21%). On average, 4.7 false-positives were found per patient in the remaining 278 examinations.

Once a PE has been localized, the affected lung region can be characterized by the portion of the arterial tree distal to the embolus. Therefore, Kiraly et al. [8] extended the terminal branches of the affected subtree until they touch the chest wall and compute the hull of this extended tree.

Pulmonary perfusion defects caused by PE can also be visualized using dual-energy CT (cf. ref. [49]). Dual-source CT offers the possibility of scanning with different energies from two different x-ray sources. Because the attenuation coefficient of iodine is dependent on the photon energy, it can be directly visualized in lung tissue with dual-source CT. In pulmonary perfusion analysis using dual-energy information, a vessel segmentation can facilitate the analysis and the visualization of its results using, e.g., a color-coded overlay. By excluding or including the vessels from/to the lung areas as the ROI, the perfusion analysis can be limited to the lung parenchyma or vasculature to detect filling artifacts.

Finally, the severity of PE can be characterized using the CT obstruction index proposed by Qanadli et al. [50], which is based on the number of obstructed arterial segments. To this end, an automatic labeling method of the pulmonary arterial tree was proposed in ref. [51]. Based on the spatial information of the segmented arteries, the different arterial segments are identified, which serves as an input to determine the Qanadli index.

9.3.2 Lung Nodule-CAD

In CT, certain types of nodules appear in a similar intensity range as blood vessels and might also be attached to the vasculature. Hence, pulmonary vessels are often the reason for false-positive detections. Wiemker et al. [52] identified vessel bifurcations, strongly bent vessels, and vessels with a rapid decrease in diameter, among others, as typical cause for false-positive markings of their CAD system. While PE-CAD applications are used to reduce false-positive detections by excluding candidates that do not belong to the vascular tree, candidates in lung nodule-CAD that are associated with blood vessels can be disregarded. However, it is not an easy task to robustly differentiate between vessels and nodules, especially for vascular nodules with complex connections to the vessel trees. This issue is addressed in ref. [53] for previously detected true-positive lung nodules specified by the user with a focus on nodule volumetry.

Beyond that, there are a few approaches known in the literature that use vessel segmentations to reduce the false-positive rate. For instance, given the nodule detection algorithm [54], Agam et al. [23] reduced the set of nodule candidates by calculating the overlap between the nodule candidates and the segmented vascular tree. Depending on the overlap threshold, they found that, based on 38 diagnostic thoracic CT studies containing a total of 83 lung nodules, it is possible to remove 38% of false-positives while only removing 5% true positives at the same time. In a different study with 58 noncontrast CT scans, Zhou et al. [20] found that shape features extracted from their vessel segmentation can support differentiating nodules and pulmonary vascular structures. More recently, Cerello et al. [55] proposed the so-called "Channeler Ant Model," a 3D object segmentation tool, to segment and remove bronchial and vascular trees in the lungs. Results of this method are available for the ANODE'09 study and can be found in ref. [56].

Additionally, it is noteworthy that there exist several nodule enhancement filters that are similarly designed like vessel enhancement filters (Sections 9.2.2 and 9.2.3). The previously mentioned work of Agam and Wu [23,57], for instance, used different enhancement filters based on the structure tensor to separately enhance vessels, junctions, and nodules. In particular, filters capable of enhancing junctions while suppressing nodules are derived. As bifurcations are a frequent cause for false-positives in lung nodule detection, other work focuses particularly on model-based junction detection [58–59].

Finally, visualization and quantitative evaluation of the spatial distribution of vessels adjacent to the tumor in consideration may be important to distinguish between benign and malignant pulmonary nodules. Quantitative evaluation, however, can be performed best using automated methods, one of which is proposed in ref. [60].

9.3.3 Airway Segmentation and Virtual Bronchoscopy

Besides utilizing the airway–artery parallelism in vessel separation (Section 9.2.5), airway segmentation can be improved by vessel guidance [61,62]. Because of partial volume effects, airways can be only robustly segmented for a very limited number of generations. Parallel arteries, however, are visible up to much higher generations. Hence, Lo et al. proposed the use of vessel segmentation to compare the orientation of an airway candidate to the orientation of its neighboring vessel [63]. In a study with 250 low-dose CT scans, they have found that incorporating the vessel orientation similarity into their appearance model-based segmentation significantly improves the outcome with, on average, a 7% increase in the total length of correctly extracted airways.

More details on airway segmentation can be found in Chapter 8. Airways, in turn, have applications in virtual bronchoscopy, measuring bronchioarterial diameter ratios for quantifying PH or characterization of bronchial diseases such as chronically inflamed airways [64], and lung fissure segmentation (Section 9.3.4).

Finally, navigation through the airways can make use of the vessel segmentation as well. Geiger et al. [65] proposed to use the fact that every bronchus is accompanied by an artery to extend the reach of virtual bronchoscopy by using peripheral arteries as surrogate pathways. Given centerline representations of the airway and the vascular tree, it should be possible to detect corresponding paths using some kind of matching strategy [13, 66, 67] and then use the proximal bronchial path and the distal arterial path combined to present, e.g., a single continuous fly-through.

9.3.4 Lung Fissures and Lung Registration

Although smaller vessels may have less direct clinical relevance, segmentation of these vessels can provide important information for tree hierarchy, lobar lung segmentation, and lung region assessment. For instance, it is very difficult to extract lung fissures directly from CT images because they are often not completely visible due to partial volume effects. The left lung has two lobes separated by a major fissure, whereas the right lung has three lobes separated by one minor (horizontal) and one major (oblique) fissure. Because lobes are functionally independent units, each lobe has its own bronchial and vascular system. Identification of these very thin separating surfaces might be beneficial for different image processing steps. It might yield landmarks for lung registration used in follow-up studies for nodule growth assessment or lung motion quantification from 4DCT images for radiation treatment planning, which need to consider the tumor movement during respiration. It allows more accurate postoperative lung function quantification in case of a lobar resection (lobectomy) planning.

Therefore, lung vessels and bronchi are typically identified and used for dividing the lung into its five lobar regions [11, 68]. To this end, Kuhnigk et al. [68] identified regions without larger vessels by computing the Euclidean distances to the segmented vessels inside the lung regions. This distance map is additionally refined using the original intensity values. In particular, distance values and intensity values are linearly combined under the assumption that fissures will exhibit relatively bright intensities in the original image, which fall at the same time into regions with locally high distance values. Finally, a multidimensional interactive watershed transform is applied to the resulting fused image. Similarly, Zhou et al. [11] first classified the airways and vessels into five lobar groups based on the bronchial tree structure. Next, the 3D distances from the centerline of each lobar region are computed for each voxel inside the lung regions. Subsequently, each voxel is classified into a specific lung lobe resulting in a Voronoi partition with its separating surfaces being the initial fissures. Finally, interlobe fissures are extracted by refining the initial fissures considering the zero-crossings of a Laplacian-filtered neighborhood around the initial surfaces.

Not only lung fissures but also major vessel bifurcations can serve as additional landmarks for deformable lung registration [69, 70]. For instance, coordinates of vessel bifurcations are derived as feature points in ref. [69] using a thinning process to extract the centerlines. Furthermore, bifurcations in very close proximity to each other are deleted. Such extracted landmarks are tracked through different time points in a set of sequential 3DCT images (4DCT) using point pattern matching with a probabilistic relaxation method. Hilsmann et al. [70] extracted so-called "pronounced" bifurcations, which are vessel bifurcations that meet certain criteria on the number of involved branches and their diameters. These bifurcations (rather than all bifurcations) are used to define point correspondences by matching the vessel trees using features extracted from the junctions. In particular, a regional shape descriptor [67] is used to find corresponding points. The latter method has been compared with a surface-tracking method and two instances of registration methods minimizing the sum of squared differences on 10 CT data sets acquired for radiation therapy in ref. [71]. In this study, all methods showed a target registration error between 2.5 and 3.3 mm. More details on lung registration can be found in Chapter 5.

9.4 Summary and Conclusions

Many different medical applications can greatly benefit from segmenting vascular structures but often have different requirements on the segmentation outcome. On the one hand, applications examining vascular diseases directly, such as CAD and visualization of PE, require a particularly accurate segmentation. On the other hand, applications that use vessel segmentation as a basis to provide planning tools for lobar resections require the extracted vascular trees to reliably represent the corresponding anatomy. In such cases, the accurate delineation of the vessel boundaries is mostly of secondary interest. Additionally, the specific clinical question under investigation influences the demands on segmentation sensitivity versus specificity. Finally, the medical condition of the patient to be examined might impose further time constraints.

In this chapter, an overview of state-of-the-art pulmonary vessel segmentation methods is given, including a unique fuzzy segmentation approach. This fully automatic approach to pulmonary vessel segmentation in CTA data is robust to varying vessel intensities depending on contrast agent, scan protocol, etc. Because of its fuzzy segmentation scheme, it can be used in different applications as it allows influencing the sensitivity and specificity of the algorithms by simply adjusting a single threshold. Vessels of different size (large and small) are segmented accurately by the use of appropriate probability-like functions. Such probability functions allow the sound incorporation of local image features such as intensity information and vesselness filter response as well as higher-level knowledge. Furthermore, it allows the efficient addition of missed subtrees with single seed points.

Future challenges in pulmonary vessel segmentation include robust vessel separation and proper validation. Until recently, there has been only very limited work done on evaluating segmentation systems caused by missing ground truths. Consequently, objective comparison of the different existing techniques is hardly possible. Besides evaluating segmentation performances with respect to image quality, pathologies, etc., the effect of the segmentation quality on subsequent processing steps would be of interest. Currently, systems such as PE-CAD are only evaluated in terms of overall sensitivity and false-positives, but it is typically not examined if, e.g., false-negative PEs are caused by the detection or the underlying segmentation step.

References

1. Kaftan, J.N., A.P. Kiraly, M. Erdt, M. Sühling, T. Aach, 2008. Fuzzy pulmonary vessel segmentation using optimized vessel enhancement filtering. *MICCAI 1st International Workshop on Pulmonary Image Analysis*, 233–242.
2. Kaftan, J.N., A.P. Kiraly, A. Bakai, M. Das, C.L. Novak, T. Aach, 2008. Fuzzy pulmonary vessel segmentation in contrast enhanced CT data. *SPIE Medical Imaging*, 6914, 69141Q.
3. Grady, L. 2006. Random walks for image segmentation. *IEEE Transactions on Pattern Analysis and Machine Intelligence* 28:1768–1783.
4. Remy-Jardin, M., J. Remy, J.R. Mayo, N.L. Müller, 2001. *CT Angiography of the Chest*. Philadelphia, PA: Lippincott, Williams & Wilkins.
5. American Heart Association. 2009. Heart disease and stroke statistics 2009 update: A report from the American Heart Association Statistics Committee and Stroke Statistics Subcommittee. *Circulation* 119, e21–e181.

6. Wildberger, J.E., A.H. Mahnken, M. Das, A. Küttner, M. Lell, R.W. Günther, 2005. CT imaging in acute pulmonary embolism: Diagnostic strategies. *European Radiology* 15:919–929.
7. Kamangar, N., M.S. McDonnell, S. Sharma, Pulmonary embolism.
8. Kiraly, A.P., E. Pichon, D.P. Naidich, C.L. Novak, 2004. Analysis of arterial subtrees affected by pulmonary emboli. *SPIE Medical Imaging* 5370:1720–1729.
9. Masutani, Y., H. MacMahon, K. Doi, 2001. Automated segmentation and visualization of the pulmonary vascular tree in spiral CT angiography: An anatomy-oriented approach based on three-dimensional image analysis. *Journal of Computer Assisted Tomography* 25:587–597.
10. Bouma, H., J.J. Sonnemans, A. Vilanova, F.A. Gerritsen, 2009. Automatic detection of pulmonary embolism in CTA images. *IEEE Transactions on Medical Imaging* 28:1223–1230.
11. Zhou, X., T. Hayashi, T. Hara, H. Fujita, R. Yokoyama, T. Kiryu, H. Hoshi, 2006. Automatic segmentation and recognition of anatomical lung structures from high-resolution chest CT images. *Computerized Medical Imaging and Graphics* 30:299–313.
12. Fetita, C., P.Y. Brillet, F.J. Prêteux, 2009. Morpho-geometrical approach for 3D segmentation of pulmonary vascular tree in multi-slice CT. *SPIE Medical Imaging* 7259:72594F.
13. Bülow, T., R. Wiemker, T. Blaffert, C. Lorenz, S. Renisch, 2005. Automatic extraction of the pulmonary artery tree from multi-slice CT data. *SPIE Medical Imaging* 5746:730–740.
14. Park, S. 2006. Artery–Vein Separation from Thoracic CTA Scans with Application to PE Detection and Volume Visualization. University of Texas at Austin, Austin, TX.
15. Bruyninckx, P., D. Loeckx, D. Vandermeulen, P. Suetens, 2009. Segmentation of lung vessel trees by global optimization. *SPIE Medical Imaging* 7259:725912.
16. Zhu, X., Z. Xue, X. Gao, Y. Zhu, S.T.C. Wong, 2009. Voles: Vascularity-oriented level set algorithm for pulmonary vessel segmentation in image guided intervention threrapy. *Proceedings of the IEEE International Symposium on Biomedical Imaging (ISBI)*:1247–1250.
17. Shikata, H., E.A. Hoffman, M. Sonka, 2004. Automated segmentation of pulmonary vascular tree from 3D CT images. *SPIE Medical Imaging* 5369:107–116.
18. Shikata, H., G. McLennan, E.A. Hoffman, M. Sonka, 2009. Segmentation of pulmonary vascular trees from thoracic 3D CT images. *International Journal of Biomedical Imaging* 2009:1–11.
19. Liu, X., D.Z. Chen, X. Wu, M. Sonka, 2008. Optimal graph-based segmentation of 3D pulmonary airway and vascular trees across bifurcations. *MICCAI 1st International Workshop on Pulmonary Image Analysis*, 103–111.
20. Zhou, C., H.-P. Chan, B. Sahiner, L.M. Hadjiiski, A. Chughtai, S. Patel, J. Wei, J. Ge, P.N. Cascade, E.A. Kazerooni, 2007. Automatic multiscale enhancement and segmentation of pulmonary vessels in CT pulmonary angiography images for CAD applications. *Medical Physics* 34:4567–4577.
21. Korfiatis, P., A. Karahaliou, L. Costaridou, 2009. Automated vessel tree segmentation: Challenges in computer aided quantification of diffuse parenchyma lung diseases. *Proceedings of the 9th International Conference on Information Technology and Applications in Biomedicine (ITAB)*, 1–4.
22. Zhou, J., S. Chang, D.N. Metaxas, L. Axel, 2007. Vascular structure segmentation and bifurcation detection. *Proceedings of the IEEE International Symposium on Biomedical Imaging (ISBI)*, 872–875.
23. Agam, G., S.G. Armato III, C. Wu, 2005. Vessel tree reconstruction in thoracic CT scans with application to nodule detection. *IEEE Transactions on Medical Imaging* 24:486–499.
24. Wu, C., G. Agam, A.S. Roy, S.G. Armato III. 2004. Regulated morphology approach to fuzzy shape analysis with application to blood vessel extraction in thoracic CT scans. *SPIE Medical Imaging* 5370:1262–1270.
25. Song, G., A. Ramirez-Manzanares, J.C. Gee, 2008. A simultaneous segmentation and regularization framework for vessel extraction in CT images. *MICCAI 1st International Workshop on Pulmonary Image Analysis*, 185–193.
26. Eiho, S., H. Sekiguchi, T. Sugimoto, S. Urayama, 2004. Branch-based region growing method for blood vessel segmentation. *XXth ISPRS Congress, ISPRS*, 796–801.

27. Lorenz, C., I.-C. Carlsen, T.M. Buzug, C. Fassnacht, J. Weese, 1997. Multi-scale line segmentation with automatic estimation of width, contrast and tangential direction in 2D and 3D medical images. *First Joint Conference Computer Vision, Virtual Reality and Robotics in Medicine and Medical Robotics and Computer-Assisted Surgery (CVRMed-MRCAS)*, 233–242.
28. Sato, Y., S. Nakajima, N. Shiraga, H. Atsumi, S. Yoshida, T. Koller, G. Gerig, R. Kikinis, 1998. Three-dimensional multi-scale line filter for segmentation and visualization of curvilinear structures in medical images. *Medical Image Analysis* 2:143–168.
29. Frangi, A.F., W.J. Niessen, K.L. Vincken, M.A. Viergever, 1998. Multiscale vessel enhancement filtering. *Medical Image Computing and Computer-Assisted Intervention (MICCAI)*, 1496. LNCS, 130–137.
30. Erdt, M., M. Raspe, M. Sühling, 2008. Automatic hepatic vessel segmentation using graphics hardware. *4th Int Workshop on Medical Imaging and Augmented Reality (MIAR)*, 5128. LNCS, 403–412.
31. Lesage, D., E.D. Angelini, I. Bloch, G. Funka-Lea, 2009. Design and study of flux-based features for 3D vascular tracking. *Proceedings of the IEEE International Symposium on Biomedical Imaging (ISBI)*, 286–289.
32. Aylward, S.R., E. Bullitt, 2002. Initialization, noise, singularities, and scale in height ridge traversal for tubular object centerline extraction. *IEEE Transactions on Medical Imaging* 21:61–75.
33. Li, K., X. Wu, D.Z. Chen, M. Sonka, 2006. Optimal surface segmentation in volumetric images—A graph-theoretic approach. *IEEE Transactions on Pattern Analysis and Machine Intelligence* 28:119–134.
34. Boykov, Y., G. Funka-Lea, 2006. Graph cuts and efficient N-D image segmentation. *International Journal of Computer Vision* 70:109–131.
35. Udupa, J.K., S. Samarasekera, 1996. Fuzzy connectedness and object definition: Theory, algorithms, and applications in image segmentation. *Graphical Models and Image Processing* 58:246–261.
36. Ciesielski, K.C., J.K. Udupa, 2010. Affinity functions in fuzzy connectedness based image segmentation I: Equivalence of affinities. *Computer Vision and Image Understanding* 114:146–154.
37. Lesage, D., E.D. Angelini, I. Bloch, G. Funka-Lea, 2009. A review of 3D vessel lumen segmentation techniques: Models, features and extraction schemes. *Medical Image Analysis*, 13:819–845.
38. Kiraly, A.P., J.P. Helferty, E.A. Hoffman, G. McLennan, W.E. Higgins, 2004. Three-dimensional path planning for virtual bronchoscopy. *IEEE Transactions on Medical Imaging* 23:1365–1379.
39. Chen, Y., C.O. Laura, K. Drechsler, 2009. Generation of a graph representation from three-dimensional skeletons of the liver vasculature. *2nd International Conference on Biomedical Engineering and Informatics (BMEI)*. IEEE, 1–5.
40. Saha, P.K., Z. Gao, S.K. Alford, M. Sonka, E.A. Hoffman, 2010. Topomorphologic separation of fused isointensity objects via multiscale opening: Separating arteries and veins in 3-D pulmonary CT. *IEEE Transactions on Medical Imaging* 29:840–851.
41. Pichon, E., C.L. Novak, A.P. Kiraly, D.P. Naidich, 2004. A novel method for pulmonary emboli visualization from high-resolution CT images. *SPIE Medical Imaging*, 5367:161–170.
42. Kiraly, A.P., C.L. Novak, D.P. Naidich, I. Vlahos, J.P. Ko, G.T. Brusca-Augello, 2006. A comparison of 2D and 3D evaluation methods for pulmonary embolism detection in CT images. *SPIE Medical Imaging* 6146:132–140.
43. Masutani, Y., H. MacMahon, K. Doi, 2002. Computerized detection of pulmonary embolism in spiral CT angiography based on volumetric image analysis. *IEEE Transactions on Medical Imaging* 21:1517–1523.
44. Zhou, C., H.P. Chan, B. Sahiner, L.M. Hadjiiski, A. Chughtai, S. Patel, J. Wei, P.N. Cascade, E.A. Kazerooni, 2009. Evaluation of computerized detection of pulmonary embolism in independent data sets of computed tomographic pulmonary angiographic (CTPA) scans. *SPIE Medical Imaging* 7260:72600B.

45. Chan, H.-P., L. Hadjiiski, C. Zhou, B. Sahiner, 2008. Computer-aided diagnosis of lung cancer and pulmonary embolism in computed tomography—A review. *Academic Radiology* 15:535–555.
46. Das, M., G. Mühlenbruch, A. Helm, A. Bakai, M. Salganicoff, S. Stanzel, J. Liang, M. Wolf, R. Günther, J. Wildberger, 2008. Computer-aided detection of pulmonary embolism: Influence on radiologists' detection performance with respect to vessel segments. *European Radiology* 18:1350–1355.
47. Dewailly, M., M. Rémy-Jardin, A. Duhamel, J.-B. Faivre, F. Pontana, V. Deken, A. Bakai, J. Remy, 2010. Computer-aided detection of acute pulmonary embolism with 64-slice multi-detector row computed tomography: Impact of the scanning conditions and overall image quality in the detection of peripheral clots. *Journal of Computer Assisted Tomography* 34:23–30.
48. Wittenberg, R., J.F. Peters, J.J. Sonnemans, M. Prokop, C.M. Schaefer-Prokop, 2010. Computer-assisted detection of pulmonary embolism: Evaluation of pulmonary CT angiograms performed in an on-call setting. *European Radiology* 20:801–806.
49. Thieme, S.F., C.R. Becker, M. Hacker, K. Nikolaou, M.F. Reiser, T.R.C. Johnson, 2008. Dual energy CT for the assessment of lung perfusion—Correlation to scintigraphy. *European Journal of Radiology* 68:369–374.
50. Qanadli, S.D., M. El Hajjam, A. Vieillard-Baron, T. Joseph, B. Mesurolle, V.L. Oliva, O. Barre, F. Bruckert, O. Dubourg, P. Lacombe, 2001. New CT index to quantify arterial obstruction in pulmonary embolism: Comparison with angiographic index and echocardiography. *American Journal of Roentgenology* 176:1415–1420.
51. Peters, R., H.A. Marqueringa, H. Doğanc, E.A. Hendriks, A. de Roosc, J.H.C. Reibera, B.C. Stoela, 2007. Labeling the pulmonary arterial tree in CT images for automatic quantification of pulmonary embolism. *SPIE Medical Imaging* 6514:65143Q.
52. Wiemker, R., P. Rogalla, T. Blaffert, D. Sifri, O. Hay, E. Shah, R. Truyen, T. Fleiter, 2005. Aspects of computer-aided detection (CAD) and volumetry of pulmonary nodules using multislice CT. *British Journal of Radiology* 78:S46–S56.
53. Kuhnigk, J.M., V. Dicken, L. Bornemann, A. Bakai, D. Wormanns, S. Krass, H.-O. Peitgen, 2006. Morphological segmentation and partial volume analysis for volumetry of solid pulmonary lesions in thoracic CT scans. *IEEE Transactions on Medical Imaging* 25:417–434.
54. Armato III, S.G., M.B. Altman, P.J.L. Riviere, 2003. Automated detection of lung nodules in CT scans: Effect of image reconstruction algorithm. *Medical Physics* 30:461–472.
55. Cerello, P., S.C. Cheran, S. Bagnasco, R. Bellotti, L. Bolanos, E. Catanzariti, G. De Nunzio, et al. 2010. 3-D object segmentation using ant colonies. *Pattern Recognition* 43:1476–1490.
56. van Ginneken, B., S.G. Armato 3rd, B. de Hoop, S. van Amelsvoort-van de Vorst, T. Duindam, M. Niemeijer, K. Murphy, et al. 2010. Comparing and combining algorithms for computer-aided detection of pulmonary nodules in computed tomography scans: the ANODE09 Study. *Medical Image Analysis* 14:707–722.
57. Wu, C., G. Agam, 2006. Probabilistic nodule filtering in thoracic CT scans. *SPIE Medical Imaging* 6144:612–620.
58. Mendonça, P.R.S., R. Bhotika, S.A. Sirohey, W.D. Turner, J.V. Miller, R.S. Avila, 2005. Model-based analysis of local shape for lesion detection in CT scans. *Medical Image Computing and Computer-Assisted Intervention (MICCAI)*, 3749. LNCS 688–695.
59. Zhao, F., P.R.S., Mendonca, R. Bhotika, J.V. Miller, 2007. Model-based junction detection algorithm with application to lung nodule detection. *Proceedings of the IEEE International Symposium on Biomedical Imaging (ISBI)*, 504–507.
60. Shikata, H., H. Kitaoka, Y. Sato, T. Johkou, H. Nakamura, S. Tamura, 2003. Quantitative evaluation of spatial distribution of line structure in the lung for computer-aided diagnosis of pulmonary nodules. *Systems and Computers in Japan* 34:58–70.
61. Sonka, M., W. Park, E.A. Hoffman, 1996. Rule-based detection of intrathoracic airway trees. *IEEE Transactions on Medical Imaging* 15:314–326.

62. Lo, P., J. Sporring, H. Ashraf, J.J.H. Pedersen, M. de Bruijne, 2008. Vessel-guided airway segmentation based on voxel classification. *MICCAI 1st International Workshop on Pulmonary Image Analysis*, 113–122.
63. Lo, P., J. Sporring, H. Ashraf, J.J.H. Pedersen, M. de Bruijne, 2010. Vessel-guided airway tree segmentation: A voxel classification approach. *Medical Image Analysis* 14:527–538.
64. Kiraly, A.P., B.L. Odry, M. Godoy, B. Geiger, C.L. Novak, D.P. Naidich, 2008. Computer-aided diagnosis of the airways: Beyond nodule detection. *Journal of Thoracic Imaging* 23:105–113.
65. Geiger, B., A.P. Kiraly, D.P. Naidich, C.L. Novak, 2005. Virtual bronchoscopy of peripheral nodules using arteries as surrogate pathways. *SPIE Medical Imaging* 5746:352–360.
66. Kaftan, J.N., A.P. Kiraly, D.P. Naidich, C.L. Novak, 2006. A novel multi-purpose tree and path matching algorithm with application to airway trees. *SPIE Medical Imaging* 6143:215–224.
67. Bülow, T., C. Lorenz, R. Wiemker, J. Honko, 2006. Point based methods for automatic bronchial tree matching and labeling. *SPIE Medical Imaging* 6143:61430O.
68. Kuhnigk, J.M., H.K. Hahn, M. Hindennach, V. Dicken, S. Krass, H.-O. Peitgen, 2003. Lung lobe segmentation by anatomy-guided 3D watershed transform. *Medical Imaging* 5032:1482–1490.
69. Tashiro, M., S. Minohara, T. Kanai, K. Yusa, H. Sakurai, T. Nakano, 2006. Three-dimensional velocity mapping of lung motion using vessel bifurcation pattern matching. *Medical Physics* 33:1747–1757.
70. Hilsmann, A., T. Vik, M. Kaus, K. Franks, J.-P. Bissonette, T. Purdie, A. Bejzak, T. Aach, 2007. Deformable 4DCT lung registration with vessel bifurcations. *Proceedings of the 21st International Congress on Computer Assisted Radiology and Surgery (CARS)*.
71. Vik, T., S. Kabus, J. von Berg, K. Ens, S. Dries, T. Klinder, C. Lorenz, 2008. Validation and comparison of registration methods for free-breathing 4D lung-CT. *SPIE Medical Imaging* 6914:69142P.

10

A Novel Level Set-Based Computer-Aided Detection System for Automatic Detection of Lung Nodules in Low-Dose Chest Computed Tomography Scans

Ayman El-Baz, Aly Farag, Georgy Gimel'farb, Robert Falk, and Mohamed Abo El-Ghar

CONTENTS

10.1 Introduction

Lung cancer remains the leading cause of mortality cancer. In 1999, there were approximately 170,000 new cases of lung cancer [1,2], one in every 18 women and one in every 12 men develop lung cancer. Early detection of lung tumors (visible on chest film as nodules) may increase the patient's chance of survival [3,4], but detecting nodules is a complicated task (see, e.g., refs. [5,6]). Nodules show up as relatively low-contrast white circular objects within the lung fields. The difficulty for computer-aided detection (CAD) schemes is distinguishing true nodules from (overlapping) shadows, vessels, and ribs.

At present, low-dose spiral computed tomography (LDCT) is of prime interest for screening (high-risk) groups for early detection of lung cancer [1,7,8]. The LDCT provides chest scans with very high spatial, temporal, and contrast resolution of anatomic structures and is able to gather a complete three-dimensional (3D) volume of a human thorax in a single breath-hold [5]. Hence, for these reasons, in recent years, most lung cancer screening programs are being investigated in the United States [8–12] and Japan [7,13–15] with low-dose helical computed tomography (LDCT) as the screening modality of choice.

The automatic screening typically involves two-stage detection of lung abnormalities (nodules). First, initial candidate nodules are selected, and then, false-positive nodules (FPNs) are partially eliminated while preserving true-positive nodules (TPNs).

At the first stage, conformal nodule filtering [16] or unsharp masking [17] can enhance nodules and suppress other structures to separate the candidates from the background by simple thresholding (to improve the separation, background trend is corrected in refs. [18–21] within image regions of interest) or multiple gray-level thresholding technique [22–24]. A series of 3D cylindrical and spherical filters are used to detect small lung nodules from high-resolution CT images [25–29]. Circular and semicircular nodule candidates can be detected by template matching [17,30,31]. However, these spherical, cylindrical, or circular assumptions are not adequate for describing general geometry of the lesions. This is because their shape can be irregular due to the spiculation or the attachments to the pleural surface (i.e., juxtapleural and peripheral) and vessels (i.e.,vascularized) [32]. In refs. [33–36], they used morphological operators to detect lung nodules. The drawbacks to these approaches are the difficulties in detecting lung wall nodules. Also, there are other pattern recognition techniques used in the detection of lung nodules such as clustering [38–40, 55], linear discriminate functions [41], rule-based classification [42], Hough transform [47], connected component analysis of thresholded CT slices [43,44], gray-level distance transform [40], and patient-specific a priori model [45].

The FPNs are excluded at the second stage by feature extraction and classification [18,19,46–49]. Such features as circularity, size, contrast [19], or local curvature [49], which are extracted by morphological techniques, and artificial neural networks (ANN) are frequently used as postclassifiers [33,48,50–54]. Also, there is a number of classification techniques used in the final stage of the nodule detection systems to reduce the FPNs, such as rule-based or linear classifier [21–23, 25, 27, 30, 38, 55, 56], template matching [45], nearest cluster [34,36], Markov random field [57]. Also, there are other extensive studies to get accurate segmentation of lung nodules. Okada et al. [58] proposed an anisotropic intensity model fitting with analytical parameter estimation. Zhao et al. [59,60] and Kostis et al. [32] proposed to segment 2D and 3D nodules based on thresholding the voxel intensity. Their algorithms accurately segment well-defined solid nodules with similar average intensities but become unreliable on the cavity or nonsolid nodules. Table 10.1 gives an overview of the different CAD models that are covered in this chapter.

The overview in Table 10.1 shows the following limitations of the existing approaches:

1. Most need to manually set some parameters to correspond to the given data.
2. Most are suitable only for segmenting solid circular or spherical nodules and fail to segment nodules of irregular shapes.
3. Most are not suitable for segmenting cavity nodules.
4. All of them are very slow due to the huge space they are searching.

In this chapter, we present a fully automatic approach to detect lung nodules. Our CAD system detects the nodules in LDCT images in three main steps: (1) segmentation of the raw scanning information to isolate the lung tissues from the rest of the structures in the chest cavity; (2) extraction of the 3D anatomic structures (e.g., blood vessels, bronchioles, alveoli, possible abnormalities) from the already segmented lung tissues; and (3) identification of the nodules by isolating the true nodules from other extracted structures. The purpose of the first two steps is to considerably reduce the searching space. The proposed approach in this paper includes a 3D deformable nodule prototype (simulated nodule) combined with a central-symmetric 3D intensity model of the nodules. The model closely approximates an empirical marginal probability distribution of image intensities in the real nodules of different size and is analytically identified from the empirical distribution.

TABLE 10.1

Overview of the Most Recent CAD Approaches

Study	FP Reduction
Kanazawa et al. [55]	Rule based
Suzuki et al. [53]	Massive training ANN
Brown et al. [45]	–
Ko and Betke [23]	–
Lee et al. [30]	MAP-based classification using five grayscale features
Tanino et al. [36]	Classification based on principle component analysis
Saita et al. [44]	Classification based on location based features
Kubo et al. [39]	Rule based
Takizawa et al. [57]	–
Weir et al. [2]	–
Wiemker et al. [31]	–
Fetita et al. [35]	–
Mekadaa et al. [21]	Rule based
Yamada et al. [40]	Rule based
Awai et al. [33]	Threshold based
Chang et al. [25]	Shape based
Enquobahrie et al. [20]	Filter based
Li and Doi [27]	–
Paik et al. [28]	–
Zhang et al. [54]	–
Zhao et al. [24]	Rule based
Mendona et al. [29]	Morphology based

Note: The data parameters used in these studies (number of scans, number of subjects, slice thickness, and radiation dose) mentioned in the "Data" column.

10.2 Methods and Data Acquisition

In our protocol, LDCT imaging is employed by a multidetector GE light speed plus scanner (General Electric, Milwaukee, WI). The LDCT was performed with the following parameters: slice thickness, 2.5 mm; reconstructed every 1.25 mm; scanning pitch, 1 mm; kilovolt, 120; milliampere, 220; field of view 36 cm.

Figure 10.1 shows the block diagram and an illustration example of the proposed approach. The system consists of the following main steps: (1) accurate statistical model describing the distribution of gray level for each CT slice; (2) lung extraction; (3) artery, vein, bronchus, bronchiole, and abnormality extraction (if it exists); (4) detection of lung abnormalities; and (5) reduction of FPNs. Note that the proposed algorithm involves two segmentation steps (steps 2 and 3) to reduce the searching space. Therefore, the probability to detect the lung nodules is increased, and also, the two steps are essential for estimating the parameters required for template model in order to decrease the number of FPNs that may be detected by the proposed approach. In this chapter, we focus on the detection step, and the details of the two segmentation steps are shown in details in ref. [61].

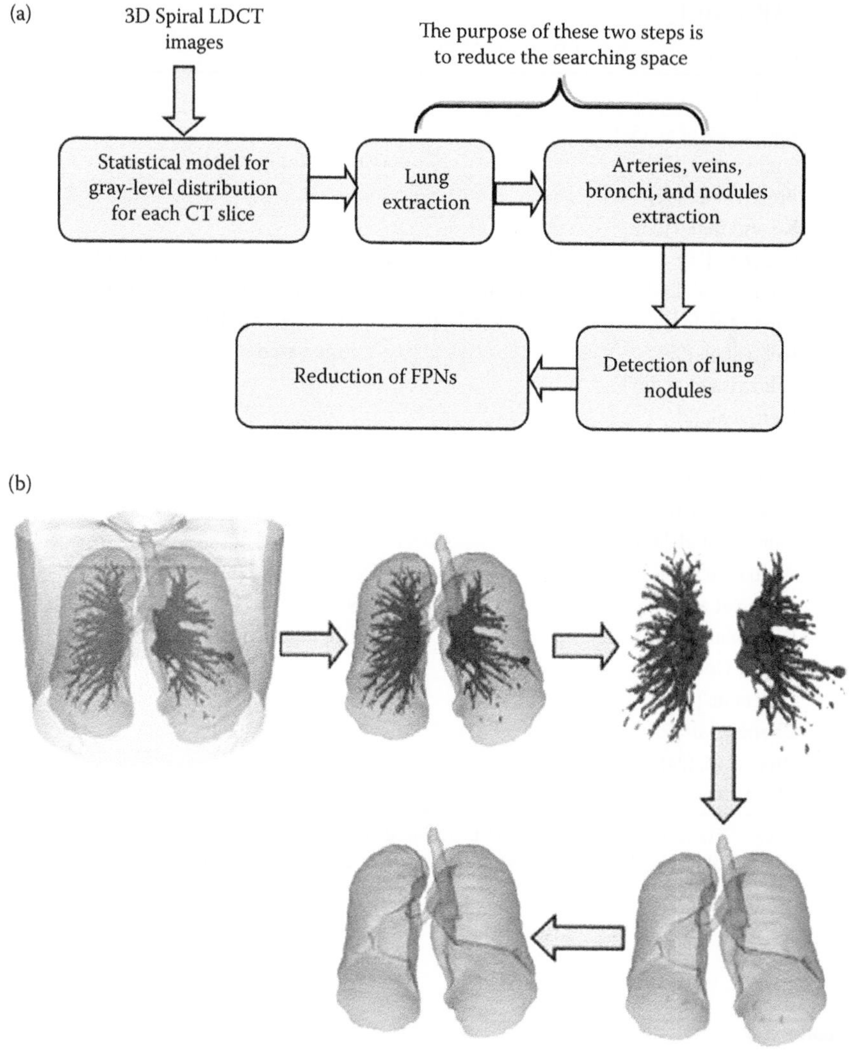

FIGURE 10.1
(See color insert.) The lung abnormality detection system: (a) block diagram and (b) illustration example.

10.3 Detecting Lung Nodules with Deformable Prototypes

The detection step extracts by shape and intensities and classifies the nodule candidates among all the 3D objects selected at the second segmentation stage.

10.3.1 Deformable Prototype of a Candidate Nodule

To extract the nodule candidates among the already selected objects like those in Figure 10.1b, we use the deformable prototypes generated by level sets [62] that have become a powerful segmentation tool in recent years. The evolving prototype's surface at time instant τ^{o} is a propagating zero-level front $\phi(i,j,z,\tau^{o}) = 0$ of a certain 4D scalar function $\phi(i,j,z,\tau)$ of 3D Cartesian coordinates (i,j,z) and time τ. Changes in φ in continuous time are given by the partial differential equation:

$$\frac{\partial\phi(i,j,z,\tau)}{\partial\tau} + F(i,j,z)\left| \quad \phi(i,j,z,\tau)\right| = 0 \tag{10.1}$$

where $F(i,j,z)$ is a velocity function and ∇ denotes the differential operator $= \left[\frac{\partial}{\partial i}, \frac{\partial}{\partial j}, \frac{\partial}{\partial z}\right]^{T}$.

The scalar velocity function controlling the front evolution depends on local geometric properties, e.g., a local curvature, $k(i,j,z)$, of the front, and on local input data parameters, e.g., a 3D gradient, $\nabla\mathbf{X}(i,j,z)$, of the segmented 3D image $\mathbf{X}$.

In practice, the difference relationship replaces the differential one of Equation 10.1, and each next value $\phi(i,j,z,\tau_{n+1})$ at discrete time instant τ_{n+1} relates to the current $\phi(i,j,z,\tau_n)$ at instant τ_n such that $\tau_{n+1} - \tau_n = \Delta\tau$ as follows:

$$\phi(i,j,z,\tau_{n+1}) = \phi(i,j,z,\tau_n) - \Delta\tau . F(i,j,z)|\nabla\phi(i,j,z,\tau_n)|$$

The velocity function F plays a major role in the propagation process. Among variants in refs. [63,64], we have chosen $F(i,j,z) = h(i,j,z)(-1 - \varepsilon k(i,j,z))$, where $h(i,j,z)$ and ε are a local consistency term and a smoothing factor, respectively. Since the level set for a segmented 3D image $\mathbf{X}$ can always be initialized inside an object, an appropriate consistency term to evolve faster to the object boundary can be as follows:

$$h(i,j,z) = \frac{d(i,j,z)}{\left(1 + \left| \quad \mathbf{X}(i,j,z)\right|\right)}$$

where $d(i,j,z)$ is the distance map inside the segmented data $\mathbf{X}$ as shown in Figure 10.2c. The objective of using the distance map term inside the consistency term $h(i,j,z)$ is to prevent the level set front from propagating through blood vessels to which the nodules may be connected. In this chapter, we used fast marching level sets method [62] to compute the

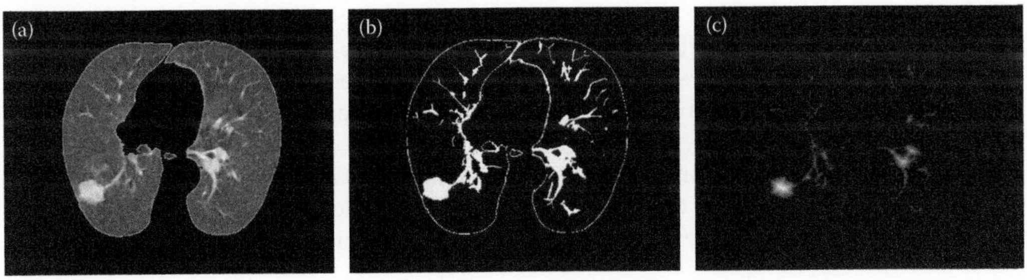

FIGURE 10.2
(a) Segmented lung region, (b) segmented arteries, veins, and lung nodule using the approach proposed in ref. [61], and (c) distance map inside the extracted arteries, veins, and lung nodule shown in (b).

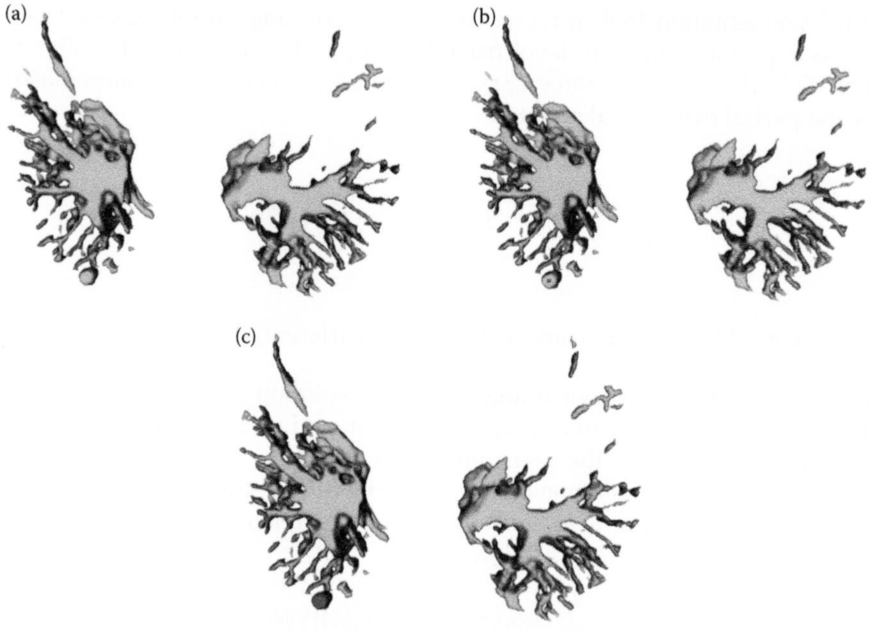

FIGURE 10.3
(See color insert.) (a) Part of the separated 3D lung objects, (b) the initialized level set shown in red, and (c) the finally extracted potential nodule candidate.

distance map shown in Figure 10.2c. Figure 10.3 shows the results of extracting a potential nodule candidate with the deformable prototype. To check whether the extracted object is really a nodule candidate, we should measure similarity between grayscale patterns in the extracted part of the initial 3D image and the intensity prototype of the nodule of that shape.

10.3.2 Similarity Measure for Grayscale Nodule Prototypes

Analysis of abnormalities in real 3D LDCT slices suggests that gray levels in central cross sections of a solid-shape 3D nodule or in a solid-shape 2D nodule roughly follow a central symmetric Gaussian spatial pattern such that the large central intensity gradually decreases toward the boundary. Moreover, the marginal gray-level distributions for all 3D objects separated from the lung tissues at the second segmentation stage (e.g., arteries, veins, bronchi, nodules of different size) are very similar to each other. The 3D Gaussian intensity pattern in each grayscale nodule prototype ensures that the marginal gray-level distribution closely approximates the empirical one for each real nodule in the LDCT data.

Let the prototype be a central-symmetric 3D Gaussian of radius R with the maximum intensity q_{max} in the center so that the gray-level $q(r)$ at any location (i,j,z) at radius $r = (i^2 + j^2 + z^2)^{1/2}$ with respect to the center (0,0,0) is given by the obvious relationship:

$$q(r) = q_{max} \exp\left(-\left(\frac{r}{\rho}\right)^2\right); \qquad 0 \le r \le R \tag{10.2}$$

The scatter parameter ρ in Equation 10.2 specifies how fast the signals decrease toward the boundary of the prototype. The maximum gray level, $q_{max} = q(0)$, and the minimum one, $q_{min} = q(R)$, on the boundary of the spherical Gaussian prototype of the radius R uniquely determine this parameter as follows:

$$\rho = R\left(\ln q_{max} - \ln q_{min}\right)^{-\frac{1}{2}} \tag{10.3}$$

Because all the prototype's points with a fixed gray value q in the continuous interval $[q_{min}, q_{max}]$ are located at the spherical surface of the radius $r(q) = \rho(\ln q_{max} - \ln q)^{1/2}$, their density is proportional to the surface area $4\pi r^2(q)$. Therefore, the marginal probability density function for such a prototype (simulated nodule or generated deformable template) is $\psi(q) = \gamma\pi r^2(q)$, where γ is the normalizing factor such that $\int_{q_{min}}^{q_{max}} \psi(q)\,\mathrm{d}q = 1$. It is easily shown that this function has the following closed form:

$$\psi(q \mid q_{min}, q_{max}) = \frac{\ln q_{max} - \ln q}{q_{max} - q_{min}(1 + \ln q_{max} - \ln q_{min})} \tag{10.4}$$

The gray-level parameters q_{max} and q_{min} are estimated from the empirical marginal distribution for each segmented 3D object, e.g., $q_{max} = 255$ and $q_{min} = 61$ (Figure 10.4) for the extracted arteries, veins, and nodule (Figure 10.1b, red).

To evaluate similarity, the gray-level nodule prototype is centered at the centroid of the volume extracted with the deformable prototype.

10.3.3 Lung Nodule Detection Algorithm

1. Separate lung regions from a given CT scan using the segmentation algorithms described in ref. [61].
2. Separate arteries, veins, bronchi, bronchioles, and lung nodules (if they exist) from the above lung regions using the same segmentation algorithms described in ref. [61].

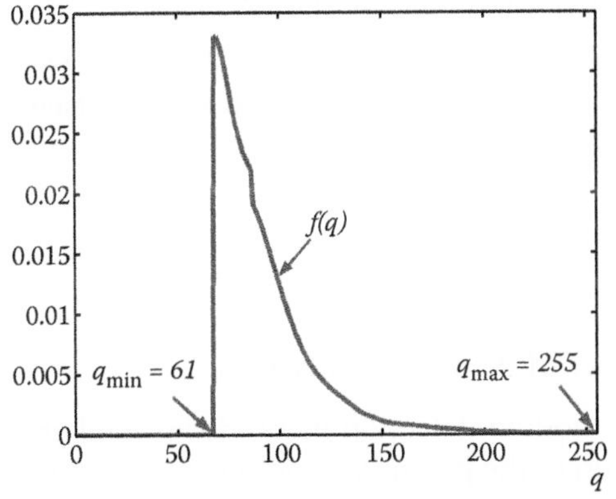

FIGURE 10.4
Empirical gray-level distribution over the extracted arteries, veins, and nodule presented in red in Figure 10.1b.

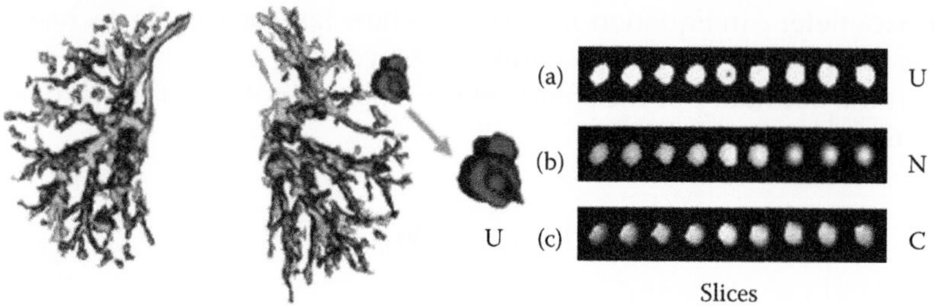

FIGURE 10.5
(See color insert.) Detected nodule candidate: (a) slices of the extracted voxel set U, (b) the gray-level prototype N, and (c) the actual gray levels C (the correlation $\text{Corr}_{C,N} = 0.886$).

3. From the empirical marginal gray-level distribution for the objects separated at step 2, calculate $q_{\min}$ and $q_{\max}$ (see an example in Figure 10.4).
4. Stack all the voxels separated at step 2.
5. Pop-up a top voxel from the stack as a seed for the deformable prototype and let this latter propagate until reaching a steady state indicating that the voxel set **U** enclosed by the final prototype constitutes an extracted object.
6. Calculate the centroid for the voxel set **U** extracted at the previous step; find the maximum and the minimum radii, $R_{\max}$ and $R_{\min}$, respectively, from the centroid of the boundary of that set; find the average radius, $R = (R_{\min} + R_{\max})/2$, and estimate the scatter parameter ρ from Equation 10.3.
7. Use Equation 10.2 to assign the prototype gray levels $N_{i,j,z}$ for each extracted voxel $(i,j,z) \in \mathbf{U}$.
8. Use the normalized cross-correlation $\text{Corr}_{C,N}$ between the actual extracted object $\mathbf{C} = [C_{i,j,z} : (i,j,z) \in \mathbf{U}]$ and its gray-level nodule prototype $\mathbf{N} = [N_{i,j,z} : (i,j,z) \in \mathbf{U}]$ as the similarity measure (see Figure 10.5).
9. If $\text{Corr}_{C,N} \geq T$, where T is a preselected similarity threshold (in our experiments below we set it to $T = 0.85$ on the empirical basis), then classify the extracted object as the potential nodule candidate (see Figure 10.6).
10. Remove all the voxels of the extracted object from the stack (see Figure 10.6).
11. If the stack is empty, then stop; otherwise, go to step 5 (see Figure 10.6).

10.4 Postclassification of Nodule Features

As with most automatic nodule detection methods, a number of FPNs are encountered during the initial selection of the potential candidates. To reduce the error rate, the potential candidates are postclassified using three shape and image features: (i) radial nonuniformity of the boundary $\max_\alpha(d(\alpha)) - \min_\alpha(d(\alpha))$, where $d(\alpha)$ is the distance in spatial direction α between the centroid and the boundary, (ii) mean gray-level (q_{avr}), and (iii) the

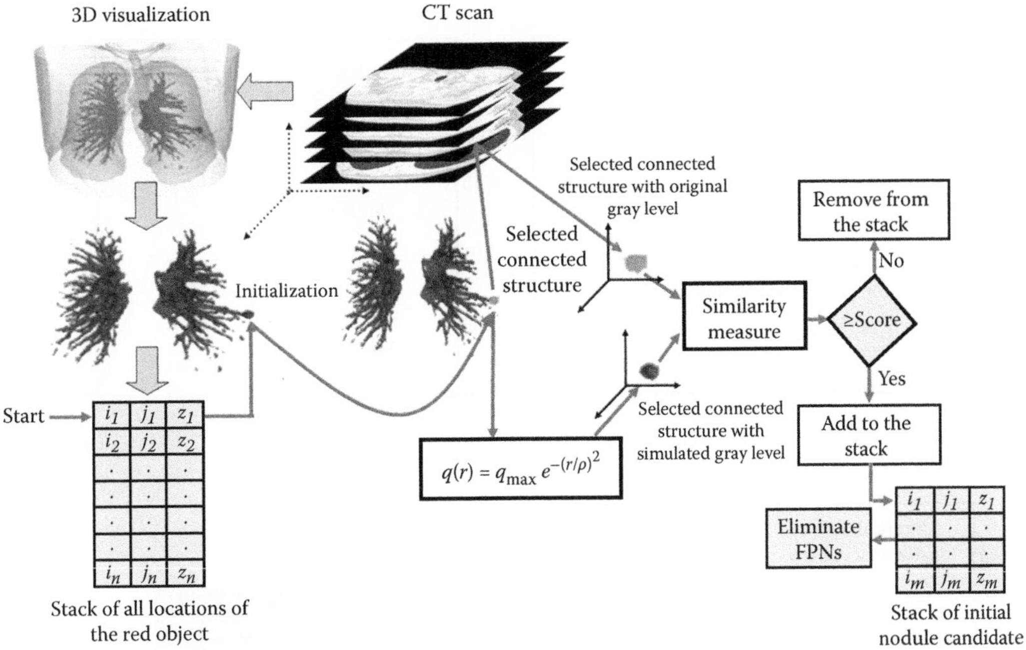

FIGURE 10.6
(See color insert.) Step-by-step illustration of the proposed CAD detection system.

10th percentile gray level for the marginal gray-level distribution for the potential candidate. A Bayesian-supervised classifier, assuming the features are statistically independent, is trained to distinguish between the FPNs and TPNs. To get more accurate probability distributions of each feature required by the classifier, we approximate empirical distributions for a given training set of the false and true nodules with linear combinations of discrete Gaussians (LCDGs) having positive and negative components. The approximation is performed with our modified expectation-maximization–based algorithms proposed in ref. [61]. Figure 10.7 shows the empirical and estimated distributions of each feature for both TPNs and FPNs.

10.5 Experimental Results and Conclusions

The proposed algorithm was tested on the same LDCT scans of 200 screened subjects. Among them, 21 subjects had abnormalities in their CT scans and 179 subjects were normal (this classification was validated by three radiologists). Each scan was 2.5 mm thin and 512 × 512 pixels. Our approach extracted 113 potential nodule candidates out of the true 119 nodules and 14 FPNs. The postclassification has reduced the number of FPNs to four but simultaneously rejected two true nodules. Thus, the final detection rate of the TPNs was 93.3% (111/119), with the FPNs rate of 3.36%. Both the rates are notably better

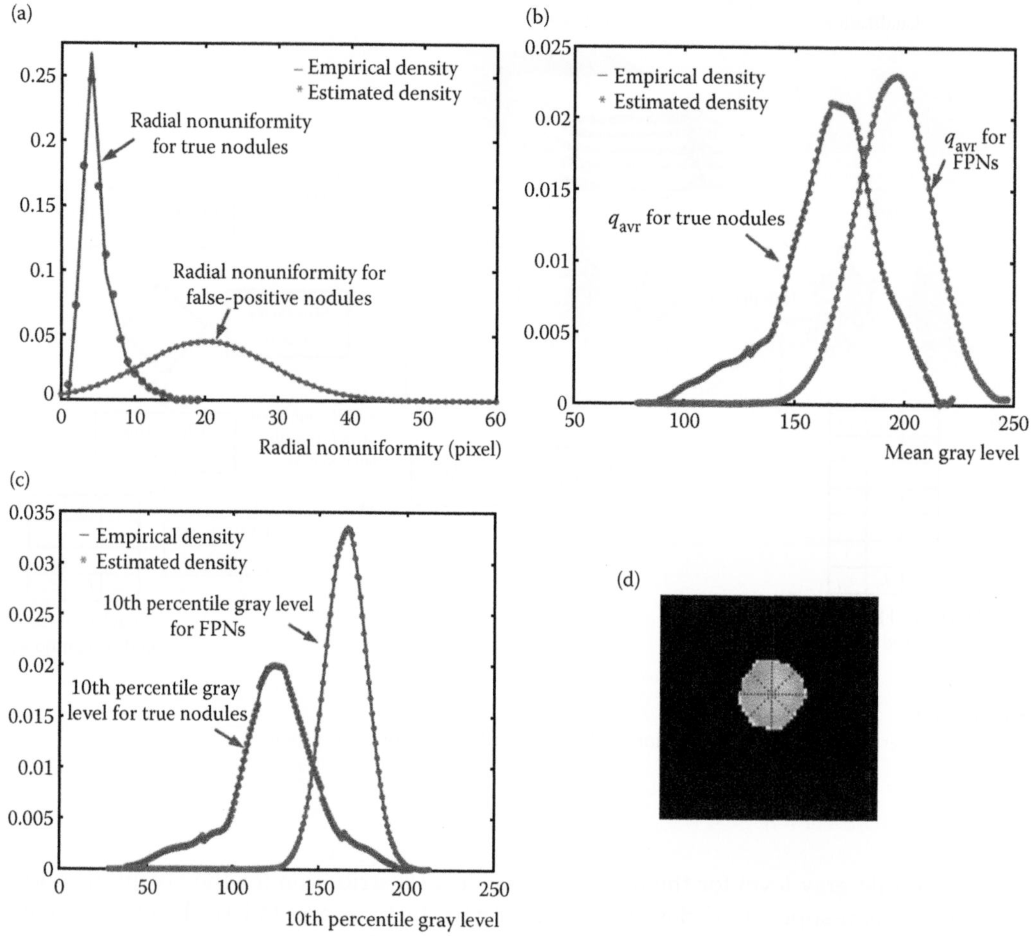

FIGURE 10.7
Estimated and empirical distributions for (a) radial nonuniformity, (b) mean gray level, (c) 10th percentile gray level, and (d) the calculation of $d(\alpha)$ at eight directions.

than 82.3% and 9.2% in ref. [65], respectively. Figures 10.8 and 10.9 show several large lung nodules detected by our approach, and a few small detected TPNs are depicted in Figure 10.10. Figures 10.11 and 10.12 show axial cross section in some detected lung nodules using the proposed approach. It is clear from Figures 10.11 and 10.12 that the cross sections of the detected nodules are not purely circular, which highlight the advantages of using level sets to generate the deformable templates that have the same shape as the true nodules. Table 10.2 presents the above results in detail.

Another way to measure and test the performance of the system is to compute the receiver operating characteristic (ROC) [66]. An ROC curve is a plot of test sensitivity (the fraction of correctly classified positive samples) on the y-axis versus its FPNs (or 1 − specificity) plotted on the x-axis. Note that specificity is defined as the fraction of correctly

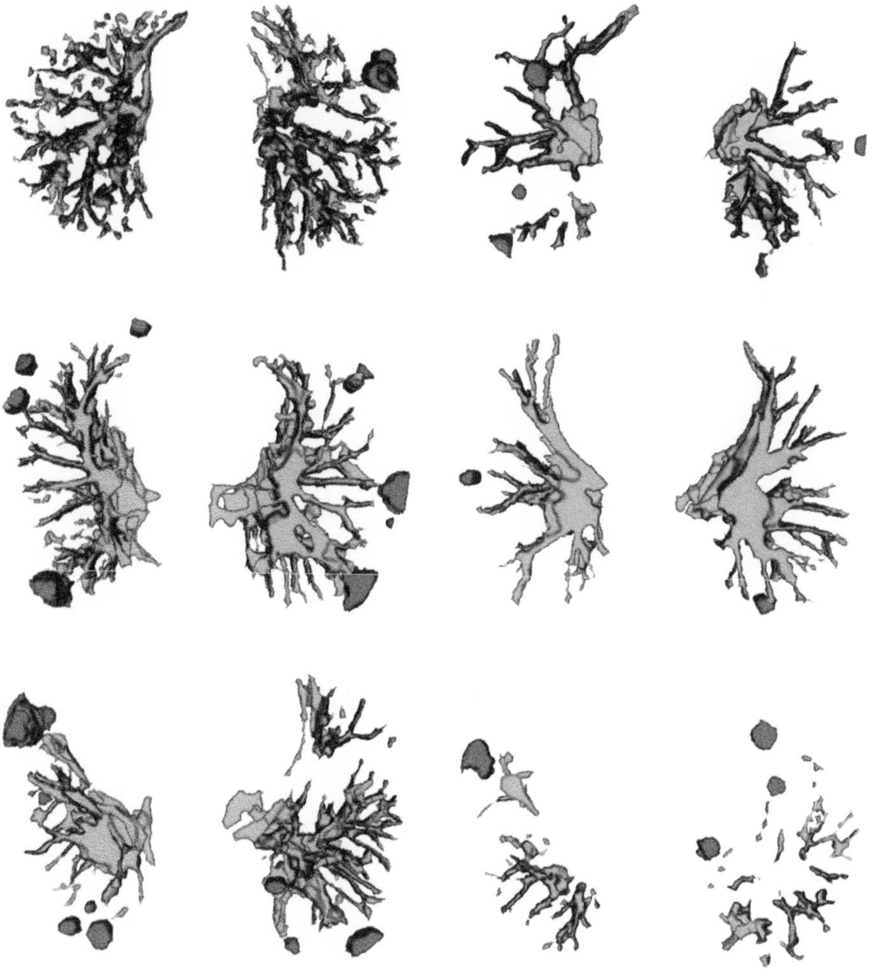

FIGURE 10.8
(See color insert.) Large candidate nodules (shown in red) detected with our approach.

classified negative samples. Each point on the graph is generated by using a different cut-point. The set of data points generated from the different cut-points is the empirical ROC curve. To change the cut-point, we change the prior probability of each class from 0 to 1 by a step of 0.01. Figure 10.13 shows the ROC of the two approaches: our present algorithm and previous one in ref. [65]. It is clear from Figure 10.12 that the area under ROC curve of our present approach is the largest (A_z = 94.3%) in comparison to the area under ROC of our previous approach [65] (A_z = 89.6%). The high sensitivity and specificity of the proposed approach is due to high accuracy of the density estimation for each feature using our LCDG model. Also, the feature that we used to discriminate between true nodules and false nodules are more separable than the features used in other existing approaches.

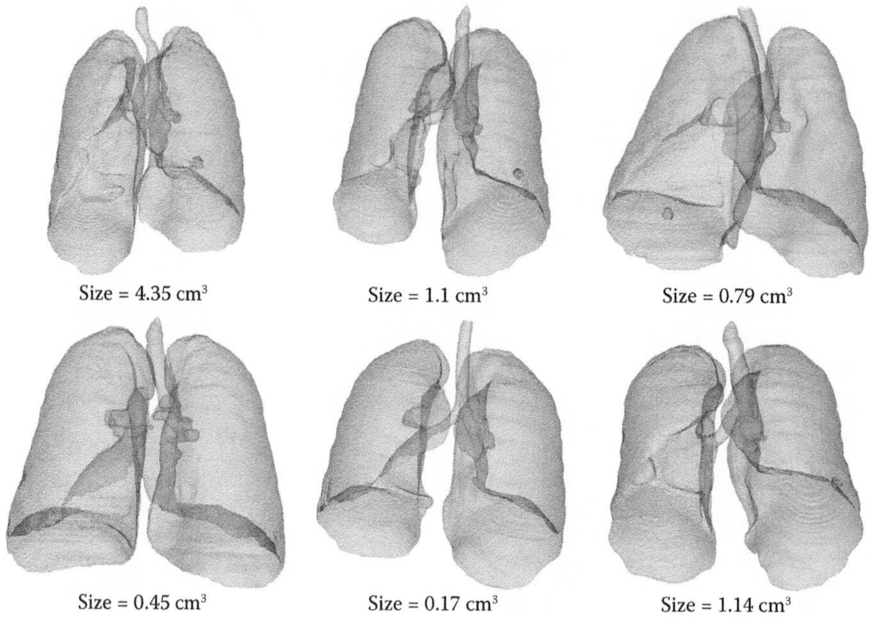

FIGURE 10.9
(See color insert.) Large candidate nodules (shown in green) detected with our approach.

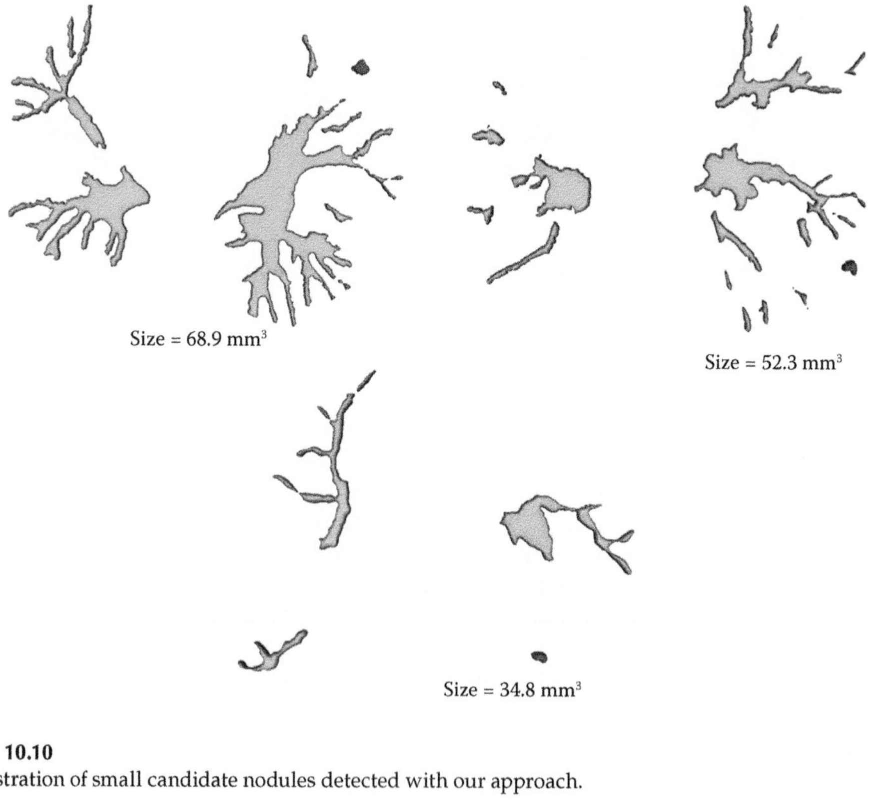

FIGURE 10.10
Demonstration of small candidate nodules detected with our approach.

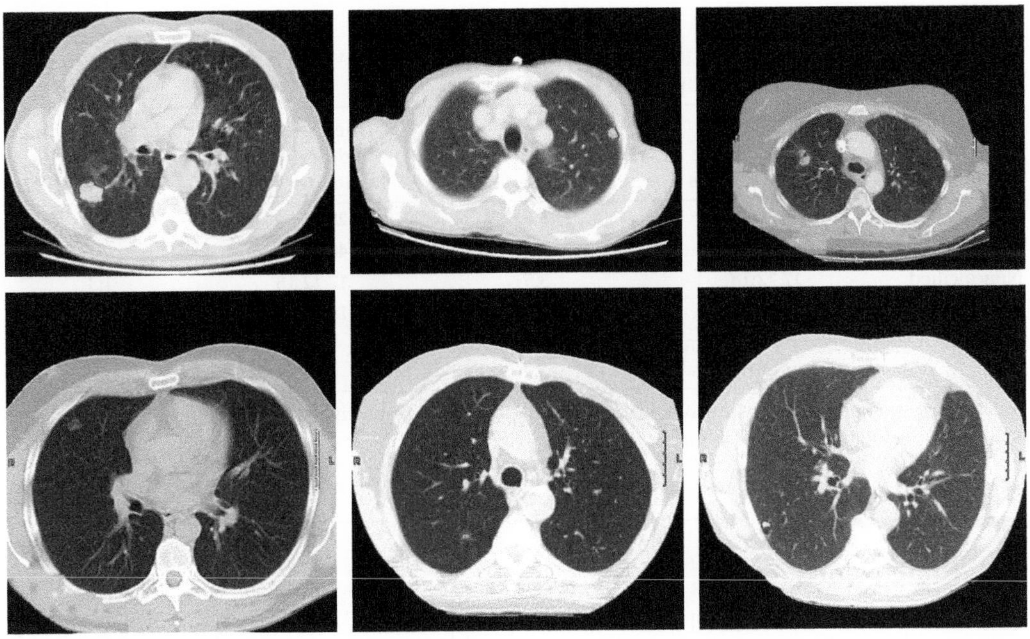

FIGURE 10.11
Axial cross section for some detected nodules.

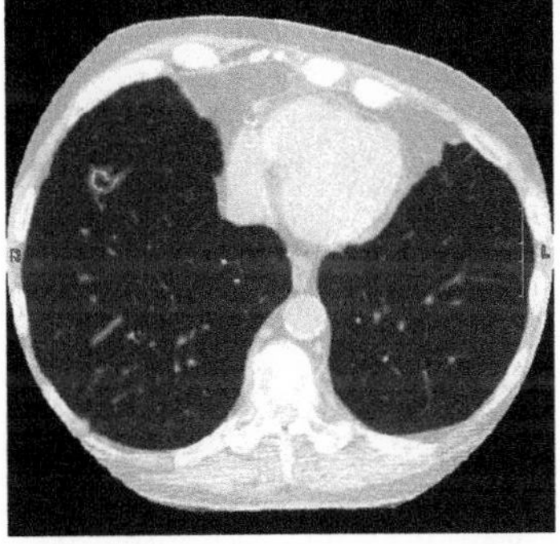

FIGURE 10.12
Axial cross section in detected cavity nodule.

TABLE 10.2

Recognition of Different Abnormalities with Our Present and Previous Algorithms [65], with Respect to the "Ground Truth" by Three Radiologists

Type of Nodules	True Detected Nodules Before Removing FPNs	False Detected Nodules Before Removing FPNs	True Detected Nodules After Removing FPNs	False Detected Nodules After Removing FPNs
Lung wall	**28**:***28***:29	**3**:***8***	**28**:***27***:29	**1**:***2***
Calcified	**49**:***46***:49	**2**:***4***	**48**:***46***:49	**0**:***1***
Noncalcified	**17**:***12***:18	**3**:***5***	**17**:***12***:18	**1**:***3***
Small	**19**:***17***:23	**6**:***25***	**18**:***15***:23	**2**:***5***
	Total TPN rate		**93.3%**:***82.3%***	
	Total FPN rate		**3.4%**:***9.2%***	

Note: Corresponding numbers are in bold, bold italic, and regular, respectively. Note that the cavity nodules are included in the "Small" category.

10.6 Conclusions

In this chapter, we introduced a fully automatic approach to detect lung nodules from spiral low-dose CT scans. The experimental results show that our new deformable level-set prototype with the analytically modeled standard intensity pattern is capable of detecting more than 90% of the true lung abnormalities. The overall time for processing the data set of size 512 × 512 × 186 is 6 and 18 min for the proposed approach and the algorithms in ref. [65], respectively, but it is still difficult to accurately detect very small lung nodules similar to bronchi and bronchioles. Our future work is focused on selecting features that distinguish between the small lung nodules and normal objects. Also, we are going to analyze the accuracy of our CAD system with respect to the ground truth on a much larger number of the real LDCT scans.

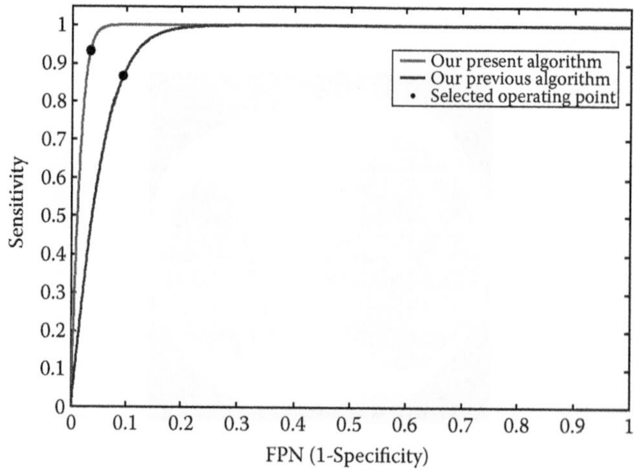

FIGURE 10.13

Comparison of two ROC curves. The ROC curve of the proposed approach (the area under the curve equal to 94.3%), and the ROC curve of the approach proposed in ref. [65] (the area under the curve equal to 89.6%).

References

1. P. M. Boiselle and C. S. White (eds.), *New Techniques in Thoracic Imaging*, Marcel Dekker, New York, 2002.
2. H. K. Weir, M. J. Thun, B. F. Hankey, L. A. G. Ries, H. L. Howe, P. A. Wingo, A. Jemal, E. Ward, R. N. Anderson, and B. K. Edwards, "Annual report to the nation on the status of cancer, 1975–2000," *Journal of the National Cancer Institute*, vol. 95, no. 17, pp. 1276–1299, 2003.
3. Alliance for Lung Cancer Advocacy, Support, and Education, *Early Detection and Diagnostic Imaging*, Lung Cancer Alliance, Washington, DC, 2001.
4. American Cancer Society, *Cancer Facts and Figures*, 2003.
5. L. Quekel, A. Kessels, R. *Goei, and J. V. Engelsh*oven, "Miss rate of lung cancer on the chest radiograph in clinical practice," *Chest*, vol. 115, no. 3, pp. 720–724, 1999.
6. F. Li, S. Sone, H. Abe, H. MacMahon, S. Armato, and K. Doi, "Lung cancers missed at low-dose helical CT screening in a general population: Comparison of clinical, histopathologic, and imaging findings," *Radiology*, vol. 225, pp. 673–683, 2002.
7. M. Kaneko, K. Eguchi, H. Ohmatsu, R. Kakinuma, T. Naruke, K. Suemasu, and N. Moriyama, "Peripheral lung cancer: Screening and detection with low-dose spiral CT versus radiography," *Radiology*, vol. 201, no. 3, pp. 798–802, December 1996.
8. O. S. Miettinen and C. I. Henschke, "CT screening for lung cancer: Coping with nihilistic recommendations," *Radiology*, vol. 221, no. 3, pp. 592–596, December 2001.
9. C. I. Henschke et al., "Early lung cancer action project: Initial finding on repeat screening," *Cancer*, vol. 92, no. 1, pp. 153–159, July 2001.
10. S. J. Swensen, J. R. Jett, T. E. Hartman, D. E. Midthun, J. A. Sloan, A. M. Sykes, G. L. Aughenbaugh, and M. A. Clemens, "Lung cancer screening with CT: Mayo Clinic experience," *Radiology*, vol. 226, no. 3, pp. 756–761, March 2003.
11. H. Rusinek, D. P. Naidich, G. McGuinness, B. S. Leitman, D. I. Mc-Cauley, G. A. Krinsky, K. Clayton, and H. Cohen, "Pulmonary nodule detection: Low-dose versus conventional CT," *Radiology*, vol. 209, no. 1, pp. 243–249, October 1998.
12. K. Garg, R. L. Keith, T. Byers, K. Kelly, A. L. Kerzner, D. A. Lynch, and Y. E. Miller, "Randomized controlled trial with low-dose spiral CT for lung cancer screening: Feasibility study and preliminary results," *Radiology*, vol. 225, no. 2, pp. 506–510, November 2002.
13. F. Li, S. Sone, H. Abe, H. MacMahon, S. G. Armato, and K. Doi, "Lung cancer missed at low-dose helical CT screening in a general population: Comparison of clinical, histopathologic, and imaging findings," *Radiology*, vol. 225, no. 3, pp. 673–683, December 2002.
14. T. Nawa, T. Nakagawa, S. Kusano, Y. Kawasaki, Y. Sugawara, and H. Nakata, "Lung cancer screening using low-dose spiral CT," *Chest*, vol. 122, no. 1, pp. 15–20, July 2002.
15. S. Sone, F. Li, Z. G. Yang, T. Honda, Y. Maruyama, S. Takashima, M. Hasegawa, S. Kawakami, K. Kubo, M. Haniuda, and T. Yamanda, "Results of three-year mass screening programme for lung cancer using mobile low-dose spiral computed tomography scanner," *British Journal of Cancer*, vol. 84, no. 1, pp. 25–32, January 2001.
16. S. C. B. Lo, M. T. Freedman, J. S. Lin, and S. K. Mun, "Automatic lung nodule detection using profile matching and back-propagation neural network techniques," *Journal of Digital Imaging*, vol. 6, no. 1, pp. 48–54, 1993.
17. F. Mao, W. Qian, J. Gaviria, and L. Clarke, "Fragmentary window filtering for multiscale lung nodule detection," *Academic Radiology*, vol. 5, no. 4, pp. 306–311, 1998.
18. T. Matsumoto, H. Yoshimura, K. Doi, M. Giger, A. Kano, H. MacMahon, M. Abe, and S. Montner, "Image feature analysis of false-positive diagnoses produced by automated detection of lung nodules," *Investigative Radiology*, vol. 27, no. 8, pp. 587–579, 1992.
19. X. Xu, S. Katsuragawa, K. Ashizawa, H. MacMahon, and K. Doi, "Analysis of image features of histograms of edge gradient for false positive reduction in lung nodule detection in chest radiographs," *Proceedings of SPIE*, vol. 3338, pp. 318–326, 1998.

20. A. A. Enquobahrie, A. P. Reeves, D. F. Yankelevitz, and C. I. Henschke, "Automated detection of pulmonary nodules from whole lung helical CT scans: Performance comparison for isolated and attached nodules," *Proceedings of SPIE*, vol. 5370, pp. 791–800, 2004.
21. Y. Mekadaa, T. Kusanagi, Y. Hayase, K. Mori, J.-I. Hasegawa, J.-I. Toriwaki, M. Mori, and H. Natori, "Detection of small nodules from 3D chest X-ray CT images based on shape features," *Computer Assisted Radiology and Surgery, CARS–03*, vol. 1256, pp. 971–976, 2003.
22. S. G. Armato, M. L. Giger, C. J. Moran, J. T. Blackburn, K. Doi, and H. MacMahon, "Computerized detection of pulmonary nodules on CT scans," *Radiographics*, vol. 19, no. 5, pp. 1303–1311, 1999.
23. J. P. Ko and M. Betke, "Chest CT: Automated nodule detection and assessment of change over timepreliminary experience," *Radiology*, vol. 218, no. 1, pp. 267–273, 2001.
24. B. Zhao, M. S. Ginsberg, R. A. Lefkowitz, L. Jiang, C. Cooper, and L. H. Schwartz, "Application of the LDM algorithm to identify small lung nodules on low-dose MSCT scans," *Proceedings of SPIE*, vol. 5370, pp. 818–823, 2004.
25. S. Chang, H. Emoto, D. N. Metaxas, and L. Axe, "Pulmonary micronodule detection from 3D chest CT," *Proceedings of International Conference on Medical Image Computing and Computer-Assisted Intervention, MICCAI-2004*, Saint-Malo, France, September 26–29, 2004, pp. 821–828.
26. H. Takizawa, K. Shigemoto, S. Yamamoto, T. Matsumoto, Y. Tateno, T. Iinuma, and M. Matsumoto, "A recognition method of lung nodule shadows in X-ray CT images using 3D object models," *International Journal of Image and Graphics*, vol. 3, pp. 533–545, October 2003.
27. Q. Li and K. Doi, "New selective enhancement filter and its application for significant improvement of nodule detection on computed tomography," *Proceedings of SPIE*, vol. 5370, pp. 1–9, 2004.
28. D. S. Paik, C. F. Beaulieu, G. D. Rubin, B. Acar, R. B. J. Jeffrey, J. Yee, J. Dey, and S. Napel, "Surface normal overlap: A computer-aided detection algorithm with application to colonic polyps and lung nodules in helical CT," *IEEE Transactions on Medical Imaging*, vol. 23, no. 6, pp. 661–675, 2004.
29. P. R. S. Mendona, R. Bhotika, S. A. Sirohey, W. D. Turner, J. V. Miller, R. S. Avila, "Model-based analysis of local shape for lesion detection in CT scans," *Proceedings of International Conference on Medical Image Computing and Computer-Assisted Intervention, MICCAI-05*, Palm Springs, CA, October 26–29, 2005, pp. 688–695.
30. Y. Lee, T. Hara, H. Fujita, S. Itoh, and T. Ishigaki, "Automated detection of pulmonary nodules in helical CT images based on an improved template-matching technique," *IEEE Transactions on Medical Imaging*, vol. 20, pp. 595–604, 2001.
31. R. Wiemker, P. Rogalla, A. Zwartkruis, and T. Blaffert, "Computer aided lung nodule detection on high resolution CT data," *Proceedings of SPIE*, vol. 4684, pp. 677–688, 2002.
32. W. J. Kostis, A. P. Reeves, D. F. Yankelevitz, and C. I. Henschke, "Three-dimensional segmentation and growth-rate estimation of small pulmonary nodules in helical CT images," *IEEE Transactions on Medical Imaging*, vol. 22, no. 10, pp. 1259–1274, October 2003.
33. K. Awai, K. Murao, A. Ozawa, M. Komi, H. Hayakawa, S. Hori, and Y. Nishimura, "Pulmonary nodules at chest CT: Effect of computer-aided diagnosis on radiologists detection performance," *Radiology*, vol. 230, no. 2, pp. 347–352, 2004.
34. T. Ezoe, H. Takizawa, S. Yamamoto, A. Shimizu, T. Matsumoto, Y. Tateno, T. Iinuma, and M. Matsumoto, "An automatic detection method of lung cancers including ground glass opacities from chest X-ray CT images," *Proceedings of SPIE*, vol. 4684, pp. 1672–1680, 2002.
35. C. I. Fetita, F. Preteux, C. Beigelman-Aubry, and P. Grenier, "3D automated lung nodule segmentation in HRCT," *Proceedings of International Conference on Medical Image Computing and Computer-Assisted Intervention, MICCAI-03*, Montreal, Quebec, Canada, November 2003, pp. 626–634.
36. M. Tanino, H. Takizawa, S. Yamamoto, T. Matsumoto, Y. Tateno, and T. Iinuma, "A detection method of ground glass opacities in chest x-ray CT images using automatic clustering techniques," *Proceedings of SPIE*, vol. 5032, pp. 1728–1737, 2003.

37. K. Kanazawa, Y. Kawata, N. Niki, H. Satoh, H. Ohmatsu, R. Kakinuma, M. Kaneko, N. Moriyma, and K. Eguchi, "Computer-aided diagnosis for pulmonary nodules based on helical CT images," *Computerized Medical Imaging and Graphics*, vol. 22, pp. 157–167, 1998.
38. M. N. Gurcan, B. Sahiner, N. Petrick, H.-P. Chan, E. A. Kazerooni, P. N. Cascade, and L. Hadjiiski, "Lung nodule detection on thoracic computed tomography images: Preliminary evaluation of a computer-aided diagnosis system," *Medical Physics*, vol. 29, no. 11, pp. 2552–2558, 2002.
39. M. Kubo, K. Kubota, N. Yamada, Y. Kawata, N. Niki, K. Eguchi, H. Ohmatsu, R. Kakinuma, M. Kaneko, M. Kusumoto, K. Mori, H. Nishiyama, and N. Moriyama, "A CAD system for lung cancer based on low dose single-slice CT image," *Proceedings of SPIE*, vol. 4684, pp. 1672–1680, 2002.
40. N. Yamada, M. Kubo, Y. Kawata, N. Niki, K. Eguchi, H. Omatsu, R. Kakinuma, M. Kaneko, M. Kusumoto, H. Nishiyama, and N. Moriyama, "ROI extraction of chest CT images using adaptive opening filter," *Proceedings of SPIE*, vol. 5032, pp. 869–876, 2003.
41. Y. Kawata, N. Niki, H. Ohmatsu, M. Kusumoto, R. Kakinuma, K. Mori, H. Nishiyama, K. Eguchi, M. Kaneko, N. Moriyama, "Computer-aided diagnosis of pulmonary nodules using three-dimensional thoracic CT images," *Proceedings of International Conference on Medical Image Computing and Computer-Assisted Intervention, MICCAI–01*, Utrecht, the Netherlands, October 14–17, 2001, pp. 1393–1394.
42. M. Betke, and J. P. Ko, "Detection of pulmonary nodules on CT and volumetric assessment of change over time," *Proceedings of International Conference on Medical Image Computing and Computer-Assisted Intervention, MICCAI–1999*, Cambridge, UK, 1999, pp. 245–252.
43. T. Oda, M. Kubo, Y. Kawata, N. Niki, K. Eguchi, H. Ohmatsu, R. Kakinuma, M. Kaneko, M. Kusumoto, N. Moriyama, K. Mori, and H. Nishiyama, "A detection algorithm of lung cancer candidate nodules on multi-slice CT images," *Proceedings of SPIE*, vol. 4684, pp. 1354–1361, 2002.
44. S. Saita, T. Oda, M. Kubo, Y. Kawata, N. Niki, M. Sasagawa, H. Ohmatsu, R. Kakinuma, M. Kaneko, M. Kusumoto, K. Eguchi, H. Nishiyama, K. Mori, and N. Moriyama, "Nodule detection algorithm based on multi-slice CT images for lung cancer screening," *Proceedings of SPIE*, vol. 5370, pp. 1083–1090, 2004.
45. M. S. Brown, M. F. McNitt-Gray, J. G. Goldin, R. D. Suh, J. W. Sayre, and D. R. Aberle "Patient-specific models for lung nodule detection and surveillance in CT images," *IEEE Transactions on Medical Imaging*, vol. 20, pp. 1242–1250, 2001.
46. M. L. Giger, N. Ahn, K. Doi, H. MacMahon, and C. E. Metz, "Computerized detection of pulmonary nodules in digital chest images: Use of morphological filters in reducing false-positive detections," *Medical Physics*, vol. 17, no. 5, pp. 861–865, 1990.
47. W. Lampeter, "ANDS-V1 computer detection of lung nodules," *Proceedings of SPIE*, vol. 555, pp. 253–261, 1985.
48. J. S. Lin, P. A. Ligomenides, Y. M. F. Lure, M. T. Freedman, and S. K. Mun, "Application of neural networks for improvement of lung nodule detection in radiographic images," *Proceedings of Computer Assisted Radiology, CARS–92*, 1992, pp. 108–115.
49. M. J. Carreira, D. Cabello, M. G. Penedo, and J. M. Pardo, "Computer aided lung nodule detection in chest radiography," *Image Analysis Applications and Computer Graphics, Berlin*, pp. 331–338, 1995.
50. S.-C. B. Lo, S.-L. A. Lou, J.-S. Lin, M. T. Freedman, M. V. Chien, and S. K. Mun, "Artificial convolution neural network techniques and applications for lung nodule detection," *IEEE Transactions on Medical Imaging*, vol. 14, pp. 711–718, August 1995.
51. J. S. Lin, S. B. Lo, A. Hasegawa, M. T. Freedman, and S. K. Mun, "Reduction of false positives in lung nodule detection using a two-level neural classification," *IEEE Transactions on Medical Imaging*, vol. 15, pp. 206–216, April 1996.
52. H. Arimura, S. Katsuragawa, K. Suzuki, F. Li, J. Shiraishi, S. Sone, and K. Doi, "Computerized scheme for automated detection of lung nodules in low-dose computed tomography images for lung cancer screening," *Academic Radiology*, vol. 11, no. 6, pp. 617–629, 2004.

53. K. Suzuki, S. G. Armato, F. Li, S. Sone, and K. Doi, "Massive training artificial neural network (MTANN) for reduction of false positives in computerized detection of lung nodules in low-dose computed tomography," *Medical Physics*, vol. 30, no. 7, pp. 1602–1617, 2003.
54. X. Zhang, G. McLennan, E. A. Hoffman, and M. Sonka, "Computerized detection of pulmonary nodules using cellular neural networks in CT images," *Proceedings of the SPIE*, vol. 5370, pp. 30–41, 2004.
55. K. Kanazawa, Y. Kawata, N. Niki, H. Satoh, H. Ohmatsu, R. Kakinuma, M. Kaneko, N. Moriyama, and K. Eguchi, "Computer-aided diagnosis for pulmo*nary nodules based on helical CT* images," *Computerized Medical Imaging and Graphics*, vol. 22, no. 2, pp. 157–167, 1998.
56. G.-Q. Wei, L. Fan, and J. Qian, "Automatic detection of nodules attached to vessels in lung CT by volume projection analysis," *Proceedings of International Conference on Medical Image Computing and Computer-Assisted Intervention, MICCAI–02*, Tokyo, Japan, September 25–28, 2002, pp. 746–752.
57. H. Takizawa, S. Yamamoto, T. Matsumoto, Y. Tateno, T. Iinuma, and M. Matsumoto, "Recognition of lung nodules from X-ray CT images using 3D Markov random field models," *Proceedings of SPIE*, vol. 4684, pp. 716–725, 2002.
58. K. Okada, D. Comaniciu, and A. Krishnan, "Robust anisotropic gaussian fitting for volumetric characterization of pulmonary nodules in multislice CT," *IEEE Transactions on Medical Imaging*, vol. 24, no. 3, pp. 409–423, March 2005.
59. B. Zhao, D. Yankelevitz, A. Reeves, and C. Henschke, "Two-dimensional multicriterion segmentation of pulmonary nodules on helical CT images," *IEEE Transactions on Medical Imaging*, vol. 22, pp. 1259–1274, 2003.
60. B. Zhao, D. F. Yankelevitz, A. P. Reeves, and C. I. Henschke, "Two-dimensional multi-criterion segmentation of pulmonary nodules on helical CT images," *Medical Physics*, vol. 26, no. 6, pp. 889–895, June 1999.
61. A. Farag, A. El-Baz, and G. Gimel'farb, "Precise segmentation of multi-modal images," *IEEE Transactions on Image Processing*, vol. 15, no. 4, pp. 952–968, April 2006.
62. J. A. Sethian, *Level Set Methods and Fast Marching Methods*, Cambridge University Press, Cambridge, MA, 1999.
63. J. Gomes and O. Faugeras, "Reconciling distance functions and level-sets," Technical *Report 3666*, INRIA, April 1999.
64. N. Paragios and R. Deriche, "Unifying boundary and region-based information for geodesic active tracking," *Proceedings of IEEE Conference on Computer Vision and Pattern Recognition*, Fort Collins, CO, June 1999, vol. 2, pp. 300–305, 1999.
65. A. A. Farag, A. El-Baz, G. Gimelfarb, R. Falk, and S. G. Hushek, "Automatic detection and recognition of lung abnormalities in helical CT images using deformable templates," *Proceedings of International Conference on Medical Image Computing and Computer-Assisted Intervention, MICCAI-05*, Saint-Malo, France, September 26–29, 2004, pp. 856–864.
66. L. Lusted, "Signal detectability and medical decision-making," *Science*, vol. 171, pp. 1217–1219, 1971.

11

Model-Based Methods for Detection of Pulmonary Nodules

Paulo R. S. Mendonça, Rahul Bhotika, and Robert Kaucic

CONTENTS

11.1 Introduction

According to the GLOBOCAN 2008 survey carried out by the World Health Organization and International Agency for Research on Cancer [13], lung cancer is the leading cause of cancer deaths worldwide, with an estimated death toll in 2004 of more than 1.4 million and with over 1.6 million new cases diagnosed. The overall survival rate of a lung cancer patient is about 14% [3,16], a figure that can be improved to anywhere between 40% and 70% for early-stage patients that undergo a lung resection (removal of part of or a whole lung) [3,14,28]. The key to this extended survival rate is early detection of the cancer, motivating the development of techniques to aid radiologists in these detection tasks.

State-of-the-art computed tomography (CT) scanners, with spatial resolutions of less than 1 mm, routinely provide images of small nodules, i.e., nodules under 3 mm in diameter, characteristic of early-stage lung cancer [34]. However, these gains in spatial resolution have led to an explosion in the sizes of the image volumes that a radiologist has to review, resulting in significant variability in radiological readings [29], as shown in Figure 11.1.

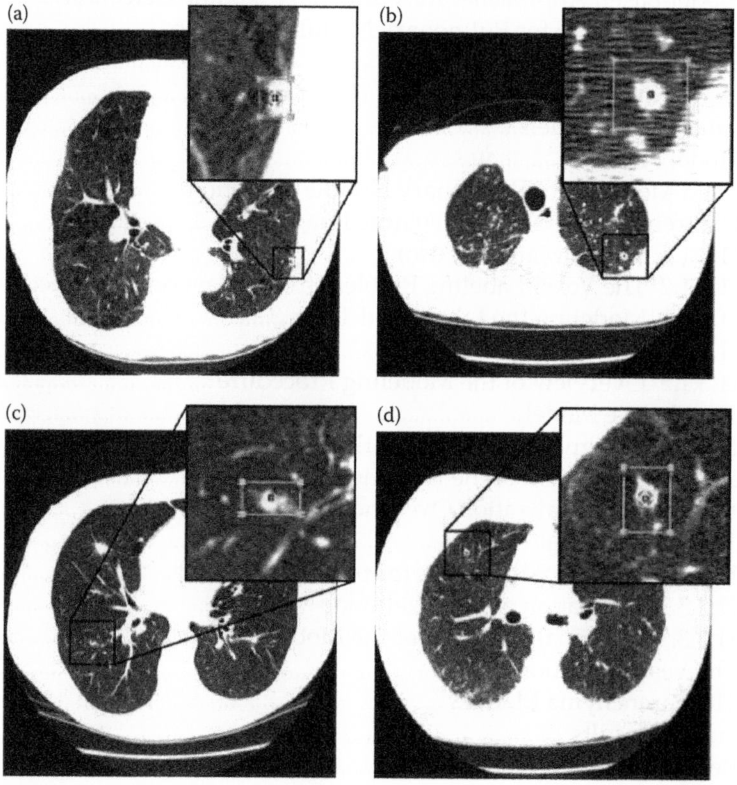

FIGURE 11.1
Four distinct examples of structures overlooked by an expert radiologist. Image (a) shows a salient structure in the lung wall. Image (b) displays a round structure in the lung apex, a region where CT images are often noisy. Images (c) and (d) show opacities in complex areas with multiple vessels and vessel junctions. The overlooking of these structures may have been intentional, i.e., the radiologist saw the structure and deliberately not marked it as relevant or as not being a nodule. However, in each case, the structure was independently classified as a nodule by two other expert radiologists, and therefore, the overlooking is more likely to have been an oversight. Such oversights are the raison d'être for the development of CAD algorithms for pulmonary nodules.

Such difficulties motivate the development of computer-aided detection (CAD) algorithms for the identification of pulmonary nodules depicted in CT images.

11.1.1 State of the Art in CAD

There is a wealth of research in the area of CAD systems applied to the detection of lung nodules in CT examinations [43]. Brown et al. [3] use simple shape- and intensity-based features of segmented regions with a fuzzy classifier. The data consisted only of selected cross sections of the lung with a thickness of 2 cm, favoring the three-dimensional (3D) segmentation technique upon which the algorithm is dependent and avoiding the difficult apex region. McCulloch et al. [25,30] obtained encouraging results with a Bayesian classifier—70% sensitivity at 8 false-positives per case operating on noisy low-dose data. Their method uses two-dimensional (2D) segmentation to generate candidates and the number of false-positives grows with the use of thinner slices in CT. The distribution of surface normals at the air–tissue interface was used as a feature for nodule detection in ref. [38]; the algorithm was tested on only eight images, and results were reported for nodules larger than the minimum size of 4 mm for which a follow-up is recommended [9]. Farag et al. [11] report numbers as high as 82.3% sensitivity with 9.2% false-positive rate, however, over 80% of their ground truth consists of nodules above 12 mm. Others have used local structure information alone to discriminate between particular shapes [41,47,49]. Other works [12] also report strong results, but the x-ray dose prescribed in those scans does not achieve the goal of a low-dose protocol [9].

11.1.2 Overview

We describe here techniques for the analysis of 3D images and demonstrate their application in assisting the detection of lung nodules in CT examinations. The proposed techniques combine geometric and intensity models with local shape analysis in order to identify pulmonary nodules in CT. The model and algorithm parameters are either learned from data—training data or data already available in medical publications—or derived from the models themselves, in which case no model fitting or optimization is performed.

At a high level, this work applies a Bayesian statistical framework to the problem of local shape and intensity analysis. It is distinct from previous works in differential shape analysis [32,41] that follow a purely deterministic approach. Great care was taken in developing rigorous statistical models to avoid the often hasty adoption of off-the-shelf Gaussian likelihoods, uniform priors, and maximum likelihood estimators; concessions to mathematical simplicity were made in generating a practical solution to the problem, but less so in the problem statement. We make specific choices of features, models, and priors, but we acknowledge that different choices are possible and that such choices are paramount to algorithm performance.

11.1.3 Model-Based Approaches for Pulmonary Nodule Detection

A model-based approach for a detection problem consists in the use of explicit mathematical models for the structure, object, or phenomenon to be detected and, possibly, to objects or structures that ought to be avoided—the confounding factors. Such models must capture the intensity, texture, shape, or any other characteristic feature of the relevant objects as presented in the data. In the particular problem of detection of pulmonary nodules in CT, it is therefore necessary to model not only nodules and possible confounding factors per se, but also how such structures are depicted in CT images. Models for nodule detection in CT will be necessarily different than models for detection in, say, positron emission tomography images. The modeling process also requires (and benefits from) the use of available domain knowledge related to the problem at hand. In the case of detection of pulmonary nodules, this means that information about the distribution of nodule size and the anatomy of the pulmonary vasculature, for example, must be employed whenever possible.

11.2 Region-Based Methods for Pulmonary Nodule Detection

Our region-based CAD system consists of two subsystems, which are schematically represented in Figure 11.2. The first subsystem consists of a multistage modeling architecture in which anatomical structures (currently corresponding to lung parenchyma, vascular structure, chest wall, and nodules) are modeled at several stages of representation. The second subsystem is a Bayesian model selection architecture in which the alternative representations of the imagery compete with one another to determine the most probable

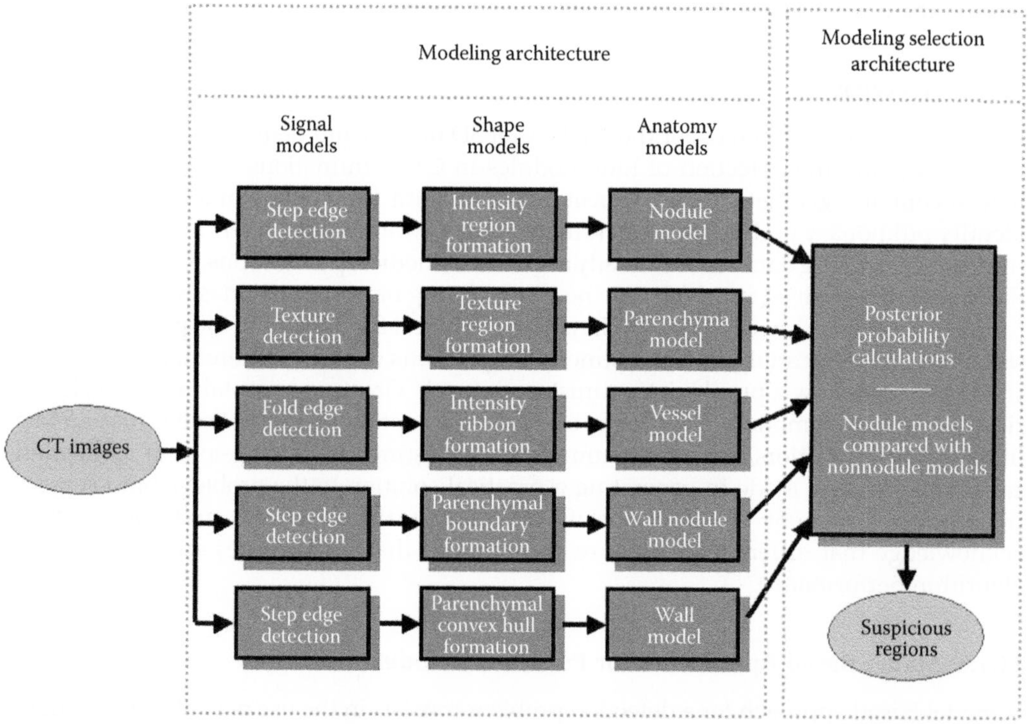

FIGURE 11.2
Model region-based block diagram. There are two main subsystems corresponding to a modeling architecture for representing structures at varying levels of representation (columns in main block) and a Bayesian model selection architecture (right block) in which alternate representations of the imagery compete with one another. Structures are modeled at the signal, shape, and anatomical/pathological level.

explanation of the underlying data. Regions best explained by a nodule model are deemed suspicious and highlighted by the system for further review by the radiologist.

The model region-based algorithm attempts to describe all normal and abnormal anatomy in the lung by starting at the lowest level of representation (image voxels) and building up more detailed models until all structures are explained. At present, the approach is based on three stages of representation: signal, shape, and anatomy, although additional stages can be added. The output of the last stage of model representation is used as input to the model selection architecture in which suspicious regions are identified. In the following paragraphs, we describe the main components of the modeling architecture corresponding to the columns of Figure 11.2: the signal models, shape models, and anatomy models. We do not attempt here to give an exhaustive treatment of all models in the architecture. Rather, we provide instructive examples of models at each level of representation.

11.2.1 Signal Models

The first stage of representation (Figure 11.2, first column) characterizes the signal formation process. In CT imagery, the signal models represent the blurring (point spread function) and noise characteristics inherent to the imaging system. These models permit the accurate detection of primitive events in the image such as intensity peaks and discontinuities. These primitives form the basis for later stages of representation. For example, in the lung nodule representation, the initial stage of modeling consists of step-edge detection using the Canny edge detector [4]. To account for noise, the image is convolved with a 2D Gaussian kernel (oriented perpendicular to the axial direction) in which the scale of the kernel can be optimally computed from the point spread function of the scanner [10]. The resulting edge elements, or edgels, are located where the magnitude of the gradient of the smoothed image is a local maximum along the gradient direction. Adjacent edgels for which the magnitude of the gradient is above a threshold are linked to produce edges. This threshold can be computed from the signal-to-noise ratio in the image and the point spread function of the scanner. The output of this stage of processing is a set of edges corresponding to locations in the image where there are large-intensity gradients. An example of the output of the edge detector can be seen on the top left corner of Figure 11.3. The first stage of vessel representation uses a fold edge detector in lieu of the step edge detector. Here, the Hessian of the image is computed to find the local maximum in the curvature of the image intensity profile (the fold). These local maxima are linked along the direction of the fold in a similar fashion as was done in the step-edge detector, and these fold edges are passed on to the next level of representation. The result of this sequence of operations is exemplified in the central image in the top row of Figure 11.3.

11.2.2 Shape Models

The next stage of representation (column 2 in Figure 11.2) captures the appearance of features in the image in terms of their intensity and shape. This representation, which provides an elementary vocabulary for describing anatomical structures, is formed by grouping the low-level features detected at the signal level. These grouped units are then suitable for modeling anatomy at the next level of representation. For example, at this level of the nodule representation, the image is segmented into regions by grouping edges from the signal model stage into regions that serve as candidate nodules for the anatomy stage of representation. The edges from the preceding signal modeling stage are grouped into closed regions by tracing along the edges and following the image gradient until a closed

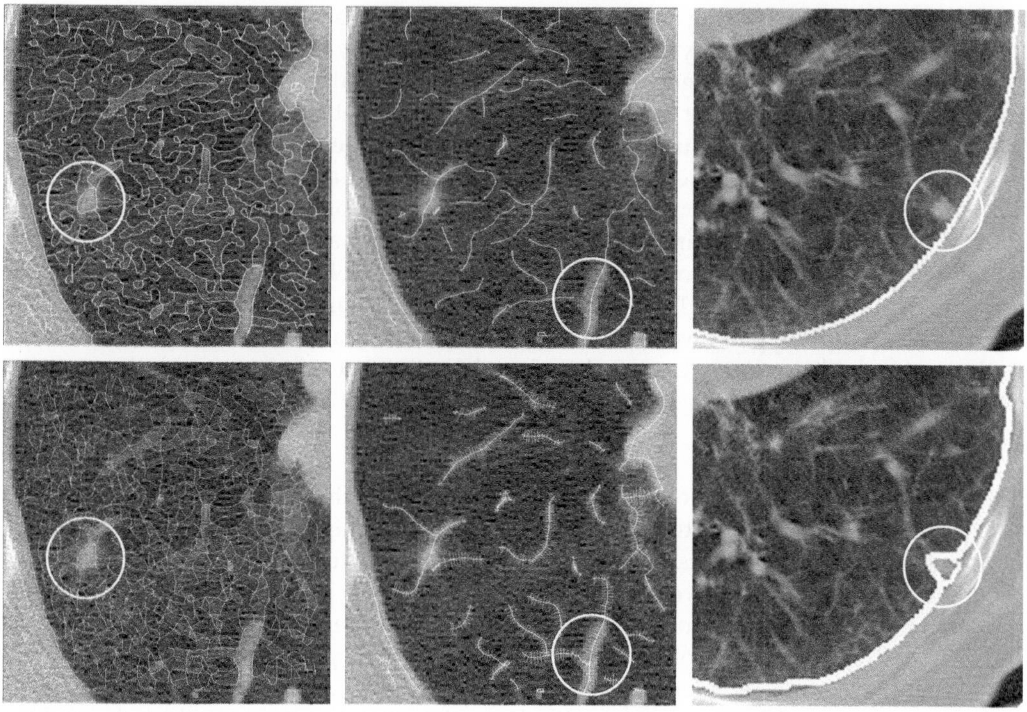

FIGURE 11.3
Examples of the signal and shape model stages of representation. The left two columns of images are the same area surrounding a lung nodule (circled in the left column) and a blood vessel (circled in the middle column). The right column shows an area surrounding a wall nodule. The upper and lower panels of the left column are the output of the step edge detection and intensity region formation, respectively, for the nodule representation. The upper and lower panels of the middle column are the output of the fold edge detection and intensity ribbon formation, respectively, for the vessel representation. The upper and lower panels of the right column are the output of the parenchymal convex hull formation and the parenchymal boundary formation, respectively.

structure can be formed. The result is a connected network of vertices and edges [48] delimiting adjacent image regions within which the voxel intensities vary slowly. Regions in the network can be queried for their properties including location, area, average density, and for the properties of their neighbors. The left panel in the bottom row of Figure 11.3 gives an example of intensity region formation near a lung nodule. At this level of the vessel representation, a similar tracing algorithm is used in the intensity ribbon formation process to group intensity ridges into models consistent with the vascular structure. These ridges correspond to the folds detected in the signal model stage previously described. Vertices are placed at branching points, resulting in a connected network of vessel-like structures. The width of these structures is determined by the location of the nearest surrounding edges. The Hessian operator is applied to the image data to extract the orientation of the principal axes of these candidate vessels. The middle panel in the bottom row of Figure 11.3 gives an example of intensity ribbon formation near a vessel. The chest wall is modeled at this level of representation as a convex surface. First, the parenchymal boundary is found by connecting large strength edges computed at the signal model level of representation. Then, a parenchymal hull is defined as the convex hull of the parenchymal boundary. The two right panels of Figure 11.3 show an example wall nodule, in which the lower panel gives the computed parenchymal boundary representing chest wall and possible wall nodules, and the upper panel shows the parenchymal hull representing the chest wall alone.

11.2.3 Anatomical Models

The last stage of representation encodes anatomical concepts by grouping and determining by parameters the elements of the shape models into anatomical units. For example, a confluence of thin, branching structures can be interpreted as a vascular network with appropriate constraints on branching and size that is consistent with lung anatomy. Concavities on the chest wall can be explained as vessels running along the pleura, scarring, or nodules. At this highest level of data representation, the anatomy models attempt to capture the salient aspects of the structure being modeled by specifying full probability distributions on voxel intensities, geometric features, and neighborhood properties. These probabilistic model specifications facilitate the model selection procedures described in the next section.

For any given model M (e.g., nodule/vessel/parenchyma), the probability distribution required later for model selection is

$$p(x,\theta|M) = \int p(x,\theta|\beta_M, M)p(\beta_M|M)\,d\beta_M \tag{11.1}$$

where the vector x contains voxel data, the vector θ contains supplementary nonvoxel features (e.g., geometry, neighborhood properties), and the vector β_M represents any nuisance parameters in the model. Equation 11.1 gives the method of marginalization of nuisance parameters to calculate the required probability distribution on the left-hand side.

As an example of applying Equation 11.1, consider the nodule model (M = Nod), which is designed to favor compact regions with intensity profiles that are high and concave down in all dimensions. Given an intensity region generated in the second level of the modeling architecture, this concept can be expressed concisely in a model exclusively on the voxel data x inside the intensity region extracted from the preceding shape modeling stage. Therefore, in the following discussion, we formulate a model $p(x|M = \text{Nod})$ rather than a larger model on voxel data and other features, $p(x,\theta|M = \text{Nod})$.

We can express this voxel data model as a second-order linear regression with normal errors in which the dependent variable is the image intensity at a given voxel, and the linear predictor is a second-order polynomial on the voxel location. Using a normal prior distribution on the nuisance regression parameters, the data model and prior distribution in Equation 11.1 can then be written

$$p(x|\beta_{\text{Nod}}, M = \text{Nod}) = N(Z\beta_{\text{Nod}}, \sigma^2 I) \text{ and } p(\beta_{\text{Nod}}|M = \text{Nod}) = N(\nu, W) \tag{11.2}$$

where $N(A, B)$ represents the multivariate normal distribution with mean A and covariance matrix B, and I is the identity matrix. In Equation 11.2, the data variance σ^2, prior mean vector η, and covariance matrix W are learnt from exemplar nodules and fixed a priori to encourage concave-down intensity profiles with proper noise characteristics. The voxel location data are encoded in Z, which contains one column for each element of the regression parameter vector β_N. In our implementation, Z contains 2D pixel locations (axial view) in a transformed coordinate system: after centering the pixel locations by subtracting the overall mean from each, we apply a rotation that would force the least-squares estimate of the interaction term in a full six-parameter paraboloid to be zero. In this new coordinate system, we construct Z with three columns: the first is a column of ones for the intercept parameter and each image dimension contributes one column of squared (transformed) pixel locations for each second-order parameter. Under these assumptions, the integral in Equation 11.1 can be shown to be a normal distribution,

$$\int p(x|M = \text{Nod}) = N(Zv, ZWZ^t + \sigma^2 I)$$

whose value for a given vector of data can be directly calculated from the definition of the normal probability density function. See ref. [7] for further information on regression analysis. Similar methods are used to define all the anatomy models on voxel data and supplementary features. For example, the vessel model is also expressed as a linear regression with image intensity as a dependent variable and transformed pixel locations as independent variables. In the vessel model, matrix Z contains two columns. Similar to the nodule model, the first is a column of ones for the intercept parameter and the second column is defined using the intensity ribbon process from the preceding shape modeling stage. For each pixel in the intensity ribbon, the pixel's squared distance from the ribbon's central axis is calculated and inserted in the second column of Z. Equation 11.2 is reused with prior parameters that are fixed a priori to encourage concave-down intensity profiles perpendicular to the intensity ribbon's central axis.

11.2.4 Model Selection

At the final stage of representation, there are a number of models that could plausibly provide an interpretation of the underlying image and supplementary features. Our approach uses Bayesian model selection [2], which prescribes that the model with highest posterior probability, given the observed data, should be selected. Bayes' theorem gives the definition of the posterior probability of a particular model M,

$$p(M|x,\theta) = \frac{p(x,\theta|M)p(M)}{\sum_m p(x,\theta|m)p(m)} \tag{11.3}$$

where $p(M)$ is the prior probability of the model before collecting image data. The denominator is a normalizing constant independent of M, which is calculated by summing the numerator over all competing models m. Structures having a large posterior probability favoring a nodule model are deemed suspicious and flagged for review. For example, the model selection for the lung nodule shown in the left column of Figure 11.3 considers three competing representations: nodule, vessel, and parenchyma. Under uniform model priors ($p(M = \text{Nodule}) = p(M = \text{Vessel}) = p(M = \text{Parenchyma}) = 1/3$), the log posterior probability ratio for the nodule versus vessel models, $p(M = \text{Nodule}|x, \theta)/p(M = \text{Vessel}|x, \theta)$, equals 52. This can be interpreted as extremely strong evidence for the nodule model over the vessel model. The log posterior ratio of nodule versus parenchyma is even larger, registering over our operational cutoff of 200. For efficiency, we do not calculate the third posterior ratio, vessel versus parenchyma, because it is not of interest for nodule detection.

11.3 Voxel-Based Methods for Pulmonary Nodule Detection

The choice of a *Bayesian* voxel labeling technique to address the problem of pulmonary nodule detection is justified for several reasons. The uncertainty inherent to the detection problems commonly faced in medical imaging is best accounted for through statistical techniques. Moreover, there often is useful medical knowledge that can be utilized to regularize or bound the solution of such problems. Bayesian methods are, therefore, a natural choice due to their ability to incorporate *informative prior probabilities (or simply priors) that encode* and account for pertinent data and metadata, such as patient family history or prior medical examinations. Besides, as aptly put in ref. [45], the use of priors forces the explicit acknowledgment of otherwise hidden assumptions.

As for the choice of a voxel labeling scheme for nodule detection, it should be contrasted with the alternative method of generating candidate detections through segmentation followed by classification of the segmented regions (ref. [30] is a good example). This is a perfectly sound approach, with potential advantages over voxel labeling—in particular, it eases the reckoning of spatial information. However, such detection systems are hostages of the segmentation step. First, the detection rate of the segmentation step places an upper bound on the detection rate of the complete system. Even if the segmentation provides a full partition of the image, in our experience, undersegmentation (common with small and vascularized nodules) and oversegmentation (common with large and complex nodules) occurs frequently. This issue could perhaps be tackled by a joint segmentation and detection algorithm, but the state of the art on such tasks [6] assumes a few discrete data sources, unsuitable to describe a space of segmentations. Voxel labeling bypasses such issues by incorporating information from neighboring pixels in a predefined way and making decisions only at a local level.

11.3.1 Differential Operators on Volume Images

A *volume image* I is defined as a twice-differentiable (C^2) mapping from a compact domain $\mathcal{V} \subset \mathbb{R}^3$ into $\mathbb{R}$. For any given k,

$$I(\mathbf{x}) = k \tag{11.4}$$

defines an isosurface $M_k \subset \mathcal{V}$ at the points $\mathbf{x}$ satisfying Equation 11.4 and $\nabla I(\mathbf{x}) \neq 0$ [36]. Moreover, the isosurface M_k is orientable, and its normal vector field is given by $\hat{\mathbf{n}} = I/\| I\|$.

A common descriptor for the local structure of an image I is its Hessian $\mathbf{H}$ [41]. Although the eigenvalues of $\mathbf{H}$ provide an intuitive measure of local structure, they do not capture the true underlying shape, which is more accurately described by the curvature of the isosurfaces defined by Equation 11.4. For example, consider an isotropic Gaussian intensity profile (see Figure 11.4). Hessian-based shape measures [41] would incorrectly signal the presence of a cylinder at the inflection points of the profile, while the principal curvatures would correctly flag the entire structure as spherical.

11.3.1.1 The Curvature Tensor

It can be shown that, at the point $\mathbf{x}$, the principal directions of the isosurface given by Equation 11.4 can be obtained directly from the implicit function through the solutions of the eigenproblem [32]

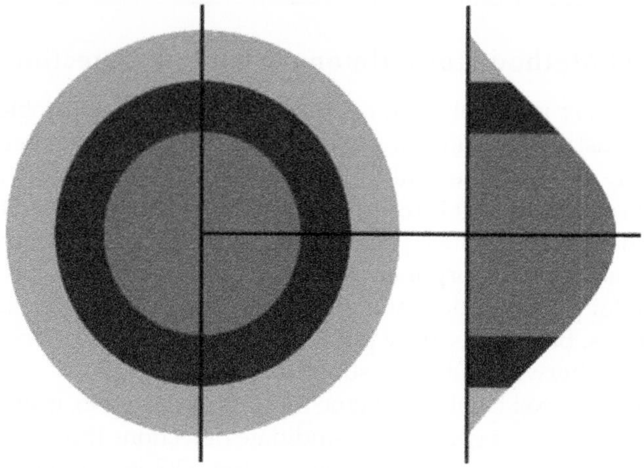

FIGURE 11.4
Cross-section and top view of Hessian responses on a 2D Gaussian profile. The Hessian response is spherical in the innermost circle, cylindrical in the dark band containing the inflection point, and void in the outer band.

$$\min_{\hat{\mathbf{v}}}/\max_{\hat{\mathbf{v}}} \frac{-\hat{\mathbf{v}}^T \mathbf{N}^T \mathbf{H} \mathbf{N} \hat{\mathbf{v}}}{\|I\|}, \quad \text{Subject to} \|\hat{\mathbf{v}}\| = 1, \tag{11.5}$$

where $\mathbf{N}$ is the 3×2 matrix of the null space of ∇I. The principal directions $\mathbf{v}_1$ and $\mathbf{v}_2$ are given by $\mathbf{v}_{1,2} = \mathbf{N}\hat{\mathbf{v}}_{1,2}$, where $\hat{\mathbf{v}}_{1,2}$ are the solutions of Equation 11.5, and the corresponding principal curvatures κ_1 and κ_2 are the eigenvalues of the 2×2 matrix $-\mathbf{N}^T\mathbf{H}\mathbf{N}/\|\nabla I\|$, with $\kappa_1 \le \kappa_2$. Matrix $\mathbf{C} = -\mathbf{N}^T\mathbf{H}\mathbf{N}/\|\nabla I\|$ is herein defined as the *curvature tensor* of the volume image.

Yoshida et al. [49] present a method to compute κ_1 and κ_2 for an implicit surface. Their technique also estimates curvatures directly from an implicit function. However, it requires the isosurfaces to be amenable to a local parameterization via Monge patches, which cannot be achieved everywhere on the surface [15]. The solution from Equation 11.5 circumvents this problem and avoids the rotation step required by Vos et al. [47].

11.3.1.2 The Voxel-Labeling Problem from a Bayesian Perspective

The symbol $P(A)$ denotes the probability of the event A in an adequate probability space. The symbol $p_X(x)$ denotes the value of the probability density of the random variable X at x. We omit the subscript X in $p_X(x)$ when doing so is not ambiguous.

Let $\{\mathcal{M}_i, i = 1, \ldots, N\}$ be a set of parametric models. Each $\mathcal{M}_i$ has parameters $\mathbf{m}_i$ in the domain $\mathbf{M}_i$. Given a choice of $\mathcal{M}_i$, if $\mathcal{D}$ can be assumed to be a set $\mathcal{D} = \{\mathcal{D}_j, j = 1, \ldots, M\}$ of independent datum $\mathcal{D}_j$ associated with voxel $\mathbf{x}$, we have, using Bayes' law, and marginalizing over the model parameters,

$$P(\mathcal{M}_i|\mathcal{D},\mathbf{x}) = \frac{P(\mathcal{M}_i|\mathbf{x})}{p(\mathcal{D}|\mathbf{x})} p(\mathcal{D}|\mathcal{M}_i,\mathbf{x}) = \frac{P(\mathcal{M}_i|\mathbf{x})}{p(\mathcal{D}|\mathbf{x})} \prod_{j=1}^{M} p(\mathcal{D}_j|\mathcal{M}_i,\mathbf{x})$$
$$= \frac{P(\mathcal{M}_i|\mathbf{x})}{p(\mathcal{D}|\mathbf{x})} \prod_{j=1}^{M} \int_{\mathbf{M}_i} p(\mathcal{D}_j|\mathbf{m}_i,\mathcal{M}_i,\mathbf{x}) p(\mathbf{m}_i|\mathcal{M}_i,\mathbf{x}) d\mathbf{m}_i. \tag{11.6}$$

The independence assumption embedded in Equation 11.6 is admittedly strong, but there is little hope that a practical solution can be achieved under weaker hypotheses. The integral in Equation 11.6 is complicated enough; without this assumption, it would be unmanageable.

In the first line of the derivation of Equation 11.6, the posterior, likelihood, and prior terms are $P(\mathcal{M}_i|\mathcal{D}, \mathbf{x})$, $p(\mathcal{D}|\mathcal{M}_i, \mathbf{x})$, and $P(\mathcal{M}_i|\mathbf{x})$, respectively. The independence assumption allows for the factorization of the likelihood term. The marginalization step underscores the distinction between the problems of detection and that of joint detection and fitting. While in the latter the parameters of the selected model are also estimated, in the former, they are simply nuisance parameters whose values are accounted for but not explicitly computed. The identity $p(\mathbf{m}_i|\mathcal{D}_j,\mathcal{M}_i,\mathbf{x}) = \frac{p(\mathbf{m}_i|\mathcal{M}_i,\mathbf{x})}{p(\mathcal{D}_j,|\mathcal{M}_i,\mathbf{x})} p(\mathcal{D}_j|m_i,\mathcal{M}_i,\mathbf{x})$ justifies referring also to $p(\mathcal{D}_j|\mathbf{m}_i, \mathcal{M}_i, \mathbf{x})$ and $p(\mathbf{m}_i|\mathcal{M}_i, \mathbf{x})$ as likelihood and prior terms, and it is to indicate these probability densities that these words are henceforth reserved. Whenever a reference to $p(\mathcal{D}|\mathcal{M}_i, \mathbf{x})$ and $P(\mathcal{M}_i|\mathbf{x})$ is made, we will avoid confusion by using the terms *data likelihood* and *model prior* instead.

11.3.1.3 Modeling the Likelihood Term

To compute the likelihood term $p(\mathcal{D}_j|\mathbf{m}_i, \mathcal{M}_i, \mathbf{x})$ in Equation 11.6, we first need to define the parametric model $\mathcal{M}_i$ and the datum $\mathcal{D}_j \in \mathcal{D}$ for the set $\mathcal{D}$ associated to the voxel $\mathbf{x}$. We consider four models: the same nodule $\mathcal{M}_1$, vessel $\mathcal{M}_2$, and parenchyma $\mathcal{M}_4$ models adopted in Section 11.2, but also a vessel junction model $\mathcal{M}_3$. The nodule, vessel, and junction models are jointly referred to as anatomical models, as they are representative of structures found in lungs. As in Section 11.2, the parenchyma model captures properties of the background lung tissue.

The above choices are reasonable if one considers the anatomy and pathology of the lungs, but what constitutes a good choice of $\mathcal{D}$ is less clear. A number of works in CAD of lung nodules [32,41] or colonic polyps [47,49] have demonstrated that differential operators such as the Hessian or the structure tensor can be efficiently used to discriminate between round and elongated structures in images. A comparison of differential operators was carried out in ref. [32], suggesting an advantage for the curvature tensor. In view of this, we choose to use principal curvatures $\kappa = (\kappa_1, \kappa_2)$, with $\kappa_1 \leq \kappa_2$, as the datum $\mathcal{D}_j \in \mathcal{D}$. This, in turn, makes geometric representations a natural choice for our anatomical models. The likelihood term $p(\mathcal{D}_j|\mathbf{m}_i, \mathcal{M}_i, \mathbf{x}) = p(\kappa|\mathbf{m}_i, \mathcal{M}_i, \mathbf{x})$ is thus defined as the probability density of the random vector $\mathbf{K}^i$, which maps a voxel $\mathbf{x}$ to a pair (κ_1, κ_2), given the geometric model $\mathcal{M}_i$ with parameters $\mathbf{m}_i$.

11.3.1.4 Modeling the Prior

At the heart of the still ongoing philosophical debate on the validity of Bayesian methods [8] is the alleged subjectivism with which prior distributions are selected. Since Jeffreys [21], however, there are firm grounds to reject such criticism, and there are now a number of objective methods to elicit prior probabilities [23]. Of these, the maximum entropy principle [20] is particularly attractive to our problem, due to its amenability to the incorporation of external information. In a nutshell, the maximum entropy principle prescribes as the prior the distribution p of maximal entropy $S = -\int p(x) \log p(x)\, dx$, subject to the available constraints, expressed in the form $\int p(x) f_k(x)\, dx = c_k$ for given functions f_k and constants c_k. We therefore obtain p through the solution of a standard variational problem.

Bringing medical scholarship into the design of the prior distribution of the model parameters is of fundamental importance in this work. A popular alternative is the learning of parameter distributions from training data [27,37], where prior knowledge is encoded in the form of prelabeled data samples. In this work, the probability distributions of the model parameters are inferred from data in the medical literature. Obviously, both approaches have merits. In many situations, particularly in more exploratory research, the very point of the work is to gain medical knowledge by understanding the parameters of a given model [17], in which case data-driven learning techniques are the best option.

Volume normalization. The procedure above computes $p(\mathbf{m}_i|\mathcal{M}_i)$, not $p(\mathbf{m}_i|\mathcal{M}_i, \mathbf{x})$. But once $p(\mathbf{m}_i|\mathcal{M}_i)$ is obtained, $p(\mathbf{m}_i|\mathcal{M}_i, \mathbf{x})$ can be found with the help of the identity $p(\mathbf{m}_i|\mathcal{M}_i, \mathbf{x}) = p(\mathbf{x}|\mathbf{m}_i, \mathcal{M}_i)p(\mathbf{m}_i|\mathcal{M}_i)/p(\mathbf{x}|\mathcal{M}_i)$. Taking a frequentist detour from our Bayesian orthodoxy, we argue that $p(\mathbf{x}|\mathbf{m}_i, \mathcal{M}_i)/p(\mathbf{x}|\mathcal{M}_i)$ is proportional to the volume $V(\mathbf{m}_i, \mathcal{M}_i)$ since, all else being equal, we are more likely to sample a voxel from the instance of $\mathcal{M}_i$ that has more voxels. Therefore, given $p(\mathbf{m}_i|\mathcal{M}_i)$, $p(\mathbf{m}_i|\mathcal{M}_i, \mathbf{x})$ can be obtained as $p(\mathbf{m}_i|\mathcal{M}_i,\mathbf{x}) = p(\mathbf{m}_i|\mathcal{M}_i)V(\mathbf{m}_i,\mathcal{M}_i) / \int_{\mathbf{M}_i} p(\mathbf{m}_i|\mathcal{M}_i)V(\mathbf{m}_i,\mathcal{M}_i)\,d\mathbf{m}_i$. This frequentist argument can also be used to determine $P(\mathcal{M}_i|\mathbf{x})$.

The Bayesian horizon. The constraints on the priors are, in general, not directly accessible from medical literature but must themselves be inferred from available information. This estimation problem could, in turn, be tackled with the introduction of hyperpriors [2], a process that should not be iterated indefinitely; the ad hoc point at which one stops is one's Bayesian horizon (a term, to our knowledge, coined by Nils Krahnstoever [26]).

11.3.1.5 Overview of the Modeling Procedure

We can now describe the general steps of the modeling procedure. All of these steps must be adapted to the particular model under consideration and are prescribed here only as general guidelines. They are (i) selection of a geometric representation for $\mathcal{M}_i$, (ii) design of the priors $p(\mathbf{m}_i|\mathcal{M}_i, \mathbf{x})$ and $P(\mathcal{M}_i|\mathbf{x})$, (iii) derivation of the likelihood $p(\kappa|\mathbf{m}_i, \mathcal{M}_i, \mathbf{x})$, and (iv) marginalization of $p(\kappa|\mathbf{m}_i, \mathcal{M}_i, \mathbf{x})$ over $p(\mathbf{m}_i|\mathcal{M}_i, \mathbf{x})$. This procedure is carried out for each of our four models, as shown in the schematic diagram in Figure 11.5.

The marginalization is further broken down into two steps: simplification of the integrand and solution of the simplified integral. The integral in Equation 11.6 is, in general, intractable, and a conservative variant of Laplace's method [24] is employed to simplify it. The procedure affects only the likelihood term, resulting in

$$p(\kappa|\mathbf{m}_i,\mathcal{M}_i,\mathbf{x}) \approx \sum_{j=1}^{J} w_j \delta(\kappa_1 - g_j(\kappa_2,\mathbf{m}_i,\mathcal{M}_i)) p_j(\kappa_2|\mathbf{m}_i,\mathcal{M}_i,\mathbf{x}),$$

where the number of terms J, the weights w_j, with $\sum_j^J w_j = 1$, the functions g_j and the densities p_j depend on $p(\kappa_1|\kappa_2, \mathbf{m}_i, \mathcal{M}_i, \mathbf{x})$. The roles of κ_1 and κ_2 may be exchanged as long as the necessary modifications in g_j and p_j are made. While most variants of Laplace's method completely replace the integral in Equation 11.6 with an integral-free term, our approximation only reduces the number of nested integrals, resulting in an expression that can be solved in closed form.

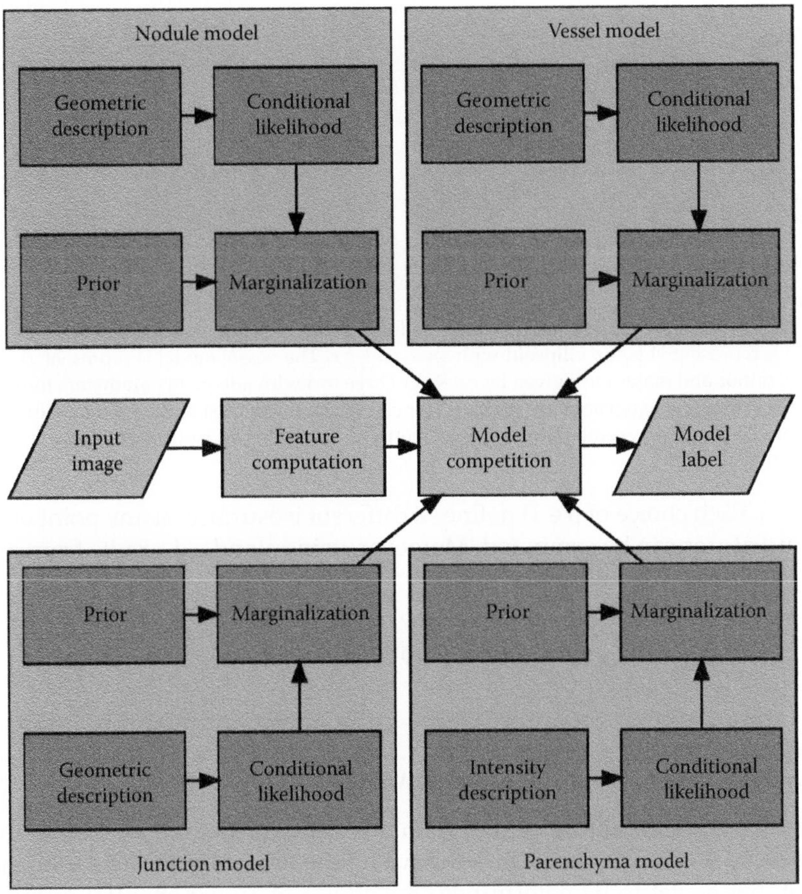

FIGURE 11.5
The steps described in Section 11.3.1.5—selection of a geometric or intensity description, design of priors, derivation of the likelihood, and marginalization—are carried out for each of our four models, in an off-line process. The actual labeling procedure consists of computation of image features at each voxel and model competition using Bayes factors.

11.3.2 The Nodule Model

The model $\mathcal{M}_1$ chosen to represent a nodule is a solid ellipsoid with similar concentric ellipsoidal isosurfaces such that the outermost isosurface has semiaxes a, b, and c with $a = b \leq c$, i.e.,

$$\mathcal{M}_1 : \Pi \times \Theta \times \Phi \to \mathbb{R}^3$$

$$(\rho, \theta, \phi) \mapsto \mathbf{x} = \begin{matrix} a\rho\cos\theta\cos\phi \\ a\rho\sin\theta\cos\phi \\ c\rho\sin\phi \end{matrix}$$

where $\Pi = [0, 1]$, $\Theta = [0, 2\pi)$, $\Phi = [-\pi/2, \pi/2]$. A pictorial description of the nodule model is shown in Figure 11.6a. The parameters of the model are $\mathbf{m}_1 = (a, c)$, with domain $\mathbf{M}_1 = \{(a, c)$

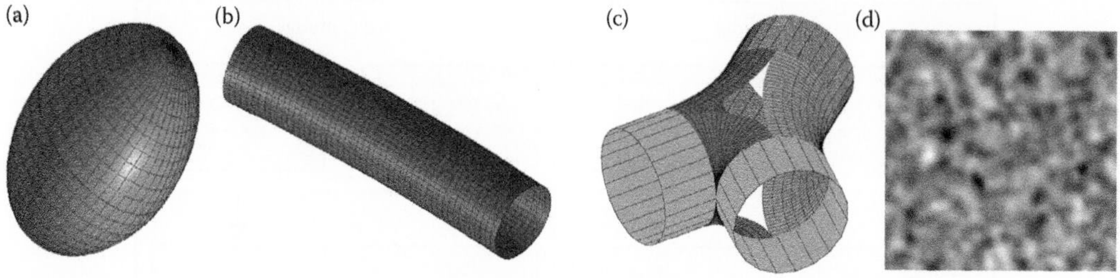

FIGURE 11.6
(See color insert.) Graphical representation of the nodule, vessel, junction, and parenchyma models. (a) The nodule model is represented by an ellipsoid with axes $a = b \leq c$. The vessel model is represented by a segment of a torus with minor and major radii given by $r \leq R$. (c) Three tori with adequate parameters form the junction model, with the cylindrical extensions are included for clarity. (d) In contrast to the previous three models, the parenchyma model is not represented through a geometric shape, but as an isotropic Gaussian random field.

$\in \mathbb{R}^2 | 0 < a \leq c\}$. Each choice of $\rho \in \Pi$ defines a different isosurface, at any point of which the principal curvatures can be computed. Moreover, using standard results from differential geometry [5], it can be shown that

$$\rho = (c/a^2)\sqrt{\kappa_1/\kappa_2^3} \text{ and } \sin^2\phi = (c^2 - a^2(\kappa_2/\kappa_1))/(c^2 - a^2). \tag{11.7}$$

11.3.2.1 Design of the Priors for the Nodule Model

Let A and C be random variables that map a nodule to the half-size of its minor and major axes (a, c). Assuming that nodules have nonnegative dimensions with an average diameter of $2/\lambda$, as yet to be determined, the choice of an exponential distribution for A is supported by both the principle of maximum entropy and data from the medical literature [44]. The same is true for the random variable C, but now the additional constraint that $0 < A \leq C$ must be satisfied. Observe that the second inequality is arbitrary: A and C are chosen from the pair (A', C'), with $0 < A' < \infty$ and $0 < C' < \infty$, so that $A \leq C$. Therefore, the maximum entropy principle can be first applied to (A', C'), resulting in a probability density for the pair (A', C') given by $p(a', c') = \lambda^2 e^{-\lambda(a'+c')}\mathbb{I}_{(0,\infty)}(a')\mathbb{I}_{(0,\infty)}(c')$, where $\mathbb{I}_X$ is the indicator function of the set X, i.e., $\mathbb{I}_X(x) = 1$ if $x \in X$ and 0 otherwise. This expression implies that A' and C' are independent, which, in the absence of contrary evidence, is the maximum entropy solution. The joint distribution for (A, C) can then be obtained via the transformation $A = \min(A', C')$, $C = \max(A', C')$, resulting in $p(\mathbf{m}_1 | \mathcal{M}_1) = p(a,c) = 2\lambda^2 e^{-\lambda(a+c)}\mathbb{I}_{\mathrm{M}_1}(\mathbf{m}_1)$. Given the volume $V(a, c) = 4\pi a^2 c/3$ of an instance of $\mathcal{M}_1$, following the procedure discussed in Section 11.3.1.4, we obtain the desired prior $p(\mathbf{m}_1 | \mathcal{M}_1, \mathbf{x})$ for $\mathbf{m}_1 = (a, c)$ as

$$p(\mathbf{m}_1 | \mathcal{M}_1, \mathbf{x}) = (8/5)\lambda^5 a^2 c e^{-\lambda(a+c)}\mathbb{I}_{\mathrm{M}_1}(\mathbf{m}_1). \tag{11.8}$$

Using data from ref. [44], a maximum likelihood estimation of λ results in $\lambda \approx 0.5$ mm^{-1}. To determine $P(\mathcal{M}_1 | \mathbf{x})$ we again used the data in ref. [44], which places the likelihood of finding a nodule in a given examination of a cohort as 60%, with average nodule volume of 0.033 ml.

11.3.2.2 Derivation of the Likelihood

Let $\mathbf{x}$ be a point in the range $\mathcal{M}_1(\Pi \times \Theta \times \Phi) = \mathbb{R}_1 \subset \mathbb{R}^3$ of $\mathcal{M}_1$, randomly chosen according to a uniform distribution on $\mathcal{R}_1$. Define now the random variables Π_1, Φ_1, and $\mathbf{K}^1 = (K_1^1, K_2^1)$, given by

$$\begin{aligned} \Pi_1 &: \mathcal{R}_1 \to \mathbb{R} \\ \mathbf{x} &\mapsto \rho(\mathbf{x}) \in \Pi, \end{aligned} \qquad \begin{aligned} \Phi_1 &: \mathcal{R}_1 \to \mathbb{R} \\ \mathbf{x} &\mapsto \phi(\mathbf{x}) \in \Phi \end{aligned} \qquad \text{and} \qquad \begin{aligned} \mathbf{K}^1 &: \mathcal{R}_1 \to \mathbb{R}^2 \\ \mathbf{x} &\mapsto \kappa(\mathbf{x}) = (\kappa_1, \kappa_2). \end{aligned}$$

The joint probability density function of Π_1 and Φ_1 can be computed from the fractional volume element $d\mathbf{x}/dV$ in polar coordinates and is given by

$$p(\rho,\phi) = (3/2)\rho^2 \cos\phi \mathbb{I}_\Pi(\rho)\mathbb{I}_\Phi(\phi). \tag{11.9}$$

Using Equation 11.9 and the Jacobian of Equation 11.7, the joint probability density $p(\kappa|\mathbf{m}_1, \mathcal{M}_1, \mathbf{x})$ of $\mathbf{K}^1$ can be computed via a simple transformation of random variables, yielding

$$p(\kappa|\mathbf{m}_1, \mathcal{M}_1, \mathbf{x}) = 3c^3\left(2a^4\sqrt{\kappa_2^9(c^2 - a^2)(c^2\kappa_1 - a^2\kappa_2)}\right)^{-1} \mathbb{I}_{\mathcal{K}_1}(\kappa), \tag{11.10}$$

where $\mathcal{K}_1 = \left\{ \kappa \in \mathbb{R}^2 \middle| \frac{a}{c^2} \le \kappa_1 \text{ and } \max\left(\kappa_1, \left(\frac{c^2\kappa_1}{a^4}\right)^{1/3}\right) \le \kappa_2 < \frac{c^2}{a^2}\kappa_1 \right\}$.

11.3.2.3 Marginalization Over the Model Parameters

The probability density in Equation 11.10 is sharply peaked (in fact, infinite) on the set $\mathcal{K}_1^\infty = \{\kappa \in \mathcal{K}_1 | c^2\kappa_1 - a^2\kappa_2 = 0\}$ and quickly falls as the distance $d(\kappa, \mathcal{K}_1^\infty)$ grows. Therefore, at the isosurface of $\mathcal{M}_1$ defined by a given ρ, the expressions

$$\kappa_1(\rho) \triangleq E[K_1^1|\rho] = \int_\Phi \kappa_1(\phi,\rho)p(\phi|\rho)\, d\phi = h_1(\rho) = (c\rho)^{-1}, \tag{11.11}$$

$$\kappa_2(\rho) \triangleq E[K_2^1|\rho] = \int_\Phi \kappa_2(\phi,\rho)p(\phi|\rho)\, d\phi = h_2(\rho) = \frac{c \arccos(a/c)}{a\rho\sqrt{c^2 - a^2}}, \tag{11.12}$$

which suppress the dependence of κ_1 and κ_2 on ϕ, are excellent approximations for the actual values of κ_1 and κ_2. From Equations 11.11 and 11.12 one can write

$$\kappa_2 \approx g(\kappa_1, \mathbf{m}_1, \mathcal{M}_1) = \kappa_1 \frac{c^2 \arccos(a/c)}{a\sqrt{c^2 - a^2}} \approx \kappa_1(4c - a)/(3a). \qquad \textit{(Taylor series)} \tag{11.13}$$

Furthermore, computing the marginal probability density $p\Pi_1(\rho)$ of Π_1 from Equation 11.9 and using the Jacobian of Equation 11.11, we obtain $p(\kappa_1|\mathbf{m}_1, \mathcal{M}_1, \mathbf{x}) = p\Pi(h_1^{-1}(\kappa_1))dh_1^{-1}$ d = $(\kappa_1)/d\kappa_1 = 3/(c^3\kappa_1^4)\mathbb{I}_{\{1/c \le \kappa_1\}}(\kappa_1)$. Using this result together with the expression for $g(\kappa_1, \mathbf{m}_1, \mathcal{M}_1)$ defined by Equation 11.13, we obtain the simplified likelihood term

$$p(\kappa|\mathbf{m}_1,\mathcal{M}_1,\mathbf{x}) \approx \frac{3\delta(\kappa_2-\kappa_1(4c-a)/(3a))}{c^3\kappa_1^4}\mathbb{I}_{[1/c,\infty)}(\kappa_1)\mathbb{I}_{[0,\kappa_2]}(\kappa_1). \tag{11.14}$$

Using the approximation in Equation 11.14 and the prior Equation 11.8, the integral in Equation 11.6 can be computed, resulting in

$$p(\kappa|\mathcal{M}_1,\mathbf{x}) \approx 4608\lambda^3 e^{-\frac{\lambda(5\kappa_1+3\kappa_2)}{\kappa_1(\kappa_1+3\kappa_2)}}\frac{\kappa_1(\kappa_1+3\kappa_2)+\lambda(5\kappa_1+3\kappa_2)}{5\kappa_1^2(\kappa_1+3\kappa_2)^3(5\kappa_1+3\kappa_2)^2}\mathbb{I}_{[0,\kappa_2]}(\kappa_1).$$

11.3.3 The Vessel Model

The vessel model $\mathcal{M}_2$ is represented as a section of a solid torus with similar concentric isosurfaces such that the outermost isosurface has minor and major radii r and R with $r \le R$, i.e.,

$$\mathcal{M}_1 : \Pi \times \Theta_0 \times \Psi \to \mathbb{R}^3$$

$$(\rho,\theta,\psi) \mapsto \mathbf{x} = \begin{matrix}(R+r\rho\cos\psi)\cos\theta \\ (R+r\rho\cos\psi)\sin\theta \\ r\rho\sin\psi\end{matrix}, \tag{11.15}$$

where $\Pi = [0, 1]$, $\Theta_0 = [0, \theta_0]$, $\Psi = [-\pi/2, 3\pi/2)$, and each choice of $\rho \in \Pi$ defines a different isosurface. A pictorial description of the vessel model is shown in Figure 11.6b. The parameters of the model are $\mathbf{m}_2 = (\theta_0, r, R)$, with domain $\mathbf{M}_2 = \{(\theta_0, r, R) \in \mathbb{R}^3 | 0 < \theta_0 < 2\pi \text{ and } 0 < r \le R\}$. The principal curvatures (κ_1, κ_2) at any point $\mathbf{x}$ in the torus can be expressed in terms of the model parameters (ρ, θ, ψ) as

$$\rho = 1/(r\kappa_2) \text{ and } \cos\psi = \kappa_1\kappa_2 R/(\kappa_2-\kappa_1). \tag{11.16}$$

11.3.3.1 Design of the Priors for the Vessel Model

The first step in determining the priors on the parameters $\mathbf{m}_2$ of the vessel model is examining available clinical data. Murray's [35] work on vessel structures provides the basis for deriving several mathematical relationships between the vessel model parameters. Two particular corollaries of Murray's law are a power-law distribution for vessel radius, $p(r) \propto 1/r^3$ [1], and a linear relationship between vessel length and diameter, $\theta_0 R \propto r$ [22], with the latter implying that the vessel volume is proportional to r^3. The volume normalization step produces a prior $p(r|\mathbf{x}) \propto 1$, which is improper. To address this issue, we assume an upper bound for r and take one further step in our Bayesian horizon. Invoking the maximum entropy principle under the appropriate constraints, we obtain as a hyperprior for r_{max} a gamma distribution with shape parameter 1 and scale parameter t, such that $E[r_{max}] = t$. We then marginalize the bounded prior over r_{max}, yielding $p(r|\mathbf{x}) = e^{-r/t}/t$, where t is the average maximum radius of a pulmonary vessel ($\approx$ 15 mm using the radius of the aorta).

Now, a probability distribution on R must satisfy the constraint $R \geq r$ and expert advice [39] indicated that pulmonary vessels tend to be straight, i.e., $R \approx \infty$, suggesting a better representation for the model parameters as ($I_R = 1/R$, r), with $0 \leq I_R \leq 1/r$. The maximum entropy distribution for I_R is simply the uniform distribution, i.e., $p(I_R|r) = r\mathbb{I}_{[0,1/r]}(I_R)$, and therefore $p(R|r) = (r/R^2)\mathbb{I}_{[r,\infty]}(R)$, which combined with $p(r|\mathbf{x})$ yields

$$p(\mathbf{m}_2|\mathcal{M}_2,\mathbf{x}) = (r/(R^2t))e^{-r/t}\mathbb{I}_{\mathbf{M}_2}(\mathbf{m}_2). \tag{11.17}$$

Finally, $P(\mathcal{M}_2|\mathbf{x})$ is proportional to the volume of the pulmonary tree (≈ 300 ml [42]).

11.3.3.2 Derivation of the Likelihood

We omit the derivation of the likelihood term, $p(\kappa|\mathbf{m}_2, \mathcal{M}_2, \mathbf{x})$ for the vessel model, because it follows exactly the same steps as that of the nodule model. The final result is

$$p(\kappa|\mathbf{m}_2,\mathcal{M}_2,\mathbf{x}) = \frac{2R/(\pi r^2)}{(\kappa_2-\kappa_1)^2\sqrt{(\kappa_2-\kappa_1)^2-(\kappa_1\kappa_2R)^2}}\mathbb{I}_{\mathcal{K}_2}(\kappa), \tag{11.18}$$

where $\mathcal{K}_2$ is the set $\mathcal{K}_2 = \kappa \in \mathbb{R}^2 \big| 1/r \leq \kappa_2 \text{ and } \frac{\kappa_2}{1-R\kappa_2} \leq \kappa_1 \leq \frac{\kappa_2}{1+R\kappa_2}$.

11.3.3.3 Marginalization Over the Model Parameters

The probability density in Equation 11.18 is infinite on the set $\mathcal{K}_2^\infty = \mathcal{K}_2^{\infty,-} \cup \mathcal{K}_2^{\infty,+}$, where $\mathcal{K}_2^{\infty,-} = \{1/r \leq \kappa_2 \text{ and } \kappa_1 = \kappa_2/(1-\kappa_2R)\}$ and $\mathcal{K}_2^{\infty,+} = \{1/r \leq \kappa_2 \text{ and } \kappa_1 = \kappa_2/(1+\kappa_2R)\}$ and falls sharply as the distance $d(\kappa,\mathcal{K}_2^\infty)$ grows. Observe that the sets $\mathcal{K}_2^{\infty,-}$ and $\mathcal{K}_2^{\infty,+}$ are disjoint, and using Equation 11.16, they can be identified with the sets $\Psi^- = [(\pi/2, 3\pi/2)$ and $\Psi^+ = (-\pi/2, \pi/2)]$ with $\Psi = \Psi^- \cup \Psi^+$. Analogous to the case of the simplified nodule model, we have, for a given ρ defining a specific isosurface,

$$\kappa_1^-(\rho) \triangleq E[K_1^1|\rho,\psi \in \Psi^-] = \frac{\int_{\Psi^-}\kappa_1(\psi,\rho)p(\psi|\rho)d\psi}{\int_{\Psi^-}p(\psi|\rho)d\psi} = h_1^-(\rho) = \frac{-2}{R\pi-2r\rho}, \tag{11.19}$$

$$\kappa_1^+(\rho) \triangleq E[K_1^1|\rho,\psi \in \Psi^+] = \frac{\int_{\Psi^+}\kappa_1(\psi,\rho)p(\psi|\rho)d\psi}{\int_{\Psi^+}p(\psi|\rho)d\psi} = h_1^+(\rho) = \frac{2}{R\pi+2r\rho}, \tag{11.20}$$

which approximate κ_1 in Ψ^- and Ψ^+, despite suppressing its dependence on ψ. There is no need to approximate κ_2, since we see from Equation 11.16 that it is already independent of ψ. From Equations 11.19 and 11.20, we obtain

$$\kappa_1^- \approx g_1(\kappa_2, \mathbf{m}_2, \mathcal{M}_2) = \frac{2\kappa_2}{2 - R\pi\kappa_2} \text{ and } w_1 = \int_{\psi^-} \rho(\psi)\, d\psi = \frac{1}{2} - \frac{2r}{3\pi R}$$

$$\kappa_1^+ \approx g_2(\kappa_2, \mathbf{m}_2, \mathcal{M}_2) = \frac{2\kappa_2}{2 + R\pi\kappa_2} \text{ and } w_2 = \int_{\psi^+} \rho(\psi)\, d\psi = \frac{1}{2} + \frac{2r}{3\pi R}.$$

Proceeding as with the nodule model and again using Equation 11.16, we have $p(\kappa_2 | \kappa_1, \mathbf{m}_2, \mathcal{M}_2, \mathbf{x}) = 2/(\kappa_2^3 r^2)\mathbb{I}_{\kappa_2 \geq 1/r}(\kappa_2)$ and finally

$$p(\kappa | \mathbf{m}_2, \mathcal{M}_2, \mathbf{x}) \approx \left(1 - \frac{4r}{3\pi R}\right)\delta\left(\kappa_1 - \frac{2\kappa_2}{2 - R\pi\kappa_2}\right) + \left(1 + \frac{4r}{3\pi R}\right)\delta\left(\kappa_1 - \frac{2\kappa_2}{2 + R\pi\kappa_2}\right)\frac{1}{\kappa_2^3 r^2}\mathbb{I}_{\kappa_2 \geq 1/r}(\kappa_2). \tag{11.21}$$

The integral in Equation 11.6 for the vessel model can now be estimated, using the approximation in Equation 11.21 and the prior in Equation 11.17, resulting in

$$p(\kappa | \mathcal{M}_2, \mathbf{x}) \approx \pi \left(\frac{\kappa_1 \left(e^{\frac{-1}{t\kappa_2}} e^{\frac{2(\kappa_1 - \kappa_2)}{t\pi\kappa_2 |\kappa_1|}} \right)}{3(\kappa_2 - \kappa_1)^3} - \frac{\mathrm{Ei}\left(\frac{-1}{t\kappa_2}\right) - \mathrm{Ei}\left(\frac{2(\kappa_1 - \kappa_2)}{t\pi\kappa_2|\kappa_1|}\right)}{2t\kappa_2(\kappa_2 - \kappa_1)^2} \right) \mathbb{I}_{\mathcal{K}_2^*}(\kappa),$$

where $\mathcal{K}_2^* = \{\kappa \in \mathbb{R}^2 | \kappa_2 \geq 0, -2\kappa_2/(\pi - 2) \leq \kappa_1 \leq 2\kappa_2/(\pi + 2)\}$ and Ei denotes the exponential integral function.

11.3.4 The Vessel Junction Model

Junction detection is an interesting problem on its own, and the derivation of the junction model is quite involved. Here, we limit ourselves to a superficial discussion of its prior and likelihood terms and refer the reader to ref. [50] for details.

By appropriately "slicing" and "stitching" three tori with parameterizations as in Equation 11.15 but different values for R, we obtain the object $\mathcal{M}_3$ depicted in Figure 11.6c. Vessel junctions are often described as the most common source of false-positives in lung CAD systems aimed at detecting nodules [40,46], and to account for that, we fill the gap between the three tori with an ellipsoid. For the joint prior of this structure, we have

$$p(\mathbf{m}_3 | \mathcal{M}_3, \mathbf{x}) = \delta(a - c_0^{3/2}/c^{1/2}) \times \frac{{}^2 c e^{-\ (c - c_0)}}{1 + \ c_0} \times \frac{e^{-r/t}}{t}\mathbb{I}_{\mathbf{M}_3}(\mathbf{m}_3),$$

where $\mathbf{m}_3 = (a, c, r)$, $c_0 = ar$, $a \approx 0.41$ (an exact form is available), $\mathbf{M}_3 = \{\mathbf{m}_3 \in \mathbb{R}^3 | r \geq 0, 0 \leq a \leq c_0 \leq c\}$, and t is the same as in Equation 11.17. For the likelihood term, we have

$$p(\kappa|\mathbf{m}_3,\mathcal{M}_3,\mathbf{x}) = (1 - \omega_2 - \omega_3)p_1(\kappa|a,c) + \omega_2 p_2(\kappa|r) + \omega_3 p_3(\kappa|r),$$

where p_1 is given by Equation 11.14, p_2 is given by Equation 11.21, with $R = r$, p_3 is also given by Equation 11.21, but with $R = r \sin\beta/(1 + \sin\beta)$, $\beta = \arccos(2^{-1/3})$, $\omega_2 \approx 0.25$ and $\omega_3 \approx 0.69$, for which exact but lengthy expressions are available. The result of the marginalization is an enormous expression that can be obtained with the aid of a symbolic computation package.

11.3.5 The Parenchyma Model

The parenchyma model does not comply with the steps provided in Section 11.3.1.2; there is no deterministic shape on which we can base its computation. Instead, we adapt recent results in the theory of Gaussian random fields [33], which directly establish the joint probability distribution of random isosurfaces of an initially spatially uncorrelated Gaussian random field after smoothing by an isotropic kernel.

As with the junction model, the full derivation of the parenchyma model is quite involved. However, the key idea is to adapt a result first derived by Mehta [31] to our applications. Theorem 3.3.1 in ref. [31] provides a "closed-form" expression for the probability density of the eigenvalues of random matrices in the Gaussian orthogonal ensemble (GOE$_n$). This is the ensemble of (n, n) real symmetric matrices $\mathbf{M}$ with probability density invariant with respect to similarity transformations $\mathbf{M} \rightarrow \mathbf{R}^T\mathbf{M}\mathbf{R}$ for any given (n, n) orthonormal $\mathbf{R}$ and such that the probability distribution of distinct entries are independent from each other. In his work, Mehta has shown that the only matrices that satisfy this invariance condition are those with independent and identically distributed Gaussian entries. We would like to apply Mehta's result to the matrix $\mathbf{C} = -\mathbf{N}^T\mathbf{H}\mathbf{N}/||\nabla I||$ in Equation 11.5, with the volume image I being a realization of an isotropic Guassian random process. As shown in ref. [33], the entries of $\mathbf{C}$ in Equation 11.5 are not independent, and therefore, Mehta's result cannot be applied directly. However, the requirement of independence was needed only to derive an expression for the joint probability density of the entries of random matrices in GOE$_n$; in our problem, the normality of $-\mathbf{N}^T\mathbf{H}\mathbf{N}$ is a trivial consequence of the assumed normality of I, and Mehta's result do apply. Therefore, the probability distribution of the eigenvalues λ_1 and λ_2 (with $\lambda_1 \leq \lambda_2$) of $-\mathbf{N}^T\mathbf{H}\mathbf{N}$ is given by

$$p(\lambda_1,\lambda_2) = \frac{\lambda_2 - \lambda_1}{2\sqrt{2}\pi(\sigma^2\rho_0^{(4)})^{3/2}}\exp\left(-\frac{3(\lambda_1+\lambda_2) - 2\lambda_1\lambda_2}{16\sigma^2\rho_0^{(4)}}\right),$$

where σ is the variance of the I at any given $\mathbf{x}$ and $\rho_0^{(4)}$ is the fourth derivative of the autocorrelation function of I at zero. (The autocorrelation function of I takes in a scalar argument because the Gaussian random field I is assumed to be isotropic.) Moreover, it can be seen that the denominator of $\mathbf{C}$, given by $||\nabla I||$, follows a χ-distribution with 3 degrees of freedom. Therefore, the probability distribution of the ratio of λ_1 and λ_2 by $||\nabla I||$ can be easily computed, yielding the final result

$$p(\kappa|\mathcal{M}_4,\mathbf{x}) = \frac{256\sigma_0^3(\kappa_2-\kappa_1)}{\pi(4+3\sigma_0^2\kappa_2^2 - 2\sigma_0^2\kappa_2\kappa_1 + 3\sigma_0^2\kappa_1^2)^3}\mathbb{I}_{0,\kappa_2}(\kappa_1).$$

11.4 Experimental Results

11.4.1 Region-Based Methods

The region-based methods for pulmonary nodule detection were evaluated using the model selection described in Section 11.2.4. Given the posterior probabilities of the individual models, the models are competed with one another using Bayes factors [2], which are equivalent to ratios of a posteriori probabilities under uniform model priors. Structures having large Bayes factors favoring the nodule model in all competitions were deemed suspicious and flagged for review.

For example, the Bayes factor comparing a nodule model of a segmented region with a vessel model of that region is defined as

$$\frac{p(x,\theta|M=N)}{p(x,\theta|M=V)} = \frac{\int p(x,\theta|\beta_N, M=N)p(\beta_N|M=N)d\beta_N}{\int p(x,\theta|\beta_V, M=V)p(\beta_V|M=V)d\beta_V} \tag{11.22}$$

where M is a model indicator (N for nodule and V for vessel), the vector x represents the image data inside the segmented region, and the vector θ represents salient geometric features of the region. In Equation 11.22, we explicitly integrate over nuissance parameters in both models β_N and β_V, respectively, using Equation 11.3.

Free response receiver operating characteristic (FROC) curves of sensitivity versus the number of false-positives per case can be plotted by sweeping over the minimum Bayes factor of all the model competitions applied to each individual putative nodule. This minimum Bayes factor can be thought of as the evidence in the region supporting the nodule model over all other models.

We give results on 50 low-dose CT lung examinations taken at 40 mA, 120 kVp, and 2.5 mm collimation with a 1.5:1 helical pitch. The data were selected from a large patient population such that 75% of the cases were required to have at least one nodule 5 mm or larger, and the remaining 25% of the cases were required to have no nodules in this size range. These cases were read by three board-certified radiologists with extensive experience in reading low-dose lung CT examinations. The readers were blinded from each other's findings. For each identified lesion, the readers recorded their subjective judgment on the severity of the lesion on a 5-point scale ranging from "definitely not cancer" to "definitely cancer". Readers were asked to perform a highly conservative reading by indicating all areas that could be possibly construed as a nodule and use the severity score to express their level of concern about each finding. We present results on all lesions detected by a majority of the readers and judged to be more severe than "definitely not cancer".

Each case was then analyzed by our model-based CAD method, and sensitivity was recorded with respect to majority-detected lesions (those detected by two or all of the three radiologists) and with respect to those majority-detected lesions not detected by all readers. This CAD sensitivity to missed lesions gives a measure of the potential for CAD to improve radiologist detection performance of suspicious lesions. In total, 35 noncalcified solid lesions greater than 5 mm in diameter were identified by a majority of the readers. Four of these 35 lesions were not identified by all readers. The model-based algorithm detected 27 of the majority-detected noncalicified solid lesions with 8.3 false-positives per

TABLE 11.1

Improvement in Radiological Sensitivity Using CAD

Reader	No. of Cases Read	No. of Majority Detected Lesions	Reader Sensitivity (%)	Reader + CAD Sensitivity (%)	Sensitivity Improvement (%)
A	50	37/43	86	93	7
B	50	41/43	95	100	5
C	50	43/43	100	100	0
CAD	50	30/43	70		
Average			93.8	97.7	3.9

Note: On average, a radiologist improves his sensitivity to majority found nodules from 94% to 98% when our CAD system is used.

case. The algorithm detected three of the four lesions not identified by all readers. Using a preliminary nonsolid nodule model, the algorithm detected 30 of the 43 total (solid and subsolid) lesions identified by a majority of readers, at the same false-positive rate as above. The algorithm detected five of the eight total lesions not identified by all readers. When CAD results were combined with radiological findings, two of the participating readers improved their sensitivity to these lesions by 4.7% and 7.0%, respectively. The third reader did not miss any majority-detected lesions. The results are summarized in Table 11.1.

One advantage of the model-based approach is that both solid and nonsolid lesions can be detected. Examples of detected nodules from both populations are shown in Figure 11.7. Lesions not detected by the model-based algorithm were generally complex lesions that did not fit well to our current nodule model and dim nonsolid lesions in areas of significant beam hardening. The majority of false-positives were due to abnormalities on the pleura (scars and fluid build-up) and convoluted vessel junctions. Examples of nodules not detected by our algorithm are shown in Figure 11.8.

11.4.2 Bayesian Voxel Labeling

The algorithm for assisting in the detection of lung nodules depicted in CT volumes using the models described in Sections 11.3.2 to 11.3.5 was implemented with the Insight Toolkit [19]. The volume image is first smoothed with a Gaussian kernel to reduce the effect of noise in the computation of derivatives. The lung volume is automatically extracted to obtain a region of interest (ROI) for all subsequent operations. Given a voxel $\mathbf{x}$ in the extracted ROI, the principal curvatures $\kappa(\mathbf{x})$ of the implicit isosurface at $\mathbf{x}$ are computed directly from the image intensities [32,47]. Given the curvatures, the probabilities $p(\kappa|\mathbf{m}_i, \mathcal{M}_i, \mathbf{x})$ are computed at each voxel $\mathbf{x}$ for each model $\mathcal{M}_i$. The probability distributions involve parameters such as the expected nodule diameter and the expected maximum vessel radius that were set to typical anatomical values. The curvatures at every voxel in a neighborhood $\mathcal{N}$ centered at $\mathbf{x}$ are used to define the set $\mathcal{D}$ and $p(\mathcal{D}|\mathcal{M}_i, \mathbf{x})$ is computed as the product $\Pi_{j \in \mathcal{N}} p(\mathcal{D}_j|\mathbf{m}_i, \mathcal{M}_i, \mathbf{x})$. The neighborhood shape is a simple cube with size set to 4 mm, the diameter of the smallest nodule of interest [9]. Finally, multiplying by the model prior probabilities, $P(\mathcal{M}_i|\mathbf{x})$, yields the individual posterior probabilities, $P(\mathcal{M}_i|\mathcal{D}, \mathbf{x})$.

The utility of explicitly modeling the junctions is illustrated via results on a synthetic image as shown in Figure 11.9. In the absence of an explicit junction model, the central

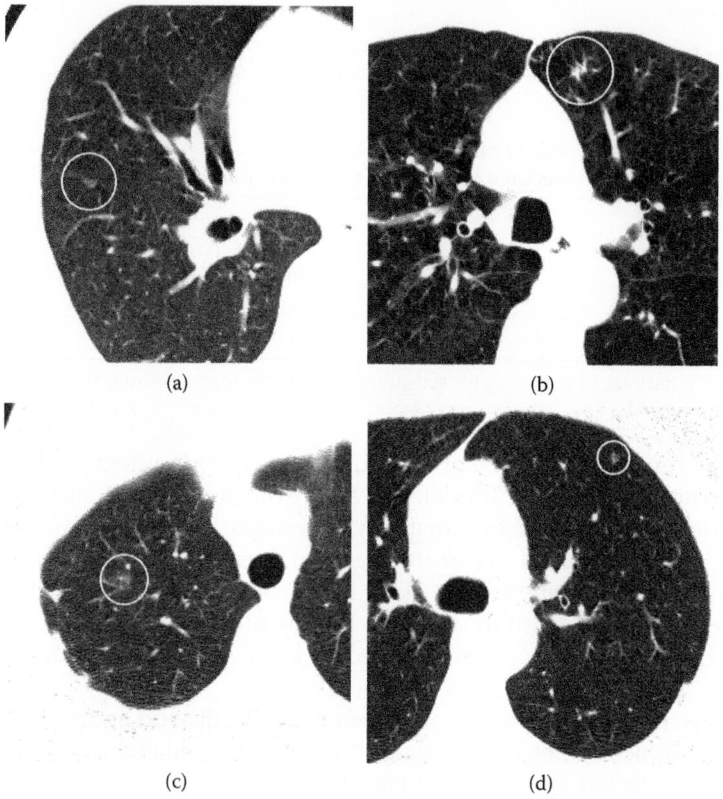

FIGURE 11.7
Detected nodules in region-based CAD. (a, b) Two solid nodules (as judged by the radiologist readers); (c, d) two nonsolid nodules. Each nodule shown here was missed by at least one reader in the multireader study.

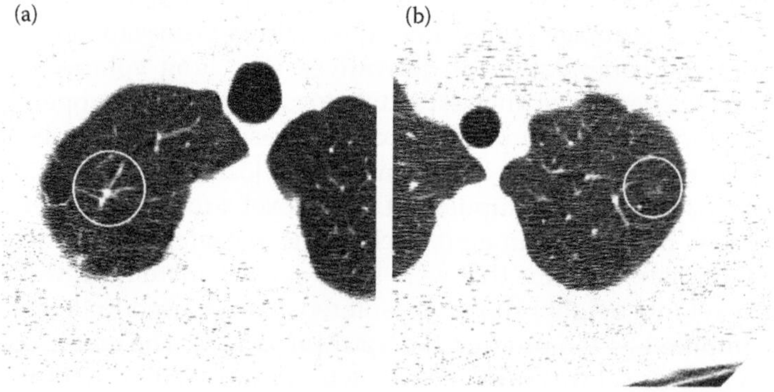

FIGURE 11.8
Missed nodules in region-based CAD. (a) Dim nonsolid nodule (average intensity −650 HU); (b) complex solid nodule. Both nodules are in the lung apex, where the proximity to the bones in the shoulders produces significant beam hardening.

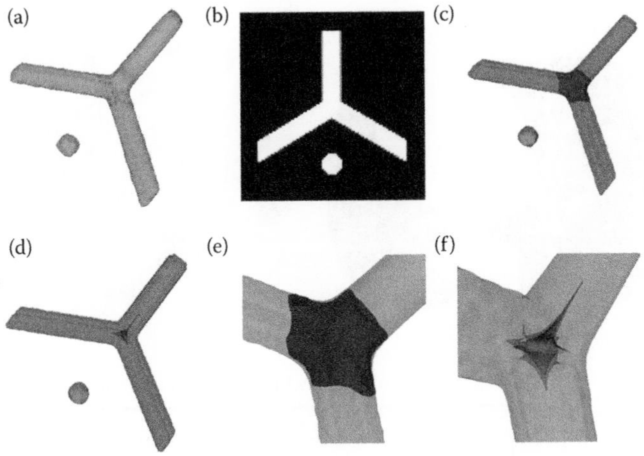

FIGURE 11.9
(See color insert.) Experiments on synthetic data. (a) 3D rendering and (b) 2D slice of a phantom vessel bifurcation. Bayesian voxel labeling results (c) with and (d) without including the junction model with zoom-in views shown in (e) and (f), respectively. Each voxel is colored according to the model with the highest probability using red for vessels, green for nodules, and blue for junctions. Note that without the junction model, (d) and (f) show nodule responses at the bifurcation center.

regions of vessel bifurcations give rise to nodule-like responses, resulting in false-positives. When the junction model is used in combination with the neighborhood integration, it wins over both the vessel and nodule models.

The posterior model probabilities can be used to design a utility function over misclassification errors (false-negatives and false-positives), but this can be difficult in the case of distinguishing between more than two alternatives or models [18]. Since the target application is in assisting radiologist in performing nodule detection, we reduce the decision problem to two classes (nodule and nonnodule) by combining all model posteriors other than $P(\mathcal{M}_1|\mathcal{D}, \mathbf{x})$ into a single probability and evaluating the Bayes factor [24] for the nodule model as $P(\mathcal{M}_1|\mathcal{D}, \mathbf{x})/P(\mathcal{M}_i \neq \mathcal{M}_1|\mathcal{D}, \mathbf{x})$. Figure 11.10a–b shows results of the Bayesian voxel labeling using this scheme on a high-resolution 0.625-mm slice thickness CT scan of a patient with over 80 nodules due to metastatic lung cancer.

Validation of the algorithm was performed against ground truth provided by three radiologists through FROC analysis. A data set of 50 low-dose CT scans of asymptomatic high-risk subjects, acquired via a low-dose protocol (40 mA s, 120 kVp, slice thickness of 1.25 mm), was used to validate the proposed algorithm. Ground truth was defined as all nodules with diameter greater or equal to 4 mm marked by at least two out of three radiologists and included 60 noncalcified solid parenchymal nodules. To perform the FROC analysis, a connected component algorithm was run to group neighboring voxels as a single unit. After applying a diameter threshold of 3 mm to remove small, clinically irrelevant detections, the average Bayes factor over the constituent voxels of each suspicious region was used as the threshold parameter to generate the FROC curve. The algorithm achieved 90% sensitivity at 5.1 false-positives per case. In comparison, the algorithm from ref. [32], which uses the ratio κ_1/κ_2 as the decision threshold, gave only 70% sensitivity at the same false-positive rate. The corresponding FROC curves are shown in Figure 11.10c. The Bayesian framework shows better specificity and achieves a much higher overall maximum sensitivity (95%).

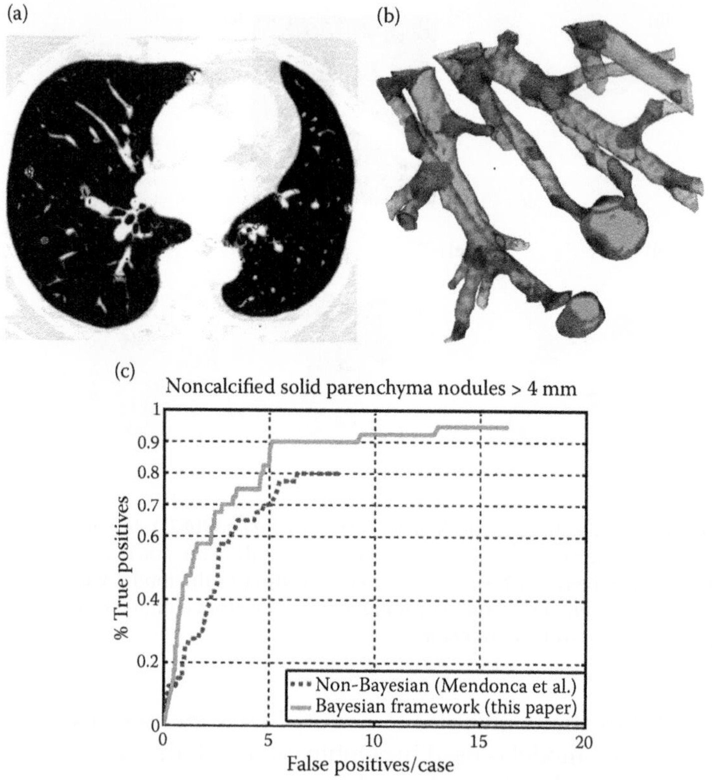

FIGURE 11.10
(See color insert.) Experimental validation. (a) A 2D slice of a high-resolution CT scan with nodule labels overlaid in green on the intensity image. (b) A 3D rendering of the voxel labeling for a small region from the same case showing nodules (green), vessels (red), and junctions (blue). (c) FROC curves comparing performance of the Bayesian voxel labeling framework to a curvature-based nonprobabilistic approach given in ref. [32].

11.5 Summary and Conclusion

We have described a general model-based program for assisting in detection of lung nodules in pulmonary CT images, following the general paradigm of (a) modeling the imaging formation process, (b) statistically modeling features of the objects of interest, i.e., the nodules themselves as well as possible confounding factors for detection, such as vessels and junctions, (c) computing the modeled features from image data, and (d) carrying out a Bayesian competition to determine the model that best explains the data. Two different modeling approaches were presented: one in which the modeling and the features computation is carried out over segmented regions within the image (region-based modeling) and the other in which the modeling and feature computation are executed for individual voxels (voxel labeling). The region-based approach benefits from coherent integration of data across neighboring voxels and can therefore make use of richer features computed over a larger image region. However, segmentation of the lung field is in itself a difficult problem and oversegmentation or undersegmentation are likely to occur. The voxel-based approach, on the other hand, is restricted to use either completely local features or features computed over fixed, arbitrary neighborhoods around each voxel. Such features are often less rich and possibly less informative than those computed over well-defined, anatomically consistent regions. However, the voxel-based approach bypasses the segmentation problem and can be implemented through nonlinear filters, albeit complex ones, applied to the image volume. Despite this differences, both methods achieve good performance on low-dose scans.

Acknowledgments

This publication was supported by GE Healthcare and the DOD and the Medical University of South Carolina under DOD Grant W81XWH-05-1-0378. Its contents are solely the responsibility of the authors and do not necessarily represent the official views of the DOD or the Medical University of South Carolina.

References

[1] S. H. Bennett, M. W. Eldridge, C. E. Puente, R. H. Riedi, T. R. Nelson, B. W. Beotzman, J. M. Milstein, S. S. Singhal, K. Horsfield, and M. J. Woldenberg. Origin of fractal branching complexity in the lung. Preprint, 2001. Available at http://www.stat.rice.edu/~riedi/UCDavisHemoglobin/fractal3.pdf.

[2] J. M. Bernardo and A. F. M. Smith. *Bayesian Theory. Wiley Series in Probability and Statistics*. Wiley, Chichester, 2004.

[3] M. S. Brown, J. G. Goldin, R. D. Suh, M. F. McNitt-Gray, J. W. Sayre, and D. R. Aberle. Lung micronodules: Automated method for detection at thin-section CT—Initial experience. *Radiology*, 226(1):256–262, Jan. 2003.

[4] J. F. Canny. A computational approach to edge detection. *IEEE Trans. Pattern Anal. Machine Intell.*, 8(6):679–698, Nov. 1986.

[5] M. P. do Carmo. *Differential Geometry of Curves and Surfaces*. Prentice-Hall, 1976.

[6] N. Dobigeon, J.-Y. Tourneret, and J. D. Scargle. Joint segmentation of multivariate astronomical time series: Bayesian sampling with a hierarchical model. *IEEE Trans. Signal Process.*, 55(2):414–423, Feb. 2007.

[7] N. R. Draper and H. Smith. *Applied Regression Analysis. Wiley Series in Probability and Statistics.* John Wiley & Sons, New York, 3rd ed., 1998.

[8] B. Efron. Bayesians, frequentists, and scientists. *J. Am. Stat. Assoc.*, 100(469):1–5, Mar. 2005. ISSN 0162-1459. doi: 10.1198/016214505000000033. Available at http://dx.doi.org/10.1198/-016214505000000033.

[9] ELCAP. International early cancer action program— Protocol, Oct. 2003. Available at http://icscreen.med.cornell.edu/ielcap.pdf.

[10] J. H. Elder and S. W. Zucker. Local scale control for edge detection and blur estimation. *IEEE Trans. Pattern Anal. Machine Intell.*, 20(7):699–716, July 1998.

[11] A. A. Farag, A. El-Baz, G. G. Gimel'farb, R. Falk, and S. G. Hushek. Automatic detection and recognition of lung abnormalities in helical CT images using deformable templates. In C. Barllot, D. R. Haynor, and P. Hellier, editors, *Medical Image Computing and Computer-Assisted Intervention, Lecture Notes in Computer Science*, no. 3217, pp. 856–864, Saint-Malo, France, Sept. 2004. Springer-Verlag.

[12] A. A. Farag, A. El-Baz, G. G. Gimel'farb, M. A. El-Ghar, and T. Eldiasty. Quantitative nodule detection in low dose chest CT scans: New template modeling and evaluation for cad system design. In J. Duncan and G. Gerig, editors, *Medical Image Computing and Computer-Assisted Intervention, Lecture Notes in Computer Science*, no. 3749, pp. 720–728, Palm Springs, CA, Oct. 2005. Springer-Verlag.

[13] J. Ferlay, H. R. Shin, F. Bray, D. Forman, C. Mathers, and D. M. Parkin. GLOBOCAN 2008: Cancer incidence, mortality and prevalence worldwide. Technical report, IARC CancerBase No. 10, Lyon, France, 2010. Available at http://www-dep.iarc.fr/.

[14] B. J. Flehinger, M. Kimmel, and M. R. Melamed. The effect of surgical treatment on survival from early lung cancer: Implications for screening. *Chest*, 101(4):1013–1018, Apr. 1992.

[15] D. A. Forsyth. Shape from texture and integrability. *Proc. 8th Int. Conf. on Computer Vision*, vol. II, pp. 447–452, Vancouver, BC, Canada, July 2001.

[16] W. A. Fry, H. R. Menck, and D. P. Winchester. The national database report on lung cancer. *Cancer*, 77:1947–1955, 1996.

[17] G. Gerig, M. Styner, M. E. Shenton, and J. A. Lieberman. Shape versus size: Improved understanding of the morphology of brain structures. In *Medical Image Computing and Computer-Assisted Intervention, Lecture Notes in Computer Science*, no. 2208, pp. 24–32, Utrecht, the Netherlands, Oct. 2001. Available at citeseer.ist.psu.edu/gerig01shape.html.

[18] X. He, C. E. Metz, B. M. W. Tsui, J. M. Links, and E. C. Frey. Three-class ROC analysis—A decision theoretic approach under the ideal observer framework. *IEEE Trans. Med. Imaging*, 25(5):571–581, May 2006.

[19] L. Ibáñez, W. Schroeder, L. Ng, and J. Cates. *The ITK Software Guide*. Insight Consortium, Nov. 2005. Available at http://www.itk.org/ItkSoftwareGuide.pdf.

[20] E. T. Jaynes. *Probability Theory: The Logic of Science*. Cambridge University Press, Cambridge, 2003.

[21] H. Jeffreys. An invariant form for the prior probability in estimation problems. *Proc. R. Soc. London A*, 186(1007):453–461, Sept. 1946.

[22] K. L. Karau, G. S. Krenz, and C. A. Dawson. Branching exponent heterogeneity and wall shear stress distribution in vascular trees. *Am. J. Physiol.—Heart Circ. Physiol.*, 280(3):1256–1263, Mar. 2001.

[23] R. E. Kass and L. Wasserman. The selection of prior distributions by formal rules. *J. Am. Statist. Assoc.*, 91(435):1343–1370, Sept. 1996.

[24] R. T. Kass and A. E. Raftery. Bayes factors. *J. Am. Statist. Assoc.*, 90(430):773–795, Sept. 1995.

[25] R. A. Kaucic, C. C. McCulloch, P. R. S. Mendonça, D. J. Walter, R. S. Avila, and J. L. Mundy. Model-based detection of lung nodules in CT exams. In H. U. Lemke, M. W. Vannier, K. Inamura, A. G. Farman, K. Doi, and J. H. C. Reiber, editors, *Computer Assisted Radiology and Surgery, International Congress Series*, vol. 1256, pp. 990–997, London, June 2003. Elsevier.

[26] N. Krahnstoever. Personal communication, 2005.

[27] J. Martin, A. Pentland, S. Sclaroff, and R. Kikinis. Characterization of neuropathological shape deformations. *IEEE Trans. Pattern Anal. Machine Intell.*, 20(2):970–112, 1998. ISSN 0162-8828. doi: http://doi.ieeecomputersociety.org/10.1109/34.659928.

[28] N. Martini, M. S. Bains, M. E. Burt, M. F. Zakowski, P. McCormack, V. W. Rusch, and R. J. Ginsberg. Incidence of local recurrence and second primary tumors in resected stage I lung cancer. *J. Thorac. Cardiovasc. Surg.*, 109(1):120–129, Jan. 1995.

[29] C. C. McCulloch, D. Yankelevitz, C. Henschke, S. Patel, E. Kazerooni, and S. Sirohey. Reader variability and computer aided detection of suspicious lesions in low-dose CT lung screening exams. *Radiology*, 226(2):37A, 2003.

[30] C. C. McCulloch, R. A. Kaucic, P. R. S. Mendonça, D. J. Walter, and R. S. Avila. Model-based detection of lung nodules in computed tomography exams. *Acad. Radiol.*, 11(3):258–266, Mar. 2004.

[31] M. L. Mehta. *Random Matrices. Pure and Applied Mathematics*, no. 142 . Elsevier, San Diego, CA, 2004.

[32] P. R. S. Mendonça, R. Bhotika, S. Sirohey, W. D. Turner, J. V. Miller, and R. S. Avila. Model-based analysis of local shape for lesion detection in CT scans. In J. Duncan and G. Gerig, editors, *Medical Image Computing and Computer-Assisted Intervention, Lecture Notes in Computer Science*, no. 3749, pp. 688–695, Palm Springs, CA, Oct. 2005. Springer-Verlag.

[33] P. R. S. Mendonça, R. Bhotika, and J. V. Miller. Probability distribution of curvatures of isosurfaces in Gaussian random fields, May 2007. Available at http://arxiv.org/pdf/math-ph/0702031.

[34] J. L. Mulshine and R. A. Smith. Lung cancer 2: Screening and early diagnosis of lung cancer. *Thorax*, 57(12):1071–1078, Dec. 2002.

[35] C. D. Murray. The physiological principle of minimum work. I. The vascular system and the cost of blood flow. *Proc. Natl. Acad. Sci.*, 12(3):207–214, Mar. 1926.

[36] B. O'Neill. *Elementary Differential Geometry*. Academic Press, New York, 1966.

[37] W. Ow and P. Golland. From spatial regularization to anatomical priors in fMRI analysis. In G. E. Christensen and M. Sonka, editors, *Int. Conf. Information Proc. Med. Imaging, Lecture Notes in Computer Science*, no. 3565, pp. 88–100, Glenwood Springs, CO, July 2005.

[38] D. S. Paik, C. F. Beaulieu, G. D. Rubin, B. Acar, R. B. Jeffrey, Jr., J. Yee, J. Dey, and S. Napel. Surface normal overlap: A computer-aided detection algorithm with application to colonic polyps and lung nodules in helical CT. *IEEE Trans. Med. Imaging*, 23(6):661–675, June 2004.

[39] K. L. Piacsek. Personal communication, 2005.

[40] G. D. Rubin, J. K. Lyo, D. S. Paik, A. J. Sherbondy, L. C. Chow, A. N. Leung, R. Mindelzun, P. K. Schraedley-Desmond, S. E. Zinck, D. P. Naidich, and S. Napel. Pulmonary nodules on multi-detector row CT scans: Performance comparison of radiologists and computer-aided detection. *Radiology*, 234(1):274–283, 2005. doi: 10.1148/radiol.2341040589. Available at http://radiology.rsnajnls.org/cgi/content/abstrct/234/1/274.

[41] Y. Sato, C. Westin, A. Bhalerao, S. Nakajima, N. Shiraga, S. Tamura, and R. Kikinis. Tissue classification based on 3D local intensity structures for volume rendering. *IEEE Trans. Visual. Computer Graphics*, 6(2):160–180, June/April 2000.

[42] S. Singhal, R. Henderson, K. Horsfield, K. Harding, and G. Cumming. Morphometry of the human pulmonary arterial tree. *Circ. Res.*, 33(2):190–197, 1973. Available at http://circres.ahajournals.org/cgi/content/abstract/33/2/190.

[43] I. Sluimer, A. Schilham, M. Prokop, and B. van Ginneken. Computer analysis of computed tomography scans of the lung: A survey. *IEEE Trans. Med. Imaging*, 25(4):385–405, 2006. ISSN 0278-0062.

[44] S. J. Swensen, J. R. Jett, T. E. Hartman, D. E. Midthun, J. A. Sloan, A.-M. Sykes, G. L. Aughenbaugh, and M. A. Clemens. Lung cancer screening with CT: Mayo Clinic experience. *Radiology*, 226(3):756–761, Nov. 2003. doi: 10.1148/radiol.2263020036. Available at http://radiology.rsnajnls.org/cgi/content/abstract/226/3/756.

[45] P. H. S. Torr. Bayesian model estimation and selection for epipolar geometry and generic manifold fitting. *Int. J. Computer Vis.*, 50(1):35–61, Oct. 2002.

[46] B. van Ginneken, B. M. ter Haar Romeny, and M. A. Viegever. Computer-aided diagnosis in chest radiography: A survey. *IEEE Trans. Med. Imaging*, 20(12):1228–1241, 2001.

[47] F. M. Vos, I. W. O. Serlie, R. E. van Gelder, F. H. Post, R. Truyen, F. A. Gerritsen, J. Stoker, and A. M. Vossepoel. A new visualization method for virtual colonoscopy. In W. J. Niessen and M. A. Viergever, editors, *Medical Image Computing and Computer-Assisted Intervention, Lecture Notes in Computer Science*, no. 2208, pp. 645–654, Berlin, 2001. Springer-Verlag.

[48] M. A. Wesley and G. Markowsky. Fleshing out projections. *IBM J. Res. Dev.*, 25(6):934–954, Nov. 1981.

[49] H. Yoshida and J. Näppi. Three-dimensional computer-aided diagnosis scheme for detection of colonic polyps. *IEEE Trans. Med. Imaging*, 20(12):1261–1274, Dec. 2001.

[50] F. Zhao, P. R. S. Mendonça, R. Bhotika, and J. V. Miller. Model-based junction detection with applications to lung nodule detection. In *IEEE Int. Symposium on Biomedical Imaging: From Nano to Macro*, pp. 504–507, Arlington, VA, Apr. 2007.

12

Concept and Practice of Genetic Algorithm Template Matching and Higher Order Local Autocorrelation Schemes in Automated Detection of Lung Nodules

Yongbum Lee, Takeshi Hara, DuYih Tsai, and Hiroshi Fujita

CONTENTS

12.1 Introduction

According to the World Health Organization,[1] it is predicted that deaths from cancer will increase from 7.4 million globally in 2004 to 11.8 million in 2030. In particular, tracheal, bronchial, and lung cancers will emerge as the sixth leading cause of death by 2030, rising from its position as the eighth leading cause in 2004. Detection of suspicious lesions in the early stages of cancer is essential to bring down the mortality rate caused by lung cancer. Computer-aided diagnosis (CAD) can play a significant role in the early detection of suspicious lesions. Several CAD schemes for lung nodules in radiographs and computed tomography (CT) have been developed.[2,3] In this chapter, we introduce two CAD schemes for the detection of lung nodules. The first scheme is a template matching (TM) technique using a genetic algorithm (GATM),[4–8] which is presented in Section 12.2. The second scheme is a pattern recognition technique based on higher order local autocorrelation (HLAC) with multiple regression,[9–13] which is discussed in Section 12.3. Finally, the relative strengths of the two approaches are summarized in Section 12.4.

12.2 TM Using a Genetic Algorithm

12.2.1 TM

Matching is one of the most basic techniques in pattern recognition. Matching algorithms can suggest what an observed pattern is by comparing it to ideal patterns. Matching algorithms are roughly categorized into two groups: TM and structure matching. In TM, an object pattern is represented as an image, which is generally referred to as a *template image* or *reference image*, whereas structure matching examines the structure of the object pattern, specifically features extracted from the image, for matching. In this study, only TM is used, not structure matching. Figure 12.1 shows how TM works. In an input (observed) image $I(i, j)$ with $M_I \times N_I$ pixels, a template (reference) image $T(i, j)$ with $M_T \times N_T$ pixels moves in a search area. The maximum size of the search area is $(M_I - M_T + 1) \times (N_I - N_T + 1)$. Within the search area, the algorithm attempts to detect the position with the highest similarity, where $M_I \geq M_T$, $N_I \geq N_T$. The template image $T(i, j)$ is centered at an arbitrary location (x, y). The center of $T(i, j)$ visits every pixel in $I(i, j)$. Euclidean distance, city block distance, and cosine distance are used to estimate similarity as follows.

A cosine distance corresponds to the correlation coefficient:

$$R(x,y) = \frac{\sum_{i=0}^{M_T-1}\sum_{j=0}^{N_T-1}\left\{I_{(x,y)}(i,j)-\bar{I}\right\}\left\{T(i,j)-\bar{T}\right\}}{\sqrt{\sum_{i=0}^{M_T-1}\sum_{j=0}^{N_T-1}\left\{I_{(x,y)}(i,j)-\bar{I}\right\}^2}\sqrt{\sum_{i=0}^{M_T-1}\sum_{j=0}^{N_T-1}\left\{T(i,j)-\bar{T}\right\}^2}}, \tag{12.1}$$

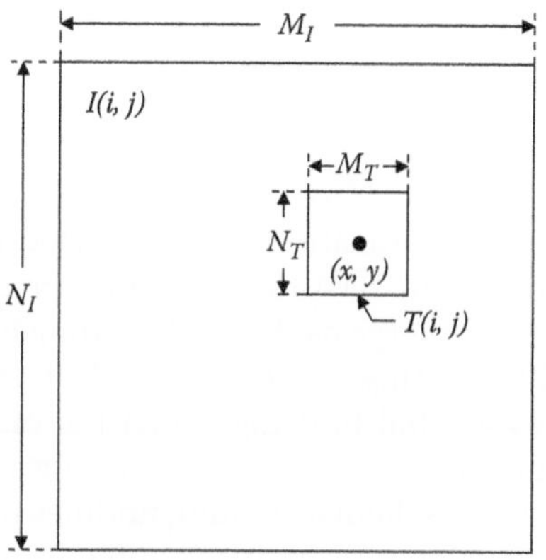

FIGURE 12.1
Schematic representation of the template matching scheme.

where

$$\bar{I} = \frac{1}{M_T N_T} \sum_{i=0}^{M_T-1} \sum_{j=0}^{N_T-1} I_{(x,y)}(i,j)$$
$$\bar{T} = \frac{1}{M_T N_T} \sum_{i=0}^{M_T-1} \sum_{j=0}^{N_T-1} T(i,j) \qquad (12.2)$$

Note that (x, y) represents an arbitrary location of a template image in the observed image, and $I_{(x, y)}(i, j)$ is a partial section image on the location (x, y) of the observed image. The size of a partial section image is equal to that of the template image. The correlation coefficient $R(x, y)$ is in the range $[-1, 1]$. A positive correlation is indicated when $0 < R(x, y) \le 1$, and a negative correlation is indicated when $-1 \le R(x, y) < 0$; when $R(x, y) = 0$, there is no correlation. The correlation coefficient is invariable under intensity transformation performed as a linear operation. This means that the correlation coefficient does not depend on the pixel values but only on the shape of the pixel-value distribution in the images. Therefore, TM using correlation is useful for matching two images that differ in contrast and brightness.

TM using city block distance or Euclidean distance for estimating similarity uses Equation 12.3 or 12.4 instead of Equation 12.1, as follows:

$$D_C(x,y) = \sum_{i=0}^{M_T-1} \sum_{j=0}^{N_T-1} \left| I_{(x,y)}(i,j) - T(i,j) \right| \qquad (12.3)$$

$$D_E(x,y) = \sqrt{\sum_{i=0}^{M_T-1} \sum_{j=0}^{N_T-1} \left\{ I_{(x,y)}(i,j) - T(i,j) \right\}^2}, \qquad (12.4)$$

where $D_C(x, y)$ and $D_E(x, y)$ are the city block distance and the Euclidean distance, respectively. These two approaches are both *minimum distance classifiers*. They both compute the distance between the template image and each part of the partial section image obtained at every pixel in the observed image. Then the smallest distance needed to detect the location with the highest similarity in the observed image is chosen. Note that these two distances are not invariable under intensity transformation performed as a linear operation. Therefore, minimum distance classifiers are sometimes not appropriate for matching two images that differ in contrast and brightness. However, minimum distance classifiers are often useful because they have a mechanism to end the computation process. This mechanism, called a sequential similarity detection algorithm (SSDA), was proposed by Barnea and Silverman[14] and is computed as follows.

Let $D_{m,n}(x, y)$ be a partial sum of the distance computed from $i = 0$ and $j = 0$ to $i = m$ and $j = n$. In SSDA, if $D_{m,n}(x, y)$ is over a certain threshold, then the computation stops and moves to the next (x, y) coordinate. The threshold value can be determined by using the minimum value found in previous sums.

12.2.2 Genetic Algorithms

A genetic algorithm (GA)[15] is a probabilistic search method based on evolutionary principles. GAs have been successfully applied to optimization problems such as wire

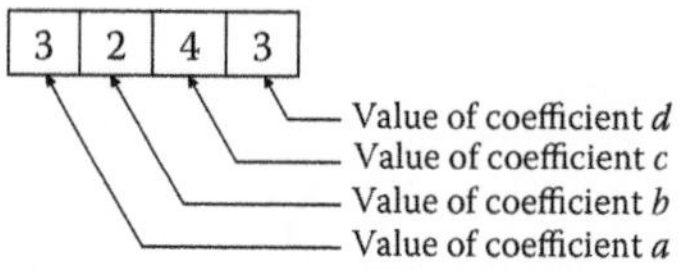

FIGURE 12.2
Chromosome composed of four genes that encode four coefficients representing a solution to the factorization problem.

routing, scheduling, adaptive control, and game playing.[16] In GA, each possible solution is regarded as an *individual*, and the set of all possible solutions is the *population*. Each individual is characterized by a *chromosome* which is composed of several numerical values that represent a single solution to the optimization problem. For example, if GA is used to solve for the factorization of the expression $12x^2 + 17x + 6$, and supposing that the solution of the factorization is of the form $(ax + b)(cx + d)$, then the four coefficients (a, b, c, d) correspond to the four *genes* that make up the chromosome (see Figure 12.2). Each individual also has information about its *fitness* with respect to the environment (see Figure 12.3). The fitness is evaluated against the solution of the original problem. The individuals repeatedly evolve by randomly manipulating their chromosomes using analogs to genetic processes including *crossover, mutation*, and *selection*. As a GA executes, the population of solutions evolves toward the optimum solution. One advantage of using a GA is that it is possible to rapidly search for an optimum solution in a wide search area because the solutions are treated as a population, which is searched in parallel while maintaining variety derived from the original solution candidates.

The general evolutionary flow for individuals in the genetic pool is described in the following steps:

Step 1. Begin with $g = 0$, where g is the number of generations considered so far.

Step 2. n individuals are generated in a genetic pool as the first generation. A genetic code for each individual is generated using random numbers. The state of the genetic pool is represented as *Pool(g)*.

Step 3. The chromosome for each individual is evaluated, i.e., the fitness is determined.

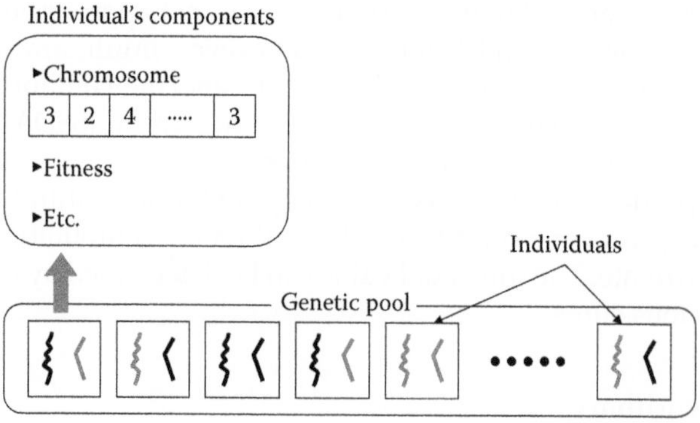

FIGURE 12.3
Individual's components and genetic pool.

Step 4. The remaining five steps are repeated until satisfying a termination condition, such as reaching a fixed number of generations.

Step 5. A parent population [*Parent(g)*] is selected from Pool(g).

Step 6. A child population [*Child(g)*] is generated from Parent(g).

Step 7. The fitness of the chromosome of each individual in Child(g) is calculated.

Step 8. The next generation [Parent(g+1)] is obtained by selecting from individuals in Parent(g) and Child(g).

Step 9. Increment $g = g + 1$; return to Step 4.

Steps 5–8 correspond to an evolutionary process for changing the population over generations. There are various methods available for evolutionary processes in GAs. One popular method is the *elite selection strategy* where selected individuals with higher fitness survive as a part of the next generation (see Figure 12.4). For instance, suppose the generation gap is defined as the ratio of survivors to deaths and represented by the variable G ($0 \leq G \leq 1$), and n is the number of individuals in the genetic pool. Then, $n(1 - G)$ individuals in the present generation would be selected and survive without genetic manipulation, and nG individuals for the next generation would be generated by genetic manipulation such as crossover and mutation. The elite selection strategy is generally superior in searching for an optimum solution. Other popular and well-studied selection methods include rank selection, roulette wheel selection, and tournament selection.

Genetic manipulation plays an important role in the evolutionary process, and it is often referred to as the *GA operator*. The GA operator is composed of selection, crossover, and mutation. Selection is used to eliminate or maintain individuals, as described in the elite selection strategy. The role of crossover is to preserve some genetic characteristics of parents in their children. Crossover is executed by exchanging a part of the chromosome of two parent individuals. There are many crossover techniques, e.g., one-point crossover (see Figure 12.5), two-point crossover (see Figure 12.6), uniform crossover (see Figure 12.7),

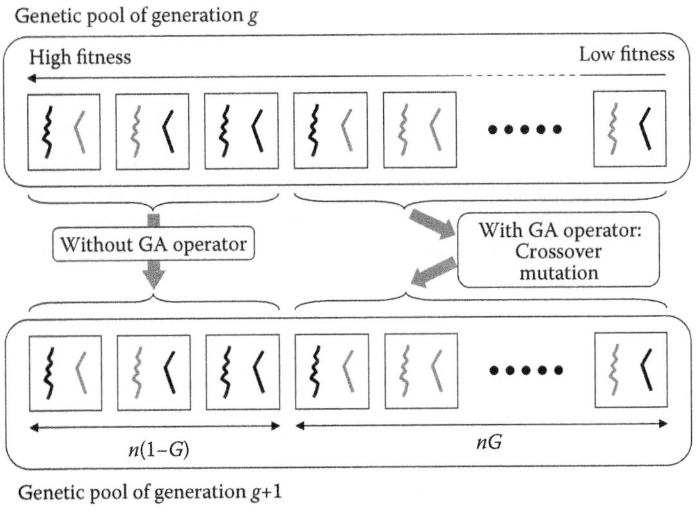

FIGURE 12.4
Elite selection strategy.

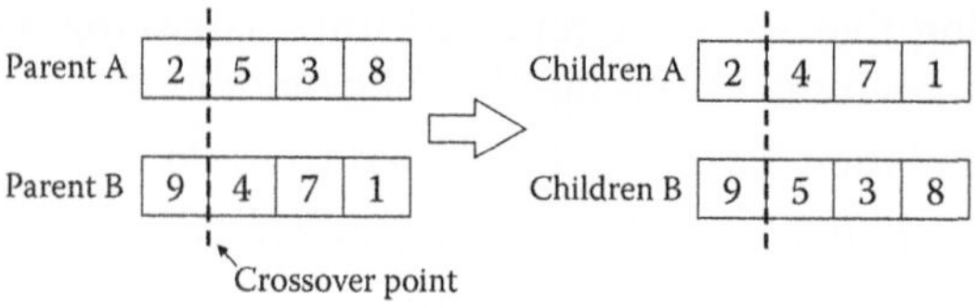

FIGURE 12.5
One-point crossover.

and so on. In one-point crossover, a single crossover point on both parents' chromosomes is selected. All data beyond that point in either chromosome are swapped between the two parent individuals. The resulting individuals are the children having the swapped chromosomes. In two-point crossover, two crossover points are selected on the parent chromosomes. Everything between the two points is swapped between the parent chromosomes. As a result, two children having swapped chromosomes are generated. The crossover point is determined randomly in any crossover. In uniform crossover, a template whose length is the same as that of the chromosome is used to indicate crossover points. The template consists of a binary number set, either 0 or 1. The binary number expresses the probability of a swap on a corresponding bit in the chromosome. Therefore, if the value of a bit in the template is 1, the corresponding bit in the chromosomes is swapped. The average of the probability in the template is typically 0.5.

Mutation is a genetic operator used to maintain genetic diversity from one generation to the next. Using a moderate probability, an arbitrary bit in a chromosome will be changed from its original state (see Figure 12.8). A common method of implementing mutation involves generating a random variable for each bit in a chromosome. Each random variable determines whether a particular bit will be modified.

12.2.3 GATM

12.2.3.1 Structure of GATM

The time needed to perform TM depends on the width of the search space and the variety in the templates. Using GA can result in a more efficient search than conventional TM. TM based on GAs is referred to as GATM.[4–8] The concept of GATM was originally proposed by Hara and Fujita[4] in 1995. Figure 12.9 shows a diagram of GATM. In GATM, supposing there are multiple templates, the GA controls the searching point (x, y) and template selection is represented by the variable s. Figure 12.10 shows the chromosome of an individual in GATM. The chromosome consists of three genes corresponding to x, y, and s. Although the

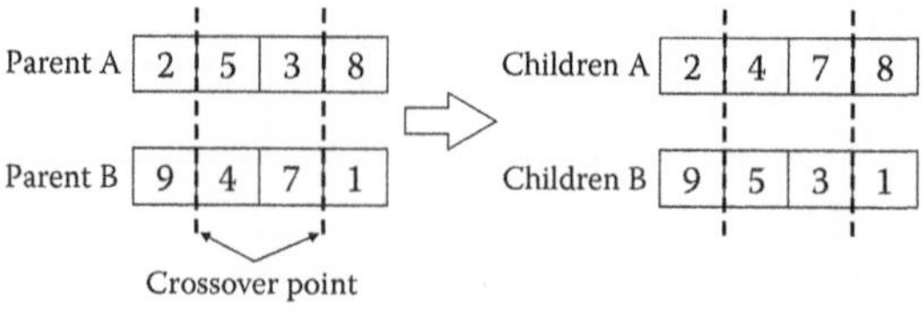

FIGURE 12.6
Two-point crossover.

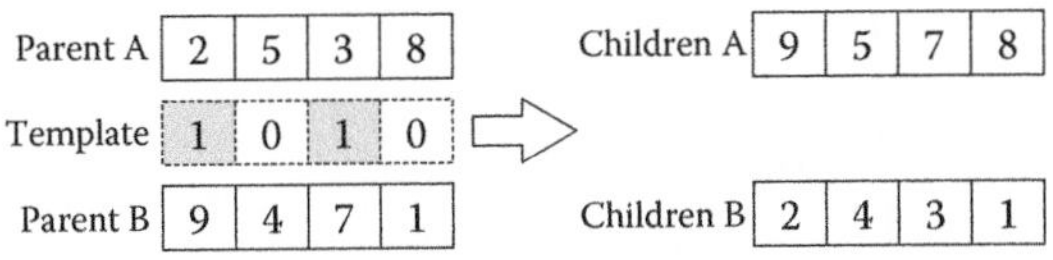

FIGURE 12.7
Uniform crossover.

gene can be coded by decimal or binary numbers, GATM generally uses binary coding. If the search space is three-dimensional (3D), the chromosome is extended to four genes with x, y, z, and s.

12.2.3.2 Setup of Simulation Studies Investigating GATM

We have previously studied the efficacy of GATM using three simulation studies[7] where GATM was used to detect artificial objects. In this section, we review the results of those simulation studies. In the simulation studies, templates corresponding to the artificial objects were placed in the search space. To simulate pulmonary nodule detection in low-dose CT images, the artificial objects were generated to resemble nodule-like objects with a Gaussian distribution (see Figure 12.11) prescribed by

$$T(x,y,z) = m \cdot e^{-(x^2+y^2+z^2)/n}, \tag{12.5}$$

where m and n are parameters representing the maximum value and the variance of the distribution.

The first search space was completely uniform, the second search space was prepared using simulated CT images, and the third search space was prepared using real CT images (see Figure 12.12). Simulated CT values of the uniform space were $-1000 + \alpha$, where the range of α was $-20 < \alpha < 20$. The simulated CT images include simulated fatty and pulmonary regions. Simulated CT values of the fatty region were 0, and simulated pulmonary regions had random CT values from -1000 to -400. The real CT images were obtained by low-dose screening CT scans.

Figure 12.13 shows a flowchart for the GA used in the simulations. Chromosomes of individuals in the initial population were generated by random. The chromosome consisted of four genes corresponding to x, y, z, and s, which were represented with 9-, 9-, 5-, and 2-bit sets, respectively. The fitness for each individual was calculated using the

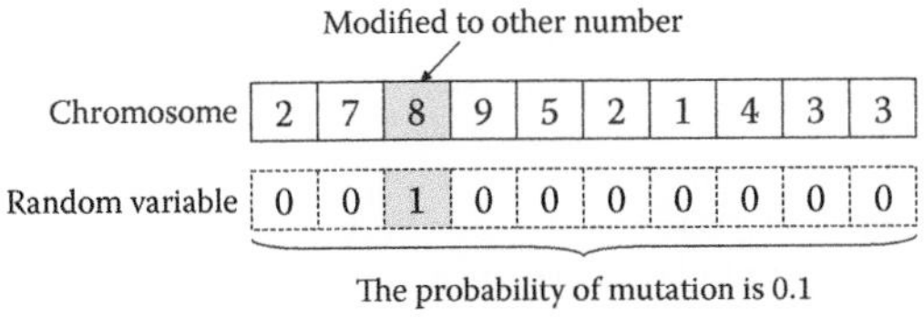

FIGURE 12.8
Mutation probability.

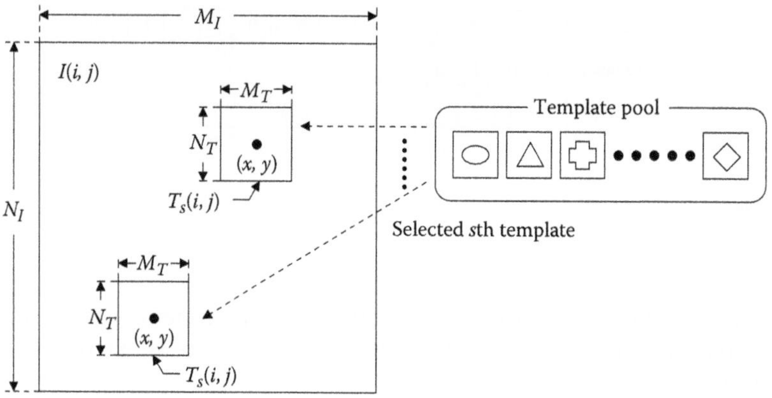

FIGURE 12.9
Schematic representation of GATM (variables x, y, and s are determined in parallel by a genetic algorithm).

correlation coefficient (Equation 12.1) corresponding to the similarity in TM. Then GA operators including selection, crossover, and mutation were applied to the population. The selection operator used the elite selection strategy, so that the lower half of the population in terms of fitness values were selected against and replaced by new individuals. The new individuals were one-point crossed over with the selected upper half of the existing generation. Mutation was executed as a bit inversion, and the probability of mutation was 10% for each bit in the chromosome. However, 10% of individuals having the highest fitness values in a generation avoided the mutation. The individual with the highest fitness in each generation was continuously carried over to the next generation regardless of any conditions. The population of one generation consisted of 300 individuals, and the maximum number of generations was 20000.

12.2.3.3 Results of the First Simulation Study Using GATM

The first simulation study was performed to investigate the potential effectiveness of GATM for search and detection of only one object. Therefore, the detection target in the first simulation was only one nodule-like object, as shown in Figure 12.11. Any one of T_1, T_2, T_3, and T_4 was randomly selected and used as a template corresponding to the detection target. The selected object was put at 14 locations (P_1–P_{14}) in the observed images O_1, O_2, and O_3, as shown in Figure 12.14. GATM was performed with 168 sets of four targets (T_1–T_4), three observed images (O_1–O_3), and 14 target locations (P_1–P_{14}).

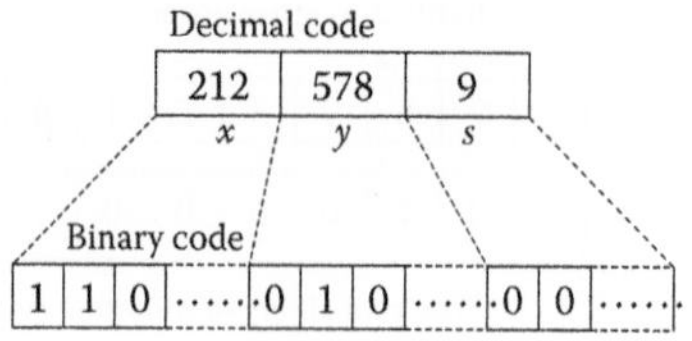

FIGURE 12.10
Decimal coded chromosome and corresponding binary coded chromosome in GATM.

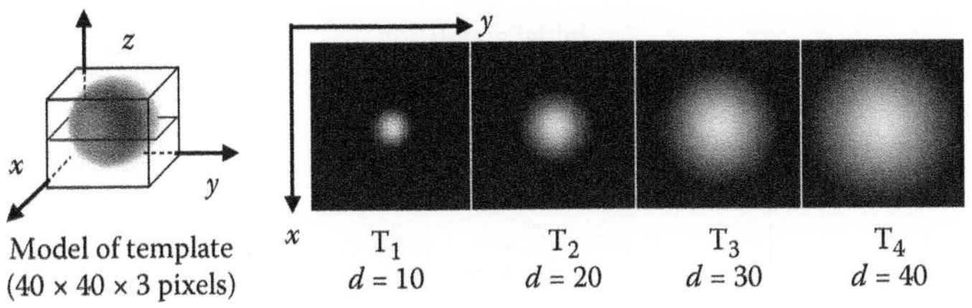

FIGURE 12.11
Templates and objects. T_1–T_4 are section images on the center of four templates. d is the diameter of the object in pixels.

In addition, to account for any dependence on the initial values given to GA, GATM was executed 30 times for each set using different random seeds to generate the initial population. If the fitness of any individual was more than 0.9, the individual was considered to be a solution, namely, the object's candidate, and then the GATM process was halted.

Tables 12.1–12.3 show the results of the first simulation. GATM was able to detect all the objects in 30 tests for observed images O_1 and O_2 (see Tables 12.1 and 12.2). The average numbers of generations generated before a successful detection for O_1 and O_2 were 230 and 675, respectively. The number of searches conducted until a successful detection was calculated by multiplying the number of generations by the number of individuals. For instance, the number of searches needed by GATM for O_2 was 657 × 300 = 197100. Note that this was just 2.5% of the entire search space (512 × 512 × 30). The detection rate in O_3 was 98.6%, not 100%, because small objects such as T_1 and T_2 were sometimes not detected (see Table 12.3). The reason for this is thought to be that the small template could detect other small objects rather than the target object. In other words, GATM has found a local maximum solution. This problem can be avoided by using a sharing technique as follows. When some individuals have gathered around a point, the point is recorded and kept as a solution candidate. Then the fitness of individuals that gathered around that point is shared and decreased. Therefore, by sharing, it is possible to obtain multiple solutions by decreasing (sharing) the fitness of a point where a sufficient number of individuals have gathered.

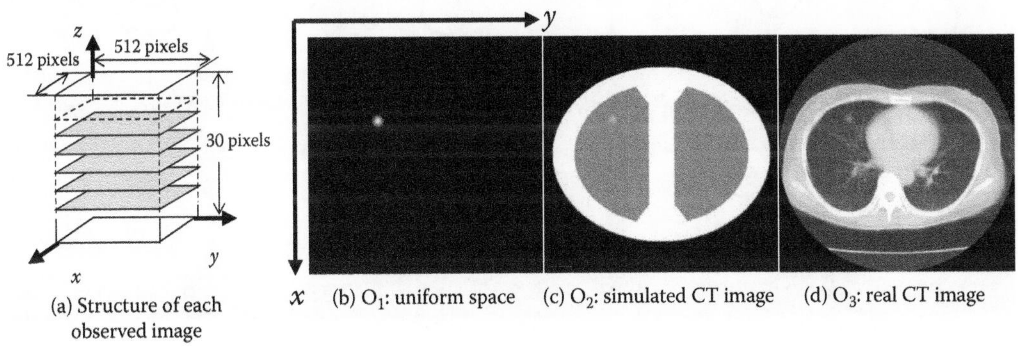

FIGURE 12.12
Three types of observed images used in the simulation studies. (b)–(d) Slice images of each observed image.

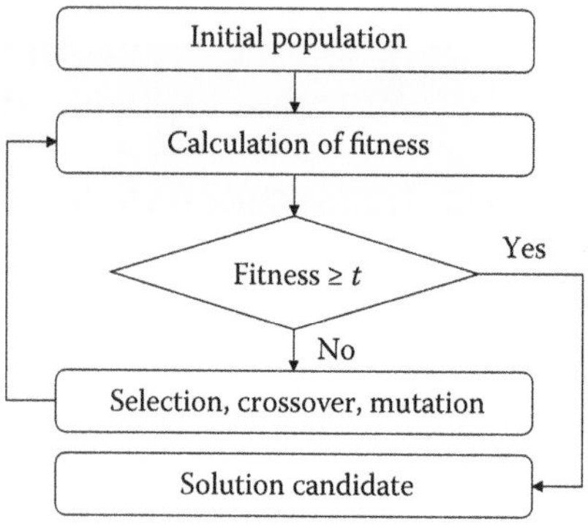

FIGURE 12.13
Flowchart of the GA process. t is a threshold with a range of $-1 \leq t \leq 1$.

GATM with sharing was applied to detect objects T_1 and T_2 in an observed image O_3. The results are shown in Table 12.4 and indicate that it was able to completely detect the object without falling into a local maximum. In this simulation, the number of searches until a successful detection of the object was 2062 (generations) × 300 (individuals) = 197100. Note that this was just 8% of the entire search space. From the first simulation, it was concluded that GATM can more rapidly detect an object as compared to conventional TM and is independent of the complexity of the observed images, target size, target location, and randomness of the initial population in GA.

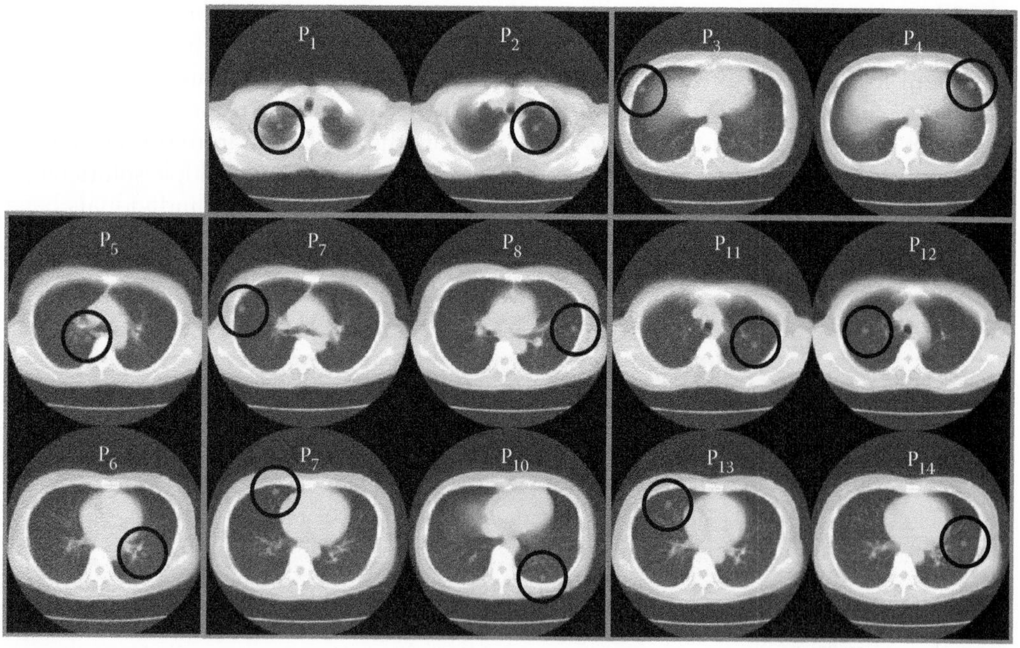

FIGURE 12.14
Fourteen locations of a simulated object T_3 embedded in chest CT images in the second simulation study. P_1, P_2: Apex pulmonis. P_3, P_4: Basis pulmonis. P_5, P_6: Around the mediastinum. P_7–P_{10}: Around the lung wall. P_{11}–P_{14}: Within the lung area.

TABLE 12.1

Results[a] of the First GATM Simulation of the Uniform Space O_1

	Apex Pulmonis		Basis Pulmonis		Around Mediastinum		Around Lung Wall				In Lung Area			
Size	P_1	P_2	P_3	P_4	P_5	P_6	P_7	P_8	P_9	P_{10}	P_{11}	P_{12}	P_{13}	P_{14}
T_1	100% (30/30)	100% (30/30)	100% (30/30)	100% (30/30)	100% (30/30)	100% (30/30)	100% (30/30)	100% (30/30)	100% (30/30)	100% (30/30)	100% (30/30)	100% (30/30)	100% (30/30)	100% (30/30)
	226	247	278	1076	387	153	557	450	869	272	380	392	95	174
T_2	100% (30/30)	100% (30/30)	100% (30/30)	100% (30/30)	100% (30/30)	100% (30/30)	100% (30/30)	100% (30/30)	100% (30/30)	100% (30/30)	100% (30/30)	100% (30/30)	100% (30/30)	100% (30/30)
	333	238	256	459	297	89	384	525	583	281	344	392	80	309
T_3	100% (30/30)	100% (30/30)	100% (30/30)	100% (30/30)	100% (30/30)	100% (30/30)	100% (30/30)	100% (30/30)	100% (30/30)	100% (30/30)	100% (30/30)	100% (30/30)	100% (30/30)	100% (30/30)
	95	115	112	133	93	80	165	161	185	121	108	102	52	80
T_4	100% (30/30)	100% (30/30)	100% (30/30)	100% (30/30)	100% (30/30)	100% (30/30)	100% (30/30)	100% (30/30)	100% (30/30)	100% (30/30)	100% (30/30)	100% (30/30)	100% (30/30)	100% (30/30)
	69	69	78	132	67	61	112	140	102	68	91	72	39	57

[a] Upper sections indicate the detection rates. Lower sections indicate the average generations produced before a successful detection.

TABLE 12.2

Results[a] of the First GATM Simulation of the Artificial CT Images O_2

	Apex Pulmonis		Basis Pulmonis		Around Mediastinum		Around Lung Wall			In Lung Area				
Size	P_1	P_2	P_3	P_4	P_5	P_6	P_7	P_8	P_9	P_{10}	P_{11}	P_{12}	P_{13}	P_{14}
T_1	100% (30/30)	100% (30/30)	100% (30/30)	100% (30/30)	100% (30/30)	100% (30/30)	100% (30/30)	100% (30/30)	100% (30/30)	100% (30/30)	100% (30/30)	100% (30/30)	100% (30/30)	100% (30/30)
	1517	841	2309	1104	661	242	1675	1655	783	635	970	737	139	426
T_2	100% (30/30)	100% (30/30)	100% (30/30)	100% (30/30)	100% (30/30)	100% (30/30)	100% (30/30)	100% (30/30)	100% (30/30)	100% (30/30)	100% (30/30)	100% (30/30)	100% (30/30)	100% (30/30)
	314	174	3361	1007	536	135	908	720	519	400	674	357	139	425
T_3	100% (30/30)	100% (30/30)	100% (30/30)	100% (30/30)	100% (30/30)	100% (30/30)	100% (30/30)	100% (30/30)	100% (30/30)	100% (30/30)	100% (30/30)	100% (30/30)	100% (30/30)	100% (30/30)
	643	799	1261	515	652	237	1194	1147	751	511	1349	616	179	556
T_4	100% (30/30)	100% (30/30)	100% (30/30)	100% (30/30)	100% (30/30)	100% (30/30)	100% (30/30)	100% (30/30)	100% (30/30)	100% (30/30)	100% (30/30)	100% (30/30)	100% (30/30)	100% (30/30)
	298	272	823	299	260	84	267	300	313	152	453	289	82	144

[a] Upper sections indicate the detection rates. Lower sections indicate average generations produced before a successful detection.

TABLE 12.3

Results[a] of the First GATM Simulation for the Helical CT Images O_3

	Apex Pulmonis		Basis Pulmonis		Around Mediastinum		Around Lung Wall				In Lung Area			
Size	P_1	P_2	P_3	P_4	P_5	P_6	P_7	P_8	P_9	P_{10}	P_{11}	P_{12}	P_{13}	P_{14}
T_1	57% (17/30)	93% (28/30)	100% (30/30)	97% (29/30)	100% (30/30)	100% (30/30)	97% (29/30)	100% (30/30)	100% (30/30)	97% (29/30)	97% (29/30)	100% (30/30)	100% (30/30)	100% (30/30)
	3205	3155	2889	1965	2203	586	1824	2993	2561	4032	4170	3560	352	2159
T_2	100% (30/30)	100% (30/30)	100% (30/30)	100% (30/30)	97% (29/30)	100% (30/30)	100% (30/30)	100% (30/30)	100% (30/30)	97% (29/30)	97% (29/30)	97% (29/30)	100% (30/30)	100% (30/30)
	5754	3556	1110	1143	3635	822	1279	1805	1152	2630	3981	3902	205	2686
T_3	100% (30/30)	100% (30/30)	100% (30/30)	100% (30/30)	100% (30/30)	100% (30/30)	100% (30/30)	100% (30/30)	100% (30/30)	100% (30/30)	100% (30/30)	100% (30/30)	100% (30/30)	100% (30/30)
	1901	872	2946	2486	1210	375	1252	608	1048	1487	612	681	137	762
T_4	100% (30/30)	100% (30/30)	100% (30/30)	100% (30/30)	100% (30/30)	100% (30/30)	100% (30/30)	100% (30/30)	100% (30/30)	100% (30/30)	100% (30/30)	100% (30/30)	100% (30/30)	100% (30/30)
	3162	1004	827	1111	968	510	545	463	293	1209	1251	560	55	464

[a] Upper sections indicate the detection rates. Lower sections indicate average generations produced before a successful detection.

TABLE 12.4

Results of GATM with Sharing for the Observed Image O_3

Size	Apex Pulmonis		Basis Pulmonis		Around the Mediastinum		Around the Lung Wall				In the Lung Area			
	P_1	P_2	P_3	P_4	P_5	P_6	P_7	P_8	P_9	P_{10}	P_{11}	P_{12}	P_{13}	P_{14}
T_1	100%	100%	100%	100%	100%	100%	100%	100%	100%	100%	100%	100%	100%	100%
	(30/30)	(30/30)	(30/30)	(30/30)	(30/30)	(30/30)	(30/30)	(30/30)	(30/30)	(30/30)	(30/30)	(30/30)	(30/30)	(30/30)
	4490	2061	1260	1268	1571	2263	1638	1580	1557	3790	2378	2292	1133	1239
T_2	100%	100%	100%	100%	100%	100%	100%	100%	100%	100%	100%	100%	100%	100%
	(30/30)	(30/30)	(30/30)	(30/30)	(30/30)	(30/30)	(30/30)	(30/30)	(30/30)	(30/30)	(30/30)	(30/30)	(30/30)	(30/30)
	4524	3541	826	1297	2644	1702	1535	740	3234	2114	2701	1584	1467	1293

12.2.3.4 Results of the Second Simulation Study Using GATM

In the second simulation study, pulmonary nodule detection in helical CT images was examined. In this simulation, the true positive fraction and the number of false positives were determined. The detection targets were eight simulated nodules, which were each sets of two of T_1, T_2, T_3, and T_4. The eight targets were embedded in helical CT images. The embedded locations were the hilus pulmonis (Q_1, Q_2), basis pulmonis (Q_3, Q_4), around the mediastinum (Q_5), around the lung wall (Q_6), and within the lung area (Q_7, Q_8), similar to Figure 12.14. Twenty cases of chest helical CT images were used as the observed images. In each case, a set of embedded locations and target sizes was determined at random. T_1, T_2, T_3, and T_4 were used as templates. Therefore, a gene composed of two bits has been added to the chromosome to select a template for the GA.

The true positive fraction and the number of false positives were estimated under a condition of $Th \leq$ fitness. *Th* is a threshold. GATM detected locations where individuals with a fitness of more than *Th* gathered as target candidates. In addition, the performances of conventional TM, GATM, and GATM with sharing were compared. The population of one generation consisted of 300 individuals, and the maximum number of generations was 15000. Table 12.5 shows the results of the second simulation study. When $Th = 0.6$, GATM with sharing was able to detect all targets in all observed images, although with 79.4 false positives per case. This performance is almost the same as that required in conventional TM; however, the number of searches needed was drastically less than that of conventional TM. The number of searches needed in the conventional TM can be calculated by multiplying the size of search space by the number of templates, namely, $512 \times 512 \times 30 \times 4$, whereas the number of searches needed by GATM was 300 (individuals) × 15000 (maximum number of generations), which is just 14% of the number of searches needed by the conventional TM. These results show that GATM with sharing is superior to GATM without sharing, and suggest that sharing is effective for detecting multiple targets.

TABLE 12.5

Results[a] of the Second Simulation Study

Condition for Detection	Conventional TM		GATM without Sharing		GATM with Sharing	
	TP Rate	FPs per Case	TP Rate	FPs per Case	TP Rate	FPs per Case
$Th = 0.3$	1.0 (160/160)	3760.1 (75201/20)	0.99 (159/160)	2653.9 (53077/20)	1.0 (160/160)	337.1 (6742/20)
$Th = 0.4$	1.0 (160/160)	1638.6 (32752/20)	0.99 (158/160)	1015.3 (20306/20)	1.0 (160/160)	333.6 (6672/20)
$Th = 0.5$	1.0 (160/160)	486.1 (9722/20)	0.99 (159/160)	249.0 (4979/20)	1.0 (160/160)	266.5 (5330/20)
$Th = 0.6$	1.0 (160/160)	99.1 (1981/20)	0.96 (153/160)	40.0 (800/20)	1.0 (160/160)	79.4 (1588/20)
$Th = 0.7$	1.0 (160/160)	10.0 (199/20)	0.89 (142/160)	2.7 (84/20)	0.96 (153/160)	8.6 (171/20)
$Th = 0.8$	1.0 (160/160)	0.6 (12/20)	0.79 (126/160)	0.2 (3/20)	0.89 (143/160)	0.5 (10/20)
$Th = 0.9$	1.0 (160/160)	0 (0/20)	0.53 (85/160)	0 (0/20)	0.84 (134/160)	0 (0/20)
$Th = 1.0$	1.0 (160/160)	0 (0/20)	0.24 (38/160)	0 (0/20)	0.73 (116/160)	0 (0/20)

[a] The condition for detection was $Th \leq$ fitness (for both GATM and conventional TM).

TABLE 12.6

Comparison of GATM and RDTM Results from the Third Simulation Study

Process Result	Detection Rate	Average of Number of Searches
RDTM	77% (23/30)	300 × 6632
GATM	100% (30/30)	300 × 95

12.2.3.5 Results of the Third Simulation Study Using GATM

The purpose of the third simulation study is to investigate GATM with random TM (RDTM), which corresponds to a random search. The probability of mutation in GATM in the previous two simulations was 10%. This probability was already high and may have led to a nearly random search because the probability of a mutation occurring for an individual with a 25-bit chromosome was $1 - (0.9)^{25} \approx 0.93$. Therefore, the third simulation was performed to compare GATM with RDTM. Both GATM and RDTM were repeated 30 times using different random seeds. In GATM, the number of individuals was 300 and the maximum number of generations was 20000. Corresponding to GATM, in RDTM, 300 locations were searched simultaneously, and the maximum number of searches was 20000. The location where the fitness or similarity was more than 0.9 was regarded as the detected target region, and then the search was halted. O_1 and T_1 were used as the observed image and the target object corresponding to the template, respectively.

Table 12.6 shows a comparison of the results obtained using RDTM and GATM. GATM had a 100% detection rate, whereas RDTM missed 7 out of 30 times. In addition, the number of searches required by RDTM was larger than that for GATM. Figure 12.15 shows a graphical comparison of the performance of GATM and RDTM. The results clearly indicated that GATM had detected the target after a low number of iterations. In contrast, theoretically, to detect the target perfectly using RDTM, the number of search iterations needed would be similar to the size of search space. Recall that the probability of mutation in the GATM was high. However, 10% of individuals having the highest fitness values in a generation avoided the mutation. This helps to explain the superiority of GATM performance as compared with RDTM.

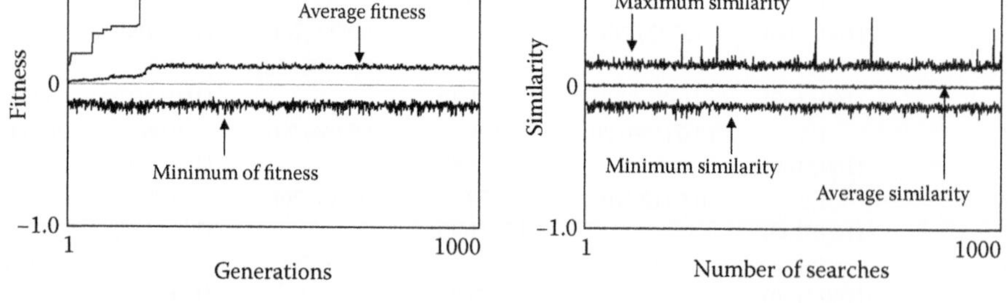

FIGURE 12.15
Comparison of search performance. (a) Relationship between the fitness number of generations for GATM. (b) Relationship between similarity and number searches for RDTM.

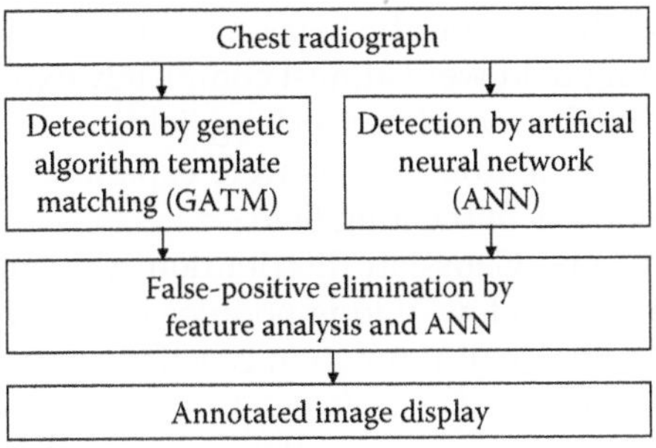

FIGURE 12.16
Overview of a CAD scheme using GATM and ANN for chest radiograms.

12.2.4 Nodule Detection by GATM in Chest Radiographs

Conventional chest radiograms have been employed as a mass screening method for lung cancer for decades; however, small lesions appearing during the first stage of cancer can cast very subtle shadows that radiologists might miss. Many computer analysis schemes for chest radiographs have been developed.[3] In this section, we review the results obtained from a CAD scheme that we developed[5] using GATM for chest radiographs. An overview of the scheme is shown in Figure 12.16. The scheme consists of two different parts: detection and false-positive elimination processing.

Many lesion candidates were indicated by two detection processes. First, a GATM was used, and second, an artificial neural network (ANN) technique was used, so as not to miss any true positives. However, some of the candidates identified likely resulted from normal shadows and were therefore false-positive findings.

Four image databases were employed to develop the CAD scheme. Table 12.7 shows the number of images in each database. Images in Group A were collected in a prefectural mass survey in Japan and included relatively easy cases with large nodules. Group B is a standard database[17,18] published by the Japanese Society of Radiological Technology. This database is excellent for evaluating CAD performance because the ease of detection for each case has already been classified into five categories and verified by receiver operating characteristic studies. Groups C and D were mass survey cases that were collected in a hospital in Japan. All the films were digitized at 0.1 or 0.175 mm with 10- or 12-bit density resolution. All of the digitized images were converted to 1024×1024 pixels with 10-bit density resolution.

The lung field was extracted to limit the region to be processed. Thresholding techniques for gray scale images were applied to extract the rough region at first. The threshold value

TABLE 12.7
Number of Chest Radiographs in Each Database

Database	No. of Normal	No. of Abnormal	Total
A	10	33	43
B	93	84	177
C	59	28	87
D	0	25	25

was determined in terms of the area of a histogram for the original images. Larger regions that corresponded to the lung field were almost completely extracted in this step. Second, smaller regions that could not be considered as lung fields were eliminated in terms of the region size. Finally, the extracted lung regions were expanded because the extracted area could not always include borders of the lung field.

In GATM, a two-dimensional Gaussian distribution was employed to generate some reference patterns because the shadow of lung nodules in radiography generally follows a distribution. The size and angle are unknown in practice, so various patterns of Gaussian distribution were generated to use as templates. A GA was employed to select a suitable template image from the various reference patterns and to show the best position in the original chest image. The individuals in GA had chromosomes represented by a binary digit system and the chromosomes were used to determine the pattern and the position of shadows by calculating the fitness of the individuals. The fitness was defined as the difference between a reference image and an observed image. Genetic operations including crossover and mutation were applied to all individuals to create new individuals in the next generation.

Figure 12.17 shows an overview of the nodule detection step based on GATM for chest radiographs. A total of 512 reference images with various sizes and angles of Gaussian distributions were prepared as shown in the left half of Figure 12.17. The chromosomes determined the positions x and y of the partial image as shown in the right half of Figure 12.17. The similarity was defined as a five-dimensional function with those parameters. The chromosomes had 42 bits that represent the recognized positions of x (10 bits: 0–1023) and y (10 bits: 0–1023), horizontal and vertical size categories of H (8 bits: #1–#8) and V (8 bits: #1–#8), respectively, and the category of the angle of reference images A (8 bits: #1–#8). The population size and generation were 120 and 200. The probability of mutation was decreased according to the generation advance, in the range of 0.25–0.01. The mutation was set up by inverting all bits at the prescribed probability. Then ranking selection and one-point crossover were employed in the GA.

The ANN-based detection method involved a feed-forward ANN with three layers. The regulated pixel values in terms of the minimum and maximum values in a partial image were entered into the ANN. The matrix size of the input image was 32 × 32 and gray scale

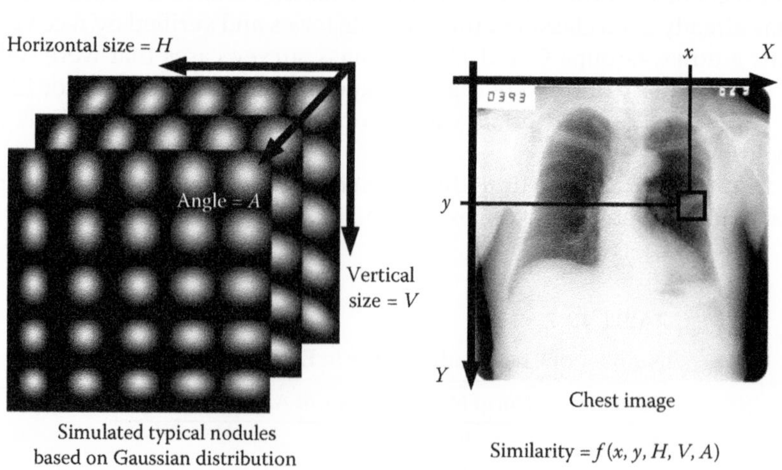

FIGURE 12.17
Overview of the nodule detection procedure based on GATM for chest radiographs.

values were converted to 0–1.0. To train ANN using the back-propagation method, 100 diagnosed shadows of 50 nodular and 50 obviously normal images were selected. In all, 2000 iterations were performed and the training error was 0.0001. By scanning the mask of 32 × 32 pixels with eight steps, the output value of the ANN was recorded, and the positions of candidates that satisfied certain conditions were retained as the detection region for nodular shadows.

Candidates that were overdetected are deemed as false positives. The images were previously analyzed and it was found that the false-positive candidates could be classified into three categories: shadows of lung margins, shadows of bones, and shadows of vessels and other features. An algorithm was developed to selectively eliminate such false-positive candidates. In the algorithm, the first classification step was based on a histogram analysis within the candidates. The candidates that include many regions outside the expanded lung field were eliminated because they appeared as low-pixel areas in the histogram. The second classification step was based on a histogram analysis of the vector images within the candidates. The *kurtosis*, which is a value indicating the sharpness of the histogram, was extracted. The final classification step was based on an analysis of entropy and the ratio of partial images inside the candidates.

In addition, another ANN was reused to eliminate false-positive candidates. The process was very similar to the ANN-based detection step. To train ANN to eliminate false-positive candidates, 100 diagnosed shadows of 50 nodular and 50 normal images were selected. The number of iterations and training error were the same as the values obtained for the detection step. The numbers of nodes of the input layer, hidden layer, and output layer were 32 × 32, 32 × 32, and 1, respectively. Normalized pixel values within partial images were calculated and entered into the ANN.

Table 12.8 shows performance metrics for each of the four image databases. The average sensitivity and the average number of false positives were 73% and about 11 per image, respectively. These values indicate that the number of false positives needs to be reduced for practical use of CAD. Figure 12.18 shows two sample images with nodules indicated by circles. The nodule candidates identified by the CAD algorithm are indicated by check marks. There were some false positives and a missed nodule, but four small nodule shadows were detected correctly.

Table 12.9 shows sensitivities by the degree of difficulty for nodule detection in databases A and B. The results in this table indicated that the CAD scheme can detect nodules that are known to be difficult to detect.

12.2.5 Nodule Detection by GATM in Thoracic CT Images

Chest CT plays an important role in not only confirming the existence of nodules but also discriminating. Many computer analysis schemes for chest CT images have been developed.[2]

TABLE 12.8

Performance Metrics for Each Radiograph Database

Database	TP	No. of FPs/img
A	75.6% (34/45)	6.3 (273/43)
B	67.8% (57/84)	15.0 (2659/177)
C	76.8% (23/30)	6.8 (589/87)
D	80.0% (20/25)	11.2 (278/25)
Total	72.8% (134/184)	11.3 (3799/334)

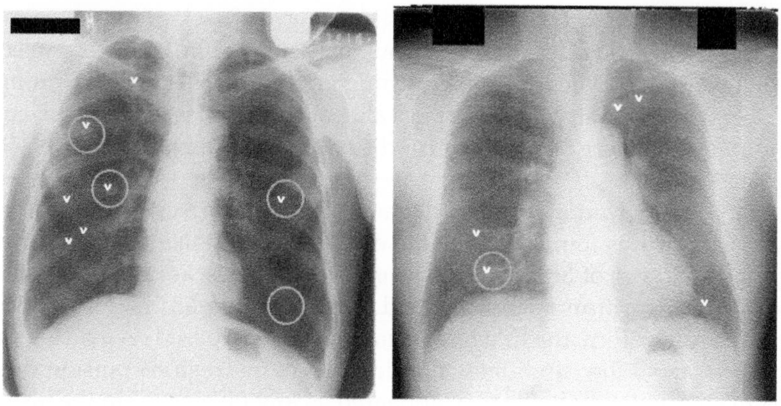

FIGURE 12.18
Two sample chest images showing superimposed computer detections (check marks) and radiologist's detections (circles).

In this section, we review the results of a CAD scheme we previously introduced[6,8] using GATM for analyzing chest CT images. A flowchart of the scheme is shown in Figure 12.19. GATM was employed to detect nodules within the lung area, whereas a conventional TM technique along the lung wall [lung wall TM (LWTM)] was also employed to detect nodules on the lung wall. Many false positives were detected by both template-matching methods, so it was necessary to eliminate them through feature analysis.

GATM was used to effectively search for the location of spherical nodules that were scattered within the lung areas. In this method, a GA was used to determine the target position in an observed image and to select an adequate template image from reference images for TM. Four artificial simulated nodules were generated using Equation 12.5. The simulated nodules were spherical models with a Gaussian distribution and consisted of three continuous slices (as shown in Figure 12.11). The diameters of the models were 10, 20, 30, and 40 pixels (where 1 pixel = 0.68 mm), respectively. The size of the reference image containing a model was 40 × 40 × 3 pixels. Using these four models, it was expected that nodules with diameters in the range 5–30 mm could be detected. Since the screening CT images are generally reconstructed with a 10-mm interval, it is difficult to extract nodules smaller than those with spherical models. In order to detect these nodules, circular models consisting of only the middle slice were introduced. Therefore, the GATM was performed twice: once using the spherical models and once using circular models as the reference image.

In the GATM, each individual had a chromosome with data not only for determining a location within the 3D space of the chest helical CT images but also for selecting an adequate reference image. Each chromosome had 25 bits, of which 23 determined the target

TABLE 12.9
Sensitivities by Degree of Difficulty for Nodule Detection

Database	Extremely Subtle	Very Subtle	Subtle	Relatively Obvious	Obvious
A	0/0	3/3	1/2	3/3	1/2
B	3/6	4/12	19/31	25/28	6/7

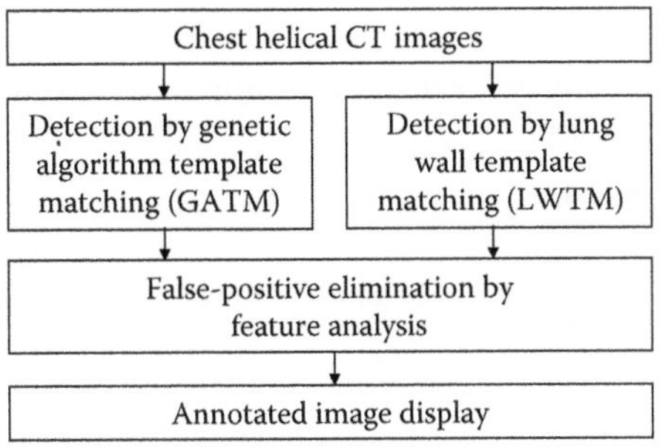

FIGURE 12.19
Flowchart for detecting lung nodules in chest CT images using GATM and other techniques.

position and two selected the reference image. Furthermore, the 23 position bits were divided into 9-, 9-, and 5-bit sets corresponding to the coordinates (x, y, z). Therefore, the GATM extracted a region from the observed image that had the same size as the reference image and whose center the chromosome determined.

The fitness of the individual was defined as the similarity calculated by the cross-correlation coefficient as shown in Equation 12.1. The GA process in this case was almost the same as shown in Figure 12.13 except that sharing was used. First, the initial population was randomly generated from a sequence of zeros and ones. Next, the fitness of each individual was calculated. Third, sharing was applied. As previously described in Section 12.2.3, sharing is a method that makes it possible to obtain multiple solutions by decreasing the fitness of a point after a sufficient number of individuals have gathered around it. It is an effective method for executing the GA in parallel as well as for detecting objects with different sizes or shapes.

Fourth, all individuals were subjected to genetic operations such as selection, (one-point) crossover, and mutation. The individual population was sorted by fitness value. The half that had lower fitness values were selected against and replaced by new individuals that had been crossed over with the half having higher fitness values. Mutation was executed as a bit inversion. The probability of mutation was 10% for each bit in the chromosome. The ten individuals having the highest fitness values in each generation avoided the mutation. The individual with the highest fitness in each generation was continuously carried over to the next generation regardless of any conditions. The processes of fitness calculation, sharing, and genetic operations constitute one generation.

The initial population consisted of 124 individuals, and the maximum number of generations was 200. After the individuals having a fitness $> f$ in each generation were extracted, the coordinates of these chromosomes were regarded as points constituting a nodule candidate. Here, f is a constant with a range of −1 to 1. This constant corresponds to whether the spherical or circular models were used as reference images.

It is possible to detect nodules on the lung wall by GATM if semicircular models are used as reference images. However, the conventional TM method was more efficient than GATM when the search was limited to the lining of the lung wall, i.e., LWTM. Each slice of the chest CT scan was used as an observed image, and semicircular models with Gaussian distribution were used as reference images. Many nodules on the lung wall appeared as an oval divided along the minor axis, in other words, semicircular as discussed above. Many of the nodules on the lung wall were small in size. Hence, two semicircular nodular

TABLE 12.10

Detection Rate in Terms of Method and Size (Successfully Detected/Total Count) and the Number of False Positives (Ratio of FPs/Case)

	True Positives				False Positives per Case	
Nodule Diameter	<10 mm	10–20 mm	>20 mm	Total	Before FP Elimination	After FP Eliminations
GATM	35/51	13/16	6/7	54/74	161.2 (3223/20)	2.9 (58/20)
LWTM	10/15	6/7	1/2	17/24	96.5 (1930/20)	2.6 (51/20)
Total	45/66	19/23	7/9	71/98	257.7 (5153/20)	5.5 (109/20)

models with Gaussian distribution were generated from a circular model. The diameters of these models were 10 and 20 pixels (where 1 pixel = 0.68 mm). This implies that if the diameter of a nodule on the lung wall is between 5 and 15 mm, it was considered as a target for detection. In the LWTM procedure, first, the rough lung area was extracted using pixel threshold and labeling techniques. The semicircular model was automatically rotated at an angle tangent to the lung wall. The rotated model was used as the reference image on the lung wall where the angle was calculated. The similarity was calculated using the correlation coefficient in Equation 12.1.

Both TM schemes encountered numerous false positives; thus, it was necessary to eliminate them. In this CAD scheme, 11 features for GATM and seven features for LWTM were employed to eliminate them.[19] The candidates detected by GATM and LWTM were classified into true positives and false positives based on a rule-based classifier using a threshold for the features.

The CAD scheme was applied to 20 chest CT scans (15 abnormal and five normal cases), which consisted of 557 slice images each with 10-mm slice thickness. A radiologist detected 98 nodules from the images. Table 12.10 shows the detection rate in terms of method and size and the number of false positives. Figure 12.20 shows the nodule candidates identified

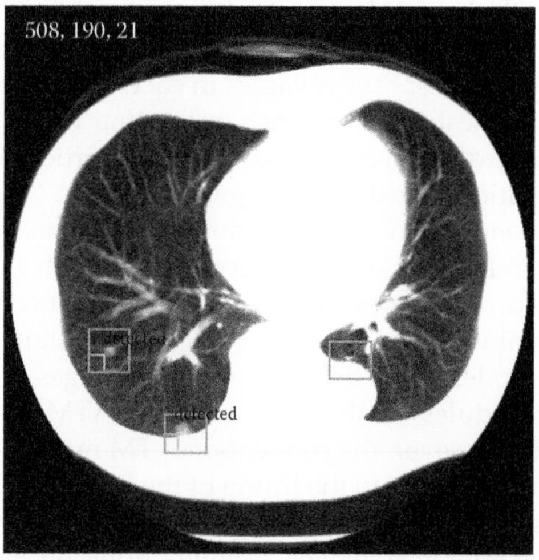

FIGURE 12.20
Nodule candidates detected by the CAD scheme, including two true positives and one false positive.

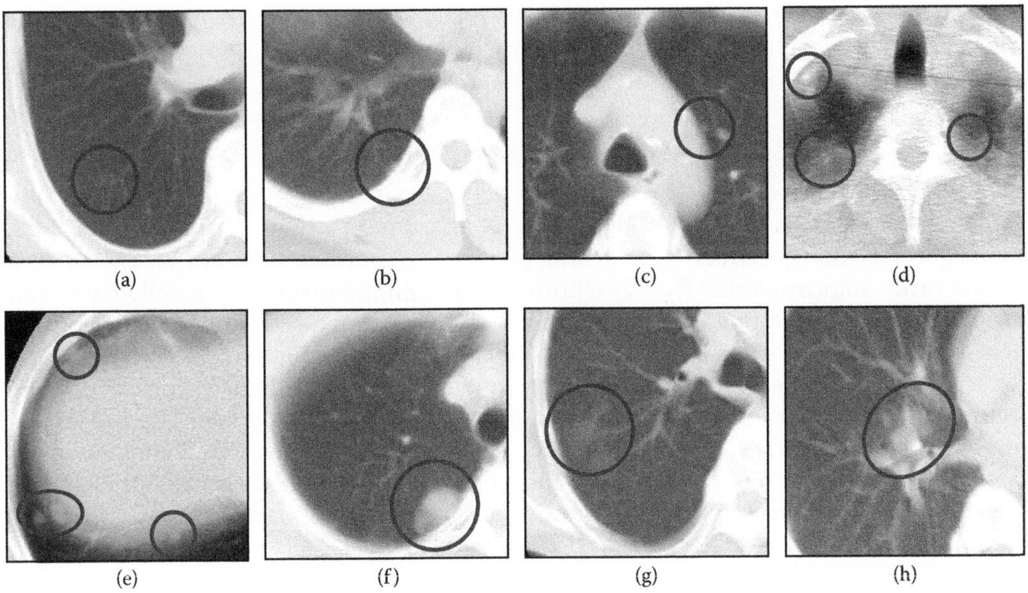

FIGURE 12.21
Undetected nodules. (a)–(c) and (e) Nodules smaller than 10 mm. (f)–(h) Nodules larger than 10 mm. (d) Both nodules; one larger and two smaller nodules.

by the CAD scheme, including two true positives and one false positive. The CAD scheme could successfully detect solitary and circular (and semicircular) nodules; however, there were some missed nodules. The missed nodules smaller than 10 mm consisted of three low-contrast nodules (see Figure 12.21a), two flat nodules on the lung wall (see Figure 12.21b), three nodules attached to the mediastinum (see Figure 12.21c), three nodules in the pulmonary apex (see Figure 12.21d), and ten nodules in the lung division (see Figure 12.21e). Similarly, missed nodules larger than 10 mm consisted of a nodule whose size was approximately 30 mm on the lung wall (see Figure 12.21f), two nodules in the pulmonary apex region (see Figure 12.21d), a low-contrast nodule (see Figure 12.21g), and two nodules attached to vessels near the bronchus (see Figure 12.21h). These nodules may be detected using an improved GATM.[20,21]

12.3 HLAC with Multiple Regression

12.3.1 HLAC

Local autocorrelation of adjacent pixels is important in image recognition. Expanded autocorrelation to higher orders is called HLAC.[22] HLAC is widely applied in image recognition,[9–13] such as face and gesture recognition,[23,24] because HLAC has several important advantages over other methods. In particular, HLAC is invariable to the location of an object. It is also not necessary to presuppose an object's model.

An HLAC is defined as follows. Let $I(r)$ be the pixel value at a reference point r; then the Nth order autocorrelation for the directional displacements $(a_1,\ldots, a_N)$ around the reference point is given by

$$x(a_1,\cdots,a_N) = \int I(r)I(r+a_1)\cdots I(r+a_N)\,dr. \tag{12.6}$$

Although an HLAC is defined by the degree N and the directional displacements $(a_1,\ldots, a_N)$, local correlations between neighboring pixels are important in an image. Therefore, a second-order autocorrelation ($N = 2$) within an area of 3 × 3 pixels is generally used, and the displacement is centered on the reference point r. Using a second-order autocorrelation, a binary image results in 25 local feature patterns from Equation 12.6, excluding the same patterns produced by the translation operation. A grayscale image procures 35 local feature patterns excluding the same patterns by the translation operation. These local features are obtained by multiplying pixel values with each other in various combinations as local patterns, as shown in Figure 12.22. Thus, the features obtained are capable of enduring a translation of the objects, and when the number of target images is two or more, the number of features of the whole image will be the sum of the targets' features. These advantages are important in recognizing and measuring images. On the other hand, an HLAC also has the disadvantage that it is difficult to accommodate a rotation of an object.

12.3.2 Multiple Regression

Multiregression analysis is a multivariate analysis technique and is composed of a criterion variable y and explanation variables $x_1,x_2,\ldots,x_p$. The expression is given by

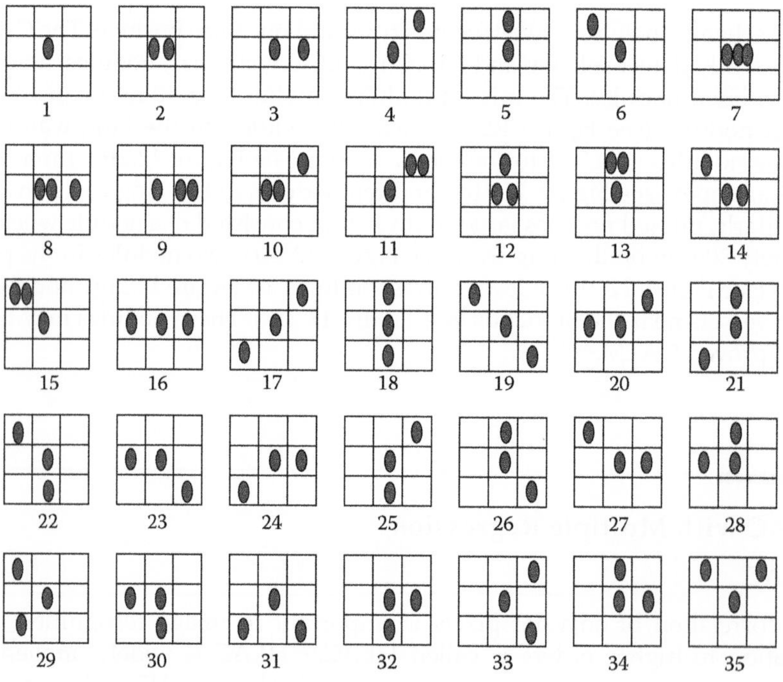

FIGURE 12.22
Local patterns used to calculate HLAC in a gray scale image.

$$Y_N = a_1 x_{1N} + a_2 x_{2N} + \cdots + a_p x_{pN} + a_0 \tag{12.7}$$

To estimate a criterion variable y, the coefficient matrix $a_0, a_1, \ldots, a_p$ must be determined, where the sum of the squares of the errors between a training signal y and an actual measurement Y is minimized. Assuming that the number of data points is N and the number of criteria variables is p, then the sum of the squares of the errors, Q, is given by

$$\begin{aligned} Q &= \{y_1 - (a_1 x_{11} + a_2 x_{21} + \cdots + a_p x_{p1} + a_0)\}^2 \\ &+ \{y_2 - (a_1 x_{12} + a_2 x_{22} + \cdots + a_p x_{p2} + a_0)\}^2 \\ &+ \cdots + \{y_N - (a_1 x_{1N} + a_2 x_{2N} + \cdots + a_p x_{pN} + a_0)\}^2 \end{aligned} \tag{12.8}$$

The simultaneous linear equation given in Equation 12.9 is obtained from partial differentials of Equation 12.8. The coefficient matrix $a_0, a_1, \ldots, a_p$ can be obtained by evaluating the set of partial differentials shown in Equation 12.9.

$$\begin{aligned} \partial Q / \partial a_1 &= 0 \\ \partial Q / \partial a_2 &= 0 \\ &\vdots \\ \partial Q / \partial a_N &= 0 \end{aligned} \tag{12.9}$$

The solution to the set of equations in Equation 12.9 is given by the set of simultaneous linear equations shown in Equation 12.10 using a variance–covariance matrix. Therefore, the coefficient matrix $a_0, a_1, \ldots, a_p$ is uniquely determined by evaluating the set of equations in Equation 12.10.

$$\begin{aligned} s_{x_1^2} a_1 + s_{x_1 x_2} a_2 + \ldots + s_{x_1 x_p} a_p &= s_{x_1 y} \\ s_{x_1 x_2} a_1 + s_{x_2^2} a_2 + \ldots + s_{x_2 x_p} a_p &= s_{x_2 y} \\ &\vdots \\ s_{x_1 x_p} a_p + s_{x_2 x_p} a_2 + \ldots + s_{x_p^2} a_p &= s_{x_p y} \end{aligned} \tag{12.10}$$

Here, $s_{x_1^2}, s_{x_2^2}, \ldots, s_{x_p^2}$ are the variances of $x_1, x_2, \ldots, x_p$, and $s_{x_m x_n}$ is the covariance between x_m and x_n. s_{xy} is a covariance between $x_1, x_2, \ldots, x_p$ and y. a_0 is derived from $a_0 = \bar{y} - (\bar{x}_1 a_1 + \bar{x}_2 a_2 + \ldots + \bar{x}_p a_p)$. $\bar{y}$ and $\bar{x}_m$ are the mean values of y and x_m, respectively.

12.3.3 Pattern Recognition Using HLAC with Multiple Regression

The unique determination of the coefficient matrix $a_0, a_1, \ldots, a_p$ is defined as the training for pattern recognition. The number of data points (N in Equation 12.7) is the number of images used in training, and the number of criteria variables p is the number of local features calculated from the HLAC (35 features in this case). In the training phase, Y is the known teacher signal. If the coefficient matrix $a_0, a_1, \ldots, a_p$ of Equation 12.7 is uniquely determined in the training phase, the actual measurement Y can be obtained by extracting the features from an unknown image.

The similarity between the unknown image and the training images is evaluated on the basis of the actual measurement Y. More specifically, if the value of Y from an unknown image is close to a teacher signal, the unknown image is recognized as resembling the training image. For example, pattern recognition using HLAC with multiple regression was applied to find the number of big and small balls in gray-level images with random noise. Figure 12.23 shows example images including large and small balls. Similar images were used as training data to determine the coefficient matrix $a_0, a_1, \ldots, a_p$ for multiple regression analysis. When the teacher signal was the number of large balls, the actual measurement value Y for the images in Figure 12.23a–c was 3.01, 3.01, and 1.01, respectively. Also when the teacher signal was the total number of large and small balls, the actual measurement value of the images in Figure 12.23a–c was 4.94, 8.98, and 8.97, respectively. These measurement values match the actual number of balls in each image.

12.3.4 Nodule Detection Using HLAC in Thoracic CT Images

An image recognition method using HLAC in 3D space has previously been developed by the authors and applied to detect lung nodules in 3D chest CT images.[10–13] In this section, a CAD scheme using both the HLAC and GATM techniques is introduced. The HLAC technique is employed chiefly to detect smaller nodules, whereas the GATM is employed chiefly to detect larger nodules. The nodule detection approach includes training and recognition.

In the training phase, the nodule patterns are analyzed using our original approach of second-order autocorrelation for features in 3D space and multiple regression analysis. Second-order autocorrelation features in 3D space are calculated using a vector calculated from the combination of voxel values in a 3 × 3 × 3 region. The number of combination patterns in a region is 235, excluding the same combination when the center of the region moves parallel. The voxel values in each combination were multiplied with each other, and the result was used as one of the elements in the feature vector.

For example, if the center of the region is given as $f_n(i, j, k)$, one of the elements of the feature vector is obtained by multiplying the three voxels $f_{-1}(i-1, j-1, k-1) \times f_0(i, j, k) \times f_{+1}(i+1, j+1, k+1)$. The number of combinations included 235 patterns when the values of f_{-1} and

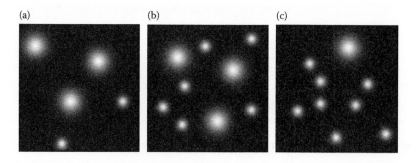

FIGURE 12.23
Images of large and small balls used for pattern recognition using HLAC with multiple regression. (a) Large: 3, small: 2, total: 5. (b) Large: 3, small: 6, total: 9. (c) Large: 1, small: 8, total: 9.

f_{+1} are at any positions around the center pixel f_0. The feature vector for a small region is defined with 235 elements summarizing each of the 235 patterns in a 3D space moving the center voxel within a small region. Using multiple regression analysis, the weighting factor for the 235 elements and one constant value are calculated to indicate training values. The training value was defined as the likelihood of the presence of a nodule. A nodular shadow yields a 3D Gaussian distribution for training output; however, a normal shadow results in a flat plane.

In the recognition phase, the following steps are performed:

1. 3D matched filtering using 3D Fourier transforms
2. Estimated image using multiple regression analysis from the 235 features
3. Calculation of mutual correlation between the training pattern and the estimated image
4. Elimination of false positives
5. Combination of detected results from GATM approach[6]
6. Final detection results

The matched filter is a band-pass filter emphasizing a special frequency band. Li et al.[25] also proposed using a similar filter technique for detecting lung nodules. The shape of the nodules can be defined as a sphere with a 3D Gaussian distribution. The frequency pattern is calculated using 9-pixel nodules (5.4 mm in diameter). The estimated image is calculated from the results of the multiple regression analysis with 235 features. The features are extracted from the region with higher values on the image after the matched filter. The output of the multiple regression analysis is a continuous value; thus, the comparison between the training pattern for multiple regression and the output also emphasizes the nodular shadows. The false positives are eliminated using the correlation value and the volume (mm^3). A GATM is also applied to detect larger nodules. A logical OR technique is employed to combine the two results.

The leave-one-out method is employed to estimate the detection performance. The detection approach using 235 features focuses on small nodules 7 mm or less in diameter. The GATM approach is designed to detect nodules between 7 and 10 mm in diameter. Nodules larger than 10 mm in diameter have been omitted in this work. Thirty-five cases (resolution: 0.585–0.703 mm, slice thickness: 0.62–0.63 mm) are analyzed. One hundred thirty-nine nodules are less than 10 mm in diameter and are not along the chest walls. Fifty-eight nodules are less than 7 mm in diameter, and 81 of the nodules are larger than 7 mm in diameter.

Table 12.11 shows the detection performance. Fifty-five of 58 small nodules (≤7 mm) and 75 of 81 large nodules (7–10 mm) are detected correctly. The numbers of false positives in 35 cases in the two-detection approach are 37 marks and 35 marks, respectively. By combining the two-detection results using a logical OR operation, the final detection rate is

TABLE 12.11

Detection Performance of the CAD Scheme Using HLAC and GATM Techniques

	True Positives	False Positives per Case
HLAC (≤7 mm)	95% (55/58 nodules)	1.1 (37 marks/35 cases)
GATM (7–10 mm)	93% (75/81 nodules)	1.0 (35 marks/35 cases)
Total	94% (130/139 nodules)	2.1 (72 marks/35 cases)

94% (130/139) true-positive fraction with 2.1% (72/35) false-positive marks per case. This result confirms the usefulness of both the HLAC and GATM techniques.

12.4 Summary

This chapter has discussed several CAD schemes for detecting lung nodules in radiographs and CT images using GATM and HLAC methods. GATM is an optimal and fast TM technique. The application of GATM to detect lung nodule in chest radiographs and CT images was shown to be useful in practice. GATM techniques could also be applied to other CAD algorithms for other medical imaging modalities and diseases, e.g., mammography and breast cancer. HLAC has many advantages for image recognition and has already been applied to other fields, e.g., face recognition. A nodule detection technique using HLAC with multiple regression was discussed and its usefulness for detecting nodules was demonstrated. We hope that these techniques contribute to early detection of lung cancer.

References

1. World Health Organization (WHO). 2008. Future trends in global mortality: major shifts in cause of death patterns. In *World Health Statistics 2008*, 29-31. http://www.who.int/entity/whosis/whostat/EN_WHS08_Full.pdf (accessed July 27, 2010).
2. Sluimer, I., A. Schilham, M. Prokop, and B.V. Ginneken. 2006. Computer analysis of computed tomography scans of the lung: a survey. *IEEE Trans. Med. Imag.* 25:385–405.
3. Katsuragawa, S., and D. Kunio. 2007. Computer-aided diagnosis in chest radiography. *Comput. Med. Imaging Graph.* 31:212–223.
4. Hara, T., and H. Fujita. 1995. Template matching of gray-scale images using a genetic algorithm. IEICE J78-D2: 385–388. (Japanese).
5. Hara, T., H. Fujita, and J. Xu. 1997. Development of automated detection system for lung nodules in chest radiograms. *Proc. IASTED Int. Conf. Intell. Inform. Syst.* (IIS97): 71–74.
6. Lee, Y., T. Hara, H. Fujita, S. Itoh, and T. Ishigaki. 1997. Nodule detection on chest helical CT scans by using a genetic algorithm. *Proc. IASTED Int. Conf. Intell. Inform. Syst.* (IIS97): 67–70.
7. Lee, Y., T. Hara, and H. Fujita. 2000. Evaluation of GA template-matching method by simulation using chest helical X-ray CT images. *Med. Imag. Inform. Sci.* 17:118–129. (Japanese).
8. Lee, Y., T. Hara, H. Fujita, S. Itoh, and T. Ishigaki. 2001. Automated detection of pulmonary nodules in helical CT images based on an improved template-matching technique. *IEEE Trans. Med. Imag.* 20:595–604.
9. Ooe, Y., N. Shinohara, T. Hara, H. Fujita, T. Endo, and T. Iwase. 2004. Development of an automated detection system for microcalcifications on mammograms by using the higher-order autocorrelation features. *Proc. SPIE* 5370:1815–1822.
10. Lee, Y., T. Nakagawa, T. Hara, H. Fujita, S. Itoh, and T. Ishigaki. 2001. Automatic detection of nodules on chest X-ray CT images using higher-order autocorrelation features. *Med. Imag. Inform. Sci.* 18:135–143. (Japanese).
11. Hara, T., M. Hirose, X. Zhou, H. Fujita, T. Kiryu, R. Yokoyama, and H. Hoshi. 2005. Nodule detection in 3D chest CT images using 2nd order autocorrelation features. *Proc. IEEE-EMBC* 2005: 6247–6249.

12. Hara, T., M. Hirose, X. Zhou, H. Fujita, T. Kiryu, H. Hoshi, R. Yokoyama, Y. Lee, and D.Y. Tsai. 2005. Nodule detection in 3D chest CT images using 2nd order autocorrelation features and GA template matching. *IEICE Tech. Rep.* 105(303):47–49.
13. Hara, T., X. Zhou, S. Okura, H. Fujita, T. Kiryu, and H. Hoshi. 2007. Nodule detection methods using autocorrelation features on 3D chest scans. *IJCARS* 2(Supplement 1):S361–S362.
14. Barnea, D.I., and H.F. Silverman. 1972. A class of algorithms for fast digital image registration. *IEEE Trans. Comput.* C-21: 179–186.
15. Goldberg, D.E. 1989. *Genetic Algorithms in Search, Optimization, and Machine Learning*. Boston, MA: Addison Wesley.
16. Michalewicz, Z. 1994. *Genetic Algorithm + Dada Structures = Evolution Programs*. Berlin, Germany: Springer-Verlag.
17. Shiraishi, J., S. Katsuragawa, J. Ikezoe, T. Matsumoto, T. Kobayashi, K. Komatsu, M. Matsui, H. Fujita, Y. Kodera, and K. Doi. 2000. Development of a digital image database for chest radiographs with and without a lung nodule: Receiver operating characteristic analysis of radiologists' detection of pulmonary nodules. *AJR* 174: 71–74.
18. Digital Image Database by Japanese Society of Radiological Technology. http://www.jsrt.or.jp/web_data/english03.php.
19. Lee, Y., D.Y. Tsai, T. Hara, H. Fujita, S. Itoh, and T. Ishigaki. 2004. Improvement in automated detection of pulmonary nodules on helical x-ray CT images. *Proc. SPIE* 5370:824–832.
20. El-Baz, A., A. A. Farag ,R. Falk, R. La Rocca. 2003. A unified approach for detection, visualization, and identification of lung abnormalities in chest spiral CT scans. *Proc. CARS* 2003: 998–1004.
21. Dehmeshki, J., X. Ye, X.Y. Lin, M. Valdvieso, and H. Amin. 2007. Automated detection of lung nodules in CT images using shape-based genetic algorithm. *Comput. Med. Imaging Graph.* 31: 408–417.
22. Mclaughlin, J.A., J. Raviv. 1968. Nth-order autocorrelations in pattern recognition. *Inform. Control* 12:121–142.
23. Kurita, T., N. Otsu, and T. Sato. 1992. A face recognition method using higher order local autocorrelation and multivariate analysis. *Proc. Int. Conf. Pattern Recognit.* 2: 213–216.
24. Kurita, T., Y. Kobayashi, and T. Mishima. 1997. Higher order local autocorrelation features of PARCOR images for gesture recognition. *Proc. Int. Conf. Image Process.* 3:722–725.
25. Li, Q., S Katsuragawa, and K. Doi. 2001. Computer-aided diagnostic scheme for lung nodule detection in digital chest radiographs by use of a multiple template matching technique. *Med. Phys.* 28: 2070–2076.

13

Computer-Aided Detection of Lung Nodules in Chest Radiographs and Thoracic CT

Kenji Suzuki

CONTENTS

13.1 Introduction

Lung cancer continues to rank as the leading cause of cancer deaths among Americans. The number of lung cancer deaths each year is greater than the combined number of breast, colon, and prostate cancer deaths. Evidence suggests that early detection of lung cancer may allow more timely therapeutic intervention and thus a more favorable prognosis for the patient (Heelan et al. 1984; Sone et al. 1998). Accordingly, lung cancer screening programs are being conducted in the United States (Henschke et al. 1999; Miettinen and Henschke 2001; Henschke et al. 2001; Swensen et al. 2003), Japan (Kaneko et al. 1996; Sone et al. 1998; Sone et al. 2001; Nawa et al. 2002), and other countries with low-dose helical computed tomography (CT) as the screening modality. Helical CT, however, generates a large number of images that must be read by radiologists. This may lead to "information overload" for the radiologists. Furthermore, radiologists may miss some cancers, which are visible in retrospect, during interpretation of CT images (Gurney 1996; Li et al. 2002). Therefore, a computer-aided diagnostic (CAD) scheme for detection of lung nodules on low-dose CT images has been investigated as a useful tool for lung cancer screening, because the CAD scheme may detect some cancers that are "missed" by radiologists (Li et al. 2002), and provide quantitative detection results as a "second opinion" to assist radiologists in improving their detection accuracy (Kobayashi et al. 1996).

Many investigators have developed a number of methods for the automated detection of lung nodules in CT scans (Giger, Bae, and MacMahon 1994; Armato et al. 1999; Armato, Giger, and MacMahon 2001; Armato et al. 2002; Armato, Altman, and La Riviere 2003; Yamamoto et al. 1994; Okumura et al. 1998; Ryan et al. 1996; Kanazawa et al. 1998; Ko and Betke 2001; Reeves and Kostis 2000; Lee et al. 2001; Gurcan et al. 2002; Brown et al. 2001; Wormanns et al. 2002; Lou et al. 1999; Li et al. 2001; Wiemker et al. 2002; Oda et al. 2002; Brown et al. 2003; McCulloch et al. 2004; Lawler et al. 2003), based on morphologic filtering (Yamamoto et al. 1994; Okumura et al. 1998), geometric modeling (Ryan et al. 1996), fuzzy clustering (Kanazawa et al. 1998), and gray-level thresholding (Giger, Bae, and MacMahon 1994; Armato et al. 1999; Armato, Giger, and MacMahon 2001; Armato et al. 2002; Ko and Betke 2001). Giger et al. (Giger, Bae, and MacMahon 1994), for example, developed an automated detection scheme based on multiple gray-level thresholding and geometric feature analysis. Armato et al. (Armato, Giger, and MacMahon 2001; Armato et al. 1999; Armato et al. 2002) extended the method to include a three-dimensional (3D) approach combined with linear discriminant analysis.

On the other hand, chest radiography is the most frequently used imaging examination for chest diseases because of its low cost, simplicity, and low radiation dose. Chest radiography has been used for detection of lung cancer because some evidence suggests that early detection of lung cancer may allow a more favorable prognosis (Heelan et al. 1984; Sobue et al. 1992). Radiologists, however, may fail to detect lung nodules in chest radiographs in up to 30% of cases that have nodules visible in retrospect (Austin, Romney, and Goldsmith 1992; Shah et al. 2003). CAD schemes for nodule detection on chest radiographs have been investigated (MacMahon et al. 1990) because the computer can improve radiologists' detection accuracy (Abe et al. 1993; Kobayashi et al. 1996). Because chest radiographs are so widely used, improvements in the detection of lung nodules in chest radiographs could have a significant impact on early detection of lung cancer.

A number of researchers have developed CAD schemes for lung nodule detection on chest radiographs. Giger et al. (Giger, Doi, and MacMahon 1988; Giger et al. 1990) developed a CAD scheme based on a thresholding technique together with a rule-based classifier, and the performance of the CAD scheme was improved by incorporation of an artificial neural network (ANN) and linear discriminant analysis, an adaptive thresholding technique, and a multiple-template matching technique by Wu et al. (Wu et al. 1994), Xu et al. (Xu et al. 1997), and Li et al. (Li, Katsuragawa, and Doi 2001), respectively. Sankar et al. (Sankar and Sklansky 1982) reported on a CAD scheme based on segmentation of nodule candidates in which they used a dynamic programming technique and image feature analysis. Lo et al. (Lo et al. 1995) developed a CAD scheme based on a convolution neural network (Lin et al. 1995), and Lin et al. (Lin et al. 1996) improved the performance of the scheme by incorporating two-level convolution neural networks. Carreira et al. (Carreira et al. 1998) devised a CAD scheme based on detection of nodule candidates with normalized cross-correlation images and classification of candidates in curvature space, and Penedo et al. (Penedo et al. 1998) improved the performance of the scheme by incorporating two-level ANNs that employed cross-correlation teaching images and input images in curvature peak space. Coppini et al. (Coppini et al. 2003) developed a CAD scheme based on biologically inspired ANNs with fuzzy coding. Vittitoe et al. (Vittitoe, Baker, and Floyd 1997) developed fractal texture characterization to improve the detection accuracy for solitary pulmonary nodules in a CAD scheme. Schilham et al. (Schilham et al. 2006) proposed a new initial nodule candidate detection method based on multiscale techniques. Campadelli et al. (Campadelli, Casiraghi, and Artioli 2006) improved the performance of a CAD scheme by introducing a new lung segmentation method. Hardie et al. (Hardie et al. 2008) proposed a CAD scheme based on a weighted multiscale convergence-index filter for initial nodule candidate detection and an adaptive distance-based threshold algorithm for candidate segmentation. Other researchers, including Lampeter et al. (Lampeter and Wandtke 1986), Floyd et al. (Floyd et al. 1996), and Mao et al. (Mao et al. 1998), reported on CAD schemes with use of various techniques.

Although current CAD schemes can be useful for detection of nodules, some limitations still exist. One of the major limitations with current CAD schemes is a relatively low sensitivity. This would impose a great limit in assisting radiologists' detection task. Besides a thresholding technique, most methods for identification of nodule candidates use a model-based approach which employs mathematical forms for detecting nodules (Yamamoto et al. 1994; Li, Sone, and Doi 2003). For example, a quoit filter (Yamamoto et al. 1994) based on mathematical morphologic filtering employs a sphere as the model of a nodule and a cylinder as a model of a vessel. A 3D selective enhancement filter (Li, Sone, and Doi 2003) employs a dot as the model of a nodule and a line as the model of a vessel. Although these techniques work perfectly on idealized nodules and vessels, they do not always work on actual nodules and vessels in CT images because actual nodules can be irregular and/or of low contrast; actual vessels can be bifurcate and/or overlap with other vessels or nodules.

Another major limitation with current CAD schemes is a relatively large number of false positives (FPs). A large number of FPs are likely to distract from the radiologist's task and thus reduce the clinical value of CAD. In addition, radiologists may lose their confidence in CAD as a useful tool. Therefore, it is important to reduce the number of FPs as much as possible while maintaining a high sensitivity.

Our purpose in this study was to develop CAD schemes for detection of lung nodules on chest radiographs and thoracic CT images.

13.2 Databases

Our Institutional Review Board approved this retrospective study. Informed consent for use of cases in this study was waived by the Institutional Review Board because patient data were de-identified. This study complied with the Health Insurance Portability and Accountability Act, and it met all standards for good clinical research according to the National Institutes of Health's and local Institutional Review Board's guidelines.

13.2.1 Database of Low-Dose CT Images

The database used in this study consisted of 101 noninfused, low-dose thoracic helical CT (LDCT) scans acquired from 71 different patients who participated voluntarily in a lung cancer screening program between 1996 and 1999 in Nagano, Japan (Sone et al. 1998; Li et al. 2002; Sone et al. 2001). The CT examinations were performed on a mobile CT scanner (CT-W950SR; Hitachi Medical, Tokyo, Japan). The scans used for this study were acquired with a low-dose protocol of 120 kVp, 25 mA (54 scans) or 50 mA (47 scans), 10-mm collimation, and a 10-mm reconstruction interval at a helical pitch of two. The pixel size was 0.586 mm for 83 scans and 0.684 mm for 18 scans. Each reconstructed CT section had an image matrix size of 512 × 512 pixels. We used 38 of 101 LDCT scans which were acquired from 31 patients as a training set for our CAD scheme. The 38 scans consisted of 1057 sections and contained 50 nodules, including 38 "missed" nodules that represented biopsy-confirmed lung cancers and were not reported or misreported during the initial clinical interpretation (Li et al. 2002). The remaining 12 nodules in the scans were classified as "confirmed benign" ($n = 8$), "suspected benign" ($n = 3$), or "suspected malignant" ($n = 1$). The confirmed benign nodules were determined by biopsy or by follow-up over a period of two years. The suspected benign nodules were determined by follow-up of less than two years. The suspected malignant nodule was determined on the basis of results of follow-up diagnostic CT studies; no biopsy results were available. We used 63 of 101 LDCT scans which were acquired from 63 patients as a test set. The 63 scans consisted of 1765 sections and contained 71 nodules, including 66 primary cancers that were determined by biopsy and five confirmed benign nodules that were determined by biopsy or by follow-up over a period of two years. The scans included 23 scans from the same 23 patients as those in the training set, which were acquired at a different time (the interval was about one year or two years). Thus, the training set consisted of 38 LDCT scans including 50 nodules, and the test set consisted of 63 LDCT scans including 71 confirmed nodules.

Figure 13.1 shows the distributions of nodule sizes for the training set and the test set in our database. The nodule size was determined by an experienced chest radiologist and ranged from 4 mm to 27 mm. When a nodule was present in more than one section, the largest size was used as the nodule size. Note that the nodules were present in a maximum of three sections. The mean diameter of the 50 nodules in the training set was 12.7 ± 6.1 mm, and that of the 71 nodules in the test set was 13.5 ± 4.7 mm. In the training set, 38% of nodules were attached to the pleura, 22% of nodules were attached to vessels, and 10% of nodules were in the hilum. As to the test set, 30% of nodules were attached to the pleura, 34% of nodules were attached to vessels, and 7% of nodules were in the hilum. Three radiologists determined the nodules in the training set as three categories such as pure ground-glass opacity (pure GGO; 40% of nodules), mixed GGO (28%), and solid nodule

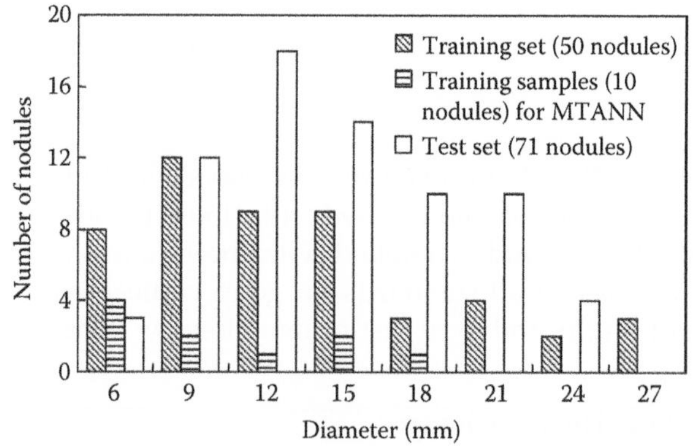

FIGURE 13.1
Distributions of nodule sizes for our database. The training set contained 50 nodules including 38 "missed" cancers, and the test set contained 71 confirmed nodules including 66 biopsy-confirmed primary cancers. (Reprinted with permission from Suzuki, K. et al., *Medical Physics*, 30, 7, 1602–1617, 2003.)

(32%); the nodules in the test set were determined as pure GGO (24%), mixed GGO (30%), and solid nodule (46%).

13.2.2 Database of Chest Radiographs

The database used in this study consisted of 91 chest radiographs containing 91 solitary pulmonary nodules with subtlety ratings of subtle, relatively obvious, and obvious from the Digital Image Database developed by the Japanese Society of Radiological Technology (Shiraishi et al. 2000), which is a publicly available database. The chest radiographs were collected from 14 medical institutions. The absence and presence of nodules in the chest radiographs were confirmed by CT. The locations of all nodules were confirmed by three chest radiologists. The criteria for inclusion in the database were: (1) no nodules larger than 35 mm, (2) no suspicious nodules which were not confirmed by CT examination, (3) no cases from the same patient, and (4) no nodules with margins which cannot be confirmed by radiologists. The chest radiographs were digitized with a 0.175-mm pixel size, a matrix size of 2048 × 2048, and a 12-bit gray-scale level. The sizes of nodules ranged from 8.9 to 29.1 mm, and the average size was 17.4 mm. The database contained 64 malignant nodules and 27 benign nodules, which were confirmed by histologic or cytologic examinations or follow-up imaging. For reduction of noise and computational efficiency, the size of the chest radiographs was reduced to 512 × 512 pixels with a 10-bit gray-scale level by use of averaging in this study.

13.3 CAD Scheme for Thoracic CT

13.3.1 Current Scheme for Lung Nodule Detection in Low-Dose CT

A flowchart for our current scheme for lung nodule detection in CT is shown in Figure 13.2. Technical details of our current scheme have been published previously (Armato, Giger, and MacMahon 2001; Armato et al. 1999; Armato et al. 2002). To summarize the

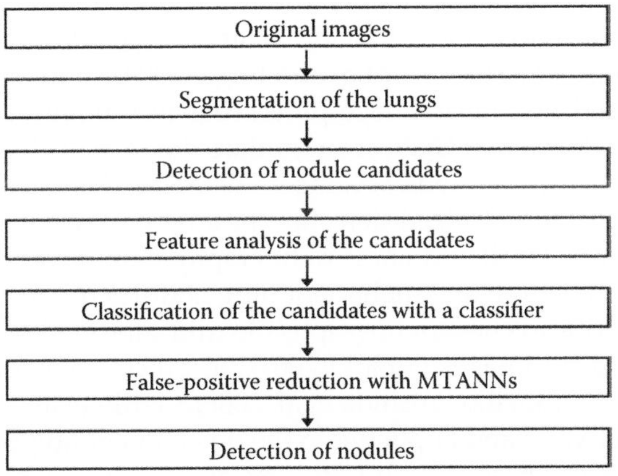

FIGURE 13.2
Flowchart for our CAD schemes for lung nodule detection in CT and chest radiography.

methodology, lung nodule identification proceeds in three phases: two-dimensional (2D) processing, followed by 3D analysis, and then the application of classifiers. A gray-level-thresholding technique is applied to a 2D section of a CT scan for automated lung segmentation. A multiple gray-level-thresholding technique is applied to the segmented lung volume. Individual structures are identified by grouping of spatially contiguous pixels that remain in the volume at each of 36 gray-level thresholds. A structure is identified as a nodule candidate if the volume of the structure is less than that of a 3-cm-diameter sphere. The categorization of nodule candidates as "nodule" or "nonnodule" is based on a combination of a rule-based classifier and a series of two linear discriminant classifiers applied to a set of nine 2D and 3D features extracted from each nodule candidate. These features include: (1) the mean gray level of the candidate, (2) the gray-level standard deviation, (3) the gray-level threshold at which the candidate was identified, (4) volume, (5) sphericity, (6) radius of the sphere of equivalent volume, (7) eccentricity, (8) circularity, and (9) compactness.

With our current CAD scheme, the multiple gray-level-thresholding technique initially identified 20,743 nodule candidates in 1057 sections of LDCT images in the training set (Armato et al. 2002). Forty-five of 50 nodules were correctly detected. Then a rule-based classifier followed by a series of two linear discriminant classifiers was applied for removal of some FPs, thus yielding a detection of 40 (80.0%) of 50 nodules (from 22 patients) together with 1078 (1.02 per section) FPs (Armato et al. 2002). The sizes of the ten false-negative nodules ranged from 5 to 25 mm, and the mean diameter was 13.2 ± 6.1 mm. In this study, we used all 50 nodules, the locations of which were identified by the radiologist, and all 1078 FPs generated by our CAD scheme in the training set, for investigating the characteristics of a massive-training ANN (MTANN) and training the MTANN. The use of radiologist-extracted true nodules with computer-generated FPs was intended to anticipate future improvements in the nodule detection sensitivity of our CAD scheme. When a nodule was present in more than one section, the section that included the largest nodule was used. When we applied our current CAD scheme to the test set, a sensitivity of 81.7% (58 of 71 nodules) with 0.98 FPs per section (1726/1765) was achieved. We used the 58 true positives (nodules from 54 patients) and 1726 FPs (nonnodules) for testing the MTANN in a validation test.

13.3.2 Architecture of Massive Training ANNs for FP Reduction

By extension of "neural filters" (Suzuki, Horiba, and Sugie 2002; Suzuki et al. 2002) and "neural edge enhancers," (Suzuki, Horiba, and Sugie 2003; Suzuki et al. 2004) which are ANN-based, supervised nonlinear image-processing techniques, 2D MTANNs (Suzuki et al. 2003) have been developed that accommodate the task of distinguishing a specific opacity from other opacities in medical images. 2D MTANNs have been applied for the reduction of FPs in the computerized detection of lung nodules in low-dose CT (Suzuki et al. 2003; Arimura et al. 2004) and chest radiography (Suzuki, Shiraishi et al. 2005), for the distinction between benign and malignant lung nodules in CT (Suzuki, Li et al. 2005), for the suppression of ribs in chest radiographs (Suzuki, Abe et al. 2006), and for enhancement of lesions in medical images (Suzuki 2009). To process 3D volumetric CT data, we developed a 3D MTANN (Suzuki, Yoshida et al. 2006; Suzuki et al. 2008) by extending the structure of the 2D MTANN and applied it to the detection of polyps in CT colonography (Suzuki, Zhang, and Xu in press; Suzuki, Rockey, and Dachman 2010; Suzuki et al. 2008; Suzuki, Yoshida et al. 2006).

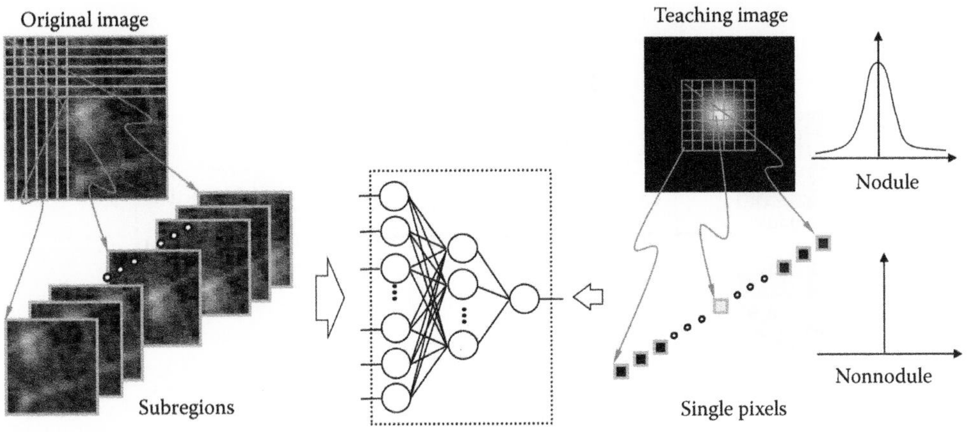

FIGURE 13.3
Architecture and training of an MTANN. (Reprinted with permission from Suzuki, K. et al., *Medical Physics*, 30, 7, 1602–1617, 2003.)

The architecture of an MTANN is shown in Figure 13.3. An MTANN consists of a linear-output multilayer ANN regression model (Suzuki, Horiba, and Sugie 2003), which is capable of operating on pixel data directly. The MTANN is trained with input CT images and the corresponding "teaching" images for enhancement of nodules and suppression of a specific type of nonnodule. The pixel values of the original CT images are linearly scaled such that –1000 Hounsfield units (HU) corresponds to 0 and 1000 HU corresponds to 1 (values below 0 and above 1 are allowed). The input to the MTANN consists of pixel values in a subregion, R_S, extracted from an input image. The output of the MTANN is a continuous scalar value, which is associated with the center pixel in the subregion, and is represented by

$$O(x,y) = NN\{I(x-i, y-j) \mid (i,j) \in R_S\}, \tag{13.1}$$

where x and y are the coordinate indices, $NN(\cdot)$ is the output of a linear-output ANN model, and $I(x,y)$ is a pixel value of the input image.

A single MTANN cannot reduce multiple types of FP sources effectively because the capability of a single MTANN is limited (Suzuki et al. 2003). To reduce various types of FPs, we extended the capability of a single MTANN and developed a mixture of expert MTANNs (Suzuki et al. 2008). The architecture of a mixture of expert MTANNs is shown in Figure 13.4. A mixture of expert MTANNs consists of several MTANNs that are arranged in parallel. Each expert MTANN is trained independently by use of a specific type of nonnodule and a common set of actual nodules. Each expert MTANN acts as an expert for distinguishing nodules from a specific type of nonnodule, e.g., MTANN no. 1 is trained to distinguish nodules from medium-sized vessels; MTANN no. 2 is trained to distinguish nodules from small-sized vessels; and so on.

The number of hidden units may be selected by use of a method for designing the structure of an ANN (Suzuki, Horiba, and Sugie 2001; Suzuki 2004). This method is a sensitivity-based pruning method, i.e., the sensitivity of the unit removal to the training error is calculated when a certain unit is removed experimentally, and the unit with the smallest training error is removed. Removing the redundant hidden units and retraining to recover the potential

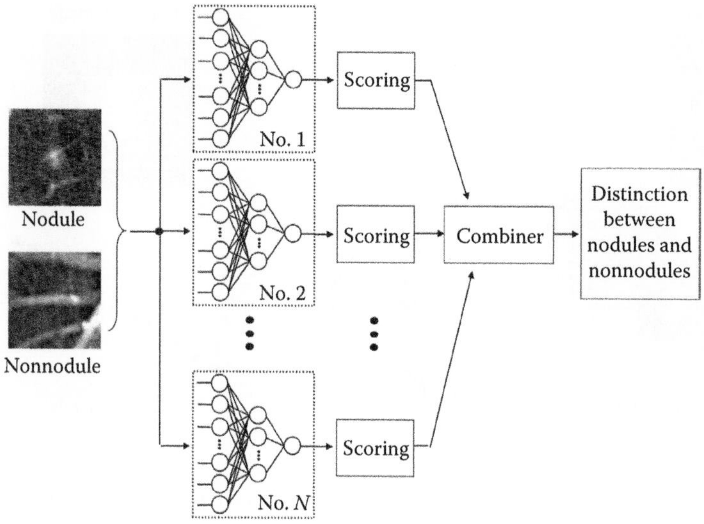

FIGURE 13.4
Architecture of a mixture of expert MTANNs for reduction of multiple types of FPs. (Reprinted with permission from Suzuki, K. et al., *Medical Physics*, 30, 7, 1602–1617, 2003.)

loss due to the removal are performed repeatedly, resulting in a reduced structure from which redundant units are removed.

13.3.3 Training Method of Expert MTANNs

For enhancement of nodules and suppression of nonnodules in CT images, the teaching image contains a 3D Gaussian distribution with standard deviation σ_T. This distribution represents the "likelihood of being a nodule" for a nodule and zero for a nonnodule:

$$T(x,y) = \begin{cases} \dfrac{1}{\sqrt{2\pi}\sigma_T}\exp\left(-\dfrac{(x^2+y^2)}{2\sigma_T^2}\right) & \text{for a nodule} \\ 0 & \text{otherwise.} \end{cases} \tag{13.2}$$

A Gaussian distribution is used to approximate an average shape of nodules. The expert MTANN involves training with a large number of subregion–pixel pairs; we call it a massive-subregion training scheme. For enriching the training samples, a training region, R_T, extracted from the input CT image is divided pixel by pixel into a large number of overlapping subregions. Single pixels are extracted from the corresponding teaching image as teaching values. The expert MTANN is massively trained by use of each of a large number of the input subregions together with each of the corresponding teaching single pixels, hence the term "massive-training ANN." The error to be minimized by training of the *n*th expert MTANN is given by

$$E_n = \frac{1}{P_n}\sum_c \sum_{(x,y)\in V_{Tn}} \left\{T_{n,c}(x,y) - O_{n,c}(x,y)\right\}^2, \tag{13.3}$$

where c is a training case number, $O_{n,c}$ is the output of the nth expert MTANN for the cth case, $T_{n,c}$ is the teaching value for the nth expert MTANN for the cth case, and P_n is the number of total training pixels in the training image for the nth expert MTANN, R_{Tn}. The expert MTANN is trained by a linear-output back-propagation (BP) algorithm (Suzuki, Horiba, and Sugie 2003). After training, the expert MTANN is expected to output the highest value when a nodule is located at the center of the subregion of the expert MTANN, a lower value as the distance from the subregion center increases, and zero when the input subregion contains a nonnodule.

13.3.4 Scoring Method for Combining Output Pixels

For combining output pixels from the trained expert MTANNs, we developed a scoring method, as shown in Figure 13.5. A score for a given nodule candidate from the nth expert MTANN is defined as

$$S_n = \sum_{(x,y)\in R_E} f_G(\sigma_n;x,y) \times O_n(x,y), \tag{13.4}$$

where

$$f_G(\sigma_n;x,y) = \frac{1}{\sqrt{2\pi}\sigma_n} \exp\left(-\frac{(x^2+y^2)}{2\sigma_n^2}\right) \tag{13.5}$$

is a Gaussian weighting function with standard deviation σ_n, and with its center corresponding to the center of the region for evaluation, R_E; and $O_n(x,y)$ is the output image of the nth trained expert MTANN, where its center corresponds to the center of R_E. The use of the Gaussian weighting function allows us to combine the responses (outputs) of a trained expert MTANN as a 2D distribution. A Gaussian function is used for scoring because the output of a trained expert MTANN is expected to be similar to the Gaussian distribution used in the teaching image. This score represents the weighted sum of the estimates for the likelihood that the image (nodule candidate) contains a nodule near the center, i.e., a higher score would indicate a nodule, and a lower score would indicate a nonnodule.

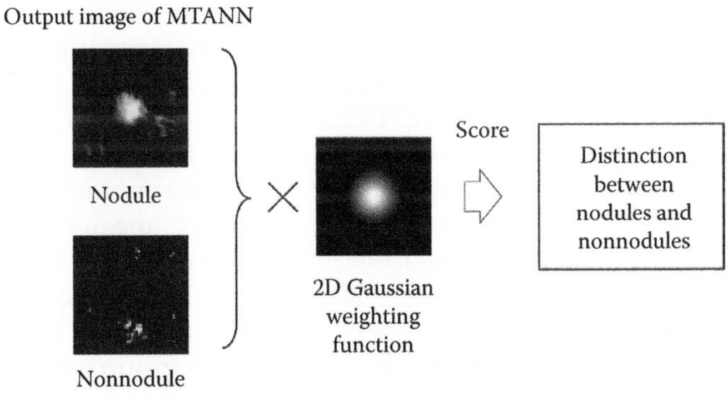

FIGURE 13.5
A scoring method for combining output pixels into a simple score for each candidate.

13.3.5 Mixing ANN for Combining Expert MTANNs

The scores from the expert MTANNs are combined by use of a mixing ANN or a logical AND operation such that different types of nonnodules can be distinguished from nodules. The mixing ANN consists of a linear-output multilayer ANN regression model with a linear-output BP training algorithm (Suzuki, Horiba, and Sugie 2003) for processing of continuous output/teaching values; the activation functions of the units in the input, hidden, and output layers are an identity, a sigmoid, and a linear function, respectively. One unit is employed in the output layer for distinction between a nodule and a nonnodule. The scores of each expert MTANN are used for each input unit in the mixing ANN; thus, the number of input units corresponds to the number of expert MTANNs, N. The scores of each expert MTANN act as the features for distinguishing nodules from a specific type of nonnodule for which the expert MTANN is trained. The output of the mixing ANN for the cth nodule candidate is represented by

$$M_c = NN[\{S_{n,c}\} | 1 \leq n \leq N], \tag{13.6}$$

where $NN(\cdot)$ is the output of the linear-output ANN model. The teaching values for nodules are assigned the value one, and those for nonnodules are zero. Training of the mixing ANN may be performed by use of a leave-one-lesion-out cross-validation scheme (Mosier 1951). After training, the mixing ANN is expected to output a higher value for a nodule and a lower value for a nonnodule. Thus, the output can be considered to be a "likelihood of being a nodule." By thresholding of the output, a distinction between nodules and nonnodules can be made. The balance between the true-positive rate and FP rate is determined by the selected threshold value. If the scores of each expert MTANN properly characterize the specific type of nonnodule for which the expert MTANN is trained, the mixing ANN combining several expert MTANNs will be able to distinguish nodules from various types of nonnodules.

13.4 CAD Scheme for Chest Radiographs

13.4.1 Our CAD Scheme

Our CAD scheme (Shiraishi et al. 2003) for lung nodule detection on chest radiographs consisted of four steps, i.e., (1) preprocessing based on a difference-image technique (Giger, Doi, and MacMahon 1988; Giger et al. 1990; Xu et al. 1997), (2) identification of initial nodule candidates by use of a multiple gray-level thresholding technique, (3) grouping of initial nodule candidates, and (4) use of rule-based and linear discriminant classifiers for reduction of FPs. The difference-image technique is a technique for enhancing lung nodules and suppressing background normal structures. The difference image was obtained by subtraction of the nodule-suppressed image from the nodule-enhanced image. Initial nodule candidates were identified on the difference image by use of a multiple gray-level thresholding technique. The initial nodule candidates were classified into 13 groups according to their pick-up threshold levels. Eight image features for each group were calculated, i.e., the effective diameter, degree of circularity, degree of irregularity, growth rate of the effective diameter, growth rate of the degree of circularity, growth rate of the degree of irregularity, run length, and contrast in the original image and the difference image. These eight image features were used as input to the rule-based and linear discriminant classifiers. With our current CAD scheme, a sensitivity of 82.4% (75/91) with 4.5 (410/91) FPs per image was achieved for the database which consisted of 91 chest radiographs. We used the 75 true positives (nodules) and the 410 FPs (nonnodules) for testing our scheme for FP reduction in this study.

13.4.2 Preprocessing for Massive Training ANN FP Reduction

The background trends in the regions of interest (ROIs) in a chest radiograph are, in general, different from those at different locations in the same image, those in a different patient's image, and those in an image acquired under a different acquisition condition. To reduce these effects, we applied a background-trend-correction technique (Katsuragawa et al. 1990) to the ROI. The background-trend-correction technique is a technique of subtracting a 2D surface that is fitted to gray levels in the ROI from the original ROI. We used a 2D nth-order polynomial as the 2D surface as follows:

$$F^n(x,y) = \sum_{k=1}^{n+1} \sum_{m=1}^{k} a_{(k-1)k/2+m} x^{k-m} y^{m-1}, \tag{13.7}$$

where a_k is the kth coefficient, and k and m are variables. The coefficients of the 2D polynomial are determined by use of the least-squares method. The background trend in the ROI is corrected by the following equation:

$$g_B(x,y) = g(x,y) - F^n(x,y). \tag{13.8}$$

Then, contrast normalization is performed on the background-trend-corrected ROI. All pixel values in the ROI are divided by the average pixel value in a circle region R_C, represented by

$$g_C(x,y) = \frac{g_B(x,y)}{\sum_{x,y \in R_C} g_B(x,y)/N}, \tag{13.9}$$

where N is the number of pixels in R_C. The diameter of the circle region was determined to be 40 pixels, which corresponds to the maximum size of nodules to be detected. The pixel values $g_C(x,y)$ of the ROI are normalized such that a pixel value of −200 is zero and a pixel value of 200 is one, which correspond to the mean for the minimum pixel values in the ROIs and the mean for the maximum pixel values in the ROIs, respectively.

13.5 Results

13.5.1 Results for Thoracic CT

The training set in our database consisted of 38 LDCT scans (a total of 1057 LDCT 512 × 512 pixel images) which included 50 nodules. Ten nodules and ten FPs were used as the training cases for the MTANN. Examples of the training cases (a region of 40 by 40 pixels is displayed as an example) are shown in Figure 13.6. An imaging scientist selected ten typical nodules as training samples from the three categories (pure GGO, mixed GGO, and solid nodule) determined by three radiologists on the basis of the visual appearance of these patterns. The distribution of nodule sizes of training cases is shown in Figure 13.1. Three of the ten nodules were attached to the pleura, three nodules were attached to vessels, and one nodule was in the hilum. A radiologist classified the FPs reported by our current CAD scheme as four major groups such as small (including peripheral) vessels (40% of FPs), medium-sized vessels (30%), soft-tissue opacities, including opacities caused by the partial volume effect between the lung region and the diaphragm (20%), and part of normal structures in the mediastinum, including large vessels in the hilum (10%). Because small (including peripheral) vessels were included in the medium-sized vessel images, we selected medium-sized vessels as the group used for training samples. The radiologist selected ten vessels with relatively high contrast from the group of medium-sized vessels because they are dominant over all medium-sized vessels.

A three-layer structure was employed as the structure of the linear-output ANN because any continuous mapping can be approximately realized by three-layer ANNs (Barron 1993; Funahashi 1989). The parameters such as the size of the local window of the MTANN, R_S, the standard deviation of the 2D Gaussian function, σ_T, and the size of the training region in the teaching image, R_T, were determined empirically based on the training set. R_S was selected to be 9 × 9 pixels. The number of units in the hidden layer was set at 25. Thus, the numbers of units in the input, hidden, and output layers were 81, 25, and 1, respectively. σ_T was determined as 5.0 pixels, which corresponds approximately to the average diameter of the nodules. R_T was selected to be 19 × 19 pixels. With the parameters above, the training of the MTANN was performed on 500,000 epochs—one epoch means one training run for one training data set—and converged with a mean absolute error of 11.2%. The training was stopped at 500,000 epochs because the performance did not increase. The training took a CPU time of 29.8 hours on a PC-based workstation (CPU: Pentium IV, 1.7 GHz), and the time for applying the trained MTANN to nodule candidates was negligibly small.

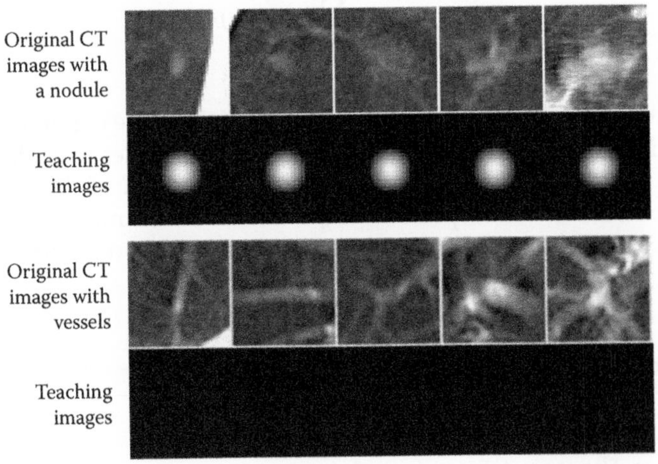

FIGURE 13.6
Illustration of nodules and nonnodules used as training cases for MTANN training and corresponding teaching images.

To investigate the basic characteristics of the trained MTANNs, we created simulated CT images that contained model nodules and model vessels (Suzuki and Doi 2005). A nodule was modeled as a sphere, and a vessel as a cylinder. The simulated images included various-sized model nodules (8.0, 14.0, and 20.0 mm in diameter) with low, medium, and high contrast (200, 400, and 600 HU), various-sized model vessels (2.0, 3.0, and 4.0 mm in diameter) with different orientations such as horizontal, vertical, and diagonal, and model nodules overlapping model vessels, as shown in Figure 13.7. We created the same-sized model nodules with different contrasts because solid opacity and GGO of the same size have different contrasts. The background level was –900 HU, which corresponds to the average background level in the lungs. In the output image of the trained MTANN, the various-sized model nodules with different contrasts are represented by light "nodular" distributions, whereas various-sized model vessels with different orientations are almost dark, and are thus removed, as shown in Figure 13.7. This result indicates that the MTANN was able to enhance sphere-like objects (model nodules) and suppress cylinder-like objects (model vessels), and that the trained MTANN would be robust against a change in scale and rotation.

To eliminate the remaining FPs, we prepared training cases for the multiple expert MTANNs. The radiologist classified the remaining FPs (nonnodules) reported by the single MTANN into seven groups such as medium-sized vessels, small (including peripheral) vessels, parts of normal structures including large vessels in the hilum, vessels with some opacities, opacities caused by the partial volume effect, abnormal opacities, and other opacities. Two major groups were divided into subgroups based on the visual appearance of patterns. The group of medium-sized vessels was divided into two subgroups such as relatively large fuzzy vessels and relatively small branching vessels. The group of small vessels was divided into two subgroups such as small (including peripheral) vessels and peripheral vessels with a light background. An imaging scientist selected ten representative nonnodules from each of the groups or the subgroups except the group of other opacities as the training samples for each MTANN; thus, the multiple expert MTANNs employed nine MTANNs.

The same ten nodules were used as training cases for all nine MTANNs. Therefore, ten nodules and 90 nonnodules were used for training of the multiple expert MTANNs.

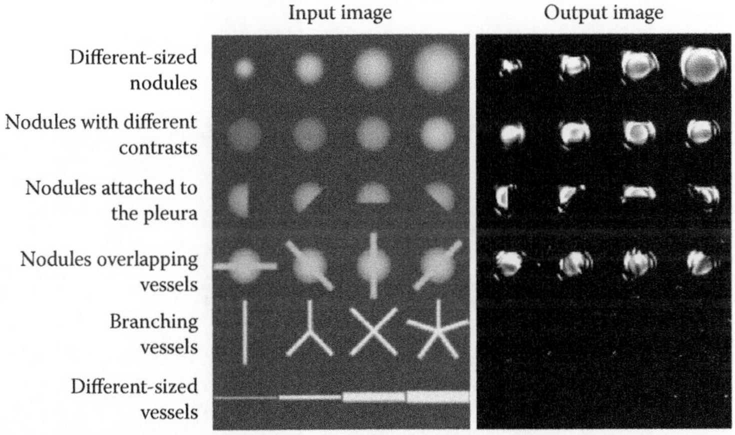

FIGURE 13.7
Simulated CT image that contains various-sized model nodules with different contrasts and various-sized model vessels with different orientations, and the corresponding output images of the MTANNs trained with 10 actual nodules and 10 actual vessel images.

The single MTANN trained with medium-sized vessels (with relatively high contrast) was used as MTANN no. 1. Nonnodules for the training of MTANN nos. 1 to 5 ranged from medium-sized vessels to small (peripheral) vessels. Nonnodules for the training of MTANN nos. 6 to 9 were large vessels in the hilum, relatively large vessels with some opacities, soft-tissue opacities caused by the partial volume effect between peripheral vessels and the diaphragm, and some abnormal opacities (focal interstitial opacities), respectively. Each MTANN was trained in the same way as a single MTANN.

The trained MTANNs were applied to 1068 FP nodule candidates not used for training. The execution time was very short, only 1.4 seconds for 1000 nodule candidates. The results for nontraining cases are shown in Figure 13.8. In the output image of the MTANN for nodules, the nodules are represented by light distributions as expected. The output images for very small (including peripheral) vessels and medium-sized vessels (with relatively high contrast) are almost uniformly dark, as shown in Figure 13.8. Because 70% of FPs are small (including peripheral) and medium-sized vessels, we can reduce a large number of FPs by using the output images of the MTANN. Output images for other types of FPs are shown in Figure 13.9. The trained MTANNs were able to suppress such various types of FPs.

The scoring method was applied to the output images of the MTANN. The standard deviation of the Gaussian function for scoring was determined as $\sigma_1 = 4.0$ by use of empirical analysis based on the training set. We used an R_E of 25 × 25 pixels. Figure 13.10 shows the distributions of the scores from four expert MTANNs for the 40 nodules and 1068 nonnodules used for testing; these were different from the ten nodules and ten nonnodules used for training. Although the two distributions overlap, it is possible to distinguish a large number of nonnodules from nodules.

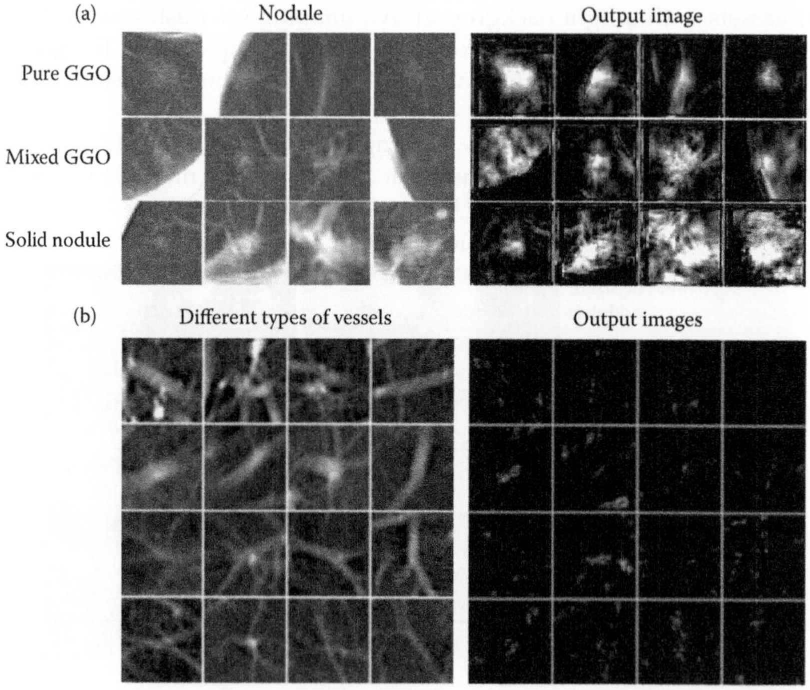

FIGURE 13.8
Illustrations of (a) nontraining actual nodules and (b) different types of vessels and the corresponding output images of the trained MTANN.

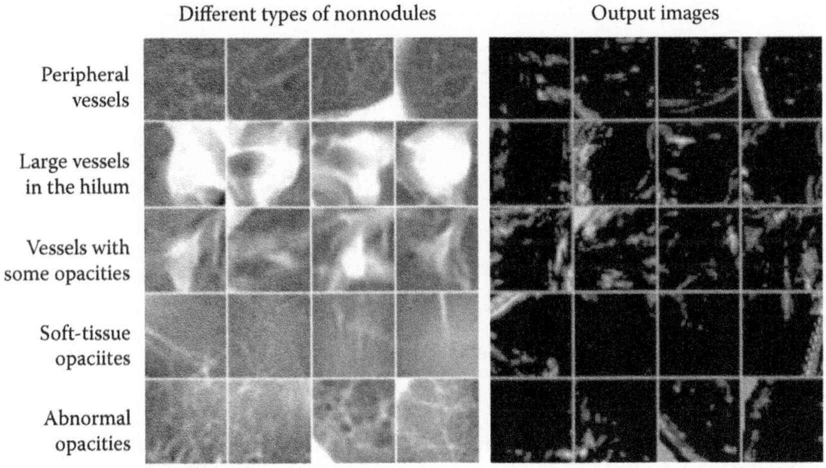

FIGURE 13.9
Illustrations of different types of nontraining nonnodules and the corresponding output images of the trained MTANN.

The performance of the single MTANN and the multiple expert MTANNs was evaluated by free-response receiver operating characteristic (FROC) curves (Bunch et al. 1978), as shown in Figure 13.11. The FROC curve represents the sensitivity as a function of the number of FPs per section at a specific operating point, which is determined by the threshold. The test set in our database consisted of 63 LDCT scans (a total of 1,765 LDCT images) and contained 71 nodules including 66 biopsy-confirmed primary cancers. The single MTANN (MTANN no. 1) and the multiple MTANNs which employed nine MTANNs were applied to the 58 true positives (nodules) and 1726 FPs (nonnodules), which were reported by our current CAD scheme for the test set. Note that none of the parameters of the single MTANN and the multiple MTANNs were changed. The FROC curves of the single MTANN and the multiple MTANNs in a validation test are shown in Figure 13.11. By using the single MTANN, we were able to remove 54% (938/1726) of FPs (nonnodules) without eliminating

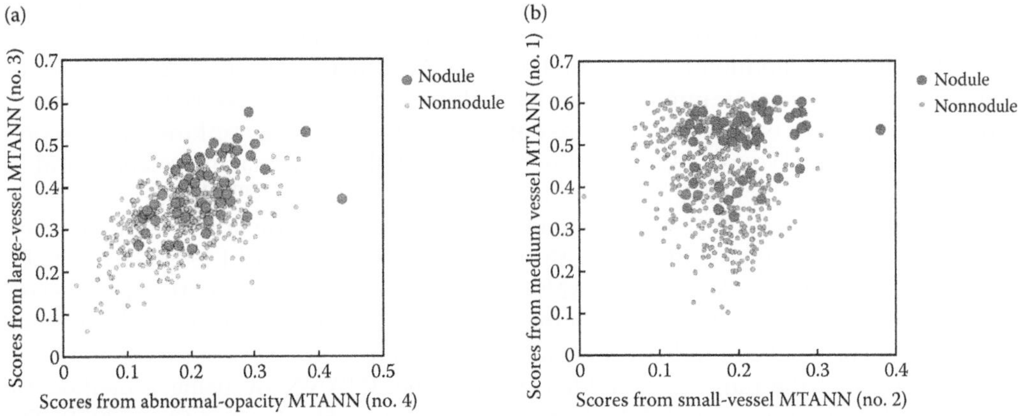

FIGURE 13.10
(See color insert.) Distributions of scores from expert MTANN nos. 1–4 for reduction of four different types of FPs. (a) Scores from MTANN nos. 1 and 2. (b) Scores from MTANN nos. 3 and 4.

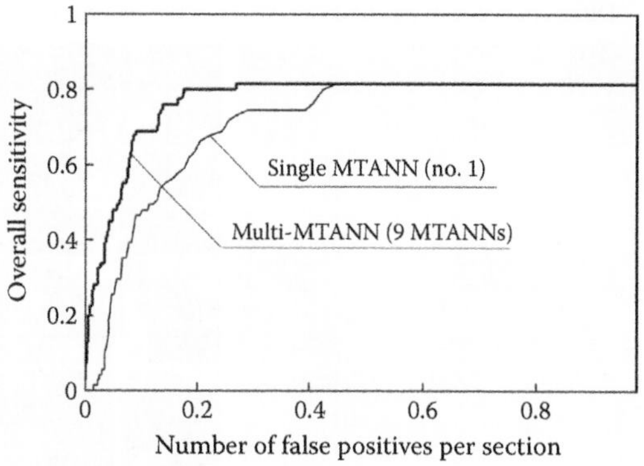

FIGURE 13.11
FROC curves of the single MTANN (MTANN no. 1) and the multiple expert MTANNs for the test set consisting of 57 true-positive nodules and 1726 FPs (nonnodules) in a validation test. (Reprinted with permission from Suzuki, K. et al., *Medical Physics*, 30, 7, 1602–1617, 2003.)

any true positives (nodules), i.e., a classification accuracy of 100% (58/58). With the multiple expert MTANNs including nine MTANNs, 83% (1424/1726) of nonnodules were removed with a reduction of one true positive, i.e., a classification sensitivity of 98.3% (57 of 58 nodules). Therefore, by use of the multiple expert MTANNs, the FP rate of our current CAD scheme was improved from 0.98 to 0.18 FPs per section (from 27.4 to 4.8 per patient) at an overall sensitivity of 80.3% (57/71).

13.5.2 Results for Chest Radiographs

Figure 13.12 illustrates the effect of the background-trend correction and the contrast normalization. Because the variations in the backgrounds and the contrast of the original ROIs are large, as shown in Figure 13.12, it is difficult to distinguish nodules from nonnodules in the original ROIs. Performing the background-trend correction and contrast normalization substantially reduced the variations in the backgrounds and the contrast, as shown in Figure 13.12. The contrast of the nodules and their backgrounds are relatively constant in the processed ROIs. It is apparent that the distinction between nodules and nonnodules in the processed ROIs is superior to that in the original ROIs.

We classified FPs (nonnodules) reported by our CAD scheme into six groups by use of a method for determining training samples for multiple expert MTANNs. With this method, training samples for each MTANN were determined based on the ranking in the scores in the FROC space. We used 12 typical nodules selected by an imaging scientist and 12 nonnodules from each of six groups as training samples for each MTANN. A three-layer structure was employed as the structure of each MTANN because any continuous mapping can be realized approximately by three-layer ANNs (Funahashi 1989; Barron 1993). The size of the subregion R_S of the MTANN, the standard deviation σ_T of the 2D Gaussian distribution, and the size of the training region R_T in the teaching image were determined empirically to be 9 × 9, 5.0, and 19 × 19 pixels, respectively.

We determined the number of hidden units of the MTANN by using a method for designing the structure of an ANN (Suzuki 2004; Suzuki, Horiba, and Sugie 2001). The method is a sensitivity-based pruning method, i.e., the sensitivity to the training error was calculated when a certain unit was removed experimentally, and the unit with the smallest training error was removed. Removing the redundant hidden units and retraining for

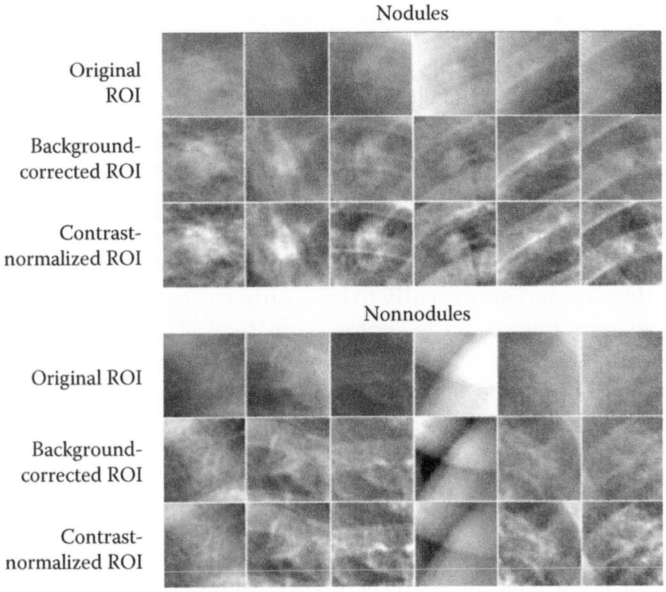

FIGURE 13.12
Illustration of the effect of the background-trend correction and the contrast normalization. (Reprinted with permission from Suzuki, K. et al., *Academic Radiology*, 12, 2, 191–201, 2005.)

recovering the potential loss due to the removal were performed alternately, resulting in a reduced structure where redundant units were removed. As a result, the number of hidden units was determined to be 20. Thus, the numbers of units in the input, hidden, and output layers were 81, 20, and 1, respectively. With the parameters above, the training of each MTANN in the multiple expert MTANNs was performed 500,000 times. The training took a CPU time of 29.8 hours on a PC-based workstation (CPU: Pentium IV, 1.7 GHz), and the time for applying the trained MTANN to nodule candidates was negligibly small.

Figure 13.13 shows nontraining nodules and the corresponding output images of the trained single MTANN no. 1. Various nodules are represented by bright distributions.

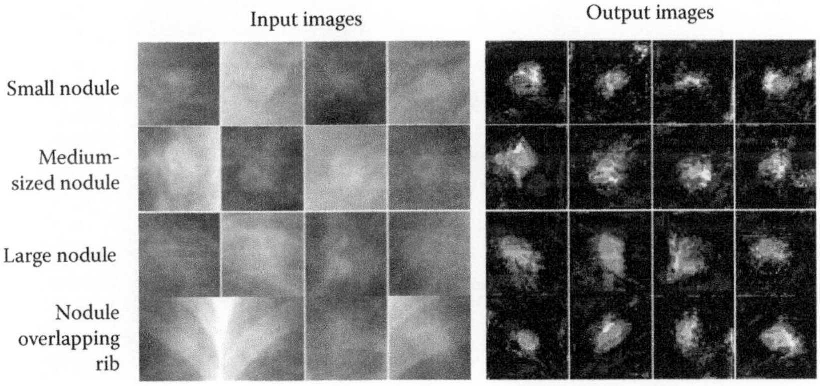

FIGURE 13.13
Illustrations of various nontraining nodules and the corresponding output images of the trained MTANN no. 1. (Reprinted with permission from Suzuki, K. et al., *Academic Radiology*, 12, 2, 191–201, 2005.)

Figure 13.14 shows nontraining, nonnodule images and the corresponding output images of each of the six MTANNs for nontraining cases. The nodules in the output images of the MTANN were represented by bright distributions near the centers of the nodules, whereas nonnodules in the corresponding group for which the MTANN was trained in the output images were mostly dark around the center, as expected. It is apparent that the distinction between nodules and nonnodules in the output images of the MTANN is superior to that in the original images. We applied the trained multiple expert MTANNs to the 75 true positives (nodules) and the 410 FPs (nonnodules) produced by our CAD scheme. The scoring method was applied to the output images of the MTANNs, where the standard deviation σ_n was determined empirically to be within the range from 4.5 to 7.7. Figure 13.15 shows the relationships between the scores from two MTANNs in the multiple expert MTANNs. The results show that each MTANN could remove different nonnodules without removal of any true positive; thus, various nonnodules could be eliminated by use of the multiple expert MTANNs. The performance of the multiple expert MTANNs was evaluated by FROC analysis, as shown in Figure 13.16. The FROC curve expresses an overall sensitivity as a function of the number of FPs per image at a specific operating point. With the multiple expert MTANNs, the number of FPs was reduced, and at a certain operating point on the FROC curve, it was reduced to 31.7% (130/410), with a reduction of one true positive. The FP rate of our original CAD scheme was improved from 4.5 to 1.4 (130/91) FPs per image at an overall sensitivity of 81.3% (74/91).

To investigate the generalization ability (performance for nontraining cases) of the multiple expert MTANNs, we evaluated the performance of the multiple expert MTANNs only with nontraining cases, i.e., the training cases of 12 nodules and 72 nonnodules were excluded from the evaluation. The performance of the multiple expert MTANNs for nontraining cases was similar to that of the multiple expert MTANNs for the complete database, as shown in Figure 13.16.

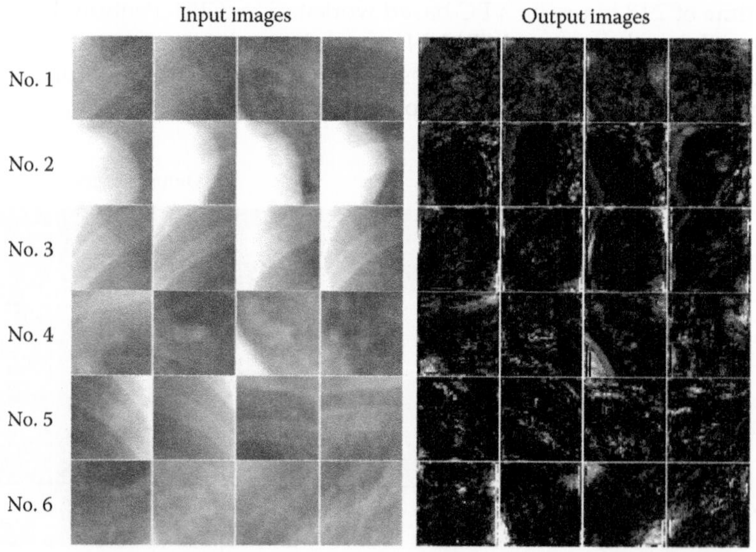

FIGURE 13.14
Illustrations of nontraining nonnodules and the corresponding output images of the trained MTANNs. (Reprinted with permission from Suzuki, K. et al., *Academic Radiology*, 12, 2, 191–201, 2005.)

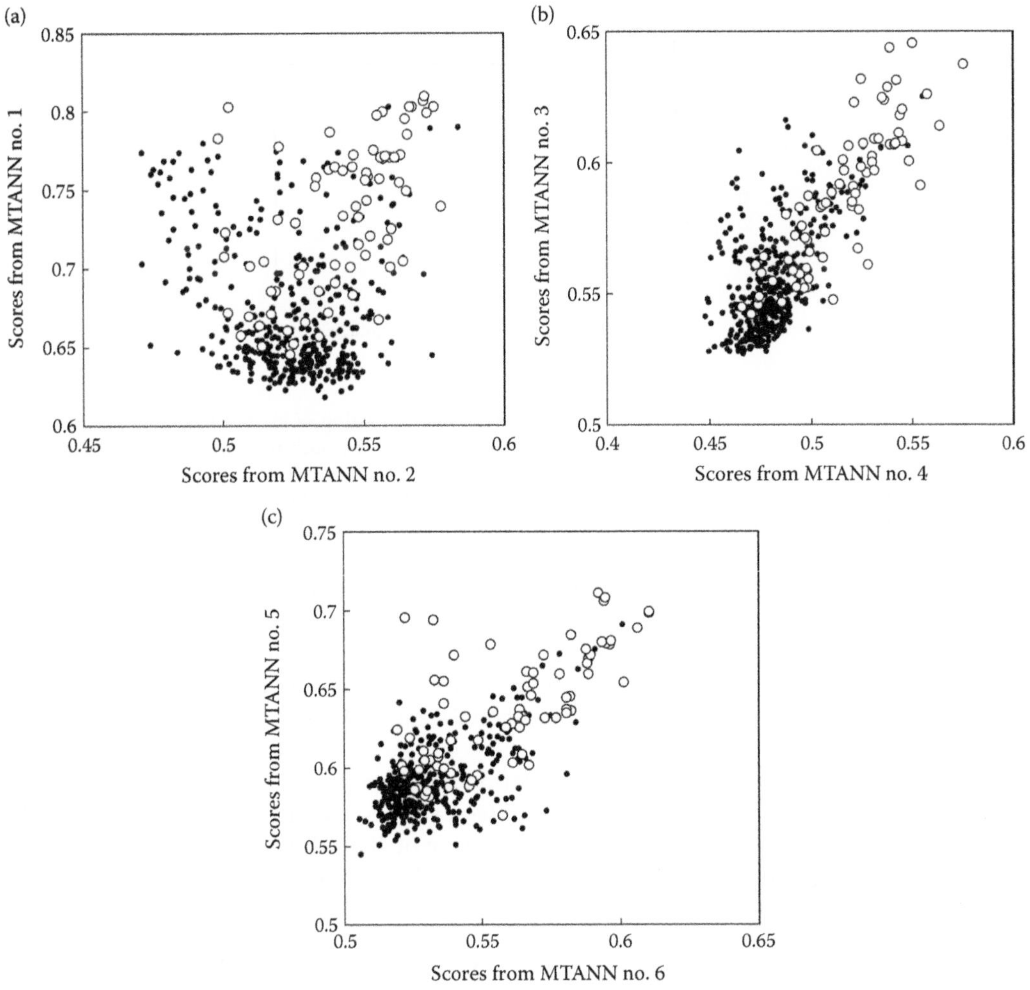

FIGURE 13.15
Relationships between scores from two MTANNs in the multiple expert MTANNs for nodules (white circles) and nonnodules (black circles). (a) Relationship between MTANN nos. 1 and 2, (b) that between MTANN nos. 3 and 4, and (c) that between MTANN nos. 5 and 6. (Reprinted with permission from Suzuki, K. et al., *Academic Radiology*, 12, 2, 191–201, 2005.)

13.6 Discussion

13.6.1 Thoracic CT CAD

Because diagnostic radiology is progressing rapidly as technology advances, a timely development of CAD schemes for diagnostic radiology is important. However, it is difficult for us to obtain a large number of training abnormal cases, particularly for a CAD scheme for diagnosis with a new modality such as a lung cancer screening with CT. The MTANN was able to be trained with such a small number of training cases. The key to this high generalization ability might be due to the division of one nodule image into

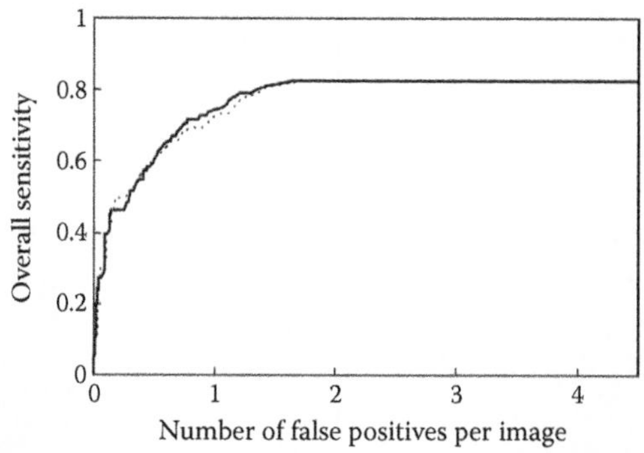

FIGURE 13.16
FROC curve (thick solid curve) of the multiple expert MTANNs consisting of six MTANNs for 75 true positives (nodules) and 410 FPs (nonnodules), and that (dotted curve) of the multiple expert MTANNs for nontraining cases, i.e., the training samples were excluded from the evaluation. The FROC curve of the multiple expert MTANNs indicates an 81.3% overall sensitivity and a reduction in the FP rate from 4.5 to 1.4 per image. (Reprinted with permission from Suzuki, K. et al., *Academic Radiology*, 12, 2, 191–201, 2005.)

a large number of subregions (Suzuki and Doi 2005). We treated the distinction between nodules and nonnodules as an image-processing task, in other words, as a highly nonlinear filter that performs both nodule enhancement and nonnodule suppression. This allowed us to train the MTANN not on a case basis, but on a subregion basis. The results might suggest that there are some consistent features of nodules in the local window.

To gain insight into such a high generalization ability of the MTANN, we investigated the effect of the number of training subregions, i.e., the size of the training region, R_T, on the performance for nontraining cases consisting of 40 nodules and 1068 nonnodules. The results show that the performance of the MTANN decreased as the number of training subregions decreased. However, there was no increase in the area under the ROC (Metz 1986) curve (AUC) (Hanley and McNeil 1983) values when the size of the training region, R_T, was increased from 19×19 to 25×25. This is the reason for employing 19×19 as the size of the training region, R_T. This result suggests that the reason for the high generalization ability of the MTANN is related to the large number of training subregions used.

To estimate roughly the number of units in the hidden layer required, a method for designing the optimal structure of an ANN (Suzuki 2004; Suzuki, Horiba, and Sugie 2001) was applied to the trained MTANN. The method is a sensitivity-based pruning method, i.e., the sensitivity to the training error was calculated when a certain unit was removed virtually, and the unit with the minimum training error was removed first. The redundant units in the hidden layer were removed on the basis of the effect of removing each unit on the training error, and then the MTANN was retrained to recover the potential loss due to this removal. Each process was performed alternately, resulting in a reduced structure where redundant units were removed. As a result, the optimal number of units in the hidden layer was determined as 22 units.

We examined the performance of the MTANN which is directly applied to the FPs reported by the multiple gray-level-thresholding technique in our current CAD scheme, instead of a combination of the rule-based and linear discriminant classifiers and the MTANN in this study. The majority of the FPs produced by the multiple gray-level-thresholding technique were relatively large vessels whose contrast was relatively high, compared to the FPs produced by our current CAD scheme including rule-based and linear discriminant classifiers. We applied MTANN no. 1 to 20,743 nodule candidates including 45 nodules identified by the multiple gray-level-thresholding technique. We achieved 5.87 FPs per section at a classification accuracy of 100%, i.e., an overall sensitivity of 90%. At an overall sensitivity of 80%, 1.85 FPs per section were achieved. The FPs eliminated by the rule-based and linear discriminant classifiers were different from those eliminated by the MTANN, although some of them overlapped. A combination of the rule-based and linear discriminant classifiers and the MTANN rather than the MTANN alone might be useful for distinction between nodules and nonnodules in a CAD scheme.

13.6.2 Chest Radiography CAD

We used 75 true-positive nodules of our original CAD scheme for testing MTANNs in this study. The performance of MTANNs on the false negatives (16 nodules) of our original scheme would be of interest. Because the false-negative nodules were relatively small and low contrast, it might also be difficult for MTANNs to maintain these false-negative nodules. However, the results of our experiments on CT images (Suzuki et al. 2003) indicated that the performance of MTANNs on the database that included computer false negatives which were small and low contrast was relatively high. Therefore, we believe that the performance of MTANNs on the false-negative nodules would be comparable to the performance on the true-positive nodules shown in this study.

13.7 Conclusion

We developed CAD schemes for lung nodule detection in thoracic CT and chest radiography. We employed an FP reduction method based on MTANNs for improving the performance of the CAD schemes. By use of the MTANNs, the FP rates of our CAD schemes for lung nodule detection on thoracic CT images and chest radiographs were improved substantially, while high sensitivities were maintained. The MTANN-based CAD schemes provide an accurate detection of lung nodules in thoracic CT and chest radiography. Therefore, our high-performance CAD schemes would be useful in improving the performance of radiologists in their detection of lung nodules in thoracic CT and chest radiographs.

Acknowledgments

The author is grateful to Heber MacMahon, MD; Kunio Doi, PhD; Samuel G. Armato III, PhD; Feng Li, MD, PhD; Shusuke Sone, MD; Hiroyuki Abe, MD, PhD; Hidetaka Arimura, PhD; Hotaka Takizawa, PhD; Qiang Li, PhD: Junji Shiraishi, PhD; Maryellen Giger, PhD; and Roger Engelmann, MS, for their valuable suggestions and contributions to this study, and to Mrs. Elisabeth F. Lanzl for improving the manuscript. The author is also grateful to Harumi Suzuki for her help with figures and graphs, and Mineru Suzuki and Juno Suzuki for cheering me up. This work was supported partially by the National Institutes of Health R01CA120549, S10 RR021039, and P30 CA14599.

References

Abe, K., K. Doi, H. MacMahon, M. L. Giger, H. Jia, X. Chen, A. Kano, and T. Yanagisawa. 1993. Computer-aided diagnosis in chest radiography. Preliminary experience. *Investigative Radiology* 28(11):987–993.

Arimura, H., S. Katsuragawa, K. Suzuki, F. Li, J. Shiraishi, S. Sone, and K. Doi. 2004. Computerized scheme for automated detection of lung nodules in low-dose computed tomography images for lung cancer screening. *Academic Radiology* 11(6):617–629.

Armato, S. G., 3rd, M. L. Giger, C. J. Moran, J. T. Blackburn, K. Doi, and H. MacMahon. 1999. Computerized detection of pulmonary nodules on CT scans. *Radiographics* 19(5):1303–1311.

Armato, S. G., 3rd, M. L. Giger, and H. MacMahon. 2001. Automated detection of lung nodules in CT scans: preliminary results. *Medical Physics* 28(8):1552–1561.

Armato, S. G., 3rd, F. Li, M. L. Giger, H. MacMahon, S. Sone, and K. Doi. 2002. Lung cancer: performance of automated lung nodule detection applied to cancers missed in a CT screening program. *Radiology* 225(3):685–692.

Armato, S. G., 3rd, M. B. Altman, and P. J. La Riviere. 2003. Automated detection of lung nodules in CT scans: effect of image reconstruction algorithm. *Medical Physics* 30(3):461–472.

Austin, J. H., B. M. Romney, and L. S. Goldsmith. 1992. Missed bronchogenic carcinoma: radiographic findings in 27 patients with a potentially resectable lesion evident in retrospect. *Radiology* 182(1):115–122.

Barron, A. R. 1993. Universal approximation bounds for superpositions of a sigmoidal function. *IEEE Transactions on Information Theory* 39(3):930–945.

Brown, M. S., M. F. McNitt-Gray, J. G. Goldin, R. D. Suh, J. W. Sayre, and D. R. Aberle. 2001. Patient-specific models for lung nodule detection and surveillance in CT images. *IEEE Transactions on Medical Imaging* 20(12):1242–1250.

Brown, M. S., J. G. Goldin, R. D. Suh, M. F. McNitt-Gray, J. W. Sayre, and D. R. Aberle. 2003. Lung micronodules: automated method for detection at thin-section CT—initial experience. *Radiology* 226(1):256–262.

Bunch, P. C., J. F. Hamilton, G. K. Sanderson, and A. H. Simmons. 1978. A free-response approach to the measurement and characterization of radiographic-observer performance. *Journal of Applied Photographic Engineering* 4:166–171.

Campadelli, P., E. Casiraghi, and D. Artioli. 2006. A fully automated method for lung nodule detection from postero-anterior chest radiographs. *IEEE Transactions on Medical Imaging* 25(12):1588–1603.

Carreira, M. J., D. Cabello, M. G. Penedo, and A. Mosquera. 1998. Computer-aided diagnoses: automatic detection of lung nodules. *Medical Physics* 25(10):1998–2006.

Coppini, G., S. Diciotti, M. Falchini, N. Villari, and G. Valli. 2003. Neural networks for computer-aided diagnosis: detection of lung nodules in chest radiograms. *IEEE Transaction on Information Technology in Biomedicine* 7(4):344–357.

Floyd, C. E., Jr., E. F. Patz, Jr., J. Y. Lo, N. F. Vittitoe, and L. E. Stambaugh. 1996. Diffuse nodular lung disease on chest radiographs: a pilot study of characterization by fractal dimension. *American Journal of Roentgenology* 167(5):1185–1187.

Funahashi, K. 1989. On the approximate realization of continuous mappings by neural networks. *Neural Networks* 2:183–192.

Giger, M. L., K. Doi, and H. MacMahon. 1988. Image feature analysis and computer-aided diagnosis in digital radiography. 3. Automated detection of nodules in peripheral lung fields. *Medical Physics* 15(2):158–166.

Giger, M. L., K. Doi, H. MacMahon, C. E. Metz, and F. F. Yin. 1990. Pulmonary nodules: computer-aided detection in digital chest images. *Radiographics* 10(1):41–51.

Giger, M. L., K. T. Bae, and H. MacMahon. 1994. Computerized detection of pulmonary nodules in computed tomography images. *Investigative Radiology* 29(4):459–465.

Gurcan, M. N., B. Sahiner, N. Petrick, H. P. Chan, E. A. Kazerooni, P. N. Cascade, and L. Hadjiiski. 2002. Lung nodule detection on thoracic computed tomography images: preliminary evaluation of a computer-aided diagnosis system. *Medical Physics* 29(11):2552–2558.

Gurney, J. W. 1996. Missed lung cancer at CT: imaging findings in nine patients. *Radiology* 199(1):117–122.

Hanley, J. A., and B. J. McNeil. 1983. A method of comparing the areas under receiver operating characteristic curves derived from the same cases. *Radiology* 148(3):839–843.

Hardie, R. C., S. K. Rogers, T. Wilson, and A. Rogers. 2008. Performance analysis of a new computer aided detection system for identifying lung nodules on chest radiographs. *Medical Image Analysis* 12(3):240–258.

Heelan, R. T., B. J. Flehinger, M. R. Melamed, M. B. Zaman, W. B. Perchick, J. F. Caravelli, and N. Martini. 1984. Non-small-cell lung cancer: results of the New York screening program. *Radiology* 151(2):289–293.

Henschke, C. I., D. I. McCauley, D. F. Yankelevitz, D. P. Naidich, G. McGuinness, O. S. Miettinen, D. M. Libby, M. W. Pasmantier, J. Koizumi, N. K. Altorki, and J. P. Smith. 1999. Early Lung Cancer Action Project: overall design and findings from baseline screening. *Lancet* 354(9173):99–105.

Henschke, C. I., D. P. Naidich, D. F. Yankelevitz, G. McGuinness, D. I. McCauley, J. P. Smith, D. Libby, M. Pasmantier, M. Vazquez, J. Koizumi, D. Flieder, N. Altorki, and O. S. Miettinen. 2001. Early lung cancer action project: initial findings on repeat screenings. *Cancer* 92(1):153–159.

Kanazawa, K., Y. Kawata, N. Niki, H. Satoh, H. Ohmatsu, R. Kakinuma, M. Kaneko, N. Moriyama, and K. Eguchi. 1998. Computer-aided diagnosis for pulmonary nodules based on helical CT images. *Computerized Medical Imaging and Graphics* 22(2):157–167.

Kaneko, M., K. Eguchi, H. Ohmatsu, R. Kakinuma, T. Naruke, K. Suemasu, and N. Moriyama. 1996. Peripheral lung cancer: screening and detection with low-dose spiral CT versus radiography. *Radiology* 201(3):798–802.

Katsuragawa, S., K. Doi, N. Nakamori, and H. MacMahon. 1990. Image feature analysis and computer-aided diagnosis in digital radiography: effect of digital parameters on the accuracy of computerized analysis of interstitial disease in digital chest radiographs. *Medical Physics* 17(1):72–78.

Ko, J. P., and M. Betke. 2001. Chest CT: automated nodule detection and assessment of change over time—preliminary experience. *Radiology* 218(1):267–273.

Kobayashi, T., X. W. Xu, H. MacMahon, C. E. Metz, and K. Doi. 1996. Effect of a computer-aided diagnosis scheme on radiologists' performance in detection of lung nodules on radiographs. *Radiology* 199(3):843–848.

Lampeter, W. A., and J. C. Wandtke. 1986. Computerized search of chest radiographs for nodules. *Investigative Radiology* 21(5):384–390.

Lawler, L. P., S. A. Wood, H. K. Pannu, and E. K. Fishman. 2003. Computer-assisted detection of pulmonary nodules: preliminary observations using a prototype system with multidetector-row CT data sets. *Journal of Digital Imaging* 16(3):251–261.

Lee, Y., T. Hara, H. Fujita, S. Itoh, and T. Ishigaki. 2001. Automated detection of pulmonary nodules in helical CT images based on an improved template-matching technique. *IEEE Transactions on Medical Imaging* 20(7):595–604.

Li, F., C. L. Novak, J. Qian, G. Kohl, and D. P. Naidich. 2001. Automatic detection of lung nodules from multi-slice low-dose CT images. *Proceedings of SPIE Medical Imaging* 4322:1828–1835.

Li, F., S. Sone, H. Abe, H. MacMahon, S. G. Armato, 3rd, and K. Doi. 2002. Lung cancers missed at low-dose helical CT screening in a general population: comparison of clinical, histopathologic, and imaging findings. *Radiology* 225(3):673–683.

Li, Q., S. Katsuragawa, and K. Doi. 2001. Computer-aided diagnostic scheme for lung nodule detection in digital chest radiographs by use of a multiple-template matching technique. *Medical Physics* 28(10):2070–2076.

Li, Q., S. Sone, and K. Doi. 2003. Selective enhancement filters for nodules, vessels, and airway walls in two- and three-dimensional CT scans. *Medical Physics* 30(8):2040–2051.

Lin, J. S., A. Hasegawa, M. Freedman, and S. K. Mun. 1995. Differentiation between nodules and end-on vessels using a convolution neural network architecture. *Journal of Digital Imaging* 8:132–141.
Lin, J. S., S. C. Lo, A. Hasegawa, M. T. Freedman, and S. K. Mun. 1996. Reduction of False Positives in Lung Nodule Detection using a Two-Level Neural Classification. *IEEE Transactions on Medical Imaging* 15(2):206–217.
Lo, S. C., S. L. Lou, J. S. Lin, M. T. Freedman, M. V. Chien, and S. K. Mun. 1995. Artificial Convolution Neural Network Techniques and Applications to Lung Nodule Detection. *IEEE Transactions on Medical Imaging* 14(4):711–718.
Lou, S. A., C. L. Chang, K. P. Lin, and T. S. Chen. 1999. Object-based deformation technique for 3-D CT lung nodule detection. Paper read at Proceedings of SPIE Medical Imaging, May.
MacMahon, H., K. Doi, H. P. Chan, M. L. Giger, S. Katsuragawa, and N. Nakamori. 1990. Computer-aided diagnosis in chest radiology. *Journal of Thoracic Imaging* 5(1):67–76.
Mao, F., W. Qian, J. Gaviria, and L. P. Clarke. 1998. Fragmentary window filtering for multiscale lung nodule detection: preliminary study. *Academic Radiology* 5(4):306–311.
McCulloch, C. C., R. A. Kaucic, P. R. Mendonca, D. J. Walter, and R. S. Avila. 2004. Model-based detection of lung nodules in computed tomography exams. Thoracic computer-aided diagnosis. *Academic Radiology* 11(3):258–266.
Metz, C. E. 1986. ROC methodology in radiologic imaging. *Investigative Radiology* 21(9):720–733.
Miettinen, O. S., and C. I. Henschke. 2001. CT screening for lung cancer: coping with nihilistic recommendations. *Radiology* 221(3):592–596.
Mosier, C. I. 1951. Problems and designs of cross-validation. *Educational and Psychological Measurement* 11:5–11.
Nawa, T., T. Nakagawa, S. Kusano, Y. Kawasaki, Y. Sugawara, and H. Nakata. 2002. Lung cancer screening using low-dose spiral CT: results of baseline and 1-year follow-up studies. *Chest* 122(1):15–20.
Oda, T., M. Kubo, Y. Kawata, N. Niki, K. Eguchi, H. Ohmatsu, R. Kakinuma, M. Kaneko, M. Kusumoto, N. Moriyama, K. Mori, and H. Nishiyama. 2002. Detection algorithm of lung cancer candidate nodules on multislice CT images. Paper read at Proceedings of SPIE Medical Imaging.
Okumura, T., T. Miwa, J. Kako, S. Yamamoto, M. Matsumoto, Y. Tateno, T. Iinuma, and T. Matsumoto. 1998. Image processing for computer-aided diagnosis of lung cancer screening system by CT (LSCT). Paper read at Proceedings of SPIE Medical Imaging.
Penedo, M. G., M. J. Carreira, A. Mosquera, and D. Cabello. 1998. Computer-aided diagnosis: a neural-network-based approach to lung nodule detection. *IEEE Transactions on Medical Imaging* 17(6):872–880.
Reeves, A. P., and W. J. Kostis. 2000. Computer-aided diagnosis of small pulmonary nodules. *Seminars in Ultrasound, CT and MR* 21(2):116–128.
Ryan, W. J., J. E. Reed, S. J. Swensen, and P. F. Sheedy. 1996. Automatic detection of pulmonary nodules in CT. Paper read at Proceedings of Computer Assisted Radiology.
Sankar, P., and J. A. Sklansky. 1982. Gestalt guided heuristic boundary follower for X-ray images of lung nodules. *IEEE Transactions on Pattern Analysis and Machine Intelligence* 4:326–331.
Shah, P. K., J. H. Austin, C. S. White, P. Patel, L. B. Haramati, G. D. Pearson, M. C. Shiau, and Y. M. Berkmen. 2003. Missed non-small cell lung cancer: radiographic findings of potentially resectable lesions evident only in retrospect. *Radiology* 226(1):235–241.
Schilham, A. M., B. van Ginneken, and M. Loog. 2006. A computer-aided diagnosis system for detection of lung nodules in chest radiographs with an evaluation on a public database. *Medical Image Analysis* 10(2):247–258.
Shiraishi, J., S. Katsuragawa, J. Ikezoe, T. Matsumoto, T. Kobayashi, K. Komatsu, M. Matsui, H. Fujita, Y. Kodera, and K. Doi. 2000. Development of a digital image database for chest radiographs with and without a lung nodule: receiver operating characteristic analysis of radiologists' detection of pulmonary nodules. *American Journal of Roentgenology* 174(1):71–74.
Shiraishi, J., H. Abe, R. Engelmann, and K. Doi. 2003. Characteristics of image database on the performance of computer-aided diagnosis for the detection of pulmonary nodules in chest radiographs. Paper read at Proceedings of SPIE Medical Imaging.

Sobue, T., T. Suzuki, M. Matsuda, T. Kuroishi, S. Ikeda, and T. Naruke. 1992. Survival for clinical stage I lung cancer not surgically treated. Comparison between screen-detected and symptom-detected cases. The Japanese Lung Cancer Screening Research Group. *Cancer* 69(3):685–692.

Sone, S., S. Takashima, F. Li, Z. Yang, T. Honda, Y. Maruyama, M. Hasegawa, T. Yamanda, K. Kubo, K. Hanamura, and K. Asakura. 1998. Mass screening for lung cancer with mobile spiral computed tomography scanner. *Lancet* 351(9111):1242–1245.

Sone, S., F. Li, Z. G. Yang, T. Honda, Y. Maruyama, S. Takashima, M. Hasegawa, S. Kawakami, K. Kubo, M. Haniuda, and T. Yamanda. 2001. Results of three-year mass screening programme for lung cancer using mobile low-dose spiral computed tomography scanner. *British Journal of Cancer* 84(1):25–32.

Suzuki, K. 2002. Efficient approximation of neural filters for removing quantum noise from images. *IEEE Transactions on Signal Processing* 50(7):1787–1799.

Suzuki, K. 2003. Neural edge enhancer for supervised edge enhancement from noisy images. *IEEE Transactions on Pattern Analysis and Machine Intelligence* 25(12):1582–1596.

Suzuki, K. 2004. Determining the receptive field of a neural filter. *Journal of Neural Engineering* 1(4):228–237.

Suzuki, K. 2004. Extraction of left ventricular contours from left ventriculograms by means of a neural edge detector. *IEEE Transactions on Medical Imaging* 23(3):330–339.

Suzuki, K. 2009. A supervised 'lesion-enhancement' filter by use of a massive-training artificial neural network (MTANN) in computer-aided diagnosis (CAD). *Physics in Medicine and Biology* 54(18):S31–S45.

Suzuki, K., and K. Doi. 2005. How can a massive training artificial neural network (MTANN) be trained with a small number of cases in the distinction between nodules and vessels in thoracic CT? *Academic Radiology* 12(10):1333–1341.

Suzuki, K., I. Horiba, and N. Sugie. 2001. A simple neural network pruning algorithm with application to filter synthesis. *Neural Processing Letters* 13(1):43–53.

Suzuki, K., I. Horiba, N. Sugie, and M. Nanki. 2002. Neural filter with selection of input features and its application to image quality improvement of medical image sequences. *IEICE Transactions on Information and Systems* E85-D(10):1710–1718.

Suzuki, K., S. G. Armato, 3rd, F. Li, S. Sone, and K. Doi. 2003. Massive training artificial neural network (MTANN) for reduction of false positives in computerized detection of lung nodules in low-dose computed tomography. *Medical Physics* 30(7):1602–1617.

Suzuki, K., F. Li, S. Sone, and K. Doi. 2005. Computer-aided diagnostic scheme for distinction between benign and malignant nodules in thoracic low-dose CT by use of massive training artificial neural network. *IEEE Transactions on Medical Imaging* 24(9):1138–1150.

Suzuki, K., J. Shiraishi, H. Abe, H. MacMahon, and K. Doi. 2005. False-positive reduction in computer-aided diagnostic scheme for detecting nodules in chest radiographs by means of massive training artificial neural network. *Academic Radiology* 12(2):191–201.

Suzuki, K., H. Abe, H. MacMahon, and K. Doi. 2006. Image-processing technique for suppressing ribs in chest radiographs by means of massive training artificial neural network (MTANN). *IEEE Transactions on Medical Imaging* 25(4):406–416.

Suzuki, K., H. Yoshida, J. Nappi, and A. H. Dachman. 2006. Massive-training artificial neural network (MTANN) for reduction of false positives in computer-aided detection of polyps: suppression of rectal tubes. *Medical Physics* 33(10):3814–3824.

Suzuki, K., H. Yoshida, J. Nappi, S. G. Armato, 3rd, and A. H. Dachman. 2008. Mixture of expert 3D massive-training ANNs for reduction of multiple types of false positives in CAD for detection of polyps in CT colonography. *Medical Physics* 35(2):694–703.

Suzuki, K., D. C. Rockey, and A. H. Dachman. 2010. CT colonography: advanced computer-aided detection scheme utilizing MTANNs for detection of "missed" polyps in a multicenter clinical trial. *Medical Physics* 30:2–21.

Suzuki, K., J. Zhang, and J. Xu. In press. Massive-training artificial neural network coupled with Laplacian-eigenfunction-based dimensionality reduction for computer-aided detection of polyps in CT colonography. *IEEE Transactions on Medical Imaging*.

Swensen, S. J., J. R. Jett, T. E. Hartman, D. E. Midthun, J. A. Sloan, A. M. Sykes, G. L. Aughenbaugh, and M. A. Clemens. 2003. Lung cancer screening with CT: Mayo Clinic experience. *Radiology* 226(3):756–761.

Vittitoe, N. F., J. A. Baker, and C. E. Floyd, Jr. 1997. Fractal texture analysis in computer-aided diagnosis of solitary pulmonary nodules. *Academic Radiology* 4(2):96–101.

Wiemker, R., P. Rogalla, A. Zwartkruis, and T. Blaffert. 2002. Computer-aided lung nodule detection on high-resolution CT data. Paper read at Proceedings of SPIE Medical Imaging.

Wormanns, D., M. Fiebich, M. Saidi, S. Diederich, and W. Heindel. 2002. Automatic detection of pulmonary nodules at spiral CT: clinical application of a computer-aided diagnosis system. *European Radiology* 12(5):1052–1057.

Wu, Y., K. Doi, M. L. Giger, C. E. Metz, and W. Zhang. 1994. Reduction of false-positives in computerized detection of lung nodules in chest radiographs using artificial neural networks, discriminant analysis, and a rule-based scheme. *Journal of Digital Imaging* 7:196–207.

Xu, X. W., K. Doi, T. Kobayashi, H. MacMahon, and M. L. Giger. 1997. Development of an improved CAD scheme for automated detection of lung nodules in digital chest images. *Medical Physics* 24(9):1395–1403.

Yamamoto, S., I. Tanaka, M. Senda, Y. Tateno, T. Iinuma, T. Matsumoto, and M. Matsumoto. 1994. Image processing for computer-aided diagnosis of lung cancer by CT (LDCT). *Systems and Computers in Japan* 25:67–80.

14

Lung Nodule and Tumor Detection and Segmentation

Jinghao Zhou and Dimitris N. Metaxas

CONTENTS

This chapter deals with detection and segmentation of the lung nodule and tumor, which can be used in various clinical applications, such as therapy response assessment. Therapy response assessment is critical for cancer patient management and new drug approval. Traditional methods to assess the response are based on measuring nodule and tumor size changes in one or two dimensions on computed tomography (CT) before and after therapy and can be biased. To investigate if changes in nodule and tumor volume can better assess therapy response, there is an urgent need to develop accurate and reproducible computer-aided tools. Automatic detection and segmentation of lung nodule and tumor is a difficult task, as lung nodule and tumor often have various sizes and irregular shapes and they can grow closer or attached to surrounding structures of similar density and intensity.

In the first part, we proposed a novel method for automatic detection and segmentation of ground glass opacity (GGO) nodule, a kind of nonsolid lung nodules. For GGO detection, we developed a classifier by boosting k-nearest neighbor (k-NN), whose distance measure was the Euclidean distance between the nonparametric density estimates of two examples. The detected GGO region was then automatically segmented by analyzing the texture likelihood map of the region.

In the second part, we proposed a novel method for automatic segmentation of large lung tumors. First, the lung areas that can be distorted by large lung tumors were segmented using robust active shape models (RASMs). Second, automatic detection and segmentation of large lung cancers used a supervised learning framework followed by the analysis of three-dimensional (3D) texture likelihood maps. Third, we presented promising results of our methods applied to different clinical applications. The proposed computer-aided methods may provide a new powerful tool for accurate and reproducible quantification of tumor volumes in lung cancer clinical trials.

14.1 Detection and Segmentation of GGO Nodule

14.1.1 Introduction

GGO is defined as hazy increased attenuation within a lung that is not associated with obscured underlying vessels but with preservation of bronchial and vascular margins [18]. It can reflect minimal thickening of the septal or alveolar interstitium, thickening of alveolar walls, or the presence of cells or fluid filling the alveolar spaces. It can represent an active disease such as pulmonary edema, pneumonia, or diffuse alveolar damage. The results of the Early Lung Cancer Action Project suggested that nodules with pure (nonsolid) or mixed (partially solid) GGO at thin-section CT are more likely to be malignant than are those with solid opacity [1]. A focal area of pure GGO on thin-section CT seems to be an early sign of bronchoalveolar carcinoma [19]. Pure GGO is useful for differentiating small localized bronchoalveolar carcinoma from small adenocarcinomas not having a replacement growth pattern [20]. Early detection and treatment of pure GGO can also improve a prognosis of lung cancer [21].

The appearances of GGO on CT images such as its shape, pattern, and boundary are very different from solid nodules. Thus, algorithms developed for segmentation of solid nodules are most likely to produce inaccurate results when applied to GGO. In ref. [22], a hybrid neural network of three single nets and an expert rule were applied to detect GGO. This method underestimated the GGO area due to its improper cut-off of the edges of GGO. Hence, this method might be used only for large GGO and might not be able to obtain accurate segmentation for small GGO. Ref. [6] detected GGO using automatic clustering techniques and focused only on GGO detection. GGO segmentation was not discussed in their work. On the other hand, ref. [13] proposed a GGO segmentation method based on Markov random field and vessel removal method based on shape analysis. However, they only focused on GGO segmentation. GGO detection was not discussed in their work.

In this chapter, we proposed a novel method for automatic detection and segmentation of GGO from chest CT images. For GGO detection, we developed a classifier by boosting k-NN, whose distance measure is the Euclidean distance between the nonparametric density estimates of two regions. The detected GGO region was then automatically segmented by analyzing the 3D texture likelihood map of the region. We also presented the statistical validation of the proposed classifier for automatic GGO detection as well as the very promising results of automatic GGO segmentation. The proposed method provided a new powerful tool for automatic detection as well as accurate and reproducible segmentation of GGO.

14.1.2 Methods

14.1.2.1 Threshold for Lung Area Segmentation

Grey-level thresholding methods were used to segment the lung area from the background in CT images [7].

14.1.2.2 Vessel and Noise Suppression with 3D Cylinder Filters

The accuracy of lung abnormalities detection might be hindered by various structures within a lung. To avoid this difficulty, we first developed a 3D cylinder filter to suppress intensity values of vessels and other elongated structures as well as noise inside a lung, while maintaining lung abnormalities intensity values intact [9]. The cylinder filter F_{cyl} is defined as

$$F_{\mathrm{cyl}}(x) = \min_{\theta}(\min_{y \in {}^{x}_{\theta}} I(y))$$

where ${}^{x}_{\theta}$ is the domain of the cylinder centered at x with orientation θ. F_{cyl} is a hybrid neighborhood proximity filter that produces strong responses to blob-like objects (i.e., GGO or large lesions). We have selected the parameters of F_{cyl} empirically and used a cylinder with the radii of 1, 2, and 3 voxels and the length of 7 voxels at 7 different orientations.

The effect of F_{cyl} is shown in Figure 14.1. Figure 14.1b shows the filter-response volume of F_{cyl} applied to Figure 14.1a. We can see from Figure 14.1b that vessels and noise are effectively suppressed while GGO remains intact. To isolate candidate GGO regions, i.e., regions of high response values, we apply a simple thresholding to the filter-response volume (Figure 14.1c). The threshold value is automatically determined by analyzing the histogram of the filter-response image, as illustrated in Figure 14.2.

14.1.2.3 Detection of GGO

To apply supervised learning framework, we first collected volumetric samples of positive (lung abnormalities) and negative (nonlung abnormalities) instances, as shown in Figure 14.3. Let Ψ_M be the region of a volumetric sample bounded by a cube. We estimated the probability density function (PDF) of the intensity values of the interior of Ψ_M. We used a

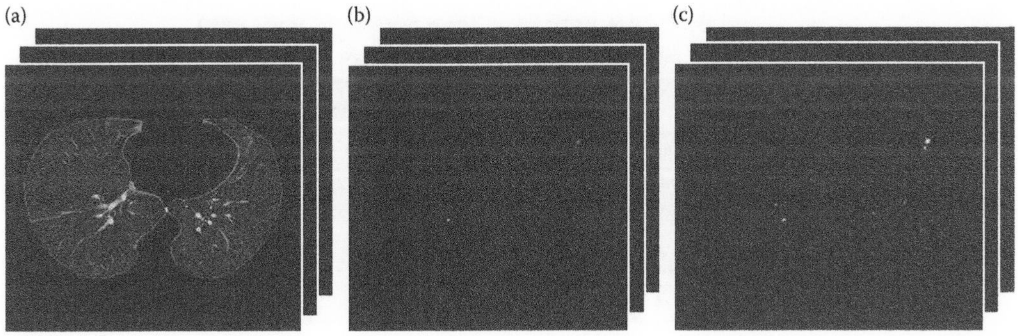

FIGURE 14.1
Effect of F_{cyl}: (a) original volume, (b) volume filtered with F_{cyc}, and (c) after thresholding.

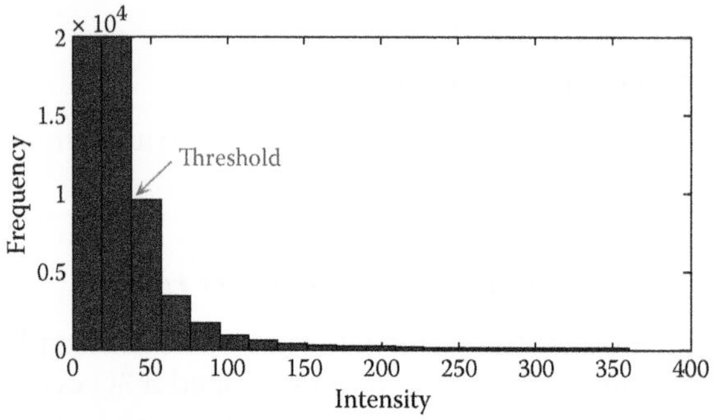

FIGURE 14.2
Histogram of a cylinder filtered volume.

nonparametric kernel-based method to approximate the PDF. Let $i, i = 0, \ldots, 255$ denote the random variable for intensity values. The intensity PDF of Ψ_M is defined by

$$P(i \mid \Psi_M) = \frac{1}{V(\Psi_M)} \iiint_{\Psi_M} \frac{1}{\sqrt{2\pi\sigma^2}} \exp\left(-\frac{(i - I(y))^2}{2\sigma^2}\right) dy \tag{14.1}$$

where $V(\Psi_M)$ denotes the volume of Ψ_M, y are the interior voxels of Ψ_M, and σ is the standard deviation of a Gaussian kernel. Figure 14.4 showed the typical intensity PDF of positive and negative instances. We could see from the figure that positive and negative instances

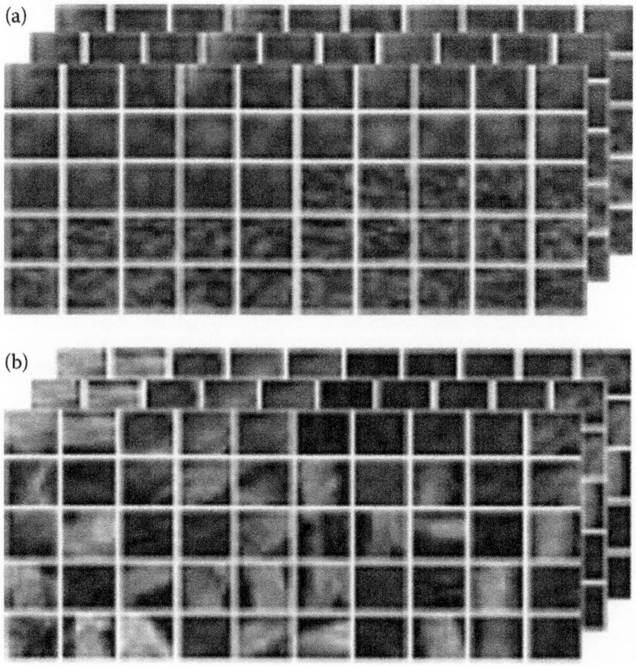

FIGURE 14.3
Volumetric samples for learning: (a) positive GGO samples and (b) negative (non-GGO) samples.

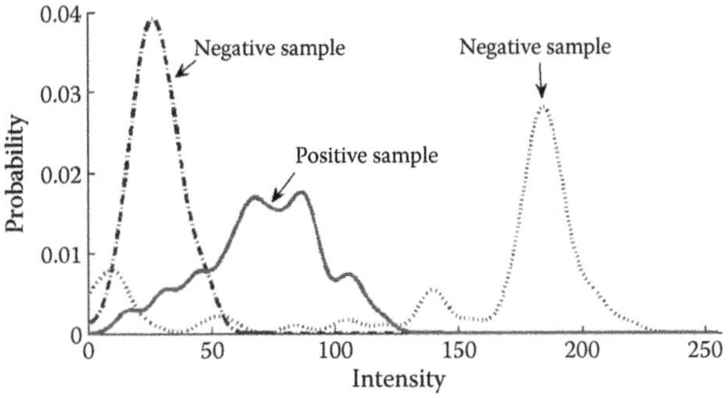

FIGURE 14.4
Typical PDFs of positive (solid line, GGO), negative (dash–dot line, typical background), and negative (dotted line, typical vessels) examples.

are well separable using the PDF. For this reason, we used as an instance the intensity PDF of the volumetric samples.

For the candidate lung abnormalities areas isolated, the learning for their classification has a discrete target function of the form $f : \mathfrak{R}^n \rightarrow V$, where V = {positive,negative}, with the label *positive* for lung abnormalities and *negative* for nonlung abnormalities areas. For k-NN, an instance x is represented as a point in n-dimensional space $\mathfrak{R}^n$ by a feature vector $\langle a_1(x), a_2(x), \ldots, a_n(x) \rangle$, where $a_i(x) = P(i|\Psi_M)$. The standard Euclidean distance is used as the distance measure between two instance vectors. Given a query instance x_q to be classified, k-NN returns $\hat{f}(x_q)$, as its estimate of $f(x_q)$, which is the most common value of f among the k training instances nearest to x_q:

$$\hat{f}(x_q) = \arg\max_{v \in V} \sum_{i=1}^{k} \delta(v, f(x_i))$$

where $x_1, \ldots, x_k$ denote the k instances from the training samples that are nearest to x_q, and $\delta(a,b) = 1$ if $a = b$ and $\delta(a,b) = 0$ otherwise. To obtain an accurate classification, k-NN requires a large training set, which results in slow classification due to the large number of distance calculations. We overcome this difficulty by boosting k-NN [15]. As in ref. [15], our purpose for boosting k-NN is to improve the speed of k-NN by reducing the number of prototype instances and thus reducing the required number of distance calculation without affecting the error rate. The details of boosting k-NN are given in ref. [15].

14.1.2.4 Segmentation of GGO Using Nonparametric Density Estimation

Because of the hazy appearance of lung abnormalities and the large overlap of intensity values between lung abnormalities and surrounding vessels, simple thresholding or edge-based segmentation methods do not produce acceptable results for lung abnormality segmentation. The proposed method applies 3D texture likelihood map method using a nonparametric density estimation for segmentation [23], followed by eigenanalysis of the Hessian matrix to accurately remove vessels overlapped with lung abnormalities [14,16].

We first extract the region of interest (ROI) surrounding a classified lung abnormalities. For each voxel in the ROI, we evaluate the likelihood of the voxel belonging to lung abnormalities by measuring 3D texture consistency between the lung abnormalities and a small spherical region (i.e., 3D texon) centered at the voxel.

Let Φ_M be the region of a volumetric sample of a classified lung abnormalities bounded by a sphere. Using Equation 14.1, we estimate the PDF of the intensity values of the interior of Φ_M, that is, $p_M = P(i|\Phi_M)$. Similarly, let Φ_T be the region of the 3D texon centered at the given voxel in the ROI. Using Equation 14.1, we also estimate the PDF of the intensity values of the interior of Φ_T, that is, $p_T = P(i|\Phi_T)$. To measure the dissimilarity between the two PDFs, we use an information theoretic distance measure called Kullback–Leibler divergence (KLD) [24]. The Bhattacharya distance, which is a symmetrized variation of KLD, between p_M and p_T is

$$B(p_M \mid\mid p_T) = -\log \rho(p_M \mid\mid p_T) = -\log \int [p_M(i)]^{\frac{1}{2}} [p_T(i)]^{\frac{1}{2}} \, di$$

We now evaluate the 3D texture likelihood of the 3D texon at every voxel in ROI. We define this likelihood using ρ, since it increases as the Bhattacharya distance between two distributions decreases. Figure 14.5b shows the 3D texture likelihood map of the volume in Figure 14.5a. The radius of 3D texons used in our chapter is 3 pixels, and the model interior texture is mostly homogeneous with some level noise. Thus, it is not necessary to consider the spatial correlation between pixels.

14.1.2.5 Removal Vessels Overlapped with Lung Abnormalities

Finally, we remove the vessels around lung abnormalities in the 3D texture likelihood map. The eigenanalysis of the Hessian matrix is a widely used method for vessel detection [14,16]. Given an image $I(x)$, the local intensity variations in the neighborhood of a point x_0 can be expressed with its Taylor expansion:

$$I(x_0 + h) \approx I(x_0) + h^T \nabla I(x_0) + h^T H(x_0) h$$

where $\nabla I(x_0)$ and $H(x_0)$ denote the gradient and the Hessian matrix at x_0, respectively. $H(x_0)$, whose components are the second-order derivatives, describes the curvature of $I(x)$ at

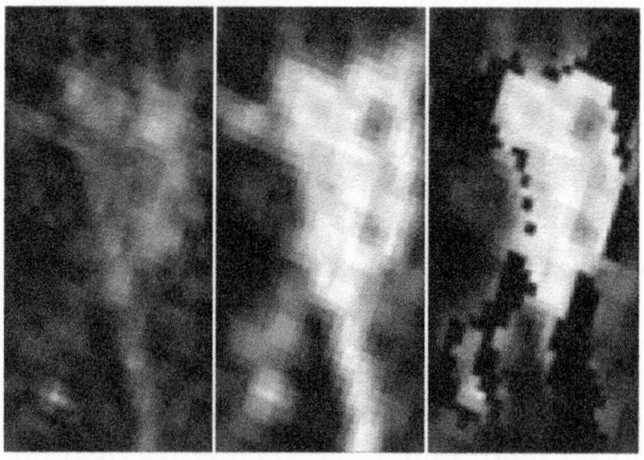

(a) (b) (c)

FIGURE 14.5
GGO segmentation: (a) ROI containing a classified GGO, (b) 3D likelihood map in ROI, and (c) 3D likelihood map in ROI after vessel removal.

TABLE 14.1
Criteria for Eigenvalues and Corresponding Shapes

Eigenvalues	Shape
$\lambda_1 \le 0, \lambda_2 \le 0, \lambda_3 \le 0$	Blob
$\lambda_1 \le 0, \lambda_2 \le 0, \lambda_3 \approx 0$	Tube
$\lambda_1 \le 0, \lambda_2 \approx 0, \lambda_3 \approx 0$	Plane
$\lambda_1 \le 0, \lambda_2 \le 0, \lambda_3 \ge 0$	Double cone

x_0. Let $\lambda_1, \lambda_2, \lambda_3$ and e_1, e_2, e_3 be the eigenvalues and eigenvectors of H such that $\lambda_1 \le \lambda_2 \le \lambda_3$ and $|e_i| = 1$. The signs and ratios of the eigenvalues provide the indications of various shapes of interest, as summarized in Table 14.1. Figure 14.5c shows the texture likelihood map after the removal of vessels in Figure 14.5b.

14.1.3 Results

14.1.3.1 Results of GGO Detection

To test the GGO detection method, we collected 600 volumetric samples (400 training samples and 200 testing samples). The samples were of size 9 × 9 × 3 voxels extracted from the CT volumes. Each sample was converted to an instance vector in $\Re^{256}$, representing its nonparametric density estimate. For the boosted *k*-NN, we used the standard Euclidean distance as the distance measure between two instances. We performed bootstrapping to estimate the generalization error of our GGO detection method [17]. We trained and tested the proposed method on bootstrap samples. After 20 steps of boosting, the test error rate converged to 3.70%. The accuracy is 96.3% for classification GGO, and the ROC curve is presented in Figure 14.6.

We also compared the boosted *k*-NN (20 boosting steps with $k = 3$) to other classifiers, i.e., *k*-NN classifier ($k = 3$), decision tree, support vector machine, neural network (one hidden layer, learning rate of 0.3), and Bayes network. Figure 14.7 summarizes the results. The multiple comparison test ($p = 0.05$) shows that the boosted *k*-NN and *k*-NN are significantly superior to other classifiers. Note that, although our purpose for boosting *k*-NN was not to improve the classification accuracy but rather to speed the classification process, the results show that boosting *k*-NN also improves the classification accuracy over *k*-NN.

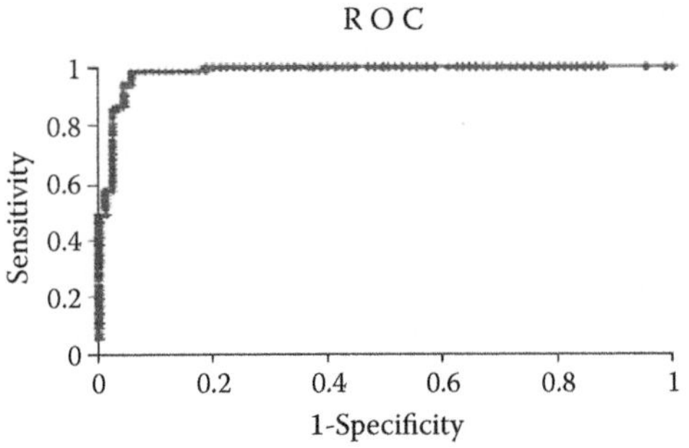

FIGURE 14.6
ROC curve measures the performance of the boosted *k*-NN method for GGO detection.

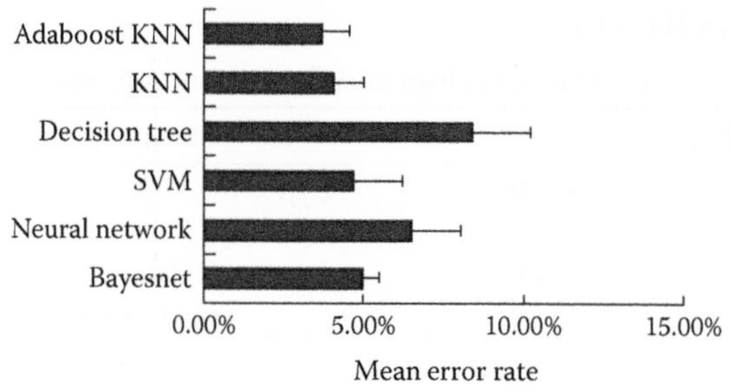

FIGURE 14.7
Comparison of the mean error rates of various classifiers by bootstrapping.

We applied the trained GGO classifier to 10 CT volumes containing 10 nodules. The CT volumes were acquired by multislice HRCT scanners with 1-mm slice collimation. The number of slices in each CT scan ranged from 23 to 29 (interpolated to 92 to 116), each of which consists of 512 × 512 pixels, with in-plane resolution ranging from 0.57 to 0.71 mm. The classifier detected the total of 11 nodules, which are all of the 10 nodules and 1 false-positive nodule.

The detected nodules were then segmented using the method described in Section 14.1.2. Figure 14.8 shows the GGO segmentation results overlaid on the original CT images and 3D reconstruction for four GGOs as examples. From the figure, we can see that the surrounding vessels are accurately removed from the GGO segmentation. Table 14.2 compares the greatest diameters, their greatest perpendicular diameters, and tumor volumes of the 10 lung GGOs from the results of the manual segmentation by experts and the automatic segmentation by the proposed method. The table shows that the mean relative error of the greatest diameter and its greatest perpendicular diameter are 2.4% and 3.2%, respectively, and shows that the mean relative error of the tumor volume is 3.2%. We also compared the overlapping ratios of the GGO regions segmented manually and automatically, which ranged from 87.5% to 95.7%. The mean overlapping ratio was 92.3%.

14.1.4 Conclusion

We proposed a novel method for the automatic detection and segmentation of GGO from chest CT images. The proposed method consists of two steps, i.e., GGO detection, followed by GGO segmentation. For GGO detection, vessels and noise were first suppressed using 3D cylinder filters. Then, candidate GGO regions were extracted by thresholding. We automatically selected the threshold by the intensity histogram analysis of the filter-response volumes. Finally, the candidate GGO regions were classified by boosting *k*-NN, whose distance measure was the Euclidean distance between the intensity PDFs of two examples. The validation of the proposed method using bootstrapping shows the mean error rate of 3.70%. Our method applied to clinical chest CT volumes containing 10 GGO nodules also showed the promising results, detecting all of the 10 nodules with one false-positive nodule.

Image texture, a function of the spatial variation in pixel intensities, is important in a variety of applications. One image analysis application of image texture is the recognition of image regions using texture properties. For example, based on textural properties, we

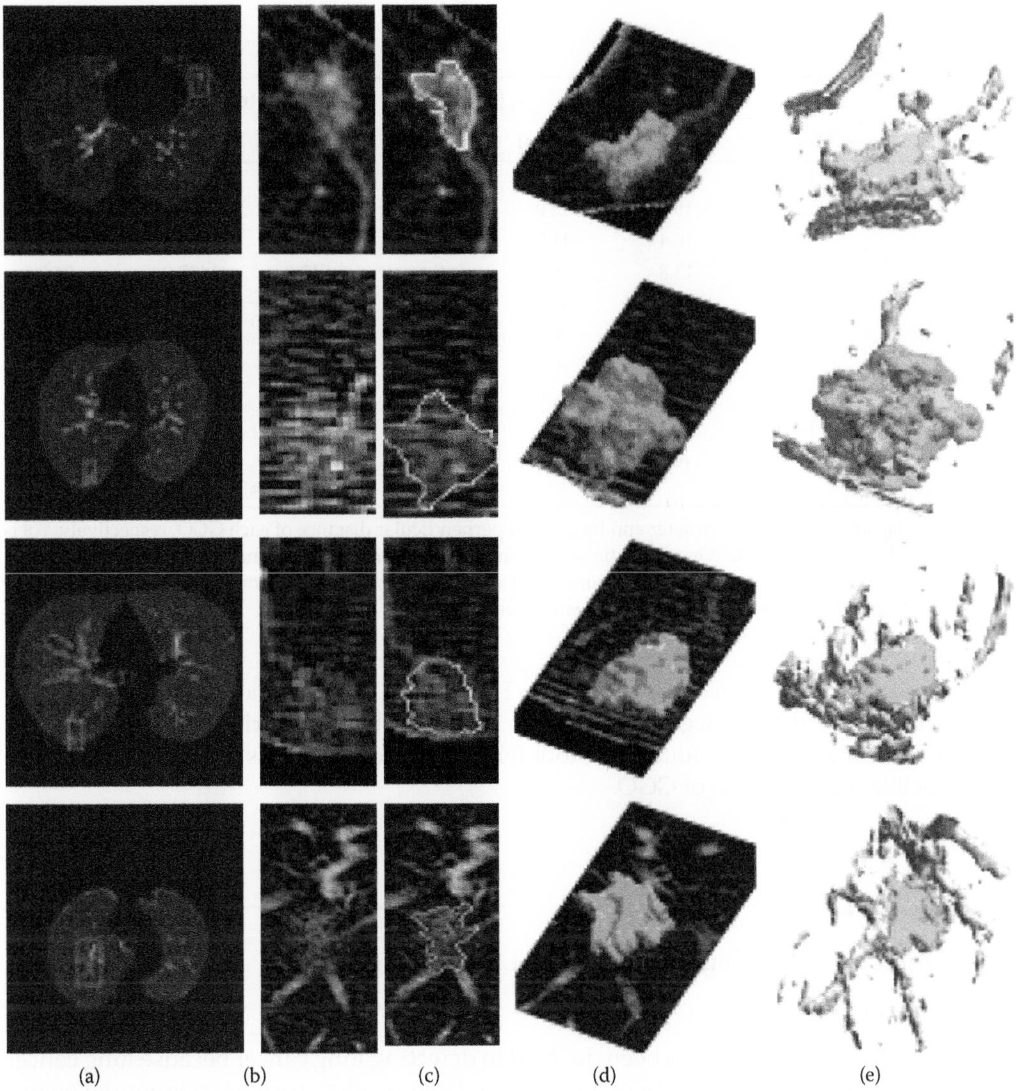

FIGURE 14.8
(See color insert.) GGO segmentation—four segmented GGO nodules are shown: (a) original CT images containing GGO nodules, (b) enlarged GGO areas, (c) segmented GGO, (d) 3D reconstruction of segmented GGO overlaid with original CT images in (a), and (e) 3D reconstruction of segmented GGO with other nearby structures.

can identify a variety of materials such as cotton canvas, straw matting, raffia, herringbone weave, and pressed calf leather. Texture is the most important visual cue in identifying these types of homogeneous regions. This is called texture classification. The goal of texture classification then is to produce a classification map of the input image where each uniform textured region is identified with the texture class it belongs to. In this chapter, the texture we used to detect the GGO is an extensive and amorphous texture called GGO [25].

Each GGO region classified was then automatically segmented by analyzing the 3D texture likelihood map of the region. We presented various results of GGO detection and

TABLE 14.2
Comparisons

Data Set	d_1 (mm)		d_2 (mm)		Vol (mm^3)		Overlap Ratio (%)
	Manual	Auto	Manual	Auto	Manual	Auto	
1	17.0	17.6	15.8	16.4	717.6	763.4	91.6
2	15.1	15.8	12.0	12.6	655.4	699.9	94.5
3	15.8	16.4	11.3	11.9	436.1	466.1	91.5
4	13.9	13.8	8.2	7.6	542.6	487.3	94.3
5	10.1	9.5	8.2	7.6	440.8	404.1	90.7
6	34.0	35.3	20.8	21.4	2610.0	2766.52	95.0
7	6.3	5.7	4.4	3.8	85.3	78.8	95.7
8	7.6	6.9	6.3	5.7	218.0	192.0	92.5
9	10.1	9.5	5.7	5.6	201.8	187.3	90.1
10	6.93	6.3	6.3	5.7	167.3	145.5	87.5
Mean error (%)	2.4		3.2		3.2		92.3

Note: d_1 and d_2 are the greatest diameter and its greatest perpendicular distance of each GGO, respectively. Vol is the volume of each GGO. Overlap ratio is the volume overlap ration of the manual segmentation results and automatic segmentation results. Manual and auto are the measurements on the manual segmentation results and the automatic segmentation results, respectively.

segmentation from clinical chest CT images. The manual segmentation of GGO has proved to be problematic due to large interobserver and intraobserver variations. The proposed method introduces a novel automatic tool for accurate detection as well as accurate and reproducible segmentation of GGO.

14.2 Detection and Segmentation of Large Lung Cancer

14.2.1 Introduction

A great amount of research has been devoted to detecting lung cancer because lung cancer is responsible for more than 25% of all cancer-related deaths every year. From the beginning of the lung cancer CT screening programs, the computer-aided diagnosis (CAD) has been a prominent field in medical image analysis–related publications. In the past years, the main research interest is on the detection of lung nodules. This is further divided into two related research areas: the measurements of nodule size and the characterization of nodule appearance. Both measurements are used to attempt to estimate of the probability of malignancy of lung tumor.

The development of the CAD systems that can be used in clinical practice requires the algorithms developed in the system to be evaluated on large numbers of cases. The collection of well-characterized clinical cases needs a huge amount of energy and expense. The availability of an open database [4] could spur advanced research work on the CAD systems. Further, it is also very important to measure the system performance in clinical field and evaluate the usefulness of CAD by radiologists.

The evaluation of therapy response is critical for determining whether a particular treatment is effective on a specific cancer type in a patient. Traditionally, the ways to assess the response are based on measuring size changes of cancer in a transverse image using CT before and after a treatment [26,27]. However, the traditional unidimensional (maximal diameter of tumor) and bidimensional (product of maximal diameter and its perpendicular maximal diameter) measurements can be biased especially when a tumor is not spherical in shape and does not change its shape in a spherical fashion. The preliminary result in a lung cancer study [28] showed that the changes in tumor volume could be determined as early as 3 weeks after a novel chemotherapy, whereas the changes of tumor volume measured in the traditional methods were significantly less sensitive in the same time period. In addition, manual delineation of tumor contours is time-consuming and lacks the reproducibility. Therefore, there is an urgent need for automatic detection and accurate segmentation methods for the volumetric assessment of therapy response.

Unlike small lung nodules, lung cancers to be treated are often large, with spiculate edges, and grow against surrounding structures such as the chest wall, the mediastinum, and blood vessels, which make automatic detection and segmentation difficult [28]. Thus, the algorithms developed for automatic detection and segmentation of small solid lung nodules are most likely to fail when applied to large lung cancers [5,8,10–12,29–32]. In those studies, larger lung lesions that were attached to the chest wall and mediastinum could be easily and mistakenly excluded from the segmented lungs in which the subsequent lesion detection would be performed [5,8,10,11]. Also, the existing segmentation algorithms often assumed that small lung nodules would possess spherical shape, which is not adequate for describing large lung cancers. Furthermore, the inability to separate a larger lesion from its surrounding structures of similar intensities was another shortcoming of the existing segmentation algorithms.

In this chapter, we propose novel methods for automatic segmentation of lung areas as well as automatic detection and segmentation of large lung cancers from CT images for the purpose of therapy response assessment. We first propose an RASM for the accurate segmentation of lung areas that are distorted and occluded by large lung cancers. Next, we develop a classifier for the detection of cancers in the segmented lung areas by boosting a *k*-NN classifier, whose distance measure is the Euclidean distance between the nonparametric density estimates of two regions. The statistical validation of the proposed classifier is also provided. Finally, the classified cancers are automatically segmented by analyzing 3D texture likelihood maps of the surrounding areas. We present the promising experimental results of our method applied to various clinical data. The proposed methods would provide a new powerful tool for automatic detection as well as accurate and reproducible segmentation of lung cancers for therapy response assessment in lung cancers.

14.2.2 Methods

14.2.2.1 RASMs for Lung Area Segmentation

Large lung cancers often grow against surrounding structures, such as the chest wall and mediastinum. Lung areas that are distorted and occluded by such lesions are hard to segment due to the similarity of the intensities between the cancers and the surrounding structures in CT images. In this section, we develop a robust method to accurately segment lung areas occluded by large cancers by improving the active shape model (ASM) framework.

An ASM represents the shapes of interest as a point distribution model [33]. Then, it constructs a shape space as a set of orthogonal basis P by applying the principal component analysis and finds an optimal shape for a new example of the shapes with principal component analysis reconstruction. Given the shape space P, the projection C of a new example shape X is given as $C = P^T\,\mathrm{d}X$, where $\mathrm{d}X = X - \bar{S}$ and $\bar{S}$ is the mean shape from the aligned shapes of the training set. Based on projection C, we can easily find a corresponding shape in the shape space as $\tilde{X} = PC + \bar{S}$. For simplicity, we denoted $\mathrm{d}\tilde{X} = PC\mathrm{d}$. Since $\bar{S}$ is constant, the accuracy of $\tilde{X}$ depends on C, which is related to $\mathrm{d}X$. In many applications, $\mathrm{d}X$ is often optimized with some low-level image features such as the gradient along normal directions to the boundary of an initial shape toward the strongest edge in the image [33].

The ASM method as described above, however, is not suitable for the accurate segmentation of lung areas with large cancers attached on their walls, since the cancers occlude the real boundary of the lung and appear as the strongest edge, as illustrated in Figure 14.9a and 14.9b. To overcome this difficulty, we develop a RASM based on the robust *M*-estimator [34]. The goal is to recover the projection C with the majority of the correct $\mathrm{d}X$ and restrain the outlier points of $\mathrm{d}X$. Mathematically, it computes C by minimizing the following robust energy function:

$$E_{\mathrm{rpac}}(C) = \min_{C} G(\|\mathrm{d}X - PC\|, \sigma) \tag{14.2}$$

where $G(x,\sigma) = x^2/(x^2 + \sigma^2)$ is the Geman–McClure error function and σ is a scale parameter that controls the convexity of the robust function. The solution for C can be obtained by an iterative gradient descent search on E_{rpca}:

$$C^{(n+1)} = C^{(n)} + \lambda \Delta C \tag{14.3}$$

where λ is a small constant that determines the step size and

$$\Delta C = \frac{\partial E_{\mathrm{rpca}}}{\partial C} = -2P(\mathrm{d}X - PC)\frac{\sigma^2}{\left(\|\mathrm{d}X - PC\|^2 + \sigma^2\right)^2}$$

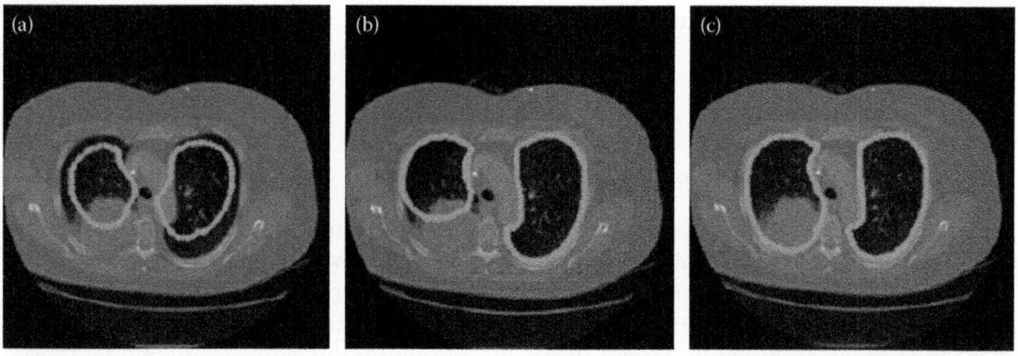

FIGURE 14.9
The segmented lung area using RASM (the bright lines are the connected contour of the ASM model): (a) large cancers attached to the chest wall and mediastinum and the initialization of the ASM, (b) ASM finding the false boundary of lung, and (c) RASM finding the correct boundary of the lung; the large white area in the left lung is a large lung cancer.

The iterative process is performed until $\left\| E_{\text{rpca}}^{(t+1)} - E_{\text{rpca}}^{(t)} \right\| < \varepsilon$, where ε is a preselected tolerance. Using the robust projection C^*, we obtain a robust shape in the shape space as

$$\tilde{X} = PC^* + \bar{S}$$

The result of this process is illustrated in Figure 14.9c, where the lung area occluded by a large lesion is accurately segmented.

14.2.2.2 Detection of Large Lung Cancers

In this section, we present a novel method for automatic detection of large lung cancers from the segmented lung areas. The method is based on 3D texture analysis using a machine learning framework, i.e., boosting the *k*-NN classifier. However, the accuracy of the detection may be hindered by various structures within a lung. Thus, we first apply a 3D cylinder filter to suppress the intensity values of vessels and other elongated structures as well as noise inside a lung while maintaining the intensity values of large lung cancers intact [9,35]. The cylinder filter F_{cyl} is defined as

$$F_{\text{cyl}}(x) = \min_{\theta}(\min_{y \in {}_{\theta}^{x}} I(y))$$

where ${}_{\theta}^{x}$ is the domain of the cylinder filter centered at x with orientation θ. F_{cyl} is a hybrid minimum neighborhood filter that produces strong responses to large blob-like objects (e.g., large cancers). In this chapter, we have selected the parameters of F_{cyl} empirically and used a cylinder with radii of 1, 2, and 3 voxels and length of 7 voxels at 7 different orientations. In Figure 14.10a and 14.10b, we can see that vessels and noise are effectively suppressed while the large lung cancers remains intact. After the filtering, we isolate the candidate regions for large lung lesions by simple thresholding (Figure 14.10c). The threshold value is automatically determined by analyzing the histogram of the filter response image [9]. Each candidate region is then classified with a learning framework described below.

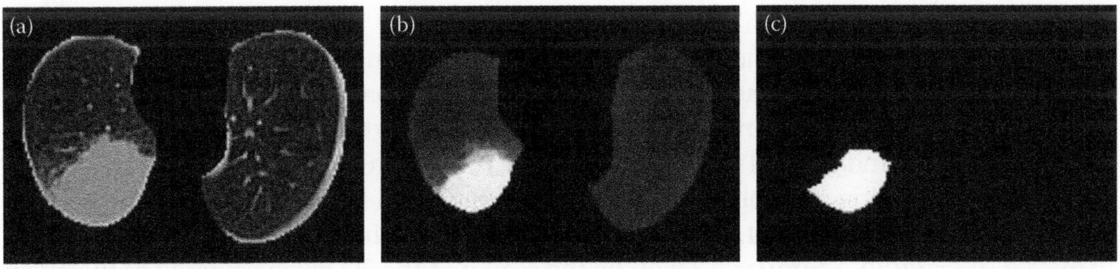

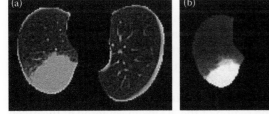

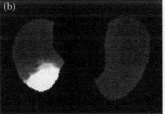

FIGURE 14.10
Effects of F_{cyl} (only one slice from the whole volume is shown): (a) original volume, (b) volume filtered with F_{cyl}, and (c) volume after thresholding.

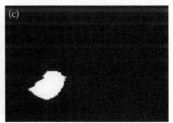

To apply a supervised learning framework, we collected volumetric samples for positive (lesion) and negative (nonlesion) examples manually. Let Ψ_M be the region of a volumetric sample bounded by a sphere. We estimate the PDF of the intensity values of the interior of Ψ_M. We use a nonparametric kernel based method to approximate the PDF. Let $i \in [0,255]$ denote the random variable for intensity values. The intensity PDF of Ψ_M is defined as

$$P(i \mid \Psi_M) = \frac{1}{V(\Psi_M)} \iiint_{\Psi_M} \frac{1}{\sqrt{2\pi\sigma^2}} \exp\left(-\frac{(i - I(y))^2}{2\sigma^2}\right) dy \tag{14.4}$$

where $V(\Psi_M)$ denotes the volume of Ψ_M, y is the voxel in the domain Ψ_M, and σ is the standard deviation of a Gaussian kernel.

For the candidate areas of large cancers isolated above, the learning for their classification has a discrete target function $f: R^n \rightarrow$ {positive,negative}, with the label *positive* for lesions and *negative* for nonlesions. For k-NN, an instance x is represented as a point in R^n by a feature vector $\langle a_1(x), a_2(x), \ldots, a_n(x) \rangle$, where $a_i(x) = P(i \mid \Psi_M)$. The Euclidean distance is used as the distance measure between two instance vectors. Given a query instance x_q to be classified, k-NN returns $\hat{f}(x_q)$ as its estimate of $f(x_q)$, which is the most common value of f among the k training instances nearest to x_q, that is, $\hat{f}(x_q) = \underset{v \in \{\text{positive,negative}\}}{\arg\max} \sum_{i=1}^{k} \delta(v, f(x_i))$, where $x_1, \ldots, x_k$ denote the k instances from training samples that are nearest to x_q and $\delta(a,b) = 1$ if $a = b$ and 0 otherwise. To obtain an accurate classification, k-NN requires a large training set, which results in slow classification due to the large number of distance calculations. We overcome this difficulty by boosting k-NN [15]. As in ref. [15], our purpose for boosting k-NN is to improve the speed of k-NN by reducing the number of prototype instances and thus reducing the required number of distance calculation without affecting the error rate.

14.2.2.3 Segmentation of Large Lung Cancers

We now segment the classified large lung cancers. Because of the hazy appearance and irregular shape of large lung cancers and the large overlap of intensity values between large lung cancers and surrounding vessels, simple thresholding and contour-based segmentation method do not provide accurate segmentation. The proposed method involves the analysis of a 3D texture likelihood map using a nonparametric density estimation [23], followed by eigenanalysis of the Hessian matrix to accurately remove vessels overlapped with large lung lesions.

We extract the ROI surrounding a classified large lung cancer based on the detection of the large lung cancers. For each voxel in the ROI, we evaluate the likelihood of the voxel belonging to a large lung cancer by measuring the 3D texture consistency between the large lung cancer and a small spherical region (i.e., 3D texon) centered at the voxel.

Let Φ_M be the region of a volumetric sample of a classified large lung cancer bounded by a sphere. Using Equation 14.4, we estimate the PDF of the intensity values of the interior of Φ_M, i.e., $p_M = P(i \mid \Phi_M)$. Similarly, let Φ_T be the region of the 3D texon centered at the given voxel in the ROI. Again using Equation 14.4, we also estimate the PDF of the interior of Φ_T, i.e., $p_T = P(i \mid \Phi_T)$. To measure the similarity between the two PDFs, we use an information theoretic distance measure called KLD [24]. The Bhattacharya distance, which is a symmetrized variation of KLD, between Φ_M and Φ_T is

$$B(p_M \,||\, p_T) = -\log \rho(p_M \,||\, p_T) = -\log \int [p_M(i)]^{\frac{1}{2}} [p_T(i)]^{\frac{1}{2}} \, di$$

We evaluate the 3D texture likelihood of the 3D texon at every voxel in ROI. We define this likelihood using ρ, since it increases as the Bhattacharya distance between two distributions decreases. The radius of a 3D neighborhood sphere used in our chapter is less than 3 voxels, and the model interior texture is mostly homogeneous with some level of noise. Thus, it is not necessary to consider the spatial correlation between voxels. Finally, we remove the remaining vessels around large lung cancers in the 3D likelihood map by using the eigenanalysis of the Hessian matrix [2,3,14].

14.2.3 Results

We have 10 chest CT images containing 16 large lung cancers. To test the proposed method, we collected 500 volumetric samples (300 training samples and 200 testing samples) from four training clinical chest CT images. The samples were of size 15 × 15 × 3 voxels from the CT volumes. Each sample was converted to an instance vector in R256, representing its nonparametric density estimate. For the boosted *k*-NN, we used the standard Euclidean distance as the distance measure between two instances as described in Section 14.2.2. We performed bootstrapping to estimate the generalization error of our large lesion detection method [17]. We trained and tested the proposed method on bootstrap samples. After 20 steps of boosting, the mean error rate converged to 3.50%. The accuracy is 96.5% for classifying large lung cancer and the ROC curve is presented in Figure 14.11.

We applied the trained classifier to all 10 CT volumes containing 16 large lung cancers. The CT volumes were acquired by multislice HRCT scanners with 5-mm slice collimation. The number of slices in each CT scan ranged from 44 to 69 (and digitally resliced to obtain cubic voxels, resulting in 130 to 205 slices), each of which are of size 512 × 512 pixels, with in-plane resolution of 0.82 mm. The classifier detected all 16 lesions successfully with no false-negatives (Figure 14.12). However, it also detected two false-positive lesions, which the trained radiologists classified as atelectases.

The detected large lung cancers were then segmented using the method described in Section 14.2.2. Figure 14.12 illustrates four representative cases of the segmented large lung cancers. The 3D reconstruction of the segmented 3D large lung cancers (middle and bottom rows) and their two-dimensional projections on one of the slices (top row) are shown in Figure 14.12. From the figure, we can also see that the surrounding vessels are accurately removed from the large lung lesions segmented. Table 14.3 compares the greatest diameters, their greatest perpendicular diameters, and tumor volumes of the 16 lung cancers from the results of the manual segmentation by experts and the automatic segmentation by the proposed method. The table shows that the mean relative error of the greatest diameter and its greatest perpendicular diameter are 2.8% and 2.2%, respectively, and shows that the mean relative error of the tumor volume is 8.4%. We also compared the overlapping ratios of the tumor regions segmented manually and automatically, which ranged from 80.9% to 97.3%. The low overlapping ratios were from cases in which the cancers were

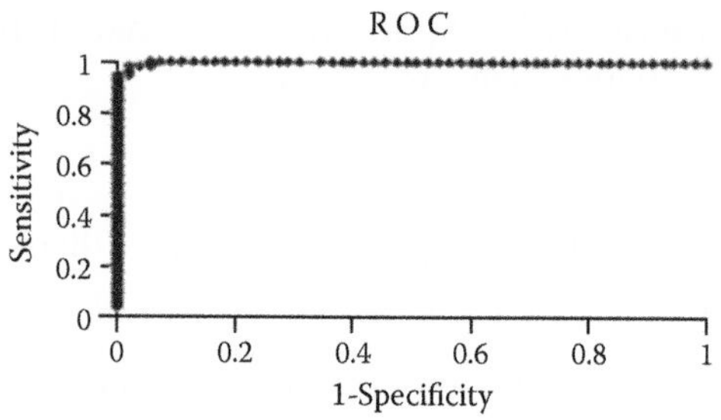

FIGURE 14.11
ROC curve measures the performance of the boosted *k*-NN method for large lung cancer detection.

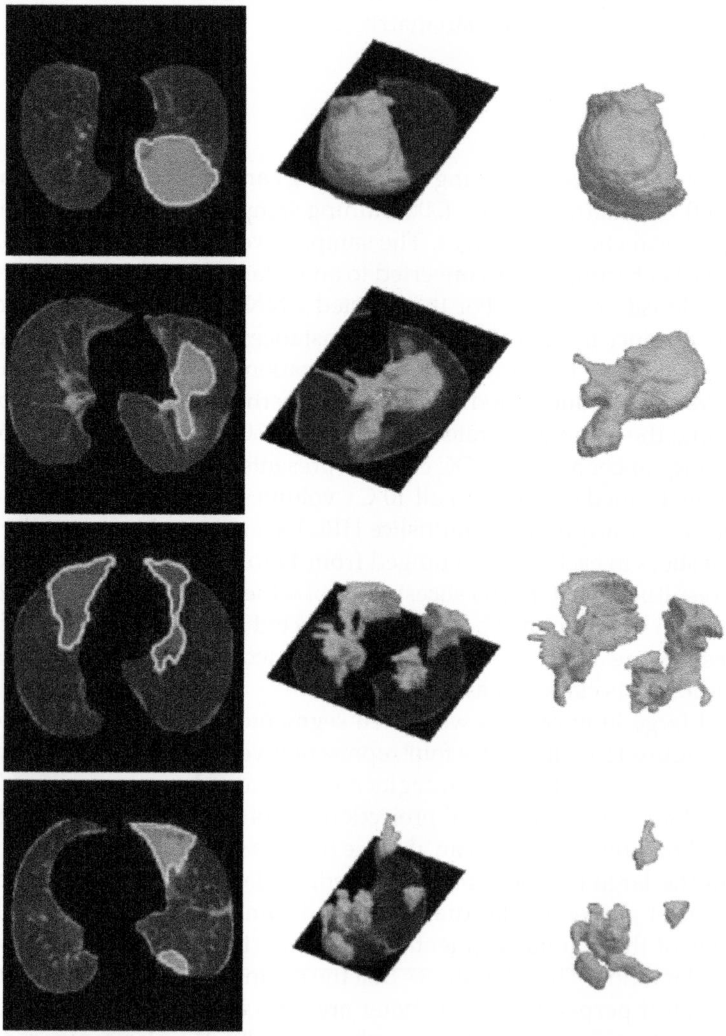

FIGURE 14.12
(See color insert.) Results: (left) segmented large lung lesions projected onto a slice and (middle and right) corresponding 3D lesions.

TABLE 14.3

Comparisons

Data Set	d_1 (mm)		d_2 (mm)		Vol (mm^3)		Overlap Ratio (%)
	Manual	Auto	Manual	Auto	Manual	Auto	
1	95	94	37	36	9676	9043	92.5
2	74	73	35	33	13357	12237	90.2
3	84	83	25	24	12704	11753	91.2
4	34	35	32	33	1643	1819	93.6
5	21	20	16	16	278	254	92.1
6	13	13	11	11	305	291	92.5
7	15	16	13	13	462	503	90.0
8	51	52	18	18	2152	2228	91.6
9	21	20	12	12	258	235	82.2
10	21	20	19	18	1402	1226	97.3
11	7	7	7	6	61	57	80.9
12	68	67	59	58	5988	5583	94.3
13	36	37	27	28	6268	6783	91.4
14	22	23	13	13	291	320	88.3
15	27	26	17	16	657	591	95.6
16	39	38	33	32	4583	4212	91.6
Mean error (%)	2.8		2.2		8.4		90.9

Note: d_1 and d_2 are the greatest diameter and its greatest perpendicular distance of each tumor, respectively. Vol is the volume of each tumor. Overlap ratio is the volume overlap ration of the manual segmentation results and automatic segmentation results. Manual and auto are the measurements on the manual segmentation results and the automatic segmentation results, respectively.

heavily occluded by blood vessels and where the expert radiologists also found difficulty. The mean overlapping ratio was 90.9%. These results demonstrate the potential of our method to correctly segment occluded lung areas as well as the accuracy of the classification and segmentation of the large lung cancers. These results demonstrate the potential of our method to correctly segment occluded lung areas as well as the accuracy of the classification and segmentation of the large lung cancers.

14.2.4 Conclusion

Lung cancers to be treated are often large and grow against surrounding structures such as chest wall, mediastinum, and blood vessels. Large lung cancers attached to such structures make it difficult to accurately segment lung areas from chest CT images, since they occlude the real boundary of the lungs and have similar intensity values as the surrounding structures. In this chapter, we proposed a novel method for automatic and accurate segmentation of lung areas that were distorted and occluded by large lung cancers using RASMs.

We also proposed a novel method for the automatic detection and segmentation of large lung cancers from chest CT images. The proposed method first extracted candidate lung cancer areas by applying the 3D cylinder filter. Then, each candidate region was classified by boosting the *k*-NN, whose distance measure was the Euclidean distance between the two intensity PDFs. We performed bootstrapping to estimate the generalization error of the method and showed the mean error rate of the method converged to 3.50%. Each cancer detected was automatically segmented by analyzing the texture likelihood map of the region.

The very promising results of our methods applied to various clinical chest CT images were also presented. Although the evaluation of therapy response is critical for determining whether a particular treatment is effective on a specific cancer type in a patient, traditional methods such as unidimensional and bidimensional measurements of tumor size are not sensitive enough to accurately evaluate the changes in tumor volumes. In addition, the manual delineation of cancer contours is time-consuming and lacks the reproducibility. The proposed methods provides a new powerful tool for automatic detection as well as accurate and reproducible segmentation of large lung cancers for therapy response assessment in lung cancers.

References

[1] Henschke, C., Yankelevitz, D., Mirtcheva, R. CT screening for lung cancer: Frequency and significance of part-solid and nonsolid nodules. *Am. J. Roentgenol.* 178 (2002) 1053–1057.

[2] Zhou, J., Chang, S., Metaxas, D.N., Axel, L. Vascular structure segmentation and bifurcation detection. *IEEE Int. Symp. Biomed. Imag.* (2007) 872–875.

[3] Zhou, J., Chang, S., Metaxas, D., Axel, L. Vessel boundary extraction using ridge scan-conversion and deformable model. *IEEE Int. Symp. Biomed. Imag.* (2006) 189–192.

[4] Armato, S.G., McLennan, G., McNitt-Gray, M.F., Meyer, C.R., Yankelevitz, D., Aberle, D.R., Henschke, C.I., Hoffman, E.A., Kazerooni, E.A., MacMahon, H., Reeves, A.P., Croft, B.Y., Clarke, L.P. Lung image database consortium: Developing a resource for the medical imaging research community. *Radiology* 232 (2004) 739–748.

[5] Brown, M.S., McNitt-Gray, M.F., Goldin, J.G., Suh, R.D., Sayre, J.W., Aberle, D.R. Patient-specific models for lung nodule detection and surveillance in CT images. *IEEE Trans. Med. Imag.* 20 (2001) 1242–1250.

[6] Tanino, M., Takizawa, H., Yamamoto, S., Matsumoto, T., Tateno, Y., Iinuma, T. A detection method of ground glass opacities in chest x-ray CT images using automatic clustering techniques. *SPIE* 5032 (2003) 1728–1737.

[7] Armato, S.G., Giger, M.L., Moran, C.J., Blackburn, J.T., Doi, K., MacMahon, H. Computerized detection of pulmonary nodules on CT scans. *Radiographics* 19 (1999) 1303–1311.

[8] Lee, Y., Hara, T., Fujita, H., Itoh, S., Ishigaki, T. Automated detection of pulmonary nodules in helical CT images based on an improved template-matching technique. *IEEE Trans. Med. Imag.* 20 (2001) 595–604.

[9] Chang, S., Emoto, H., Metaxas, D.N., Axel, L. Pulmonary micronodule detection from 3D chest CT. *Med. Image Comput. Computer-Assisted Intervention* 3217 (2004) 821–828.

[10] Takizawa, H., Yamamoto, S., Matsumoto, T., Tateno, Y., Iinuma, T., Matsumoto, M. Recognition of lung nodules from x-ray CT images using 3D Markov random field models. *SPIE* 4684 (2002) 716–725.

[11] Armato, S.G., Giger, M.L., MacMahon, H. Automated detection of lung nodules in CT scans: Preliminary results. *Med. Phys.* 28 (2001) 1552–1561.

[12] Kostis, W., Reeves, A., Yankelevitz, D., Henschke, C. Three-dimensional segmentation and growth rate estimation of small pulmonary nodules in helical CT images. *IEEE Trans. Med. Imag.* 22(10) (2003) 1259–1274.

[13] Zhang, L., Fang, M., Naidich, D.P., Novak, C.L. Consistent interactive segmentation of pulmonary ground glass nodules identified in CT studies. *SPIE* 5370 (2004) 1709–1719.

[14] Lorenz, C., Carlsen, I.C., Buzug, T., Fassnacht, C., Weese, J. Multi-scale line segmentation with automatic estimation of width, contrast and tangential direction in 2D and 3D medical images. *Proceedings of the First Joint Conference on Computer Vision, Virtual Reality and Robotics in Medicine and Medial Robotics and Computer-Assisted Surgery*, vol. 1205 (1997) 233–242.

[15] Freund, Y., Schapire, R. Experiments with a new boosting algorithm. *13th International Conference on Machine Learning* (1996) 148–156.

[16] Danielsson, P.E., Lin, Q. Efficient detection of second-degree variations in 2D and 3D images. *J. Vis. Commun. Image Represent.* 12 (2001) 255–305.

[17] Efron, B. Estimating the error rate of a prediction rule: Improvement on crossvalidation. *J. Am. Stat. Assoc.* 78 (1983) 316–331.

[18] Austin, J., Muller, N., Friedman, P.E.A. Glossary of terms for CT of the lung: Recommendations of the Nomenclature Committee of the Fleischner Society. *Radiology* 200 (1996) 327–331.

[19] Jang, H., Lee, K., Kwon, O., Rhee, C., Shim, Y., Han, J. Bronchioloalveolar carcinoma: Focal area of ground-glass attenuation at thin-section CT as an early sign. *Radiology* 199 (1996) 485–488.

[20] Kuriyama, K., Seto, M., Kasugai, T., Higashiyama, M., Kido, S., Sawai, Y., Kodama, K., Kuroda, D. Ground-glass opacity on thin-section CT: Value in differentiating subtypes of adenocarcinoma of the lung. *Am. J. Roentgenol.* 173 (1999) 465–469.

[21] Watanabe, S., Watanabe, T., Arai, K., Kasai, T., Haratake, J., Urayama, H. Results of wedge resection for focal bronchioloalveolar carcinoma showing pure ground-glass attenuation on computed tomography. *Ann. Thorac. Surg.* 73 (2002) 1071–1075.

[22] Heitmann, K., Kauczor, H.U., Mildenberger, P., Uthmann, T., Perl, J., Thelen, M. Automatic detection of ground glass opacities on lung HRCT using multiple neural networks. *Eur. Radiol.* 7 (1997) 1463–1472.

[23] Huang, X., Qian, Z., Huang, R., Metaxas, D. Deformable-model based textured object segmentation. *EMMCVPR* (2005) 119–135.

[24] Ali, S., Silvey, S. A general class of coefficients of divergence of one distribution from another. *J. R. Stat. Soc.* 28 (1966) 131–142.

[25] Kauczor, H.U., Heitmann, K., Heussel, C.P., Marwede, D., Uthmann, T., Thelen, M. Automatic detection and quantification of ground-glass opacities on high-resolution CT using multiple neural networks: Comparison with a density mask. *Am. J. Roentgenol.* 175 (2000) 1329–1334.

[26] Miller, A., Hogestraeten, B., Staquet, M., et al. Reporting results of cancer treatment. *Cancer* 47 (1981) 207–214.

[27] Therasse, P., Arbuck, S., Eisenhauer, E., et al. New guidelines to evaluate response to treatment in solid tumors. *J. Natl. Cancer Inst.* 92 (2000) 205–216.

[28] Zhao, B., Schwartz, L., Moskowitz, C., Ginsberg, M., Rizvi, N., Kris, M. Lung cancer: Computerized quantification of tumor response—Initial results. *Radiology* 241 (2006) 892–898.

[29] Zhao, B., Gamsu, G., Ginsberg, M., Jian, L., Schwartz, L. Automatic detection of small lung nodules on CT utilizing a local density maximum algorithm. *J. Appl. Clin. Med. Phys.* 4(3) (2003) 248–260.

[30] Zhao, B., Yankelevitz, D., Reeves, A., Henschke, C. Two-dimensional multicriterion segmentation of pulmonary nodules on helical CT images. *IEEE Trans. Med. Imag.* 22(10) (2003) 1259–1274.

[31] Boscolo, R., Brown, M., McNitt-Gray, M. Medical image segmentation with knowledge-guided robust active contours. *RadioGraphics* 33 (2002) 437–448.

[32] Ko, J.P., Rusinek, H., Jacobs, E.L., Babb, J.S., Betke, M., McGuinness, G., Naidich, D.P. Small pulmonary nodules: Volume measurement at chest CT phantom study. *Radiology* 228 (2003) 864–870.

[33] Cootes, T., Taylor, C., Cooper, D., Graham, J. Active shape models—Their training and application. *Comp. Vis. Imag. Under.* 61(1) (1995) 38–59.

[34] De La Torre, F., Black, M. A framework for robust subspace learning. *Int. J. Comput. Vis.* 54(1–3) (2003) 117–142.

[35] Zhou, J., Chang, S., Metaxas, D.N., Zhao, B., Schwartz, L.H., Ginsberg, M.S. Automatic detection and segmentation of ground glass opacity nodules. *International conference on Medical Image Computing and Computer Assisted Intervention* (MICCAI), 2006.

15

Texture Classification in Pulmonary CT

Lauge Sørensen, Mehrdad J. Gangeh, Saher B. Shaker, and Marleen de Bruijne

CONTENTS

15.1 Introduction

Computed tomography (CT) images of the human lungs show intensity variations that form certain repeated patterns, also referred to as texture. Some of these variations are due to noise and artifacts, but others are due to properties of the imaged tissue. Abnormal lung tissue can often be distinguished from healthy lung tissue based on its texture. The texture of the abnormal lung tissue depends on the type and severity of the abnormality. Three examples of regions of lung tissue extracted from CT are presented in Figure 15.1, an example of normal, healthy lung tissue in Figure 15.1(a) and two examples of abnormal lung tissue, in this case emphysema, in Figures 15.1(b) and 15.1(c). The normal lung tissue exhibits a noisy, gray pattern with thin, bright structures, which are mainly vessels and airway walls. The abnormal lung tissue is in this case characterized by black blobs, due to missing lung tissue, of varying sizes within the normal appearing tissue.

There exists no generally agreed-upon definition of texture, and the definitions provided in the literature often depend on the particular application at hand [15, 37]. When referring to texture in this chapter, we loosely mean *a distribution of measure(s) of local structure,*

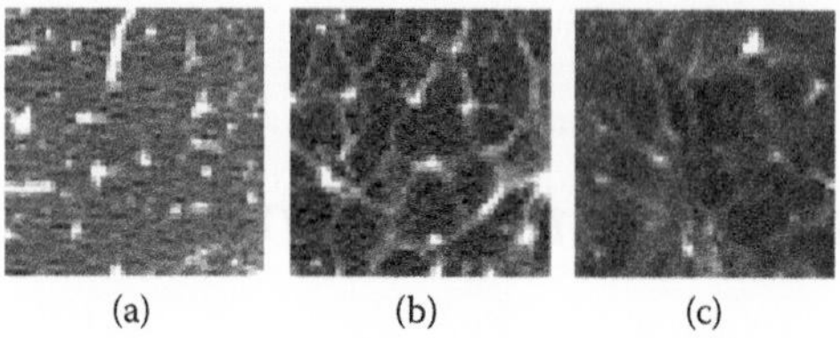

FIGURE 15.1
51 × 51 pixel regions, from CT images, with examples of normal and emphysematous lung tissue. The displayed image intensities are linearly scaled between −1024 Hounsfield units (HU) (black) and −300 HU (white).

as measured in a region. In the extreme case, the measure is the pixel values, and we simply have the histogram of intensity values computed in the region. Purely intensity-based descriptors may, however, not be sufficient to discriminate abnormal lung tissue as illustrated in Figure 15.2. Even though the textural appearance of the two example patterns is rather different, the intensity histograms look very similar. This chapter focuses on texture classification in pulmonary CT, and all the considered texture descriptors, except for the purely intensity-based descriptors presented in Section 15.2.1, use interactions among pixels and should therefore be able to discriminate between the two example patterns.

Several popular texture descriptors used in the medical image analysis literature for texture-based classification of abnormal lung tissue, e.g., for discriminating between textures of the types shown in Figure 15.1, are described and evaluated within the same classification framework. The descriptors are evaluated in a case study of emphysema classification in CT regions of interest (ROIs). However, the presented descriptors can also be used for other texture analysis tasks as well, including texture segmentation and texture synthesis [15, 37]. Further, a classification system capable of classifying abnormality can serve as a basis for different medical image analysis tasks such as texture-based detection or quantification of abnormality in complete scans [18, 28, 30, 32, 34].

Section 15.2 describes the different texture descriptors, and Section 15.3 presents the classification problem, the experimental setup including the general classification system

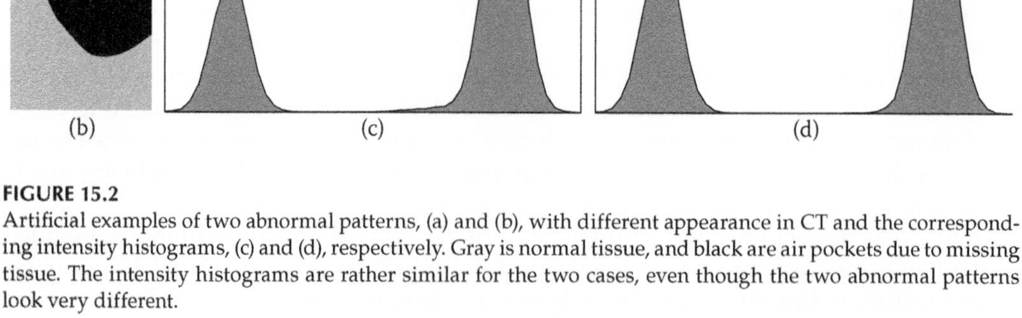

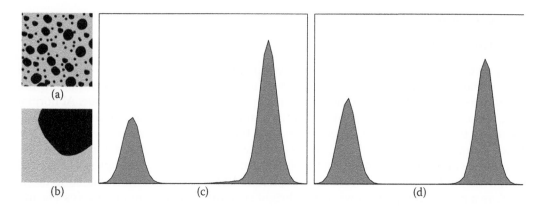

FIGURE 15.2
Artificial examples of two abnormal patterns, (a) and (b), with different appearance in CT and the corresponding intensity histograms, (c) and (d), respectively. Gray is normal tissue, and black are air pockets due to missing tissue. The intensity histograms are rather similar for the two cases, even though the two abnormal patterns look very different.

used for all descriptors, as well as the obtained results. Finally, Section 15.4 concludes the chapter.

15.2 Texture Descriptors

There exist many texture descriptors in the image processing and pattern recognition literature; see refs. [8, 15, 16, 37], for example. Many of these have also been used for texture-based classification in pulmonary CT [2, 7, 18, 20, 21, 27, 29–34, 38, 39, 45], and in this chapter, we focus on the descriptors most often used for this purpose. The following descriptors are considered:

- the intensity histogram (INT), Section 15.2.1, used in refs. [2, 18, 20, 21, 27, 29, 30, 33, 34, 38, 39, 45];
- local binary patterns (LBPs), Section 15.2.2, used in refs. [32–34];
- a Gaussian filter bank (GFB), Section 15.2.3, different variants used in refs. [27, 29–31, 34];
- gray-level co-occurrence matrices (GLCMs), Section 15.2.4, used in refs. [2, 18, 20, 21, 34, 38, 39, 45];
- gray-level run-length matrices (GLRLMs), Section 15.2.5, used in refs. [2, 18, 20, 21, 34, 38, 39, 45];
- and finally, textons, Section 15.2.6, used in ref. [7].

We focus on 2D versions of the texture descriptors since the evaluation is performed on a data set of two-dimensional CT images. However, possible 3D versions will also be discussed briefly in the end of the chapter in Section 15.4. Where possible, we consider rotation invariant versions of the descriptors since this property is often enforced in texture-based classification in CT. See refs. [2, 18, 30, 34, 39], for example.

The representations obtained using the different texture descriptors of the central 31 × 31 pixel parts of the two example regions in Figure 15.1(a) and Figure 15.1(b) are shown in the following subsections to illustrate how the different descriptors represent the information in the two regions.

15.2.1 Intensity Histogram

The intensity histogram (INT) is a simple descriptor of independent pixel information in the image, and either the full histogram or summarizing measures can be used. Several studies use moments of the intensity distribution as features [2, 18, 20, 21, 34, 38, 39, 45] or of the distribution of smoothed intensities [27, 29, 34], while others use the full histogram of (smoothed) intensities [30, 33, 34]. The most commonly used summarizing measures are as follows: the mean intensity, or first moment

$$\langle I \rangle = \frac{1}{N_p} \sum_{i=1}^{N_p} I(\mathbf{x}_i) \tag{15.1}$$

where I is an image region, $\mathbf{x}_i$ is pixel within the region, and N_p is the number of pixels in the region; and the standard deviation of the intensity, or square root of the second central moment

$$\sigma(I) = \sqrt{\frac{1}{N_p - 1}\sum_{i=1}^{N_p}(I(\mathbf{x}_i) - \ (I))^2}. \tag{15.2}$$

Further, a measure of asymmetry called skewness, or the third standardized central moment

$$skew(I) = \frac{1}{N_p}\sum_{i=1}^{N_p}\frac{I(\mathbf{x}_i) - \ (I)}{\sigma(I)}^{3} \tag{15.3}$$

as well as a measure of peakedness called kurtosis, or the fourth standardized central moment

$$kurtosis(I) = \frac{1}{N_p}\sum_{i=1}^{N_p}\frac{I(\mathbf{x}_i) - \ (I)}{\sigma(I)}^{4} - 3, \tag{15.4}$$

are often used.

Both the full intensity histogram as well as the four mentioned moments will be considered in the experiments.

Figure 15.3 shows intensity histograms computed from the example regions in Figure 15.1(a) and Figure 15.1(b). As expected, there is more mass in the low-intensity part of the histogram of the emphysema region compared to the histogram computed from the normal lung tissue.

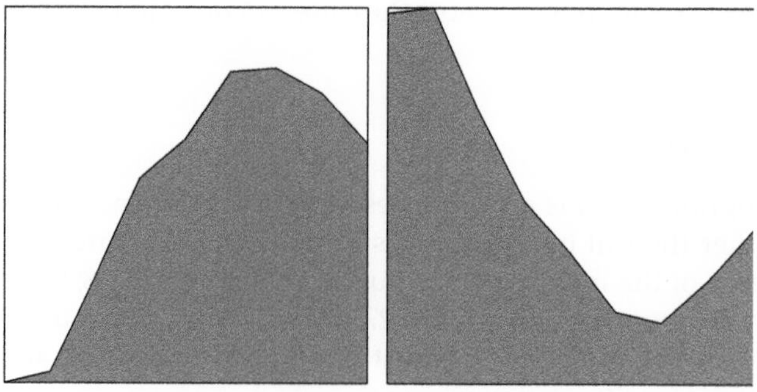

(a) (b)

FIGURE 15.3
Intensity histograms. (a) is computed from the region in Figure 15.1(a) and (b) is computed from the region in Figure 15.1(b). The histograms are quantized into $N_b = 9$ bins.

15.2.2 Local Binary Patterns

Local binary patterns (LBPs) were originally proposed by Ojala et al. as a gray-scale invariant measure for characterizing local structure in a 3 × 3 pixel neighborhood [16]. Later, a more general formulation was proposed that further allowed for multiresolution analysis, rotation invariance, and vast dimensionality reduction by considering only so-called "uniform" patterns [17].

The LBPs are obtained from an image region I by thresholding samples in a local neighborhood with respect to each center pixel intensity and are given by

$$LBP(\mathbf{x};R,P) = \sum_{p=0}^{P-1} H(I(\mathbf{x}_p) - I(\mathbf{x}))2^p \tag{15.5}$$

where $\mathbf{x}$ is the center pixel, $\mathbf{x}_p = [-R\sin(2\pi p/P), R\cos(2\pi p/P)]^T + \mathbf{x}$ are P local samples taken at a radius R around $\mathbf{x}$, and $H(\cdot)$ is the Heaviside function. By choosing a fixed sample position on the circle as the "leading bit," the thresholded samples can be interpreted as bits, and a P bit binary number, the LBP code, can be computed. The LBP codes computed in each pixel in the region are accumulated into a histogram, the LBP histogram, where each unique LBP code corresponds to a particular histogram bin. Different local structures in the region, such as edges, corners, spots, etc., are assigned different LBP codes, and the LBP histogram, therefore, captures many structures in one unified framework. The number of samples, P, governs the number of bins in the LBP histogram, e.g., $P = 8$ results in $2^8 = 256$ bins. By varying the radius R and the number of samples P, the structures are measured at different scales, and this way, LBP allows for measuring large-scale structures without smoothing effects as would, for example, occur with Gaussian-based filters. As long as the relative ordering among the gray-scale values in the samples does not change, the output of Equation 15.5 stays the same; hence, LBPs are invariant to any monotonic gray-scale transformation.

Rotation invariance can be achieved by "rotating the circle" until the lowest possible binary number is found

$$LBP^{ri}(\mathbf{x};R,P) = \min(ROR(LBP(\mathbf{x};R,P),i)) \tag{15.6}$$

for $i = 0, \ldots, P-1$. $ROR(b, i)$ performs i circular bit-wise right shifts on the P-bit binary number b. Equation 15.6 assigns the same LBP code to similar structures of different orientations, which also has the effect of reducing the dimensionality of the LBP histogram, e.g., to 36 bins for $P = 8$.

The dimensionality of the LBP histogram can further be reduced by only considering the so-called "uniform" patterns, which are local structures giving rise to, at most, two bitwise changes in the LBP code, and assign the remaining structures a designated "noise" code. This is done in the following way:

$$LBP^{riu2}(\mathbf{x};R,P) = \begin{cases} \sum_{p=0}^{P-1} H(I(\mathbf{x}_p) - I(\mathbf{x})) & \text{if } U(LBP(\mathbf{x};R,P)) \leq 2 \\ P+1 & \text{otherwise} \end{cases}, \tag{15.7}$$

where

$$U(LBP(\mathbf{x};R,P)) = \left|H(I(\mathbf{x}_{P-1}) - I(\mathbf{x})) - H(I(\mathbf{x}_0) - I(\mathbf{x}))\right| + \sum_{p=1}^{P-1} \left|H(I(\mathbf{x}_p) - I(\mathbf{x})) - H(I(\mathbf{x}_{p-1}) - I(\mathbf{x}))\right| \quad (15.8)$$

counts the number of bit transitions, from 0 to 1 or from 1 to 0, that are encountered when traversing the P thresholded samples on the circle. The resulting LBP histogram contains 10 bins for $P = 8$.

Since LBPs, by design, are invariant to any monotonic intensity transformation, important discriminative information may be left out when applied in CT. The joint LBP and intensity histogram has been proposed as a solution to this problem [32–34], resulting in a histogram where one dimension measures structure, whereas the other dimension measures at which densities the different structures occur. The histogram is obtained by computing the LBP codes in all pixels in the image, according to Equation 15.6 or 15.7, and forming the joint histogram between the resulting LBP codes and the intensities in the cor-

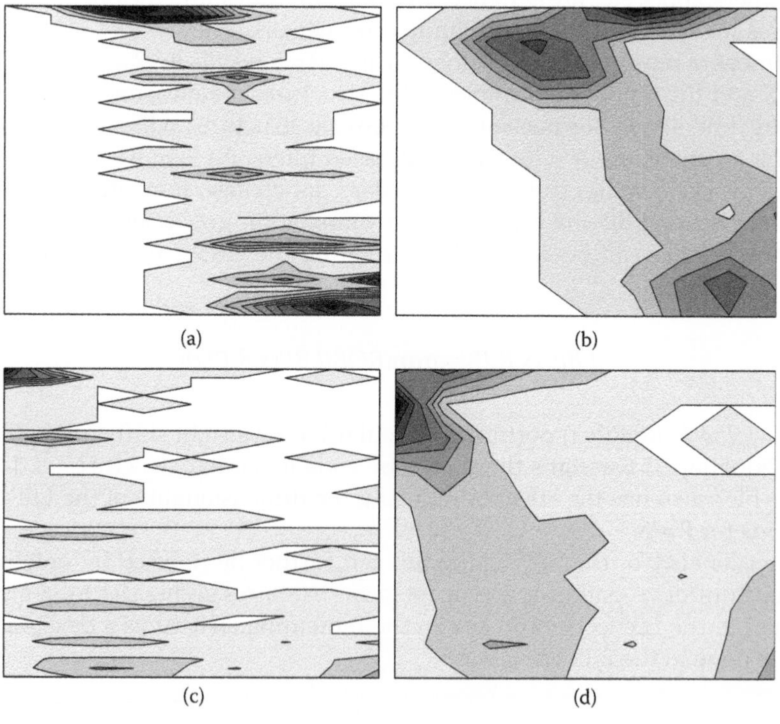

FIGURE 15.4
Joint LBP and intensity histograms using $N_b = 9$. (a) and (b) are computed from the region in Figure 15.1(a) using $LBP2^{ri}(\cdot; 1,8)$ and $LBP2^{riu2}(\cdot; 1,8)$, respectively, and (c) and (d) are computed from the region in Figure 15.1(b) using $LBP2^{ri}(\cdot; 1,8)$ and $LBP2^{riu2}(\cdot; 1,8)$. Intensity is in the horizontal direction, and LBP code is in the vertical direction. Black is high density whereas white is low density.

responding center pixels $I(\mathbf{x})$. We denote these operators $LBP2^{ri}$ and $LBP2^{riu2}$, respectively. These are the operators that we will be using in the experiments.

Figure 15.4 shows joint LBP and intensity histograms computed from the example regions in Figure 15.1(a) and Figure 15.1(b) using $LBP2^{ri}(\cdot; 1, 8)$ and $LBP2^{riu2}(\cdot; 1, 8)$. The LBPs, or local structures, generally reside at lower intensities for emphysema compared to healthy tissue, which is to be expected.

15.2.3 Gaussian Derivative-Based Filter Bank

Filtering an image region using a bank of filters and representing the resulting filter response images using histograms or moments is another commonly employed texture descriptor [40, 47]. We evaluate a multiscale Gaussian filter bank (GFB) comprising filters based on the Gaussian function and its derivatives [36]. The filtering is done by convolving the image region with the two-dimensional Gaussian function

$$G(\mathbf{x};\sigma) = \frac{1}{2\pi\sigma^2}\exp\left(-\frac{\|\mathbf{x}\|_2^2}{2\sigma^2}\right) \tag{15.9}$$

where σ is the standard deviation, or scale, and $||\cdot||_2$ is the L_2-norm. Increasing σ results in the region being increasingly blurred, which allows analysis of the image structure at larger scales.

Letting L_x and L_y denote the first-order derivatives of the convolved image region $L = I * G(\mathbf{x}; \sigma)$, and L_{xx}, L_{yy}, and L_{xy} denote the second-order derivatives, the four base filters in the GFB considered in this chapter are as follows: the Gaussian function itself (Equation 15.9); gradient magnitude

$$\|\nabla G(\mathbf{x};\sigma)\|_2 = \sqrt{L_x^2 + L_y^2}; \tag{15.10}$$

the Laplacian of the Gaussian

$$\nabla^2 G(\mathbf{x}; \sigma) = L_{xx} + L_{yy}; \tag{15.11}$$

and Gaussian curvature

$$K(\mathbf{x};\sigma) = L_{xx}L_{yy} - L_{xy}^2. \tag{15.12}$$

These four filters are used in ref. [33, 34] and are common descriptors of local structure invariant to rotation. The Gaussian function itself is included in order to allow the GFB descriptor to take CT density information into account [29, 33, 34].

From a filtered CT image region, a filter response histogram can be computed and used to characterize the texture [30, 31, 33, 34]. Alternatively, moments can be used [28, 29]. We experiment with both approaches in this chapter and use the four moments defined in Section 15.2.1, namely, the mean (Equation 15.1), standard deviation (Equation 15.2), skewness (Equation 15.3), and kurtosis (Equation 15.4) of the filter responses computed in the region, as well as the full filter response histograms.

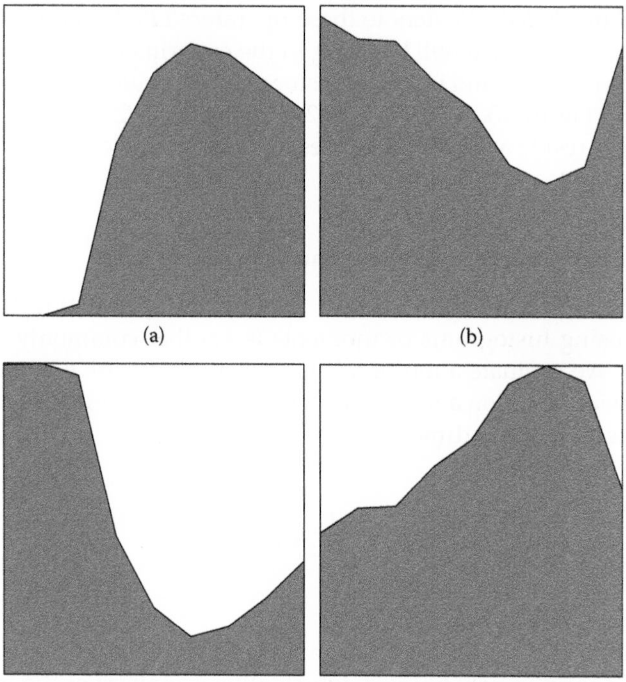

FIGURE 15.5
GFB filter response histograms where the filter responses are quantized into $N_b = 9$ bins. (a) and (b) are computed from the region in Figure 15.1(a) using G(·; 0.5) and $||\nabla G(\cdot; 1)||_2$, respectively, and (c) and (d) are computed from the region in Figure 15.1(b) using G(·; 0.5) and $||\nabla G(\cdot; 1)||_2$.

Figure 15.5 shows GFB filter response histograms computed from the example regions in Figure 15.1(a) and Figure 15.1(b) using the two different filters $G(\cdot, 0.5)$ and $||\nabla G(\cdot, 1)||_2$. As expected, there is more mass in the low-intensity part of the histogram computed from the emphysema region compared to the histogram computed from the normal lung tissue; see Figure 15.5(a) and Figure 15.5(c). The emphysema region is also characterized by having edges at a different strength, due to transitions from air pockets to lung tissue, compared to the normal lung tissue; see Figure 15.5(b) and Figure 15.5(d).

15.2.4 Gray-Level Co-Occurrence Matrices

Summarizing measures computed from a gray-level co-occurrence matrix (GLCM) are classical texture features [8]. An element $p(i, j; \theta, d)$ of a GLCM computed from an image region I expresses the number of times a pixel **x** with gray-level i occurs jointly with a pixel **y** with gray-level j in I, where **y** is positioned relative to **x** according to a displacement vector defined be an angle θ and a distance d. In this chapter, we consider symmetric GLCMs, meaning that $p(i, j; \theta, d) = p(j, i; \theta, d)$. Of the summarizing measures originally proposed in [8], the three most commonly used are: angular second moment or uniformity of energy (UE)

$$UE(p;\theta,d) = \sum_{i=1}^{N_b} \sum_{j=1}^{N_b} p(i,j;\theta,d)^2 \tag{15.13}$$

where N_b is the number of bins that the gray-levels in the region are quantized into; inertia or contrast (C)

$$C(p;\theta,d) = \sum_{i=1}^{N_b}\sum_{j=1}^{N_b} |i-j|^2\, p(i,j;\theta,d); \qquad (15.14)$$

and homogeneity or inverse difference moment (IDM)

$$IDM(p;\theta,d) = \sum_{i=1}^{N_b}\sum_{j=1}^{N_b} \frac{p(i,j;\theta,d)}{1+|i-j|^2}. \qquad (15.15)$$

These measures are all used in refs. [2, 18, 20, 21, 34, 38, 39, 45]. We further include correlation (CORR)

$$CORR(p;\theta,d) = \sum_{i=1}^{N_b}\sum_{j=1}^{N_b} \frac{(i - {}_i)(j - {}_j)p(i,j;\theta,d)}{\sigma_i\sigma_j} \qquad (15.16)$$

where ${}_i = \sum_{i=1}^{N_b}\sum_{j=1}^{N_b} ip(i,j;\theta,d)$ and $\sigma_i = \sqrt{\sum_{i=1}^{N_b}\sum_{j=1}^{N_b} p(i,j;\theta,d)(i - {}_i)^2}$ are the GLCM mean and the GLCM standard deviation, respectively. Note that since symmetric GLCMs are considered, $\mu_i = \mu_j$ and $\sigma_i = \sigma_j$. $CORR(\cdot;\theta, d)$ is used in refs. [18, 34, 38, 39, 45].

The two parameters θ and d govern the GLCM, and different values of these parameters result in different GLCMs capturing spatial pixel intensity relations in various directions and at various ranges. Some studies average the summarizing measures across different displacements, which brings down the dimensionality of the descriptor and makes it scale and rotation invariant; see refs. [2, 18], for example. We evaluate the common approach of using summarizing measures but also experiment with using the full GLCMs. Both the summarizing measures and the full GLCMs are averaged across angle, to achieve rotation invariance, but not across distance.

GLCMs for two different displacements computed from the example regions in Figure 15.1(a) and Figure 15.1(b) are shown in Figure 15.6. The GLCMs are more peaked, due to smaller differences between neighboring pixel intensities, and the mass is shifted towards the lower intensities for the emphysema case compared to the healthy tissue case.

15.2.5 Gray-Level Run-Length Matrices

Summarizing measures computed from a gray-level run-length matrix (GLRLM) are another set of classical texture features [8]. An element $p(i, j; \theta)$ of a GLRLM computed from an image region I expresses the number of times j consecutive pixels of the same gray-level i, in a given angle or direction θ, occur in I. The five most commonly used summarizing measures of GLRLMs are short run emphasis (SRE)

$$SRE(p;\theta,MRL) = \frac{1}{N_r}\sum_{i=1}^{N_b}\sum_{j=1}^{MRL} \frac{p(i,j;\theta)}{j^2} \qquad (15.17)$$

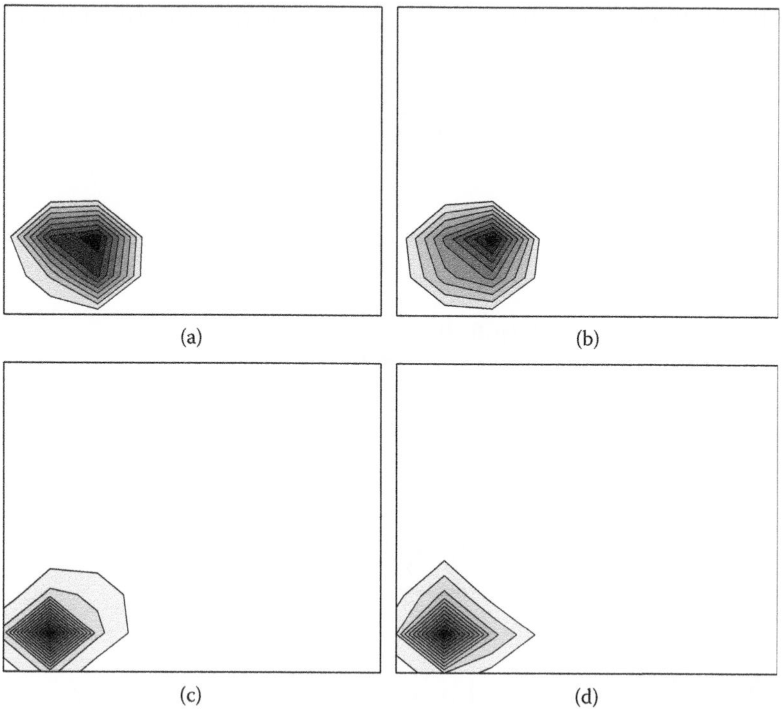

FIGURE 15.6
GLCMs with intensities quantized into $N_b = 9$ bins. (a) and (b) are computed from the region in Figure 15.1(a) using $p(\cdot,\cdot;90,1)$ and $p(\cdot,\cdot;135,2)$, respectively, and (c) and (d) are computed from the region in Figure 15.1(b) using $p(\cdot,\cdot;90,1)$ and $p(\cdot,\cdot;135,2)$. Black is high density whereas white is low density.

where N_b is the number of bins that the gray levels in the region are quantized into, MRL is the maximum run length considered, and $N_r = \sum_{i=1}^{N_b} \sum_{j=1}^{MRL} p(i,j;\theta)$ is the total number of runs in the image; long run emphasis (LRE)

$$LRE(p;\theta,MRL) = \frac{1}{N_r} \sum_{i=1}^{N_b} \sum_{j=1}^{MRL} p(i,j;\theta) j^2; \tag{15.18}$$

gray-level nonuniformity (GLN)

$$GLN(p;\theta,MRL) = \frac{1}{N_r} \sum_{i=1}^{N_b} \left(\sum_{j=1}^{MRL} p(i,j;\theta) \right)^2; \tag{15.19}$$

run-length nonuniformity (RLN)

$$RLN(p;\theta,MRL) = \frac{1}{N_r} \sum_{j=1}^{MRL} \left(\sum_{i=1}^{N_b} p(i,j;\theta) \right)^2; \tag{15.20}$$

and run percentage (RP)

$$RP(p;\theta, MRL) = \frac{1}{N_p} \sum_{i=1}^{N_b} \sum_{j=1}^{MRL} p(i, j;\theta) \tag{15.21}$$

where N_p is the number of pixels in the region. These five measures are used in refs. [2, 18, 20, 21, 34, 38, 39, 45]. The angle of the runs, θ, and the number of bins, N_b, that the intensities are quantized into, are the only parameters for the computation of the GLRLM. The maximum run length considered, *MRL*, is an extra parameter for the computation of the summarizing measures, and *MRL* effectively truncates the GLRLM in the run-length direction. Also note that N_r is influenced by *MRL* since this is the total number of runs in the truncated GLRLM. Most studies average the summarizing measures across angle, which decreases the dimensionality of the descriptor and makes it rotation invariant. We evaluate the common approach of using summarizing measures but also experiment with using the full GLRLMs. Both the summarizing measures and the full GLRLMs are averaged across angle.

GLRLMs computed from the example regions in Figure 15.1(a) and Figure 15.1(b) are shown in Figure 15.7. The emphysema case contains longer runs at a lower intensity, which is related to areas with missing lung tissue, compared to the healthy case.

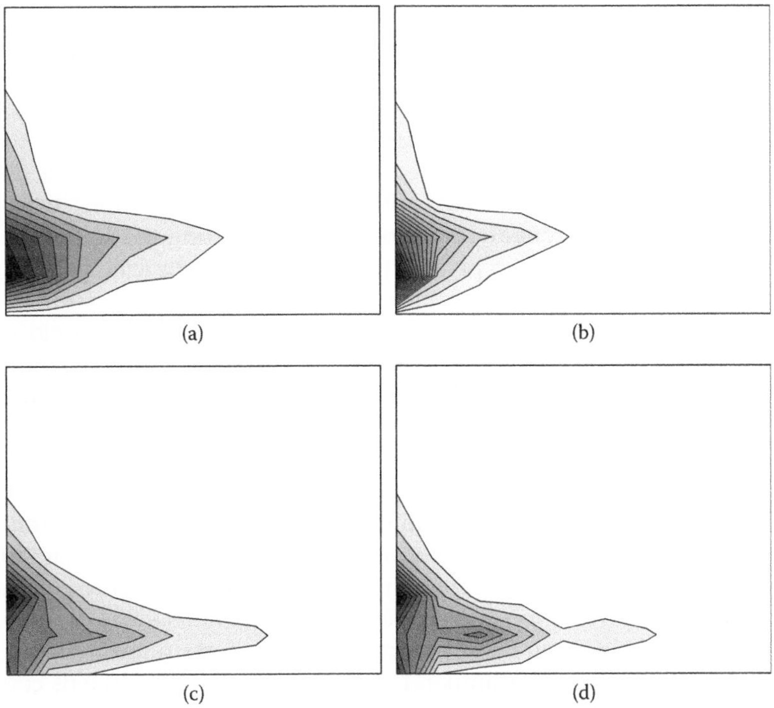

FIGURE 15.7
GLRLMs with intensities quantized into $N_b = 9$ bins and a maximum run length of MRL = 10. (a) and (b) are computed from the region in Figure 15.1(a) using $p(\cdot,\cdot;0)$ and $p(\cdot,\cdot;135)$, respectively, and (c) and (d) are computed from the region in Figure 15.1(b) using $p(\cdot,\cdot;0)$ and $p(\cdot,\cdot;135)$. Intensity is in the vertical direction, and run length is in the horizontal direction. Black is high density whereas white is low density.

15.2.6 Textons

Textons were first introduced by Julesz in his influential paper [10] as fundamental primitives capable of representing texture. Based on Julesz' theory, Leung and Malik developed a complete texture classification system [13]. They defined 2D textons as the cluster centers in filter bank responses, which made it possible to generate textons from the images automatically as the prototypes representing the source textures. These textons formed a codebook from which a texton histogram could be constructed for each image using a similarity measure. This work was further improved by Schmid [23, 24], Cula and Dana [3], and Varma and Zisserman [41–43]. The texton histogram computed from an image is a fully data-driven texture descriptor. This is different from the other descriptors considered in this chapter, which are based on prespecified rules for which only the associated parameters are optimized on the training data.

There are three main representations associated with the texton-based approach in the literature, filter banks [3, 13, 42], raw pixel representation [43], and Markov random field representation, where the probability of the central pixel value is conditioned on the pixel values in the neighboring pixels [43]. However, irrespective of the representation used to describe local image information, the descriptor construction consists of two stages: construction of a texton codebook and computation of a texton frequency histogram.

To construct the texton codebook, small-sized local patches of size $TS \times TS$ are randomly extracted from each image region in the training set and converted to an appropriate representation. The patches are subsequently aggregated over all images in a class and clustered using a clustering algorithm. The cluster centers obtained form a codebook of textons representing the class of textures. The size of the final codebook thus depends on the number of cluster centers N_c as well as the number of classes. For example, for a three-class problem with 30 cluster centers per class, $3 \times 30 = 90$ textons are generated in the codebook. The texton codebook is used to compute texton histograms, both for the training data and the test data.

The texton frequency histogram is defined as a histogram of the same size as the size of the codebook where each bin is associated with one of the learned textons in the codebook. The histogram is computed from an image region by extracting patches of the same size as the textons, one centered on each pixel in the region. Each extracted patch is converted to the same representation as is used in the texton codebook and compared to all textons in the codebook using a similarity measure. The bin corresponding to the closest texton is updated with a count. The final histogram is normalized.

In this chapter, the textons are based on a raw pixel representation, and the codebook thus consists of cluster centers in a feature space of dimension $TS \times TS$ where each dimension corresponds to the intensity in a certain pixel. The texton frequency histogram is therefore variant to both rotation and scale. Clustering is performed using the k-means algorithm [9], and the Euclidean distance in the feature space is used as a similarity measure between the small patches, both in k-means and in the texton histogram formation.

Figure 15.8 shows texton histograms from the example regions in Figure 15.1(a) and Figure 15.1(b). It is not straightforward to interpret the texton histograms, since the ordering of the bins is not meaningful. Each bin merely corresponds to a certain texton in the codebook, and neighboring bins need not be similar. For $N_c = 10$, the leftmost 10 bins correspond to cluster centers computed from the healthy samples in the training set, the center 10 bins correspond to one type of emphysema, and the rightmost 10 bins correspond to another type of emphysema. As can be seen, the histograms computed from the healthy region contain most mass in the leftmost part, and the histograms computed from the emphysema region contain most mass in the central part, which is the correct emphysema type.

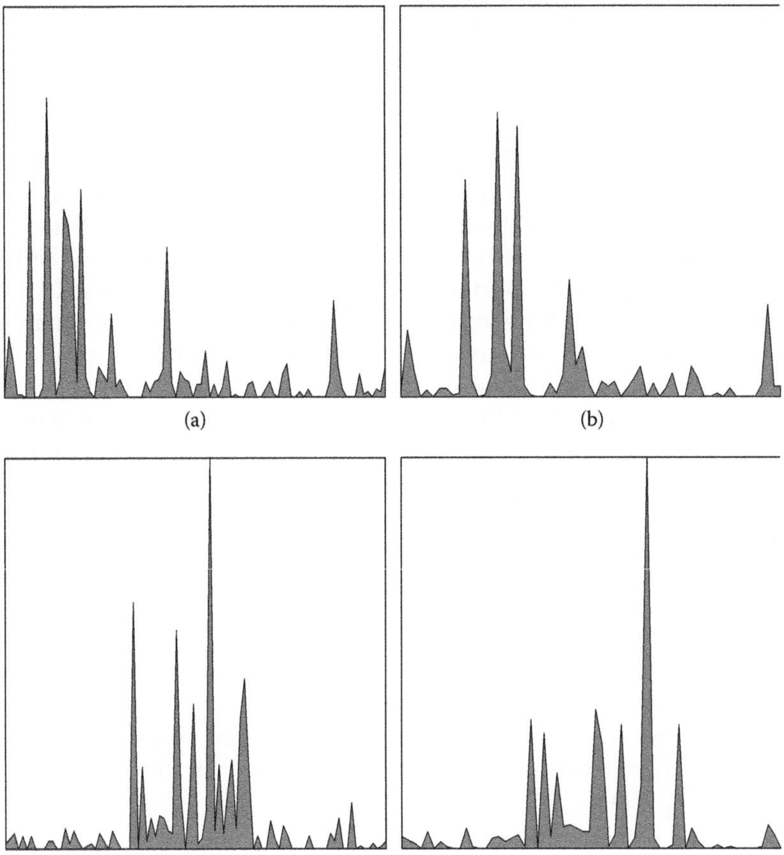

FIGURE 15.8
Texton histograms using $TS = 3$. (a) and (b) are computed from the region in Figure 15.1(a) with $N_c = 30$ and $N_c = 20$, respectively, and (c) and (d) are computed from the region in Figure 15.1(b) using $N_c = 30$ and $N_c = 20$.

15.3 Evaluation

The experiments are performed in Matlab® using in-house developed code as well as publicly available implementations of some of the descriptors. LBPs are computed using lbp.m* and getmapping.m†. GLCMs are computed using version 6.2 of Mathworks's own Image Processing Toolbox for Matlab. GLRLMs are computed using the Gray Level Run Length Matrix Toolbox‡.

* Version 0.3.2 obtained from http://www.ee.oulu.fi/mvg/page/lbp_matlab.
† Version 0.1.1 obtained from http://www.ee.oulu.fi/mvg/page/lbp_matlab.
‡ Version 1.0 obtained from http://www.mathworks.com/matlabcentral/fileexchange/17482-gray-level-run-length-matrix-toolbox.

15.3.1 A Case Study: Classification of Emphysema in CT

The different texture descriptors are evaluated and compared on the classification of different types of emphysema in CT regions of interest (ROIs). Emphysema is one of the main components of chronic obstructive pulmonary disease (COPD), the fourth leading cause of morbidity and mortality in the United States alone, which is predicted to rise from its ranking in 2000 as the 12th most prevalent disease worldwide to the 5th, and from the 6th most common cause of death worldwide to the 3rd, by 2020 [1, 22]. Automated emphysema classification may lead to better subtyping, diagnosis, and understanding of the development of emphysema but, more importantly, also to a better assessment of COPD.

Emphysema lesions, or bullae, are visible in CT images as areas of abnormally low attenuation values close to that of air and are often characterized according to their subtype and extent. Subtyping is performed based on the morphology, or textural appearance, of the emphysema patterns and can according to a common definition be classified into three subtypes or patterns [44]. These subtypes are the following: centrilobular emphysema (CLE), defined as multiple small low-attenuation areas; paraseptal emphysema (PSE), defined as multiple low-attenuation areas in a single layer along the pleura often surrounded by interlobular septa that is visible as thin white walls; and panlobular emphysema (PLE), defined as a low-attenuation lung with fewer and smaller pulmonary vessels. Examples of emphysema, more specifically CLE, as well as normal tissue (NT), are shown in Figure 15.1.

Current quantitative analysis of emphysema from CT relies only on the intensity information in individual pixels [25] and is not able to distinguish between the two abnormal patterns in Figure 15.2. This includes measures such as the relative area, also called emphysema index, and the percentile density [25]. In recent years, various studies have looked into using richer texture descriptors for improving classification of emphysema [2, 7, 18, 20, 21, 29–34, 38, 39, 45].

15.3.2 Data

The data come from an exploratory study carried out at the Department of Respiratory Medicine, Gentofte University Hospital [26], and consist of CT images of the thorax acquired using General Electric equipment (LightSpeed QX/i; GE Medical Systems, Milwaukee, WI, USA) with four detector rows. A total of 75 high-resolution CT (HRCT) slices were acquired by scanning 25 subjects in the upper, middle, and lower lung. The CT scanning was performed using the following parameters: in-plane resolution 0.78×0.78 mm, slice thickness 1.25 mm, tube voltage 140 kV, and tube current 200 mAs. The slices were reconstructed using an edge-enhancing (bone) algorithm.

An experienced chest radiologist and a CT-experienced pulmonologist each assessed the leading pattern, either NT, CLE, or PSE, in each of the 75 slices, and consensus was obtained in cases of disagreement. This resulted in 26 NT slices, 21 CLE slices, and 28 PSE slices. 168 nonoverlapping 31×31 pixel ROIs were subsequently manually annotated in the HRCT slices by indicating the center position of the ROIs. The following three classes were considered: NT (59 observations), CLE (50 observations), and PSE (59 observations). The 168 labeled CT ROIs is the data set used throughout the evaluation, and this is also the data set used in ref. [34].

15.3.3 Classification Setup

All texture descriptors are applied using the same classification setup, which consists of a supervised classifier, the k nearest neighbor classifier (kNN) [5, 9], where k is optimized on the training set. When a descriptor comprises several features or several feature histograms, an optimal subset is found by feature selection using the training set.

The *k*NN classifier is a flexible density-based classifier that makes no assumptions about the distribution of the data samples. Both unimodal and multimodal class distributions are automatically handled, as well as multiple classes, as is the case in the experiments carried out in this chapter. Further, both a vector space representation of the objects as well as a distance representation of the objects can easily be handled by *k*NN. This is practical in the experiments conducted since two representations are considered for each texture descriptor, where possible: directly using the distances computed between full histograms, e.g., distances between full GLCMs, and classification in a feature vector space where the objects are represented by summarizing measures computed from the histograms, e.g., using Equations 15.13, 15.14, 15.15, and 15.16 computed from the GLCMs.

An ROI **x** is classified by estimating the posterior probabilities $P(C_i|\mathbf{x})$ of the m different classes C_i, $i = 1, \ldots, m$, given that the input object is **x**, using the moderated *k*NN estimate [11]

$$P(C|\mathbf{x}) = \frac{k_c(\mathbf{x}) + 1}{k + m} \tag{15.22}$$

where $k_c(\mathbf{x})$ is the number of neighbors of **x** belonging to class C among the k nearest neighbors. The parameter k determines how many prototypes are used in the estimation of $P(C|\mathbf{x})$, and k effectively determines the smoothness of the decision boundary of the classifier. A larger k leads to a smoother decision boundary. The moderated *k*NN posterior estimate [11] is used since classifier combination [9] of the output of different descriptors will be investigated later in the chapter.

The *k*NN estimate in Equation 15.22 produces a soft classification output. A hard classification, i.e., a specific labeling of objects, is done by maximum a posteriori (MAP) classification [9], where an input object **x** is assigned to class C_i if

$$P(C_i|\mathbf{x}) > P(C_j|\mathbf{x}) \text{ for all } j \neq i. \tag{15.23}$$

The NT class is selected in case of a draw.

The distance between the objects used in *k*NN is computed differently depending on the representation. When using texture descriptors based on summarizing measures, the "traditional" approach to pattern recognition is taken [6], and the *k*NN classifier is applied in a feature vector space where each ROI is a point, positioned according to its corresponding feature values. We use the L_2-norm between the feature vectors as object distances in the *k*NN classifier

$$d_m(\mathbf{x}, \mathbf{y}) = \sqrt{\sum_{i=1}^{n} (x_i - y_i)^2} \tag{15.24}$$

where ROI **x** is represented by a vector of n measures $\mathbf{x} = [x_1, x_2, \ldots, x_n]^T$. When a texture descriptor based on one or several histograms is used, classification can be based on direct distance computations between the histograms. This can be seen as a "featureless" representation where object distances are used directly in classification [6]. The L_1-norm is used as histogram distance measure, which is equivalent to the histogram intersection, a traditional histogram distance measure in computer vision [35]. When the texture descriptor is based on several histograms, the distances between the individual histograms are combined by summation, giving rise to the following combined histogram distance measure

$$d_h(\mathbf{x},\mathbf{y}) = \sum_{i=1}^{N_f} \sum_{j=1}^{N_b} \left| f_{ij}(\mathbf{x}) - f_{ij}(\mathbf{y}) \right| \tag{15.25}$$

where $f_{ij}(\cdot)$ is the jth bin of the ith histogram, N_f is the number of histograms in the texture descriptor, and N_b is the number of histogram bins.

In cases where the descriptor consists of a set Y of several summarizing measures or histograms, these are optimized on the training data by feature selection. Here the goal is to find a subset $X \subseteq Y$ that is optimal according to some objective function. In this work, sequential forward selection (SFS) [9], a greedy combinatorial optimization search strategy, is used with the classification accuracy of the kNN classifier using the current representation X^i as objective function. One starts with an empty set $X^0 = \emptyset$ and iteratively evaluates each of the candidate measures or histograms x in conjunction with the existing subset $x \cup X^{i-1}$, $x \in Y \setminus X^{i-1}$ according to the objective function. The best performing combination of the current subset X^{i-1} and candidate feature $\hat{x}$ is retained producing $X^i = \hat{x} \cup X^{i-1}$. This procedure is iterated until the classification error converges.

15.3.4 Training and Parameter Selection

There are several parameters to set in the classification system, some of which are fixed, while the remaining are optimized on the training data. An ROI size of 31 × 31 pixels is used in all experiments for all texture descriptors. The number of histogram bins used when quantizing intensity in LBPs, GLCMs, GLRLMs, and INT, or when quantizing filter responses in the GFB, is fixed according to the following rule: $N_b = \sqrt[3]{N_p}$ where N_p is the number of pixels in the ROI. In all experiments, we have $N_b = \sqrt[3]{31^2} = 9$ bins. In INT, GFB, and for the intensity part of LBPs, we employ an adaptive binning principle similar to that of [16]; the total feature distribution across all ROIs in the training set is made approximately uniform. Consequently, densely populated areas in feature space are quantized with a high resolution, while sparse areas are quantized with a low resolution. In INT and GFB, the summarizing measures are computed from the original CT intensities and filter responses, respectively. In GLCMs and GLRLMs, the intensities are traditionally quantized using a fixed bin width, and we therefore use this scheme for these descriptors. For textons, no quantization of the intensities is performed. All histograms are normalized to sum to one, and all summarizing measures are centered and scaled to unit variance.

k in the kNN classifier is optimized using cross-validation, where the following k's are considered: $k = 1, 3, \ldots, \sqrt{n}$ where n is the number of prototypes in the kNN classifier, and the upper limit on k is depicted by the usual square root rule [11].

Table 15.1 lists the texture descriptors together with the descriptor-specific parameter values that are considered in the experiments. The texture descriptors described in Sections

TABLE 15.1

The Texture Descriptors Together with Their Corresponding Parameters and the Parameter Values Considered

Descriptor	Parameters	Number of Features	Feature Dimension
LBP	$(R, P)^{ri} = \{(1, 8), (2, 8), (3, 8)\}$	8	$\{36 \times 9, 10 \times 9, 18 \times 9, 26 \times 9\}$
	$(R, P)^{riu2} = \{(1, 8), (2, 16), (3, 24), (4, 24), (5, 24)\}$		
	$N_b = 9$		
$GFB^{h/m}$	$\sigma = \{0.5, 1, 2, 4\}$	$16/16 \times 4$	9/1
	$N_b = 9$		
$GLCM^{h/m}$	$\theta = \{0, 45, 90, 135\}$ (averaged)	$5/5 \times 4$	$9 \times 9/1$
	$d = \{1, 2, 3, 4, 5\}$		
	$Nb = 9$		
$GLRLM^{h/m}$	$\theta = \{0, 45, 90, 135\}$ (averaged)	1/5	$9 \times 10/1$
	$MRL = 10$		
	$N_b = 9$		
$INT^{h/m}$	$N_b = 9$	1/4	9/1
TEXTONS	$N_c = \{10, 20, 30, 40, 50\}$	5×4	$\{30, 60, 90, 120, 150\}$
	$TS \times TS = \{3 \times 3, 5 \times 5, 7 \times 7, 9 \times 9\}$		

Note: The parameters are (R, P) (LBP radius and number of samples pair, different pairs are considered for rotation invariant and uniform LBP indicated by ^{ri} and ^{riu2}.), σ (GFB scale), θ (angle in GLCMs and GLRLMs), d (distance in GLCMs), *MRL* (maximum run length in GLRLMs), N_c (number of cluster centers per class in textons), $TS \times TS$ (texton size), N_b (number of histogram bins, used both for quantizing image gray levels in LBPs, GLCMs, GLRLMs, and INT, and for quantizing filter responses in the GFB). "Number of features" is the number of candidate histograms or summarizing measures in the descriptor. An optimal subset of these is found using SFS. "Feature dimension" is the dimensionality of one candidate "feature" considered in SFS. For histograms, this is the number of bins. For summarizing measures, this is one. When both full histograms and summarizing measures are considered for a particular descriptor, this is indicated by $^{h/m}$, and the corresponding number of features and feature dimension(s) are shown for both representations separated by a forward slash.

15.2.1, 15.2.2, 15.2.3, 15.2.4, 15.2.5 and 15.2.6, which we term *INT, LBP, GFB, GLCM, GLRLM,* and *TEXTONS*, respectively, are applied. Where applicable, full histograms as well as summarizing measures are used, indicated by ^{h} and ^{m}. LBPs and textons are applied only as histograms. In *GLCM* and *GLRLM*, both the full matrices and the summarizing measures are averaged across the four angles θ = {0, 45, 90, 135} as is often done in the literature. However, we do not average across distances in *GLCM*. In *LBP*, we consider $LBP2^{ri}$ and $LBP2^{riu2}$ with different pairs of parameters (R, P).

The performance is estimated using leave-one-out error estimation at the subject level. In each of the 25 leave-out trials, all ROIs from the test subject are held out, and the classification system using the different texture descriptors is trained on the remaining data. The remaining subjects are separated into a training set and a validation set. In this separation, balanced class distributions are ensured by placing half the subjects from each class in the training set and the rest in the validation set. k in the kNN classifier is optimized using cross-validation with the ROIs in the training set as prototypes, and the classification accuracy on the validation set is used as a performance criterion. SFS is applied within this cross-validation procedure to find an optimal subset in the texture descriptor, either a set of histograms or of summarizing measures, for each value of k considered. Subsequently, the ROIs in the test set are classified with the training set ROIs as prototypes using the

TABLE 15.2

Results of the Leave-One-Out Error Estimation at Subject Level

Descriptor	CA
LBP	92.9
GFB^h	95.2
$GLCM^h$	92.3
$GLRLM^h$	89.9
INT^h	91.1
TEXTONS	92.3
GFB^m	75.6
$GLCM^m$	92.9
$GLRLM^m$	86.9
INT^m	78.0

Note: CA: classification accuracy.

optimal k and the optimal histogram or measure subset obtained using SFS. Note that INT^h and $GLRLM^h$ consist of only one histogram, and SFS is not applied in these cases.

15.3.5 Classification Results

The texture descriptors are evaluated by MAP classification accuracy (CA), the performance of the different descriptors is reported in Table 15.2, and the p-values of comparing the MAP classification outputs of the different descriptors are reported in Table 15.3. We also inspect the CA as a function of the size of the training set. This is done by varying the number of subjects in the training set, and for each size, do 10 repeated leave-one-subject-out error estimations with a randomly drawn training set of that particular size. As previous, the classes are balanced in the data splits, and the same randomly drawn training sets are used for all descriptors. The whole learning framework is applied in the same way as

TABLE 15.3

p-Values of Comparing the MAP Classification Outputs of the Different Texture Descriptors Using McNemar's Test [4]

	LBP	GFB^h	$GLCM^h$	$GLRLM^h$	INT^h	*TEXTONS*	GFB^m	$GLCM^m$	$GLRLM^m$	INT^m
LBP	-	-	-	-	-	-	-	-	-	-
GFB^h	0.386	-	-	-	-	-	-	-	-	-
$GLCM^h$	1.000	0.332	-	-	-	-	-	-	-	-
$GLRLM^h$	0.359	0.066	0.502	-	-	-	-	-	-	-
INT^h	0.546	0.146	0.773	0.831	-	-	-	-	-	-
TEXTONS	1.000	0.228	0.773	0.522	0.752	-	-	-	-	-
GFB^m	**$<10^{-4}$**	**$<10^{-4}$**	**$<10^{-4}$**	**$<10^{-4}$**	**$<10^{-4}$**	**$<10^{-4}$**	-	-	-	-
$GLCM^m$	0.814	0.423	1.000	0.404	0.646	1.000	**$<10^{-4}$**		-	-
$GLRLM^m$	0.078	**0.006**	0.124	0.458	0.265	0.124	**0.002**	**0.044**	-	-
INT^m	**$<10^{-4}$**	**$<10^{-4}$**	**$<10^{-4}$**	**0.002**	**$<10^{-4}$**	**$<10^{-4}$**	0.596	**$<10^{-4}$**	**0.021**	-

Note: Significant p-values, i.e., $p < 0.05$, are highlighted in bold font.

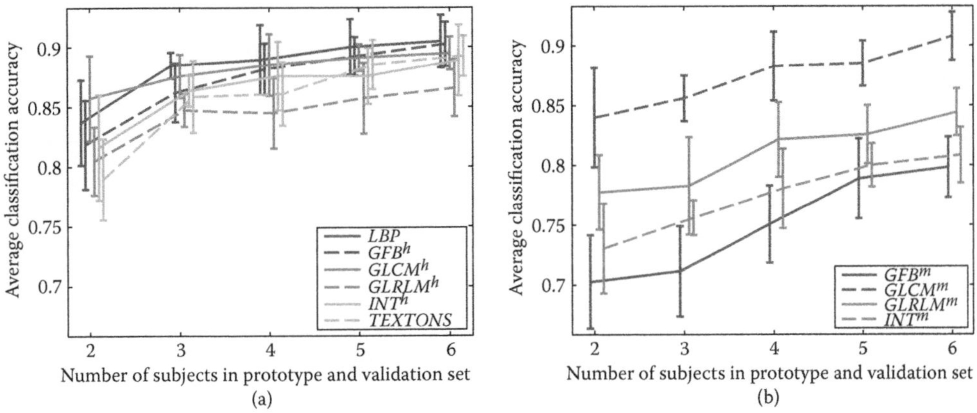

FIGURE 15.9
Learning curves for the different texture descriptors. The average ± the standard deviation of the CA from 10 random trials is reported.

described previously, including optimization of k and feature selection on the training set, for each of the 10 repeated leave-one-out trials. The average curves ± the standard deviation across the 10 trials are shown in Figure 15.9.

15.3.6 Selected Parameters

The number of times a particular k is selected in the leave-one-out estimation is reported in Table 15.4 for the different descriptors. Further, the histograms or measures that are most often selected in SFS in the leave-one-out estimation are reported in Table 15.5 for the different descriptors. Note that this does not reflect which "features" are in the same subsets in the different leave-out trials, only how often a "feature" is selected independently. Nothing is reported for INT^h and $GLRLM^h$, as these descriptors comprise only one histogram.

TABLE 15.4
Optimized ks in the kNN Classifier for the Different Descriptors in the Leave-One-Out Experiments at Subject Level

Descriptor	Value of k in kNN
LBP	1 (100%)
GFB^h	1 (80%) 3 (12%) 5 (8%)
$GLCM^h$	1 (92%) 5 (4%) 7 (4%)
$GLRLM^h$	5 (72%) 1 (28%)
INT^h	1 (68%) 3 (20%) 5 (8%) 7 (4%)
TEXTONS	1 (100%)
GFB^m	9 (44%) 1 (40%) 3 (12%) 5 (4%)
$GLCM^m$	1 (68%) 3 (24%) 9 (8%)
$GLRLM^m$	1 (72%) 3 (20%) 5 (4%) 9 (4%)
INT^m	1 (44%) 5 (24%) 3 (16%) 7 (8%) 9 (8%)

Note: 100% means that the value was selected in all 25 leave-out trials.

TABLE 15.5

The Four Most Frequently Selected Histograms or Summarizing Measures in the SFS Procedure for the Different Texture Descriptors

Descriptor	Features			
LBP	$LBP2^{ri}(\cdot; 1, 8)$ (64%)	$LBP2^{riu2}(\cdot; 4, 24)$ (36%)	$LBP2^{ri}(\cdot; 2, 8)$ (28%)	$LBP2^{riu2}(\cdot; 1, 8)$ (28%)
GFB^h	$G(\cdot, 0.5)$ (100%)	$\|\nabla G(\cdot, 1)\|_2$ (76%)	$\|\nabla G(\cdot, 0.5)\|_2$ (40%)	$K(\cdot, 0.5)$ (16%)
$GLCM^h$	$p(\cdot,\cdot; 2)$ (76%)	$p(\cdot,\cdot; 4)$ (12%)	$p(\cdot,\cdot; 3)$ (8%)	$p(\cdot,\cdot; 5)$ (4%)
TEXTONS	$\{TS = 3, N_c = 30\}$ (48%)	$\{TS = 3, N_c = 20\}$ (44%)	$\{TS = 5, N_c = 30\}$ (40%)	$\{TS = 5, N_c = 20\}$ (24%)
GFB^m	$\mu(G(\cdot, 0.5))$ (68%)	$\mu(G(\cdot, 1))$ (44%)	$\mu(G(\cdot, 4))$ (44%)	$skew(G(\cdot, 0.5))$ (32%)
$GLCM^m$	$CORR(\cdot; 1)$ (52%)	$UE(\cdot; 1)$ (44%)	$CORR(\cdot; 3)$ (44%)	$C(\cdot; 1)$ (28%)
$GLRLM^m$	$RLN(\cdot)$ (100%)	$RP(\cdot)$ (96%)	$LRE(\cdot)$ (80%)	$GLN(\cdot)$ (72%)
INT^m	$\mu(\cdot)$ (100%)	$skew(\cdot)$ (60%)	$\sigma(\cdot)$ (36%)	$kurtosis(\cdot)$ (8%)

Note: Individual occurrences are reported, but the histograms/measures are usually part of a larger subset. 100% means that the histogram or measure was selected in all 25 leave-out trials.

15.3.7 Combining Information

Several different texture descriptors have been evaluated, giving rise to several different classifiers, one for each descriptor. These different classifiers may capture different, but complementary, information in the ROIs. This motivates the idea of using classifier combination [9] for combining the information captured by the different descriptors into an overall classification. The outputs of the different classifiers are combined using a fixed combination rule, or combiner. This classifier combination scheme, where all the individual classifiers are invoked independently, is the most commonly used in the literature [9]. Three combiners are considered [9, 12]: the majority voting rule, the mean rule, and the product rule. In majority voting, MAP classification (Equation 15.23) is applied prior to voting. The mean and the product rule are both applied directly on the posteriors. Three setups are considered, one using only the histogram-based descriptors, i.e., *LBP*, GFB^h, $GLCM^h$, $GLRLM^h$, INT^h, and *TEXTONS*; one using only the summarizing measure-based descriptors, i.e., GFB^m, $GLCM^m$, $GLRLM^m$, INT^m; and one using all descriptors. Table 15.6 lists the resulting classification accuracies. Combining descriptors slightly increases

TABLE 15.6

Results of Classifier Combination

Descriptor Set	Combiner	CA
Histograms	Majority voting	94.6
	Mean	94.6
	Product	94.6
Summarizing measures	Majority voting	86.3
	Mean	87.5
	Product	86.9
Histograms + summarizing measures	Majority voting	95.2
	Mean	95.8
	Product	95.8

Note: CA: classification accuracy.

performance in two cases; the product rule and the mean rule applied to all descriptors achieves CA = 95.8%, which means that one more sample is correctly classified than with the best performing individual descriptor, GFB^h, which achieved CA = 95.2%. However, these differences are not significant.

We also experimented with an alternative way of combining information from different descriptors by considering all histograms or measures collectively in the classification system. In this case, all descriptors are candidates in the feature selection. Using full histograms achieved CA = 92.9%, and using summarizing measures achieved CA = 86.9%. Further, a combination of $GLCM^{h/m}$, $GLRLM^{h/m}$, and $INT^{h/m}$ was experimented with. This represents a descriptor that is used in several studies in the literature [2, 18, 20, 21, 38, 45]. This resulted in CA = 93.5% and CA = 87.5%, for histograms and summarizing measures, respectively.

15.4 Discussion and Conclusion

This chapter reviewed several popular texture descriptors in the literature for tissue classification in pulmonary CT, with a focus on emphysema classification.

Most of the evaluated descriptors performed well. The considered data set is small, and there were therefore few significant differences between the descriptors in general and none between the descriptors that performed well. The results suggest for using full histogram approaches, i.e., *LBP*, GFB^h, $GLCM^h$, and *TEXTONS* performed similarly and slightly better than *GLRLM* and *INT* while significantly better than using moments of distributions as was used in GFB^m and INT^m. No descriptor stood out as the single best one. The GFB using full filter response histograms, GFB^h, achieved the highest accuracy, CA = 95.2%; see Table 15.2. However, this was not significantly different from any of the competing full histogram descriptors; see Table 15.3. The data used here are the same as are used in [34], but the results are slightly different due to differences in the classification setup. In [34], the ROI size was also optimized on the training data, for example. However, the GFB using full histograms and LBPs both performed well and were not significantly different according to the results in this chapter, and this was also the result in ref. [34].

Two descriptors that are still commonly used, GFB^m and INT^m, performed significantly worse than all the remaining descriptors; see Tables 15.2 and 15.3. The two descriptors were not significantly different from each other, which is explained by the fact that the four most often selected summarizing measures in GFB^m are based on blurred intensities (see Table 15.5), i.e., the two descriptors capture similar information.

Summarizing measures, which are heavily used in the literature, did not work well for all descriptors. The results of the conducted experiment show that using moments instead of full histograms for INT and GFB discards important discriminative information for the investigated classification task, as indicated by the significant degradation in performance when comparing INT^h to INT^m and GFB^h to GFB^m; see Tables 15.2 and 15.3. For the classical texture descriptors, GLCMs and GLRLMs, the common approach of using summarizing measures, instead of full matrices, works well.

The data set used in the experiment is small, and as can be seen from the learning curves in Figure 15.9, all descriptors could benefit from more training data, i.e., none of the curves converge. Some descriptors perform well already at small data sizes, and these descriptors are *LBP*, $GLCM^h$, and $GLCM^m$. However, descriptors such as GFB^h and *TEXTONS* approach a good performance as the data size increases and may prove even better for more data than are available in this experiment. Allowing many options in the feature selection, such as in GFB where many filters are considered, also increases the demand on the training data size in order to avoid overtraining. This may also be reflected in the learning curves.

The descriptors should also be judged based on other criteria than classification performance. One criterion is the complexity of the descriptor. Histogram-based descriptors are generally richer in information at the expense of increased complexity, while summarizing measures reduce the dimensionality, and hence the complexity. The crucial point here is whether important discriminative information is lost in this process, and this was clearly the case for some descriptors in the conducted experiments. The complexity of the different descriptors can be seen in Table 15.1, where the dimensionality of the individual components of the descriptors, i.e., number of bins in the individual histograms for the histogram-based descriptors, is listed in the fourth column. In general, *LBP* is the most complex descriptor, followed by *TEXTONS*. This should also be judged in light of how many and which "features" are selected in SFS, and as can be seen in Table 15.5, $LBP2^{ri}(\cdot; 1, 8)$ that has 36×9 bins is frequently selected.

The data considered in this chapter was HRCT slices, and hence, the focus was on 2D descriptors. However, since volumetric CT images are becoming state of the art, it is important to consider whether the descriptors are applicable in 3D. INT and GFB can be, and have already been [30, 31], directly extended to 3D without any increase in complexity. Note, however, that more samples are available for estimating histograms and that the number of histogram bins therefore can be increased. GLCMs and GLRLMs have also already been extended and applied in 3D [45]. In this case, the number of angles, and thereby matrices, increases. However, when averaging across angle, the complexity stays the same. As for GFB and INT, the intensity can be quantized into more bins due to more available samples for histogram estimation. It is not straightforward how to extend LBPs to 3D. Two approximate extensions of LBP to 3D are presented in ref. [46], with the specific application being temporal texture data in computer vision. The first approach forms a helical path in the temporal direction. This idea could be applied in volumetric CT, e.g., by forming helical paths in various directions and combining the resulting LBPs. The second approach in ref. [46] computes 2D LBPs in three orthogonal planes and concatenates these. Other studies consider samples on a sphere centered on the voxel of interest [14, 19]. In these cases, there is no natural ordering of the samples as is the case when considering a circle. The complexity increases in all approaches. The texton approach considered in this chapter uses a raw pixel representation, and increasing the dimensionality to 3D has the effect of increasing the feature space where both the clustering and the texton codebook similarities are computed. This need not increase the complexity of the descriptor, i.e., the number of cluster centers, but it puts increasing demand on more training data in order to reliably estimate cluster centers.

It may seem somewhat surprising that the combination of $GLCM^m$, $GLRLM^m$, and INT^m, often used in the literature [2, 18, 20, 21, 38, 45], performed worse than $GLCM^m$ alone. This is because SFS is a greedy combinatorial optimization procedure that can get stuck in local optima, in this case due to elements from the descriptors INT^m or $GLRLM^m$ being selected early in the optimization process. Care should therefore be taken when using a feature selection scheme. The same argument holds for the results obtained when performing feature selection on the combined set of all descriptors, which also performed worse than several of the individual descriptors. Combining the texture descriptors by classifier combination in a parallel scheme using a fixed combiner improved results slightly, with CA = 95.8%, when all descriptors, both histograms and summarizing measures, were considered in conjunction with the product or the mean rule; see Table 15.6. However, this was not significantly better than the best performing individual descriptor, GFB^h. We expect classifier combination to be more beneficial in problems with more complicated and diverse texture classes than the ones encountered when classifying emphysema in CT.

In conclusion, several popular texture descriptors in the medical image analysis literature for texture-based emphysema classification in pulmonary CT were reviewed and evaluated within the same classification framework. The evaluation was performed on an emphysema CT ROI classification task. No descriptor was significantly better than all other descriptors. In general, full histogram representations performed better than moments of histograms, and intensity and run-length features alone seemed to perform less well than the more complex texture descriptors. There were indications that combining the classification output of several classifiers, each based on a different texture descriptor, is beneficial. However, the increase in performance was not significant for the considered classification task.

References

[1] Barnes, P. J. 2000. Chronic obstructive pulmonary disease. *The New England Journal of Medicine*, 343(4):269–280.

[2] Chabat, F., G.-Z. Yang, and D. M. Hansell. 2003. Obstructive lung diseases: texture classification for differentiation at CT. *Radiology*, 228(3):871–877.

[3] Cula, O. G., and K. J. Dana. 2004. 3D texture recognition using bidirectional feature histograms. *International Journal of Computer Vision*, 59(1):33–60.

[4] Dietterich, T. G. 1998. Approximate statistical test for comparing supervised classification learning algorithms. *Neural Computation*, 10(7):1895–1923.

[5] Duda, R. O., P. E. Hart, and D. G. Stork. 2000. *Pattern Classification* (2nd ed.). Wiley-Interscience.

[6] Duin, R. P. W., D. de Ridder, and D. M. J. Tax. 1998. Featureless pattern classification. *Kybernetika*, 34(4):399–404.

[7] Gangeh, M. J., L. Sørensen, S. B. Shaker, M. S. Kamel, M. de Bruijne, and M. Loog. 2010. A texton-based approach for the classification of lung parenchyma in CT images. In T. Jiang, N. Navab, J. P. W. Pluim, and M. A. Viergever (eds.), *Medical Image Computing and Computer Assisted Intervention*, volume 6363 of *Lecture Notes in Computer Science*, pp. 596–603. Springer.

[8] Haralick, R. M. 1979. Statistical and structural approaches to texture. *Proceedings of the IEEE*, 67(5):786–804.

[9] Jain, A. K., R. P. W. Duin, and J. Mao. 2000. Statistical pattern recognition: a review. *IEEE Transactions Pattern Analysis and Machine Intelligence*, 22(1):4–37.

[10] Juelsz, B. 1981. Textons, the elements of texture-perception, and their interactions. *Nature*, 290(5802):91–97.

[11] Kittler, J., and F. M. Alkoot. 2002. Moderating k-NN classifiers. *Pattern Analysis and Applications*, 5(3):326–332.

[12] Kuncheva, L. I. 2004. *Combining Pattern Classifiers: Methods and Algorithms*. Wiley-Interscience,.

[13] Leung, T., and J. Malik. 2001. Representing and recognizing the visual appearance of materials using three-dimensional textons. *International Journal of Computer Vision*, 43(1):29–44.

[14] Liao, S., and A. C. S. Chung. 2009. Non-rigid image registration with uniform spherical structure patterns. In J. L. Prince, D. L. Pham, and K. J. Myers (eds.), *Information Processing in Medical Imaging*, volume 5636 of *Lecture Notes in Computer Science*, pp. 163–175. Springer.

[15] Mirmehdiand, M., X. Xie, and J. Suri (eds.). 2008. *Handbook of Texture Analysis*. Imperial College Press.

[16] Ojala, T., M. Pietikäinen, and D. Harwood. 1996. A comparative study of texture measures with classification based on featured distributions. *Pattern Recognition*, 29(1):51–59.

[17] Ojala, T., M. Pietikäinen, and T. Mäenpää. 2002. Multiresolution gray-scale and rotation invariant texture classification with local binary patterns. *IEEE Transactions Pattern Analysis and Machine Intelligence*, 24(7):971–987.

[18] Park, Y. S., J. B. Seo, N. Kim, E. J. Chae, Y. M. Oh, S. D. Lee, Y. Lee, and S.-H. Kang. 2008. Texture-based quantification of pulmonary emphysema on high-resolution computed tomography: comparison with density-based quantification and correlation with pulmonary function test. *Investigative Radiology*, 43(6):395–402.

[19] Paulhac, L., P. Makris, and Y.-J. Ramel. 2008. Comparison between 2D and 3D local binary pattern methods for characterisation of three-dimensional textures. In A. C. Campilho and M. S. Kamel (eds.), *Image Analysis and Recognition*, volume 5112 of *Lecture Notes in Computer Science*, pp. 670–679. Springer.

[20] Prasad, M., A. Sowmya, and I. Koch. 2008. Designing relevant features for continuous data sets using ICA. *International Journal of Computational Intelligence and Applications*, 7(4):447–468.

[21] Prasad, M., A. Sowmya, and P. Wilson. 2009. Multi-level classification of emphysema in HRCT lung images. *Pattern Analysis and Applications*, 12(1):9–20.

[22] Rabe, K. F., S. Hurd, A. Anzueto, P. J. Barnes, S. A. Buist, P. Calverley, Y. Fukuchi, C. Jenkins, R. Rodriguez-Roisin, C. van Weel, J. Zielinski, and Global Initiative for Chronic Obstructive Lung Disease. 2007. Global strategy for the diagnosis, management, and prevention of chronic obstructive pulmonary disease: GOLD executive summary. *American Journal of Respiratory and Critical Care Medicine*, 176(6):532–555.

[23] Schmid, C. 2001. Constructing models for content-based image retrieval. In *IEEE Conference on Computer Vision and Pattern Recognition*, pp. 39–45. IEEE Computer Society Press.

[24] Schmid, C. 2004. Weakly supervised learning of visual models and its application to content-based retrieval. *International Journal of Computer Vision*, 56(1-2, Sp. Iss. SI):7–16.

[25] Shaker, S. B., A. Dirksen, K. S. Bach, and J. Mortensen. 2007. Imaging in chronic obstructive pulmonary disease. *COPD*, 4(2):143–161.

[26] Shaker, S. B., K. A. von Wachenfeldt, S. Larsson, I. Mile, S. Persdotter, M. Dahlbäck, P. Broberg, B. Stoel, K. S. Bach, M. Hestad, T. E. Fehniger, and A. Dirksen. 2008. Identification of patients with chronic obstructive pulmonary disease (COPD) by measurement of plasma biomarkers. *The Clinical Respiratory Journal*, 2(1):17–25.

[27] Sluimer, I. C., M. Prokop, I. Hartmann, and B. van Ginneken. 2006. Automated classification of hyperlucency, fibrosis, ground glass, solid and focal lesions in high resolution CT of the lung. *Medical Physics*, 33(7):2610–2620.

[28] Sluimer, I. C., A. Schilham, M. Prokop, and B. van Ginneken. 2006. Computer analysis of computed tomography scans of the lung: a survey. *IEEE Transactions on Medical Imaging*, 25(4):385–405.

[29] Sluimer, I. C., P. F. van Waes, M. A. Viergever, and B. van Ginneken. 2003. Computer-aided diagnosis in high resolution CT of the lungs. *Medical Physics*, 30(12):3081–3090.

[30] Sørensen, L., P. Lo, H. Ashraf, J. Sporring, M. Nielsen, and M. de Bruijne. 2009. Learning COPD sensitive filters in pulmonary CT. In G.-Z. Yang, D. J. Hawkes, D. Rueckert, J. A. Noble, and C. J. Taylor (eds.), *Medical Image Computing and Computer Assisted Intervention*, volume 5761 of *Lecture Notes in Computer Science*, pp. 699–706. Springer.

[31] Sørensen, L., M. Loog, P. Lo, H. Ashraf, A. Dirksen, R. P. W. Duin, and M. de Bruijne. 2010. Image dissimilarity-based quantification of lung disease from CT. In T. Jiang, N. Navab, J. P. W. Pluim, and M. A. Viergever (eds.), *Medical Image Computing and Computer Assisted Intervention*, volume 6361 of *Lecture Notes in Computer Science*. Springer.

[32] Sørensen, L., S. B. Shaker, and M. de Bruijne. 2008. Texture based emphysema quantification in lung CT. In M. Brown, M. de Bruijne, B. van Ginneken, A. Kiraly, J.-M. Kuhnigk, C. Lorenz, K. Mori, and J. Reinhardt (eds.), *Proc. of The First International Workshop on Pulmonary Image Analysis*, pp. 5–14.

[33] Sørensen, L., S. B. Shaker, and M. de Bruijne. 2008. Texture classification in lung CT using local binary patterns. In D. N. Metaxas, L. Axel, G. Fichtinger, and G. Székely (eds.), *Medical Image Computing and Computer Assisted Intervention*, volume 5241 of *Lecture Notes in Computer Science*, pp. 934–941. Springer.
[34] Sørensen, L., S. B. Shaker, and M. de Bruijne. 2010. Quantitative analysis of pulmonary emphysema using local binary patterns. *IEEE Transactions on Medical Imaging*, 29(2):559–569.
[35] Swain, M. J., and D. H. Ballard. 1991. Color indexing. *International Journal of Computer Vision*, 7(1):11–32.
[36] ter Haar Romeny, B. M. 1997. Applications of scale-space theory. *Gaussian Scale-Space Theory*, pp. 3–19. Kluwer Academic Publishers.
[37] Tuceryan, M., and A. K. Jain. 1998. Texture analysis. *The Handbook of Pattern Recognition and Computer Vision* (2nd ed.), pp. 207–248. World Scientific Publishing.
[38] Uppaluri, R., E. A. Hoffman, M. Sonka, P. G. Hartley, G. W. Hunninghake, and G. McLennan. 1999. Computer recognition of regional lung disease patterns. *American Journal of Respiratory and Critical Care Medicine*, 160(2):648–654.
[39] Uppaluri, R., T. Mitsa, M. Sonka, E. A. Hoffman, and G. McLennan. 1997. Quantification of pulmonary emphysema from lung computed tomography images. *American Journal of Respiratory and Critical Care Medicine*, 156(1):248–254.
[40] van Ginneken, B., and B. M. ter Haar Romeny. 2003. Multi-scale texture classification from generalized locally orderless images. *Pattern Recognition*, 36(4):899–911.
[41] Varma, M., and A. Zisserman. 2003. Texture classification: are filter banks necessary? In *IEEE Conference on Computer Vision and Pattern Recognition*, pp. 691–698. IEEE Computer Society.
[42] Varma, M., and A. Zisserman. 2005. A statistical approach to texture classification from single images. *International Journal of Computer Vision*, 62(1-2):61–81.
[43] Varma, M., and A. Zisserman. 2009. A statistical approach to material classification using image patch exemplars. *IEEE Transactions Pattern Analysis and Machine Intelligence*, 31(11):2032–2047.
[44] Webb, W. R., N. L. Müller, and D. P. Naidich. 2001. *High-Resolution CT of the Lung* (3rd ed.). Lippincott Williams & Wilkins.
[45] Xu, Y., M. Sonka, G. McLennan, J. Guo, and E. A. Hoffman. 2006. MDCT-based 3-D texture classification of emphysema and early smoking related lung pathologies. *IEEE Transactions on Medical Imaging*, 25(4):464–475.
[46] Zhao, G., and M. Pietikäinen. 2007. Dynamic texture recognition using local binary patterns with an application to facial expressions. *IEEE Transactions Pattern Analysis and Machine Intelligence*, 29(6):915–928.
[47] Zhu, S. C., Y. Wu, and D. Mumford. 1998. Filters, random fields and maximum entropy (frame): towards a unified theory for texture modeling. *International Journal of Computer Vision*, 27(2):107–126.

16

Computer-Aided Assessment and Stenting of Tracheal Stenosis

Rômulo Pinho, Kurt G. Tournoy, and Jan Sijbers

CONTENTS

16.1 Introduction

Tracheal stenosis is an unnatural narrowing of the trachea with traumatic, neoplastic, or idiopathic causes that, despite being relatively rare, can be life threatening (Spittle and McCluskey, 2000). Until now, tracheal resection surgery remains the preferred choice of treatment. In this modality, the narrowed part of the trachea is removed and the ends are sutured together (Elliott et al. 2003; Grillo et al. 1995). When the stenosis is too long or when the patient status does not permit a surgical procedure, stent implants can render a successful solution to the stricture (Venuta et al. 2004; Saito and Imamura, 2005). Stents are tubular structures, currently made of silicone or metallic alloys, used to return normal breathing function to a patient by pushing the narrowed regions of the trachea. Since they are usually implanted with bronchoscopes, they reduce the surgical risk to the patient, especially when compared with tracheal resection (Ching-Yang et al. 2007; Mandour et al. 2003; Miyazawa et al. 2004).

The choice of treatment is a direct result of the assessment of the stenosis. It means that, when assessing the stenoses, it is important to correctly determine their location, length, and degree of narrowing (Boiselle et al. 2008). Traditionally, stenoses have been assessed with rigid or flexible bronchoscopy (Carretta et al. 2006; Nouraei et al. 2006). These methods, however, are invasive, often require patient sedation, and render subjective results, which depend on the expertise of the specialist in charge. Bronchoscopic methods may not even serve their purpose if the stricture is too narrow to allow the passage of the bronchoscope itself. If a stent is to be used in the treatment, the assessment also determines its dimensions (external diameter and length) and deployment location.

With advances in the imaging field, image analysis has increasingly been used as a complementary tool for the assessment of stenosis and computed tomography (CT) is often the imaging modality of choice. A variety of methods have been proposed to assess stenosis using CT image analysis and processing. Lee et al. (2005) reviewed the use of multislice CT analysis in prestenting and poststenting scenarios. Shitrit et al. (2005) and Hoppe et al. (2004) showed that virtual bronchoscopy can be used in training as well as in real cases. A precondition to a successful treatment with stents is that the size and diameter of the tubes must be correctly estimated; otherwise, problems such as stent migration and improper mucus clearance often occur (Venuta et al. 2004; Saito and Imamura, 2005; Prasad et al. 2002; Carretta et al. 2006). Further improvements to traditional assessment methods have been proposed. In many cases, the cross-sectional diameter or area profile of the trachea is extracted from the CT images and plotted on a graph (Graham et al. 2000; Sorantin et al. 2002; Kiesler et al. 2007; Triglia et al. 2002). Ballester et al. (2009) proposed a graphical user interface in which the physician manually places a stent in the CT image of the patient. Despite these improvements, tracheal stenosis assessment and stent choice remain, to date, operator-dependent operations.

This chapter describes and discusses traditional and computer-aided methods for the assessment and stenting of tracheal stenosis. In particular, a new method proposed by Pinho et al. (2010) is described in detail. This method uses deformable shape models to estimate the healthy trachea of patients (i.e., in case stenosis was not present) and segment the narrowed tracheas from their chest CT scans. Healthy and narrowed versions of the trachea are compared in order to automatically detect the stenoses and their parameters. The parameters are eventually used in the automatic suggestion of patient-specific stents.

In the remainder of the chapter, the reader is first provided with a brief clinical background on the anatomy of the trachea and the main characteristics of stenosis and stents (Section 16.2). Section 16.3 reviews traditional methods for assessment of stenosis, whereas Section 16.4 discusses computer-aided techniques. The method presented by Pinho et al. (2010) is described in Section 16.5, and the chapter is concluded in Section 16.6.

16.2 Clinical Background

16.2.1 Anatomy of the Trachea

The tracheobronchial tree constitutes the airway below the vocal cords. Consisting of a hierarchical group of tubular structures, the trachea is the primary tube of this tree. It functions as a conduit for ventilation and clearance of secretions.

The shape of the healthy trachea may present considerable variation. Changing with age, it gradually goes from funnel-shaped in infancy to ovoid in adulthood. The radial shape is normally ovoid anteroposteriorly but can also appear ovoid in the sagittal direction, be circular or, less frequently, slightly triangular. Unique and unexplained distortions may occur as well (Grillo et al. 1995). The length goes from 9 to 12 cm in adults, measured from the lower border of cricoid cartilage down to the top of the carinal spur, while the average laterolateral diameter is between 1.3 and 2.2 cm (Webb et al. 2000; Grillo et al. 1995).

The trachea is composed of 18 to 22 anteriorly located horseshoe-shaped cartilaginous open circles, whose ends are posteriorly connected by a soft membrane. It bifurcates approximately at the sternal angle into the left and right main bronchi, and the carina is the ridge separating their openings. On CT, the tracheal wall is usually visible as a 1- to 3-mm soft tissue stripe, delineated internally by air in the tracheal lumen and externally by mediastinal fat, the lungs, larger vessels, and the esophagus. The posterior tracheal wall appears thinner and more variable in contour, since it lacks cartilage. It can appear convex, concave, or flat. During expiration, CT typically shows significant anterior bulging of the posterior membrane, but the anterior and lateral walls change little (Webb et al. 2000). Figure 16.1 provides illustrations of the tracheal anatomy.

16.2.2 Tracheal Stenosis

Tracheobronchial stenosis is defined as focal or diffuse narrowing of the tracheal lumen (Figure 16.2). By far, the most common cause of tracheal stenosis is trauma, specifically internal trauma, usually occasioned by any type of intubation (Grillo, 2004; Boiselle et al. 2008; Lee and Boiselle, 2008). There are other potential causes of tracheal stenosis, including inflammatory diseases, benign or malignant neoplastic conditions, and extrinsic

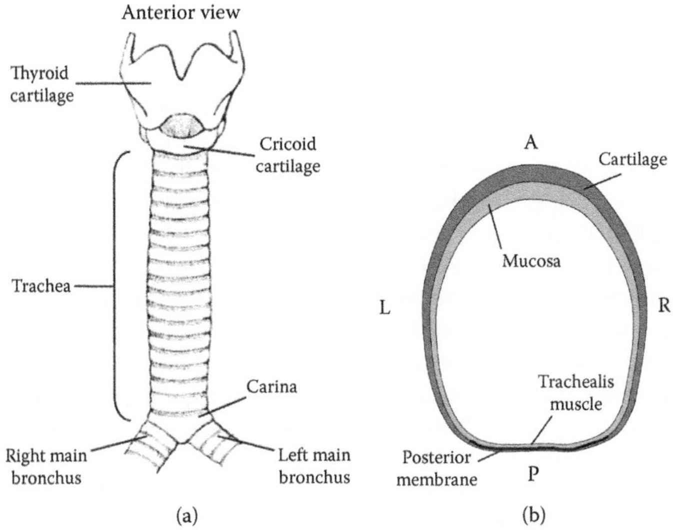

FIGURE 16.1
Different views of the trachea and its composing structures: (a) illustration of the whole trachea and (b) schematic view of an axial cross section.

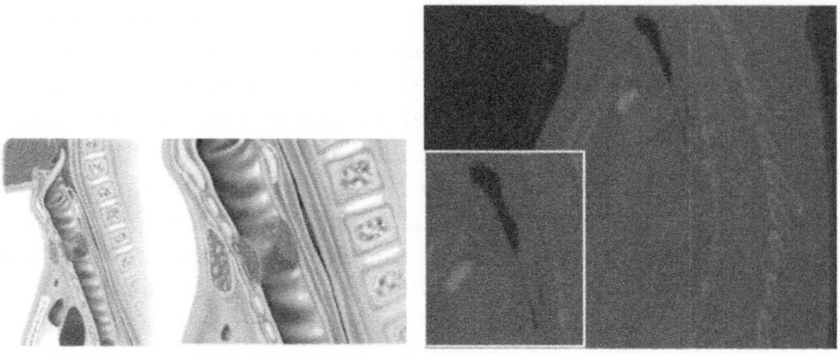
(a) (b)

FIGURE 16.2
(a) A schematic view of stenosis. (Courtesy of Dr. P. Delaere, Center for Larynx, Trachea and Hypopharynx Reconstruction, Katholieke Universiteit Leuven, Belgium.) (b) A real case showing one sagittal slice of a chest CT scan.

pressure. In addition, idiopathic narrowing of the trachea is not completely uncommon, predominantly appearing in women (Grillo et al. 1995).

Typical symptoms of tracheal stenosis include shortness of breath, coughing, and stridor. The narrowing may be seen in various different shapes. It typically extends from 1.5 to 2.5 cm in length (Webb et al. 2000), but cases of long-segment tracheal stenosis have also been reported (Elliott et al. 2003). It has also been reported that the shape of the stricture is usually associated with its causes (Lee and Boiselle, 2008; Webb et al. 2000).

16.2.3 Tracheal Stents

The medical term *stent* was introduced by Charles R. Stent, a British dentist who developed a device that supported the healing of gum grafts. The term has since been used to refer to any device designed to maintain the integrity of hollow tubular structures (Saito and Imamura, 2005; Freitag, 2000). Tracheal stents are tubular structures, currently made of silicone or metallic alloys, used to return normal breathing function to the patient by pushing the narrowed regions of the trachea (Ching-Yang et al. 2007; Mandour et al. 2003; Miyazawa et al. 2004). Examples of the different materials, shapes, and sizes of coated and uncoated stents are shown in Figure 16.3.

Although airway resection and reconstruction is most often the preferred therapy for both benign and malignant lesions, a variety of factors, including long stenosis, failed previous repair, metastatic or unresectable malignancy, or even patient refusal,may dictate nonsurgical management. In these cases, bronchoscopic treatment is indicated, and the use of stents is also an option. There are three indications for the use of stents: support of weakened tracheal walls due to tracheal malacia, re-establishment of the full tracheal lumen in case of extrinsic pressure, and sealing of fistulas toward the esophagus or pleural cavity (Freitag, 2010; Venuta et al. 2004; Saito and Imamura, 2005; Stephens and Wood, 2000; Ching-Yang et al. 2007; Mandour et al. 2003; Miyazawa et al. 2004).

Good results from airway stenting largely depend on patient selection, but satisfactory to excellent results are generally achieved in most patients undergoing airway stenting (Saito and Imamura, 2005). The tubes have also been used in tracheal reconstruction surgeries to aid the support and recovery of the reconstructed areas (Stamenkovic et al. 2007).

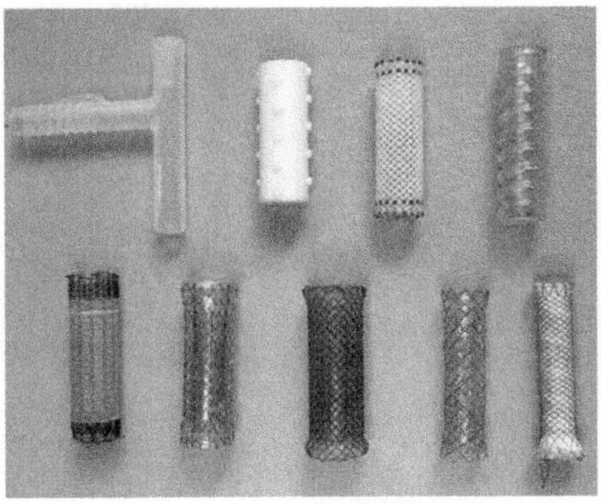

FIGURE 16.3
Typical tracheal stents. (top, left to right) Montgomery T stent, Dumon stent, Polyflex stent, and Noppen stent. (bottom, left to right) Ultraflex stent, Aero stent, Eco Nanjing stent, Hanaro stent, and Tae woong stent. (From Freitag, copyright ERS, 2010. With permission.)

In addition, stents are valuable complementary tools to other healing techniques and can provide prolonged palliation. More important, it is the only bronchoscopic technique to provide a solution for extrinsic compression (Wood et al. 2003).

The size of the stent should be adjusted according to the normal diameter proximal and distal to the area of stenosis. A narrow stent risks displacement and will be separated from the tracheal wall with failure of incorporation into the mucosa. A wider stent may lead to wall necrosis or excessive elongation with proximal or distal airway obstruction. Stents that are too long, in turn, can impede mucus clearance. Stent choice thus depends on the characteristics of the stenosis and on a physician's training and experience. Devices such as the AeroSizer® (Merit Medical Systems, South Jordan, UT) have even been created to aid in the stent sizing process. A rule of thumb is that the stent should extend 0.5 cm at each end of the stenosis (Freitag, 2010; Venuta et al. 2004; Graham et al. 2000; Ching-Yang et al. 2007; Grillo, 2004; Wood et al. 2003; Mostafa, 2003). Lee et al. (2010) reported that a stent alert card detailing the type and dimensions of the stent and its location in the tracheobronchial tree should be given to the patient. It should also indicate the appropriate size of endotracheal tube to be used if emergent intubation is required with the stent in site.

In our clinical routine, the healthy diameter of a patient's trachea is guessed from the images available. Image sources include bronchoscopy, CT, and three-dimensional (3D) reconstructions. The start and end points and the degree of narrowing of the stenosis are then visually estimated from this guess. In general, stents can be the treatment of choice for strictures with a degree of narrowing between 25% and 75%.

16.3 Traditional Methods for Airway Assessment

16.3.1 Rigid Bronchoscopy

The technique and clinical application of bronchoscopy was introduced by the German doctor Gustav Killian in 1897, when he first employed an endoscope to examine the airways. His tool was in fact an esophagoscope, which he used to remove a piece of pork bone

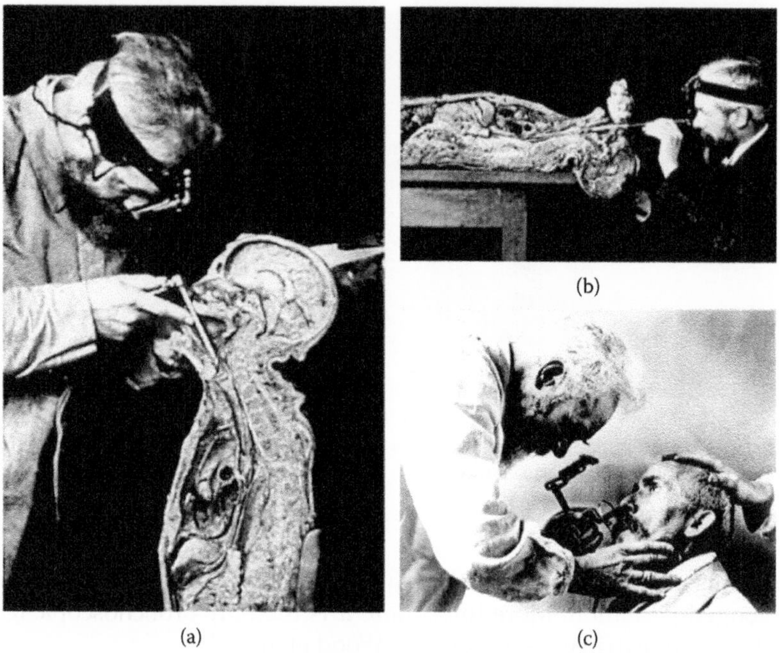

FIGURE 16.4
Dr. Gustav Killian and the first rigid bronchoscope. ((a and b) From Becker and Marsh, copyright Karger, Basel, 2000. With permission. (c) From public domain: http://en.wikipedia.org/wiki/File:Killian.jpg.)

stuck in the right main bronchus of a 63-year-old man (Becker and Marsh, 2000). Figure 16.4 shows pictures of Dr. Killian and his pioneering technique.

A rigid bronchoscope is thus a straight, hollow, metal tube through which a rigid fiber-optic device is placed, providing access to the central airways. The tube can only be inserted through the mouth and requires general anesthesia. It was the standard procedure for airway assessment until the 1970s, when the flexible bronchoscope was introduced. Today, it remains the procedure of choice for the removal of foreign objects from the airways or when a larger biopsy is needed. The rigid bronchoscope is also essential for the insertion of silicone or other stents, since it provides the necessary working channel for the insertion and removal of the tubes (Prakash, 1999).

16.3.2 Flexible Bronchoscopy

In the late 1960s, Dr. Shigeto Ikeda introduced the flexible bronchoscope, which aimed to reach further segments of the airway and to have a constant light source at the distal tip of the tube to enhance illumination of the visited areas. Later, in the late 1980s, Dr. Ikeda was also the one to introduce the videobronchoscope, which projected magnified images of the airways on a display (Miyazawa, 2000). The flexible bronchoscope became common since its introduction, and today, it is the most used invasive technique in the study of the airways (Prakash, 1999). Figure 16.5 shows Dr. Ikeda using the flexible bronchoscope.

The flexible bronchoscope is a thin flexible device that carries an optic fiber to conduct light from an external light source. It also contains an optical system to enable the visualization of the airway structures through an eyepiece or an image display. Auxiliary tools can also be inserted through the tube, commonly used for the collection of samples and

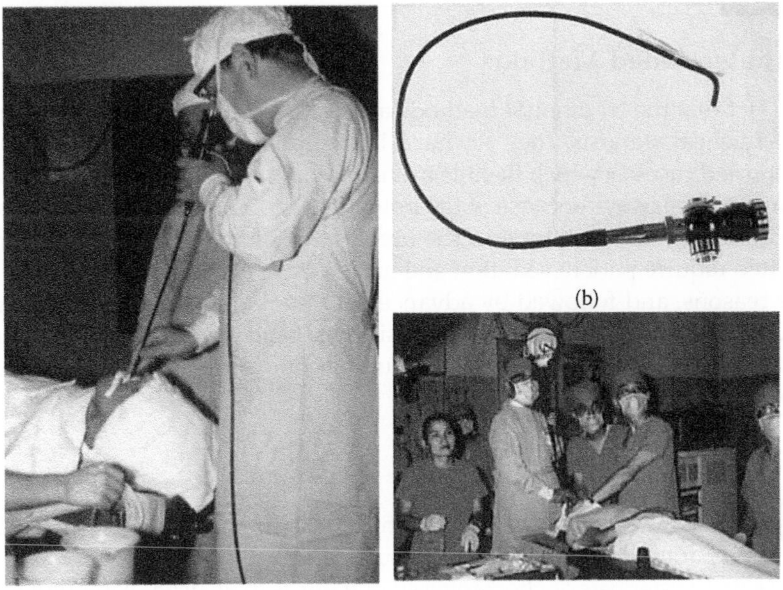

(b)

(a) (c)

FIGURE 16.5
(a) Dr. Shigeto Ikeda, (b) the flexible bronchoscope, and (c) the video bronchoscope in the operating theater. (From Miyazawa, T., copyright Karger, Basel, 2000. With permission.)

therapy. Besides the ability of reaching further areas of the airways, one advantage of the flexible bronchoscope over the rigid bronchoscope is that it generally requires only local anesthesia and mild patient sedation if necessary (Prakash, 1999; Miyazawa, 2000).

As an example of the employment of flexible videobronchoscopy in the assessment of the airways, Czaja et al. (2007) used a computer program through which the recorded images could be measured. Figure 16.6 shows the application in use. A probe with known dimensions was used in the calibration of the program, and the areas of interest could then be measured by manual delineation.

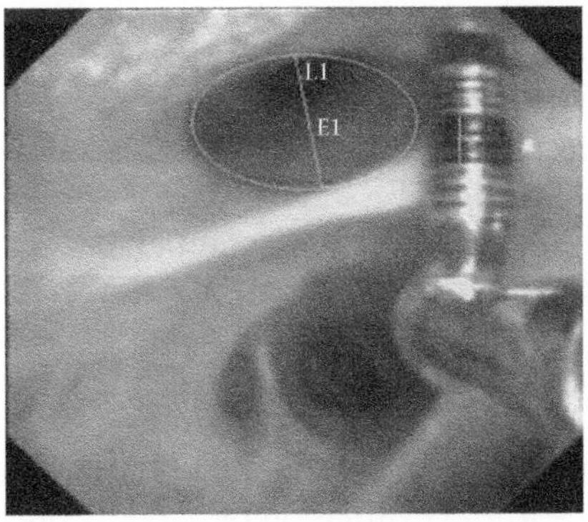

FIGURE 16.6
Airway measurement using the flexible bronchoscope. (From Czaja, P., et al. copyright Karger, Basel, 2007. With permission.)

16.4 Computer-Aided Methods

Despite the fact that the traditional methods above are still the gold standard in the management of tracheal stenosis, they do have limitations. Stephens and Wood (2000), for instance, reported cases in which flexible bronchoscopes were avoided in the evaluation of critically narrowed airways because of the potential for occlusion of the narrowed tracheal lumen. Furthermore, as mentioned in the previous section, both flexible and rigid bronchoscopy often require patient sedation and are invasive procedures by nature.

For these reasons, and followed by advances in imaging technology, noninvasive computer-aided methods for assessment of stenosis have been developed to substitute or complement the traditional techniques. Next, a number of different computer-aided methods are described and discussed.

16.4.1 Manual Methods

In the category of manual methods, the physician directly interacts with the images acquired for the patient evaluation. No computer methods are employed to aid the physician in assessing the stenosis or choosing a stent if one is to be used. Although radiography can still be used as an imaging modality, volume imaging is the preferred choice, with CT being the most often modality.

Williamson et al. (2010) and McLaughlin et al. (2008) employed a novel imaging technique called anatomical optical coherence tomography (aOCT) in the measurement of the tracheal caliber. Optical coherence tomography (OCT) is a light-based imaging technique in which receptors capture how much the light emitted from a source has been absorbed or scattered inside the analyzed tissue. aOCT is a modification of conventional OCT designed to allow macroscopic imaging of hollow organs. Light is emitted from a very thin probe (approximately 2 mm) passing through a flexible bronchoscope inside the trachea. The probe rotates at around 2.5 Hz, tracing an axial image of the airway. Longitudinal displacement of the probe inside the trachea eventually yields 3D reconstructions. Figure 16.7 shows examples of the acquired images. An advantage of aOCT over other imaging techniques is that it can be used for long periods, enabling physiological as well as anatomical analyses.

Callanan et al. (1997) were the first to use magnetic resonance imaging (MRI) to assess tracheal stenosis following tracheotomy in a study with 18 patients. The diameter of the trachea was measured in sagittal images at five separate intervals from the cricoid. If stenosis was noted, the narrowing was quantified as the percentage of reduction in the diameter relative to the regions immediately above and below the stenotic segment. The authors claimed that MRI was indeed an interesting imaging modality for the assessment of stenosis, providing good image quality and, compared with CT, it has the advantage of not subjecting the patient to ionizing radiation.

Despite the apparent advantages of MRI, the superior resolution and contrast of CT images and the much faster scanning times make CT the preferred imaging modality for tracheal and airway analysis. Lee et al. (2005), for example, used CT image analysis in the prestent and poststent placement settings. They emphasized how multislice CT provides invaluable information in the initial evaluation of patients presenting airway obstruction, being an important complementary tool to bronchoscopy. They further showed that CT aids planning of stent implants by clearly delineating the anatomy, pathology, and severity of the airway obstructions. As an added benefit, CT images show the relationship between

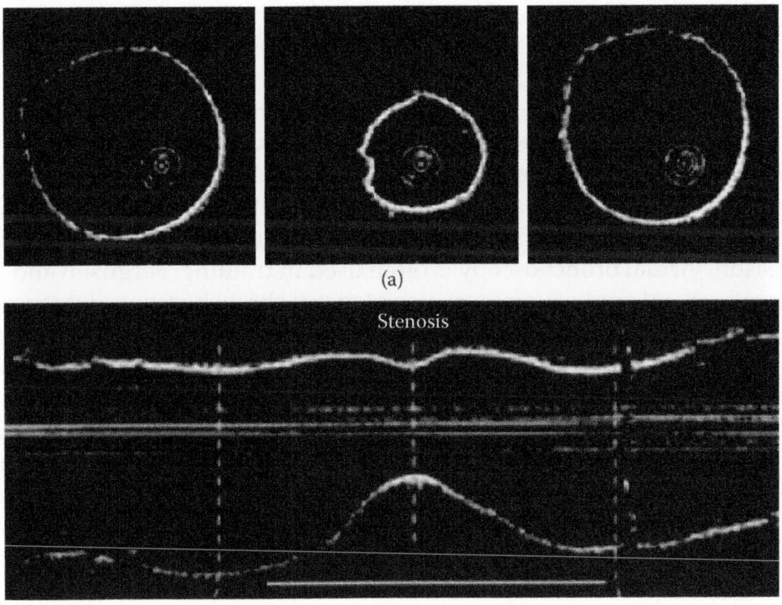

(a)

(b)

FIGURE 16.7
aOCT images of the trachea. (a) Cross sections obtained at different locations of the trachea. (b) Longitudinal displacement of the light probe along the trachea shows stenosis (the dashed lines correspond to the cross sections in (a)). (From Williamson, J.P., et al. copyright *ERS Journals*, 2010. With permission.)

the central airways and the adjacent structures, which are not visible with the bronchoscope. In the poststent placement procedures, multislice CT proved to enable accurate detection of stent complications, including migration, size discrepancies, and fracture. The authors also referred to other successful cases reported in the literature.

More recently, Parida and Gupta (2008) demonstrated good correlation in assessment of stenosis between spiral CT with 3D reconstructions (SCT-3DI) and bronchoscopy. In this imaging modality, a 3D model of the trachea is generated from the CT data (see Figure 16.8). This improves over traditional multislice CT analysis, providing the physician with

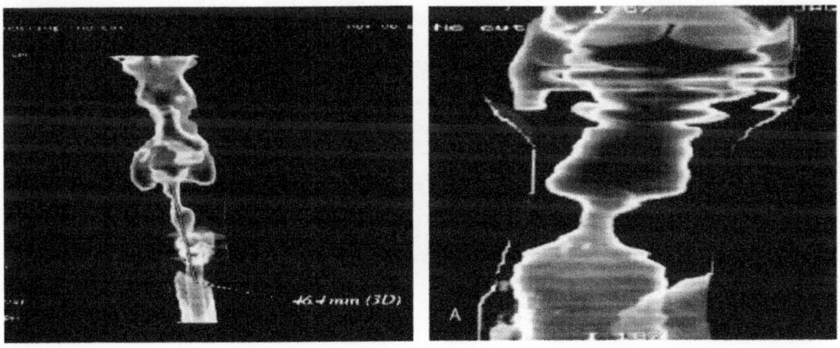

(a) (b)

FIGURE 16.8
3D models of the trachea obtained with SCT-3DI. (From Parida, P.K., and Gupta, A.K., copyright Elsevier, 2008. With permission.)

volumetric information. The authors also reported that in 16 out of 30 cases, bronchoscopy could not measure the length of the stenosis due to severe narrowing. With SCT-3DI, all cases could be measured.

Another improvement obtained with image analysis is the use of virtual bronchoscopy, in which a virtual camera is controlled by the physician through a 3D reconstruction of the airways obtained from CT. In this way, bronchoscopy is simulated in a completely virtual environment. Such a technique has the advantage of being similar in procedure to rigid or flexible bronchoscopy, with which the physician tends to be familiar, but without being invasive.

For this reason, virtual bronchoscopy is often used in training. Ferguson and McLennan (2005) reviewed several application scenarios of virtual bronchoscopy, demonstrating current and future trends for the procedure. They described, for instance, how images captured with the bronchoscope can be correlated with those of virtual bronchoscopy. This augments the physician's view and enables the visualization of structures that would otherwise be hidden when using only bronchoscopy. In airway analysis, Shitrit et al. (2005) and Triglia et al. (2002) showed significant correlation between results obtained with virtual bronchoscopy and flexible bronchoscopy in the assessment of tracheal stenosis. Hoppe et al. (2004) also demonstrated that virtual bronchoscopy can even be used to grade stenosis of the airways down to the segmental levels. Figure 16.9 gives examples of the use of virtual bronchoscopy.

Finally, Ballester et al. (2009) recently proposed an interesting system for tracheal surgery planning and choice of stents. A graphical user interface (see Figure 16.10) enables the user to visualize the CT data, 3D reconstructions of the trachea, and volume-rendered images altogether. The stents are then chosen from a prebuilt database containing computer-aided detection models of commercially available tubes. These are manually overlaid on the images so that the physicians can have a better idea of how the stent will interact with the tracheal wall and neighboring regions. The 3D reconstructions of trachea were also used for biomechanical airflow simulation studies before and after stent insertion.

All these methods have certainly proved the benefits of image analysis in the assessment of the airways and especially of tracheal stenosis. Yet, they are all still very reliant on the expertise of the operator in charge. The next section reviews methods that incorporate sophisticated algorithms aiming to reduce this operator dependency.

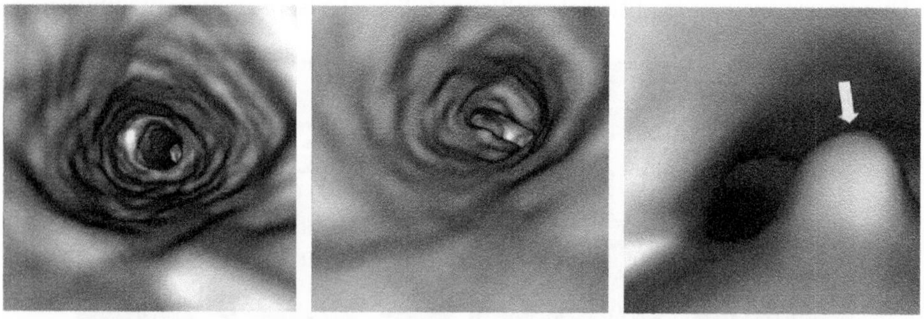

(a) (b)

FIGURE 16.9
Virtual bronchoscopy. (a) Normal (left) and narrowed (right) tracheas as seen with the virtual camera. (From Shitrit et al. copyright American College of Chest Physicians, 2005. With permission.) (b) Stenosis caused by tumor seen at the main bronchus. (From Hoppe, H., et al. copyright American College of Chest Physicians, 2004. With permission.)

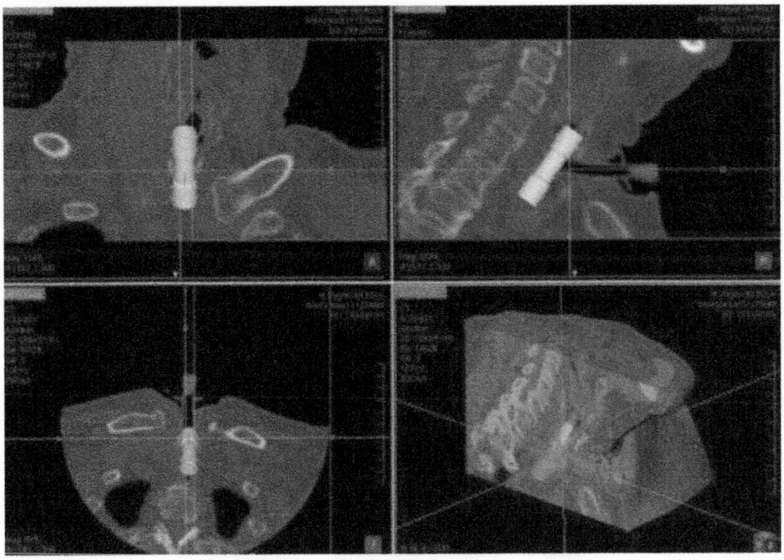

FIGURE 16.10
Graphical user interface for the planning of stent insertions. The stents are taken from a database and manually placed in the image. (From Ballester, M.A.G., et al. copyright Springer Berlin, 2009. With permission.)

16.4.2 Semiautomatic Methods

To the best of our knowledge, all semiautomatic algorithms devoted to the assessment of tracheal stenosis share the same characteristic. Namely, their output is a graph or some other interface to convey to the clinician the variation in the cross-sectional diameter or area of the trachea. What is different between these algorithms is how they achieve such results, which may involve more or less user intervention.

The first step in this process is the segmentation of the trachea from the CT image data and, possibly, its conversion to a 3D surface. Graham et al. (2000) presented a study with eight patients in which several image-based techniques employed to assess and measure the airways. They employed the software presented by D'Souza et al. (1996) and Hoffman et al. (1992) to segment the airways and extract their center lines. In the software, segmentation is semiautomatically performed on a slice-by-slice basis: rays cast from a user-defined point near the barycenter of the airway lumen determine the location of inner and outer airway walls. This information is also used to segment the lumen with region growing. Figure 16.11 illustrates some results obtained with these methods.

Triglia et al. (2002) also segmented the trachea on a slice-by-slice basis but used two-dimensional (2D) active contours (Kass et al. 1988) to delineate the axial boundary between the tracheal wall and the lumen. In their approach, user intervention is potentially reduced by selecting only the first and last slices of the trachea, segmenting the first slice, and letting the algorithm use the result of each slice as the starting point for the next. After the segmentation, new contours perpendicular to the surface's center line are computed and used in the definition of a smooth B-spline surface. The operator then marks on the center line the start and end of the stenosis, which are used to compute the length of the narrowing. The degree of narrowing is finally computed as the ratio of the cross-sectional area of the selected tracheal segment to the area of a reference healthy section also selected by the

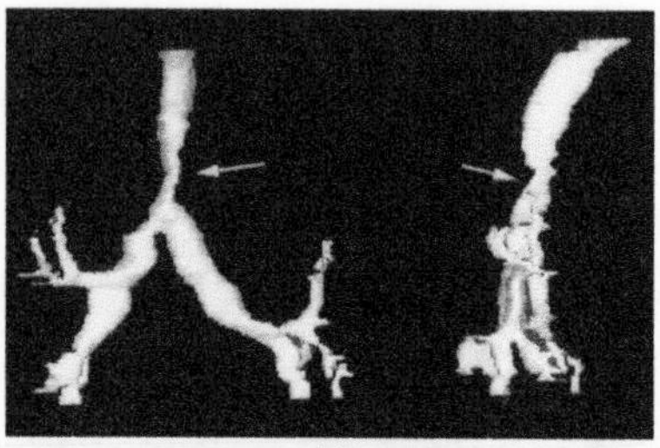

(a)

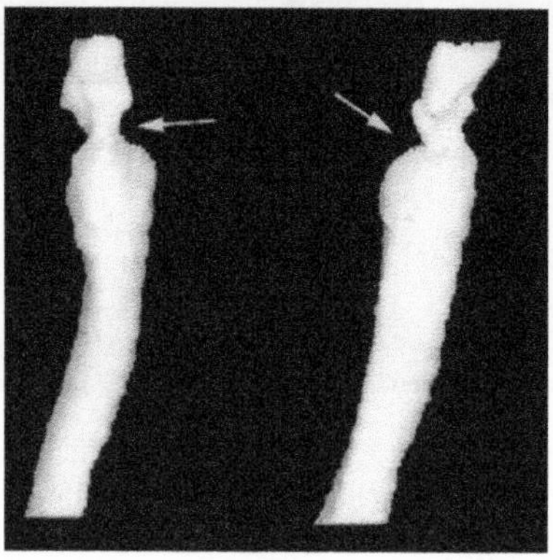

(b)

FIGURE 16.11
Examples of 3D reconstructions of the trachea and airways showing stenosis. (From Graham, S.M., et al. copyright W.B. Saunders, 2000. With permission.)

operator. The area or diameter profile of the entire trachea can further be displayed on a graph, accompanied by a visualization of the 3D surface. Figure 16.12 shows a couple of steps of this algorithm.

In the studies of Valdés-Cristerna et al. (2000) and Valdés-Cristerna and Yáñez-Suárez (2003), a 3D contour model was employed in the segmentation of the trachea. This improves Triglia et al.'s (2002) procedure by eliminating the surface generation step, since the 3D model already tends to yield a smooth 3D surface by definition. Triglia et al. (2002) also reported difficulties in the slice-by-slice segmentation whenever the narrowing was too severe and the tracheal lumen was barely visible in the image. In these cases, the missing tracheal section had to be reconstructed manually, which can obviously introduce errors. Although the 3D contour model can potentially overcome this problem, Valdés-Cristerna et al. (2000) and Valdés-Cristerna and Yáñez-Suárez (2003) did not report any result related to such situation. The tracheal area profile was once again plotted on a graph, but details on this process were not given either.

In the method presented by Sorantin et al. (2002, 2006), the cross-sectional area profile of the trachea is obtained by first segmenting the trachea with a region growing method using fuzzy connectedness (Udupa and Samarasekera, 1996). Next, a thinning algorithm (Palágyi and Kuba, 1998) is applied to the segmentation result to extract the trachea's center line. Both steps may require postprocessing by user intervention. As in the other discussed approaches, the tracheal area profile is plotted on a graph, and the start and end of

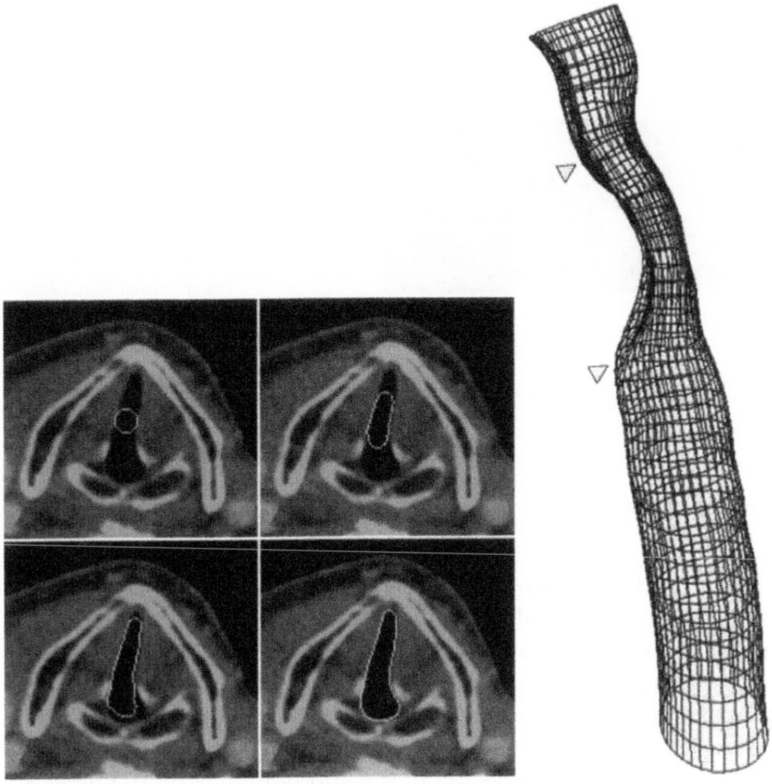

(a) (b)

FIGURE 16.12
(a) Segmentation of an axial CT slice using active contours. (b) 3D surface obtained from the segmentation with user markers indicating the start and end of the stenosis. (From Triglia, J.-M., et al. copyright Annals Publishing Company, 2002. With permission.)

the stenosis are determined by the operator based on this graph and its relationship with the 3D reconstruction of the trachea. The degree of narrowing is chosen as a percentage of the minimum cross-sectional area relative to the area of the trachea at the start and end points of the stenosis. Kiesler et al. (2007) later used this method for the assessment of three patients. Figure 16.13 illustrates the method and its results.

The improvements brought about by all these techniques over the manual methods are undeniable. Nonetheless, the methods above share another common characteristic: the analysis of the result graph and the determination of the parameters of the stenosis are still, to a large extent, operator-dependent. Although the visualization of the tracheal area profile on a graph does ease the assessment, it is the operator that decides where the stricture starts and ends, and the degree of narrowing is eventually computed from these parameters. In addition, in the case of stent choice, it is not completely clear from the graphs how much the stent should push the tracheal wall, that is, how to decide the appropriate stent diameter to be employed. In the end, it is the physician that still needs to guess the healthy tracheal shape from the available results in order to choose the correct stent.

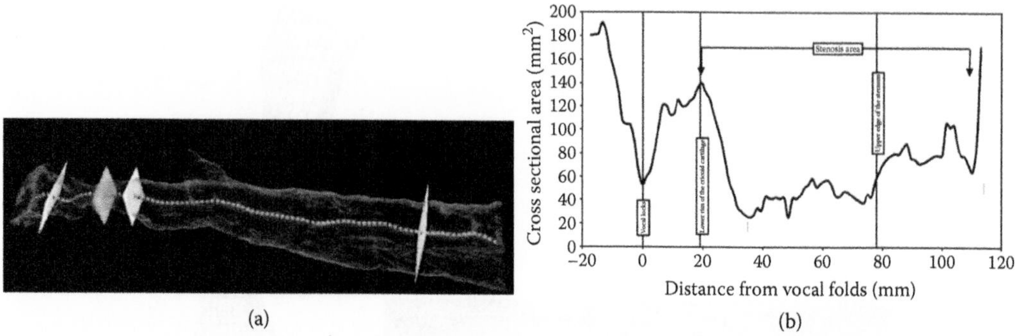

FIGURE 16.13
(a) The trachea with the center line and cross sections whose areas are computed. (b) The area profile along the trachea. (From Kiesler, K., et al. copyright Springer, New York, 2007. With permission.)

16.4.3 Deformable Models

This section describes a new method to further improve the assessment and stenting of tracheal stenosis based on deformable models of shape. In this method, a statistical shape model (Cootes et al. 1995) of healthy tracheas is used to estimate the shape of a patient's trachea in case stenosis was not present. From there, an adapted active contour model (Kass et al. 1988) is used to segment the narrowed trachea from the patient's CT scan. Both healthy and narrowed versions of the trachea are then used in the automatic detection of the stenosis and its parameters (start, end, degree of narrowing). These parameters are finally used for an automatic suggestion of the appropriate outer diameter and length of the stent. The details of this approach are given in the following.

16.4.3.1 Estimation of Healthy Tracheas

An active shape model (ASM), as defined by Cootes et al. (1995), is a statistical model of shapes whose objective is to capture the geometric variation present in a set of training shapes. This model is then capable of generating new shape instances that are constrained by the statistical variation of the training set, referred to as the allowable shape domain. As a result, a defining characteristic of ASMs, an advantage with respect to other deformable models, is that they can only generate shapes that resemble those in the training set.

This characteristic is the motivation to use an ASM of healthy tracheas to estimate the shape of a patient's trachea if stenosis was not present. Since the model contains only instances of healthy tracheas, local geometric variations typical of stenosis cannot be generated. In this way, the physician can have visual and mathematical guidance of what shape the trachea should have after treatment, with either surgery or stent implants.

The steps involved in the construction of the ASM and its registration to a patient's CT scan are described in the following.

Training set. An ASM is built from a set of training shapes. In medical imaging, these are usually obtained through segmentation. In the case of the trachea, any algorithm that can segment the tube from beginning (region right below the cricoid) to end (region of the carina) will do. In particular, Pinho et al. (2009) proposed an adaptive airway segmentation algorithm capable of yielding such results. Furthermore, this algorithm also obtains an approximation of the trachea's center line.

The points (or landmarks) defining the boundary of the shapes of the training set must have a one-to-one correspondence so that the ASM captures correct shape variations. The correspondences along the center lines obtained with the segmentation algorithm above are achieved with arc-length parametrization. From the center lines, smooth 3D representations of the boundaries of the tracheas can be obtained by regularly sampling the segmentations around the center line points. This procedure eventually yields the required point correspondence.

Active shape model. After establishing the correspondences between the N shapes of training set, each shape $\mathcal{S}_i$ has its set of landmarks $\mathcal{X}_i$ converted into a $3n$-dimensional vector $\mathbf{x}_i = (x_{i11}, x_{i12}, x_{i13}, \ldots, x_{in1}, x_{in2}, x_{in3})^T$. The tracheas are then aligned with respect to location and pose and normalized with respect to scale, such that $|\mathbf{x}_i| = 1$. Principal component analysis extracts the eigenvectors, $\mathbf{p}_i$, and eigenvalues, λ_i, of the covariance matrix of all $\mathbf{x}_i$'s. The eigenvectors, also referred to as the main modes of variation of the training set, are grouped in an orthonormal matrix $\mathbf{P}_{3n \times N}$. New healthy tracheas can be generated with this model, called a *point distribution model*, by linearly combining the mean shape with a weighted version of the eigenvector matrix **P**, that is,

$$\mathbf{x} = \bar{\mathbf{x}} + \mathbf{Pb}. \tag{16.1}$$

Vector $\mathbf{b} = (b_1, b_2, \ldots, b_N)^T$ is the set of parameters of the model and represents the contribution of each eigenvector. Since λ_i represents the variance of the training set along the eigenvector $\mathbf{p}_i$, the range $[-3\sqrt{\lambda_i}, +3\sqrt{\lambda_i}]$ is a suitable limit for b_i (Cootes et al. 1995).

In general, only the first t modes corresponding to a certain percentage of the total variance present in the point distribution model are used. The rest of the modes are considered as noise (Cootes et al. 1995). As an example, Figure 16.14 shows the first six modes of variation computed for a training set of 38 healthy

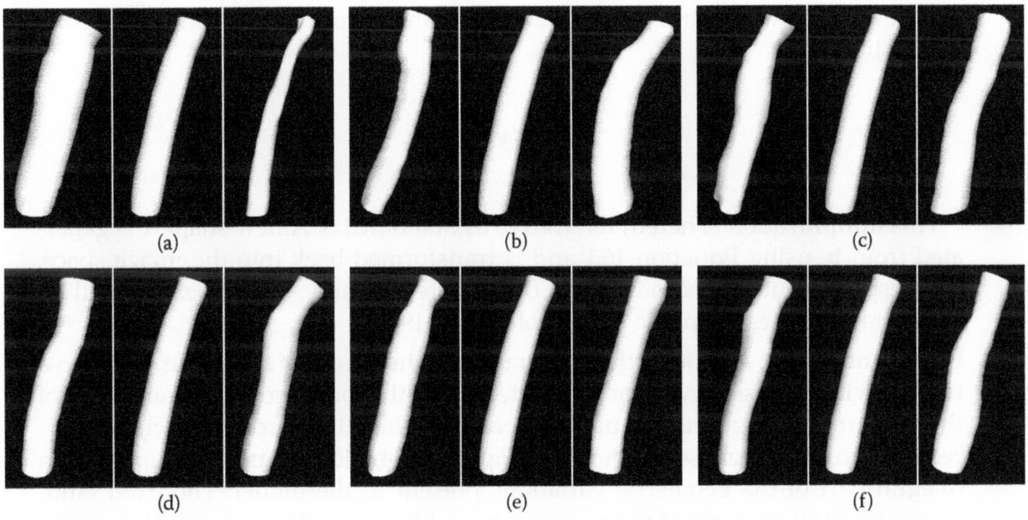

FIGURE 16.14
(a–f), The first six modes of variation of an example ASM built with 38 healthy tracheas. Each figure shows the (middle) average shape, (left) $-3\sqrt{\lambda_i}$, and (right) $+3\sqrt{\lambda_i}$ along the mode.

tracheas. The average shape is shown in the middle, and the shapes corresponding to $\pm 3\sqrt{\lambda_i}$ appear next to it. The mode with largest variation indicates changes in the caliber. The second mode represents global bending, and from then onward, different levels of local bending or twisting.

ASM registration. ASMs can be registered to an object of the class they represent by adjusting the parameter vector **b**. When the ASM is registered to an image, the registration is usually implemented as an iterative edge based search. Fitting an ASM of healthy tracheas to a stenotic trachea is a challenge in itself. The difficulty lies in the fact that the narrowed regions of the trachea may have a strong influence on the fitting process. To avoid such an influence, the registration of the ASM of healthy tracheas is subdivided in steps. It consists of an initialization step (whose aim is to scale, orient, and place the mean shape so that it is near the target in the image), followed by rigid and nonrigid registration stages. In the latter two, the landmarks of the shape generated by the model, **x**, are moved along their normals toward high gradients corresponding to edges of the target, generating a candidate shape **y**. In the rigid registration, the average shape of the model is rigidly aligned with the target trachea in the image. The nonrigid registration is described next.

Pose and shape registration. In the second stage of the ASM registration, a nonrigid registration, which optimizes pose and shape, is started, and the landmarks of the shape generated by the model at the current iteration are displaced along their normals. Once the candidate shape **y** is projected into model space, which aligns **y** with the average shape, a new set $\hat{\mathbf{b}}$ that defines the best fit of the model to **y** is obtained by minimization of the squared error between **y** and **x**, represented by the following error function:

$$\xi(\mathbf{b}) = (\mathbf{y} - \mathbf{x})^{\mathrm{T}}(\mathbf{y} - \mathbf{x}). \tag{16.2}$$

Expanding Equation 16.2 with Equation 16.1 and minimizing ξ with respect to **b** results in:

$$\hat{\mathbf{b}} = \mathbf{P}^{\mathrm{T}}(\mathbf{y} - \bar{\mathbf{x}}). \tag{16.3}$$

This minimization is herein referred to as StandardLS. A new shape $\hat{\mathbf{x}}$ is generated from $\hat{\mathbf{b}}$, using Equation 16.1 and is transformed back into the image space. The displacement of landmarks and the update of $\hat{\mathbf{b}}$ and $\hat{\mathbf{x}}$ are repeated until no significant changes are made to $\hat{\mathbf{x}}$ (Cootes et al. 1995).

Fixed landmarks. Although the registration of the model of healthy tracheas to a trachea with stenosis tends not to be affected by the local geometric variations of the stricture, the registration may still produce globally narrowed tracheas. This result is possible because, as shown in Figure 16.14, global narrowing may be an integral part of the geometric variations present in the model. The fixed landmarks registration method overcomes this problem by setting a restriction on the displacement of landmarks during the search for high gradients, which defines the candidate shape **y**. Namely, if the candidate locations are not within a short threshold distance $d > 0$ from $\mathbf{x}$, the corresponding landmarks of $\mathbf{y}$ remain fixed, while the other landmarks are allowed to move as usual.

Let $\hat{\mathbf{x}}^{(k)} = \bar{\mathbf{x}} + \mathbf{P}\hat{\mathbf{b}}^{(k)}$ be the shape generated by the model at iteration k of the non-rigid registration. Let $\mathbf{y}^{(k+1)}$ be the candidate shape generated by displacing the landmarks of $\hat{\mathbf{x}}^{(k)}$, assuming that $\mathbf{y}^{(k+1)}$ has already been projected into model space and aligned with $\bar{\mathbf{x}}$. Using the fixed landmarks principle, the parameters $\hat{\mathbf{b}}^{(k+1)}$ are given by

$$\hat{\mathbf{b}}^{(k+1)} = \mathbf{P}^T(\mathbf{y}^{(k+1)} - \bar{\mathbf{x}})\Big|_{\mathcal{L}'} + \mathbf{P}^T(\hat{\mathbf{x}}^{(k)} - \bar{\mathbf{x}})\Big|_{\mathcal{L}''}, \tag{16.4}$$

in which $\mathcal{L}'$ is the set of landmarks for which the displacement with respect to $\hat{\mathbf{x}}^{(k)}$ was longer than d, whereas $\mathcal{L}''$ are the landmarks that remained fixed because the displacement was shorter than or equal to d.

Equation 16.4 therefore shows that $\hat{\mathbf{b}}^{(k+1)}$ is determined by both the displaced landmarks $\mathbf{y}^{(k+1)}|_{\mathcal{L}'}$ and the landmarks $\hat{\mathbf{x}}^{(k)}|_{\mathcal{L}''}$, which remained fixed. Consequently, when computing

$$\hat{\mathbf{x}}^{(k+1)} = \bar{\mathbf{x}} + \mathbf{P}\hat{\mathbf{b}}^{(k+1)}, \tag{16.5}$$

$\hat{\mathbf{x}}^{(k+1)}$ will be the best fit, in a least squares minimization sense, to $\mathbf{y}^{(k+1)}|_{\mathcal{L}'}$ and $\hat{\mathbf{x}}^{(k)}|_{\mathcal{L}''}$. Figure 16.15 illustrates the whole concept. Provided that there are enough healthy areas around regions with stenosis, the fixed landmarks force the shape generated by the model to remain far from those regions, while enabling correct matches at

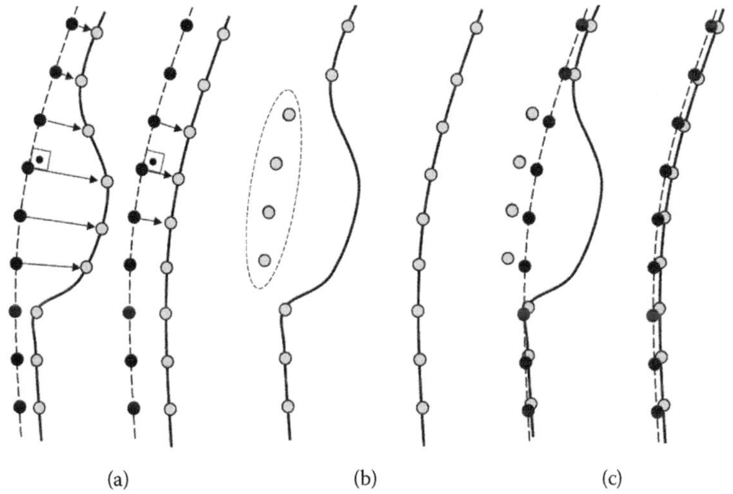

FIGURE 16.15
The fixed landmarks concept: (a) $\hat{\mathbf{x}}^{(k)}$ (dashed) is attracted by high gradients of the stenotic trachea in the image (thick lines)—the arrows indicate the landmark displacements $dy^{(k+1)}$; (b) the set of landmarks that remain fixed, $\hat{\mathbf{x}}^{(k)}|_{\mathcal{L}''}$, because the displacement was longer than d. (c) $\hat{\mathbf{x}}^{(k+1)}$—the fixed landmarks keep the shape far from the stenotic area.

the healthy areas. As the shape deforms iteratively, it progressively assumes the form of the desired healthy trachea, guided by the regions where correct matches occur.

16.4.3.2 Segmentation of Narrowed Tracheas

ACMs, commonly known as snakes, are curves defined within an image domain that are able to move under the influence of internal forces derived from the curve itself and of external forces derived from the image data. The internal and external forces are defined in such a way that the curve will register to an object boundary or other desired features within an image. As defined by Kass et al. (1988), a snake can be represented in 2D by a curve $\mathbf{v}(s) = (x(s),y(s))$, $s \in [0,1]$, responding to an energy functional of the form:

$$E = \int_0^1 [\kappa E_{int}(\mathbf{v}(s)) + (1-\kappa)E_{ext}(\mathbf{v}(s))]\, ds, \quad (16.6)$$

where $\kappa \in [0,1]$ is a weighting factor.

The internal energy E_{int} commonly restricts the deformations taking into account curvature and elasticity. Considering elasticity, the functional prevents the curve from breaking apart, maintaining its continuity. As for elasticity, the internal energy avoids the appearance of sharp corners. The external energy represents the gradient of an image I convolved with a Gaussian function G at scale σ, which causes the curve to be attracted by contours with high image gradients.

The objective is then to minimize Equation 16.6, making the system a force balance equation of the form:

$$\mathbf{F}_{\text{int}} + \mathbf{F}_{\text{ext}} = 0, \quad (16.7)$$

where

$$\mathbf{F}_{\text{int}} = -\nabla E_{\text{int}} \quad (16.8)$$

and

$$\mathbf{F}_{\text{ext}} = -\nabla E_{\text{ext}}. \quad (16.9)$$

The minimization is solved iteratively, often in the discrete domain after discretization of $\mathbf{v}(s)$. The expected result is a curve that matches the high gradients of the image while being restricted by the internal constraints, according to the assigned weighting factors.

A classical problem with ACMs, however, is initialization. The starting curve should be placed near the features to be detected in the image; otherwise, the capture range of the external energy may not extend enough to attract the curve. In addition, in the absence of external energies, the internal energies cause the curve to shrink into itself.

Several methods have been proposed to overcome the limitations of the original ACM formulation. Cohen (1991), for instance, added a balloon force to the energy formulation that pushes the curve outwards in the direction of its normals, avoiding it to shrink. Later,

Cohen and Cohen (1993) proposed to increase the capture range of the external energy by using a force based on a map of distances from any point in the image to the nearest edge. The gradient vector flow of Xu and Prince (1998) and the recent magnetostatic active contour model of Xie and Mirmehdi (2008) are other good examples of methods that affect the external force.

The concepts above naturally extrapolate to 3D and can easily be adapted to a discrete domain. Within the context of the proposed application, a discrete surface is defined as $\mathcal{S} = (\mathcal{X},\mathcal{T})$, where $\mathcal{X}$ is the set of points or landmarks, with $\mathbf{x}_{v_j}$, $j = 1,\ldots,n$, a point in this set, and $\mathcal{T}$ is the set of triangles connecting the points of $\mathcal{X}$.

The ACM is initialized with the estimation of the healthy shape of the trachea obtained with the ASM above. In this way, the initial shape tends to be near enough to the boundary of the narrowed trachea in the image. The deformation algorithm then iteratively loops through all the points in $\mathcal{X}$, applying the ACM forces locally, until no significant deformation has been made to the surface. Below, the internal and external forces are briefly presented.

External force. The ideas first presented by Cohen and Cohen (1993) are adapted to create an external force to guide the deformation of the surface. At first, the original image, I, is thresholded to segment air (at –200 Hounsfield units), after which the result is inverted. This will generate two binary images, I_{B1} and I_{B2}. Next, a 3–4–5 chamfer distance transform is applied to each binary image, yielding two distance maps, I_{D1} and I_{D2}, respectively. Both distance transforms are combined into a new distance map $I_D = I_{D1} + I_{D2}$.

Eventually, the external force term of Equation 16.7 applied to the landmark $\mathbf{x}_{v_j}$ of $\mathcal{X}$ is defined as

$$\mathbf{F}_{\mathrm{ext}_j} = -\frac{|\ I_D(\mathbf{x}_{v_j})|}{M}\ I_D(\mathbf{x}_{v_j}), \tag{16.10}$$

where M is the maximum gradient magnitude in I_D.

Internal forces. The internal force $\mathbf{F}_{\mathrm{int}}$ controls stretching and bending, in such a way that the surface is continuous (does not break apart) and remains smooth (has no sharp corners). The force tries to keep the landmarks equally spaced and tries to minimize the local Gaussian curvature of the surface. It is given by

$$\mathbf{F}_{\mathrm{int}_j} = \gamma\ \mathbf{F}_{\mathrm{elast}_j} + (1-\gamma)\mathbf{F}_{\mathrm{be}} \tag{16.11}$$

where γ is a weighting factor.

$\mathbf{F}_{\mathrm{elast}_j}$ is the elastic force applied to $\mathbf{x}_{v_j}$ of $\mathcal{X}$, defined as:

$$\mathbf{F}_{\mathrm{elast}_j} = D_j \frac{\mathbf{d}_{\mathrm{elast}_j}}{|\mathbf{d}_{\mathrm{elast}_j}|}, \tag{16.12}$$

where the directional component $\mathbf{d}_{\mathrm{elast}_j}$ moves the landmark toward a central point relative to its neighbors. The scalar component D_j, in turn, is a normalized measure of how much $\mathbf{x}_{v_j}$ deviates from this central point.

The bending force $\mathbf{F}_{\text{bend}_j}$ is given by

$$\mathbf{F}_{\text{bend}_j} = K_{G_j} \frac{\mathbf{d}_{\text{bend}_j}}{|\mathbf{d}_{\text{bend}_j}|}, \tag{16.13}$$

where $\mathbf{d}_{\text{bend}_j}$ is either equal to $\mathbf{d}_{\text{bend}_j}$ or it moves $\mathbf{x}_{\text{v}_j}$ along its normal if the landmark is not located at the open ends of the surface. In either case, the directional component moves $\mathbf{x}_{\text{v}_j}$ in such a way that the discrete Gaussian curvature computed at the landmark is minimized. The scalar component K_{G_j} is a normalized measure of how much the curvature at $\mathbf{x}_{\text{v}_j}$ deviates from zero.

Finally, for each iteration k of the deformation algorithm of the ACM, the landmarks of the surface are updated as follows:

$$\mathbf{x}_{\text{v}_j}^{(k)} = \mathbf{x}_{\text{v}_j}^{(k-1)} + \kappa \mathbf{F}_{\text{int}_j} + (1-\kappa)\mathbf{F}_{\text{ext}_j}. \tag{16.14}$$

16.4.3.3 Quantification of Stenosis

Once healthy and narrowed versions of the trachea are obtained, the assessment of the stenosis is straightforward. This is achieved by comparing the cross-sectional area profile of the two surfaces along their center lines. The narrowed surface is first intersected with the planes corresponding to the boundary contours of the healthy surface. The area of the generated set of contours is then compared with the area of the set of contours of the healthy surface. If a decrease in the area ratio between healthy and narrowed tracheas is detected, there is an indication that stenosis is present. Two thresholds must be set in this process: L_0 determines the minimum length of the detected stenosis and avoids very short segments to be considered; $R_0 \in [0,1]$ determines the maximum area ratio to be considered, balancing false-positive and detection rates of stenosis. Thus, the path that is longer than L_0 along which the area ratio is smaller than R_0 is recorded, which determines the start and end of the stenosis. The point with the lowest ratio is finally chosen as the one that determines the degree of narrowing of the stricture.

Examples of the stenosis assessment for six patients obtained with the method above are shown in Figure 16.16. Note that the detected parameters of the stenosis conform to the diagnostic details shown in the figure.

16.4.3.4 Choice of Stents

The stent parameters are directly obtained from the algorithm above. The caliber of the stent is the average diameter of all contours of the estimated healthy surface along the extent of the stenosis. The deployment location is equal to the start point. Finally, the length of the stent is the path length between the start and end points. Figure 16.17 shows examples of predicted stents for the patients of Figure 16.16. The stents are directly derived from the computed parameters of the stenosis, as described above. They cover the stenosis according to the threshold ratio R_0 set for the detection of stenosis and provide a plausible healthy caliber for the narrowed trachea.

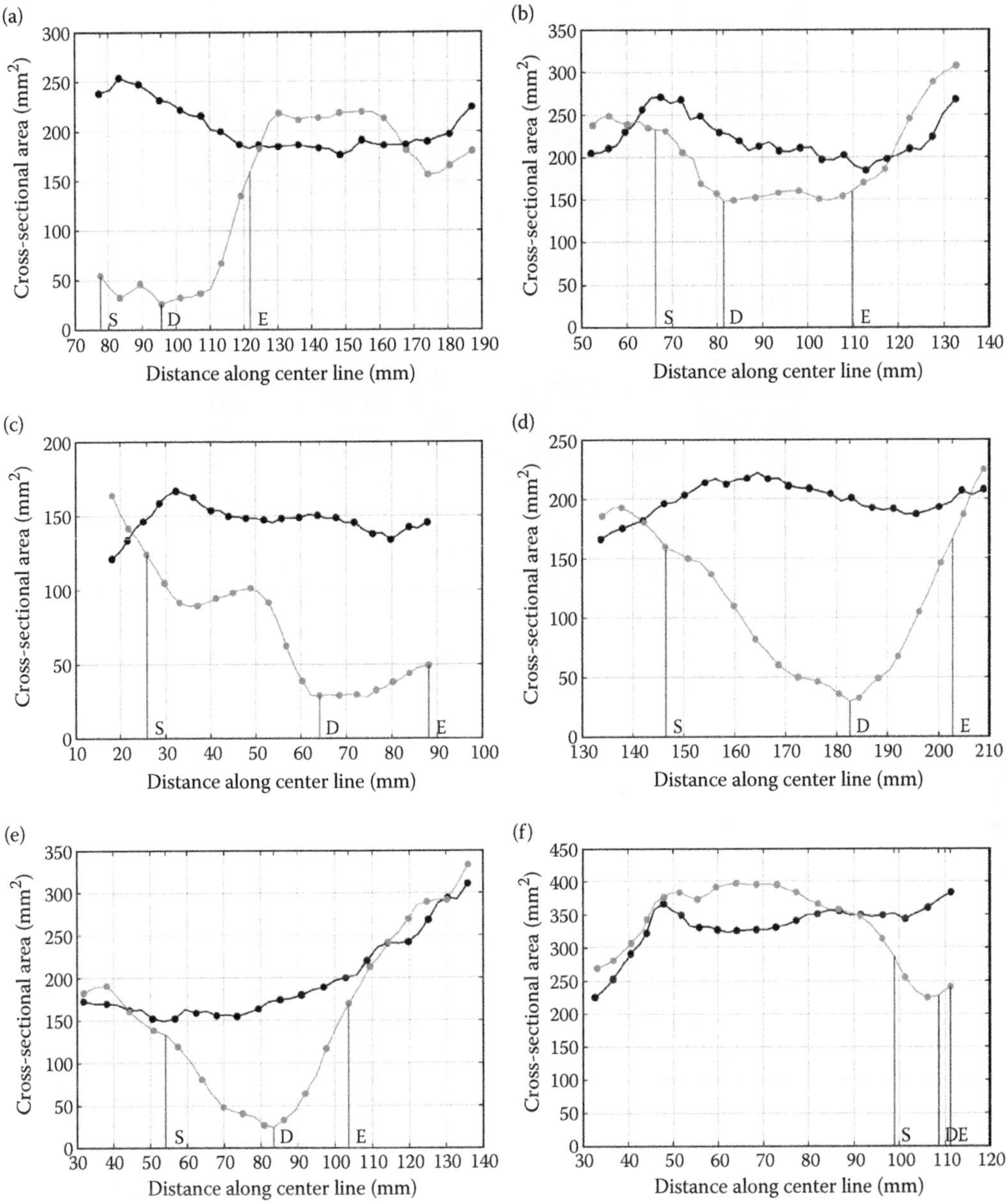

FIGURE 16.16
Examples of stenosis quantification for six patients. The vertical lines indicate the detected start, point of maximum degree, and end of the stenosis. The *x*-axis represents the distance along the center line of the trachea, where 0 marks the top (region around the cricoid).

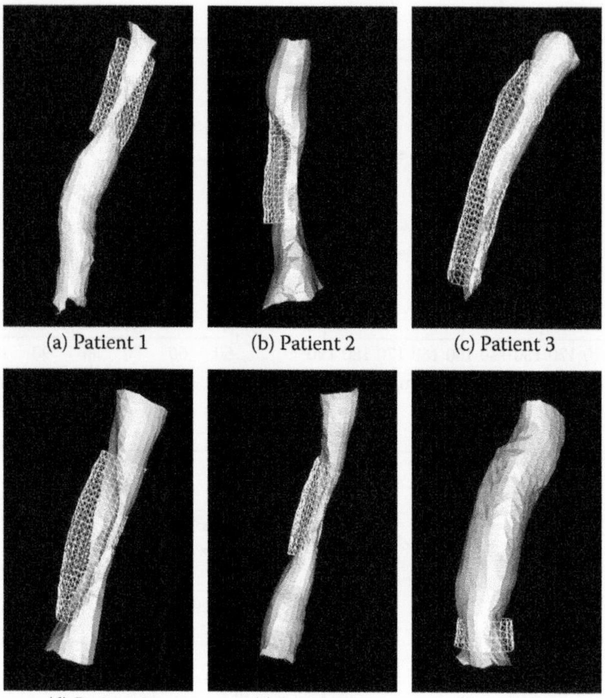

FIGURE 16.17
Visualization of the stents computed for the six patients in the examples.

16.5 Conclusions

Correct assessment of tracheal stenosis and subsequent choice of the length and diameter of stents are important preoperative steps in the management of the strictures. Assessment of tracheal stenosis and choice of tracheal stents, however, have long been very operator-dependent tasks. This chapter reviewed traditional and computer-aided methods for the assessment of tracheal stenosis and choice of stents. It has been shown that image analysis is a powerful noninvasive tool to complement the traditional bronchoscopic methods. In addition, computer-aided methods can greatly reduce the subjectivity and operator dependency usually observed in the assessment of tracheal stenosis. In particular, this chapter also described in detail a novel method to automatically assess stenoses and predict the diameter and length of stents using deformable models of shape.

References

M. A. G. Ballester, A. P. del Palomar, J. L. L. Villalobos, L. L. Rodríguez, O. Trabelsi, F. Pérez, Á. G. Cañamaque, E. B. Cortés, F. R. Panadero, M. D. Castellano, and J. H. Jover. Surgical planning and patient-specific biomechanical simulation for tracheal endoprostheses interventions. *Medical Image Computing and Computer-Assisted Intervention—MICCAI 2009, Lecture Notes in Computer Science*, vol. 5762, pp. 275–282. Springer, New York, 2009.

H. D. Becker and B. R. Marsh. History of the rigid bronchoscope. In C. T. Bolliger and P. N. Mathur, editors, *Interventional Bronchoscopy*, vol. 30, pp. 2–15. Karger, Basel, 2000.

P. M. Boiselle, J. Catena, A. Ernst, and D. A. Lynch. Tracheobronchial stenoses. In P. M. Boiselle and D. Lynch, editors, *CT of the Airways*, pp. 121–149. Humana Press–Springer, New York, 2008.

V. Callanan, K. Gillmore, S. Field, and A. Beaumont. The use of magnetic resonance imaging to assess tracheal stenosis following percutaneous dilatational tracheostomy. *Journal of Laryngology and Otology*, 111(10):953–957, 1997.

A. Carretta, G. Melloni, P. Ciriaco, L. Libretti, M. Casiraghi, A. Bandiera, and P. Zannini. Preoperative assessment in patients with postintubation tracheal stenosis. *Surgical Endoscopy*, 20(6):905–908, 2006.

W. Ching-Yang, L. Yun-Hen, H. Ming-Ju, W. Yi-Chen, L. Ming-Shian, K. Po-Jen, and L. Hui-Ping. Airway stents in management of tracheal stenosis: Have we improved? *ANZ Journal of Surgery*, 77:27–32(6), 2007.

L. Cohen and I. Cohen. Finite-element methods for active contour models and balloons for 2-d and 3-d images. *IEEE Transactions on Pattern Analysis and Machine Intelligence*, 15(11):1131–1147, Nov. 1993.

L. D. Cohen. On active contour models and balloons. *Computer Vision, Graphics, and Image Processing: Image Understanding*, 53(2):211–218, 1991.

T. F. Cootes, C. J. Taylor, D. H. Cooper, and J. Graham. Active shape models: Their training and application. *Computer Vision and Image Understanding*, 61(1):38–59, 1995.

P. Czaja, J. Soja, P. Grzanka, A. Çmiel, A. Szczeklik, and K. Sładek. Assessment of airway caliber in quantitative videobronchoscopy. *Respiration*, (74):432–438, 2007.

N. D. D'Souza, J. M. Reinhardt, and E. A. Hoffman. ASAP: Interactive quantification of 2d airway geometry. *Medical Imaging 1996: Physiology and Function from Multidimensional Images*, vol. 2709, pp. 180–196. SPIE, 1996.

M. Elliott, D. Roebuck, C. Noctor, C. McLaren, B. Hartley, Q. Mok, C. Dunne, N. Pigott, C. Patel, A. Patel, and C. Wallis. The management of congenital tracheal stenosis. *Advances in Pediatric ORL. Proceedings of the 8th International Congress of Pediatric Otorhinolaryngology. International Congress Series*, 1254:321–334, 2003.

J. S. Ferguson and G. McLennan. Virtual bronchoscopy. *Proceedings of the American Thoracic Society*, 2(6):488–491, 2005.

L. Freitag. Tracheobronchial stents. In C. T. Bolliger and P. N. Mathur, editors, *Interventional Bronchoscopy*, vol. 30, pp. 171–186. Karger, Basel, 2000.

L. Freitag. Airway stents. *Interventional Pulmonology*, vol. 48, pp. 190–217. ERS, 2010.

S. M. Graham, G. McLennan, G. F. Funk, H. T. Hoffman, T. M. McCulloch, J. Cook-Granroth, and E. A. Hoffman. Preoperative assessment of obstruction with computed tomography image analysis. *American Journal of Otolaryngology*, 21(4):263–270, 2000.

H. C. Grillo. *Surgery of the Trachea and Bronchi*. BC Decker, 2004.

H. C. Grillo, D. M. Donahue, D. J. Mathisen, J. C. Wain, and C. D. Wright. Postintubation tracheal stenosis: Treatment and results. *Journal of Thoracic and Cardiovascular Surgery*, 109(3):486–493, 1995.

E. A. Hoffman, D. Gnanaprakasam, K. B. Gupta, J. D. Hoford, S. D. Kugelmass, and R. S. Kulawiec. Vida: An environment for multidimensional image display and analysis. *Biomedical Image Processing and Three-Dimensional Microscopy*, vol. 1660, pp. 694–711. SPIE, 1992.

H. Hoppe, H.-P. Dinkel, B. Walder, G. von Allmen, M. Gugger, and P. Vock. Grading airway stenosis down to the segmental level using virtual bronchoscopy. *Chest*, 125 (2):704–711, 2004.

M. Kass, A. Witkin, and D. Terzopoulos. Snakes: Active contour models. *International Journal of Computer Vision*, V1(4):321–331, 1988.

K. Kiesler, M. Gugatschka, E. Sorantin, and G. Friedrich. Laryngo-tracheal profile: A new method for assessing laryngo-tracheal stenoses. *European Archives of Oto-Rhino-Laryngology*, 264(3):251–256, 2007.

K. S. Lee and P. M. Boiselle. Tracheal and bronchial neoplasms. In P. M. Boiselle and D. Lynch, editors, *CT of the Airways*, pp. 151–190. Humana Press–Springer, New York, 2008.

K. S. Lee, W. Lunn, D. Feller-Kopman, A. Ernst, H. Hatabu, and P. M. Boiselle. Multislice CT evaluation of airway stents. *Journal of Thoracic Imaging*, 20(2):81–88, 2005.

P. Lee, E. Kupeli, and A. C. Mehta. Airway stents. *Clinics in Chest Medicine*, 31(1):141–150, 2010.

M. Mandour, M. Remacle, P. van de Heyning, S. Elwany, A. Tantawy, and A. Gaafar. Chronic subglottic and tracheal stenosis: Endoscopic management vs. surgical reconstruction. *European Archives of Oto-Rhino-Laryngology*, 260(7):374–380, 2003.

R. A. McLaughlin, J. P. Williamson, M. J. Phillips, J. J. Armstrong, S. Becker, D. R. Hillman, P. R. Eastwood, and D. D. Sampson. Applying anatomical optical coherence tomography to quantitative 3d imaging of the lower airway. *Optics Express*, 16(22):17521–17529, 2008.

T. Miyazawa. History of the flexible bronchoscope. In C. T. Bolliger and P. N. Mathur, editors, *Interventional Bronchoscopy*, vol. 30, pp. 16–21. Karger, Basel, 2000.

T. Miyazawa, Y. Miyazu, Y. Iwamoto, A. Ishida, K. Kanoh, H. Sumiyoshi, M. Doi, and N. Kurimoto. Stenting at the flow-limiting segment in tracheobronchial stenosis due to lung cancer. *American Journal of Respiratory and Critical Care Medicine*, 169(10):1096–1102, 2004.

B. Mostafa. Endoluminal stenting for tracheal stenosis. *European Archives of Oto-Rhino-Laryngology*, 260(9):465–468, 2003.

S. A. R. Nouraei, D. W. McPartlin, S. M. Nouraei, A. Patel, C. Ferguson, D. J. Howard, and G. S. Sandhu. Objective sizing of upper airway stenosis: A quantitative endoscopic approach. *Laryngoscope*, 116(1):12–17, 2006.

K. Palágyi and A. Kuba. A 3d 6-subiteration thinning algorithm for extracting medial lines. *Pattern Recognition Letters*, 19:613–627, 1998.

P. K. Parida and A. K. Gupta. Role of spiral computed tomography with 3-dimensional reconstruction in cases with laryngeal stenosis–a radioclinical correlation. *American Journal of Otolaryngology*, 29(5):305–311, 2008.

R. Pinho, S. Luyckx, and J. Sijbers. Robust region growing based intrathoracic airway tree segmentation. *2nd International Workshop on Pulmonary Image Analysis*, pp. 261–271, London, September 2009.

U. B. S. Prakash. Advances in bronchoscopic procedures. *Chest*, 116(5):1403–1408, 1999.

M. Prasad, J. P. Bent, R. F. Ward, and M. M. April. Endoscopically placed nitinol stents for pediatric tracheal obstruction. *International Journal of Pediatric Otorhinolaryngology*, 66(2):155–160, 2002.

Y. Saito and H. Imamura. Airway stenting. *Surgery Today*, 35(4):265–270, 2005.

D. Shitrit, P. Valdsislav, A. Grubstein, D. Bendayan, M. Cohen, and M. Kramer. Accuracy of virtual bronchoscopy for grading tracheobronchial stenosis: Correlation with pulmonary function test and fiberoptic bronchoscopy. *Chest*, 128(5):3545–3550, 2005.

E. Sorantin, C. Halmai, B. Erdôhelyi, K. Palágyi, L. Nyúl, L. K. Ollé, B. Geiger, F. Lindbichler, G. Friedrich, and K. Kiesler. Spiral-CT–based assessment of tracheal stenoses using 3-D skeletonization. *IEEE Transactions on Medical Imaging*, 21(3):263–273, 2002.

E. Sorantin, D. Mohadjer, L. Nyúl, K. Palágyi, F. Lindbichler, and B. Geiger. New advances for imaging of laryngotracheal stenosis by post processing of spiral-CT data. In W. Hruby, editor, *Digital (R)Evolution in Radiology—Bridging the Future of Health Care*, pp. 297–308. Springer, New York, 2006.

N. Spittle and A. McCluskey. Lesson of the week: Tracheal stenosis after intubation. *British Medical Journal*, 321(7267):1000–1002, 2000.

S. Stamenkovic, R. Hierner, P. De Leyn, and P. Delaere. Long-segment tracheal stenosis treated with vascularized mucosa and short-term stenting. *Annals of Thoracic Surgery*, 83(3):1213–1215, 2007.

J. Stephens, Kenton E. and D. E. Wood. Bronchoscopic management of central airway obstruction. *Journal of Thoracic and Cardiovascular Surgery*, 119(2):289–296, 2000.

J.-M. Triglia, S. Marciano, B. Nazarian, G. Moulin, I. Sudre-Levillain, and A. Giovanni. Virtual laryngotracheal endoscopy based on geometric surface modeling using spiral computed tomography data. *Annals of Otology, Rhinology and Laryngology*, 111(1):36–43, 2002.

J. K. Udupa and S. Samarasekera. Fuzzy connectedness and object definition: Theory, algorithms, and applications in image segmentation. *Graphical Models and Image Processing*, 58 (3):246–261, 1996.

R. Valdés-Cristerna and O. Yáñez-Suárez. Active contours and surfaces with cubic splines for semi-automatic tracheal segmentation. *Journal of Electronic Imaging*, 12(1):81–96, 2003.

R. Valdés-Cristerna, O. Yáñez-Suárez, and V. Medina. Trachea segmentation in CT images using active contours. *Engineering in Medicine and Biology Society, 2000. Proceedings of the 22nd Annual International Conference of the IEEE*, vol. 4, pp. 3184–3187, 2000.

F. Venuta, E. A. Rendina, and T. de Giacomo. Airway stenting. Available at http://www.ctsnet.org/sections/clinicalresources/thoracic/expert_tech-1.html (accessed Nov. 2004).

E. M. Webb, B. M. Elicker, and W. R. Webb. Using CT to diagnose nonneoplastic tracheal abnormalities: Appearance of the tracheal wall. *American Journal of Roentgenology*, 174 (5):1315–1321, 2000.

J. P. Williamson, J. J. Armstrong, R. A. McLaughlin, P. B. Noble, A. R. West, S. Becker, A. Curatolo, W. J. Noffsinger, H. W. Mitchell, M. J. Phillips, D. D. Sampson, D. R. Hillman, and P. R. Eastwood. Measuring airway dimensions during bronchoscopy using anatomical optical coherence tomography. *European Respiration Journal*, 35(1):34–41, 2010.

D. E. Wood, Y.-H. Liu, E. Vallieres, R. Karmy-Jones, and M. S. Mulligan. Airway stenting for malignant and benign tracheobronchial stenosis. *Annals of Thoracic Surgery*, 76(1):167–174, 2003.

X. Xie and M. Mirmehdi. MAC: Magnetostatic active contour model. *IEEE Transactions on Pattern Analysis and Machine Intelligence*, 30(4):632–646, 2008.

C. Xu and J. Prince. Snakes, shapes, and gradient vector flow. *IEEE Transactions on Image Processing*, 7(3):359–369, 1998.

17

Appearance Analysis for the Early Assessment of Detected Lung Nodules

Ayman El-Baz, Georgy Gimel'farb, Robert Falk, Mohamed Abo El-Ghar, and Jasjit Suri

CONTENTS

17.1 Introduction

Pulmonary nodules are the most common manifestation of lung cancer, which is the principal cause of cancer-related deaths [1]. Fast and accurate classification of the nodules is of major importance for medical computer-aided diagnostic (CAD) systems.

A nodule is an approximately spherical volume of higher-density tissue visible in an x-ray lung image [2]. Large malignant nodules (generally defined as greater than 1 cm in diameter) are easily detected with any traditional imaging equipment and then diagnosed by needle biopsy or bronchoscopy. However, diagnostic options for small malignant nodules are limited due to difficulties in their accessibility, especially if they are located deep in the tissue or away from the large airways. Therefore, additional imaging and CAD techniques are needed. The popular direction of detecting small cancerous nodules is to analyze their growth rate over time. This chapter introduces a new approach to characterize the detected nodules based on their visual appearance.

Our long-term goal is to develop accurate and reliable CAD tools for early diagnosis of lung cancer. The fully automatic nodule detection system introduced in ref. [3] has an accuracy up to 93.3% on an experimental database of 200 real chest low-dose computed tomography (LDCT) data sets with 36,000 two-dimensional (2D) slices. The automatic stochastic segmentation in ref. [4] separates the lung tissues from the chest on the same database with an accuracy up to 99.7%, and the automatic segmentation proposed in ref. [5] extracted the lung nodules from the normal lung tissues with an accuracy of 98.7% (Figure 17.1). This

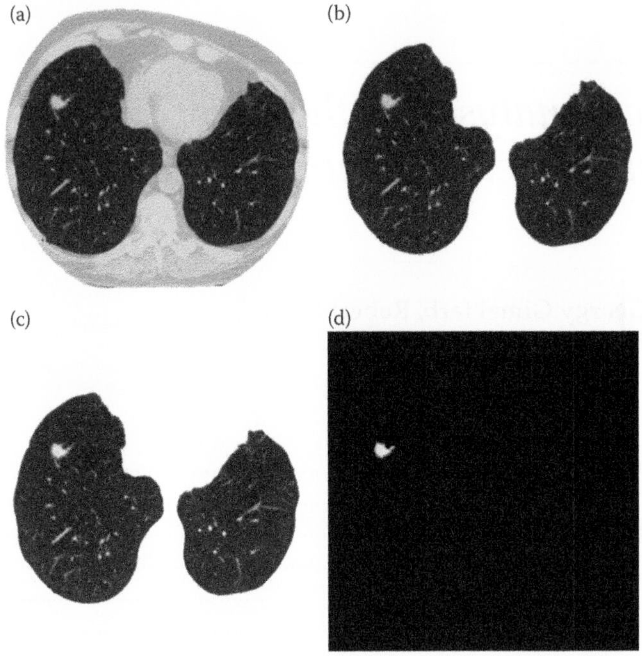

FIGURE 17.1
Data processing before the proposed appearance analysis: (a) to (d) An LDCT slice, the lung segmentation [4], the segmented lung areas equalized in line with ref. [6], and the segmented lung nodule [5].

chapter focuses on the next CAD stage, namely, on the nodule appearance analysis for accurate classification of benign and malignant nodules.

17.1.1 Previous Work

Today's techniques for detecting small cancerous nodules rely mostly on estimating their growth rate. Tracking the temporal nodule behavior is a challenging task because of changes in the patient's position at each data acquisition, as well as the effects of heartbeats and respiration. To accurately measure how the nodules are developing over time, all of these motions should be compensated for by registering the LDCT data sets taken at different time points. Many methods have been proposed for solving medical image registration problems (see, e.g., ref. [7]) and excluding the lung motions [8]. Moreover, it has been reported that computer-assisted volume measurements are more reliable for small pulmonary nodules than the measurements made by human experts [9]. But still the accuracy of nodule classification based on the growth rate remains below clinical requirements. To the best of our knowledge, this chapter is the first to characterize the detected nodules by modeling and analyzing their visual appearance. Such an analysis does not involve image registration.

The chapter is organized as follows. Section 17.2 introduces a prior translation and rotation invariant Markov-Gibbs random filed (MGRF) appearance model and an automatic procedure for selecting most characteristic pixel or voxel neighborhoods. Experimental results to validate the proposed model and conclusions are presented in Sections 17.3 and 17.4.

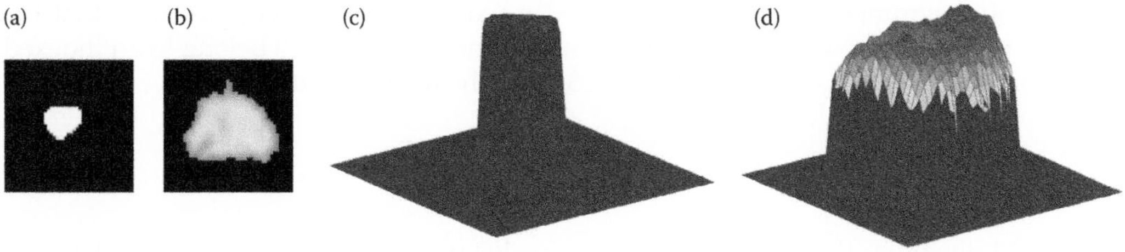

FIGURE 17.2
(See color insert.) (a, b) 2D and (c, d) 3D visualization of Hounsfield values over an axial cross section of a (a, c) benign and (b, d) malignant nodule.

17.2 MGRF-Based Prior Appearance Model

To exclude a presegmentation image alignment, the visual appearance of both small 2D and large three-dimensional (3D) malignant lung nodules in an LDCT chest image is modeled with a generic translation and rotation invariant second-order MGRF. Its voxelwise and central-symmetric pairwise voxel potentials account for differences between the Hounsfield values (i.e., gray levels, or intensities) of the nodules. Possible monotone (order-preserving) intensity changes, e.g., due to different sensor characteristics, are taken into account by equalizing [6] lung areas on every segmented LDCT data set as shown in Figure 17.1.

Figure 17.2 presents axial cross sections of two lung nodules suggesting that spatial distribution of the Hounsfield values is much less smooth for a malignant nodule compared with a benign one. The MGRF model describes peculiarities of the visual appearance of the malignant nodules in terms of pairwise spatial co-occurrences of the equalized Hounsfield values.

Let (x,y,z) be Cartesian point coordinates in a 3D lattice $\mathbf{R} = [(x,y,z) : x = 0,\ldots,X-1; y = 0,\ldots,Y-1, z = 1,\ldots,Z-1]$ supporting 3D images $\mathbf{g} = [g_{x,y,z} : (x,y,z) \in \mathbf{R}; g_{x,y,z} \in \mathbf{Q}]$ with a finite set of intensities $\mathbf{Q} = \{0,\ldots,Q-1\}$. The translation and rotation invariant MGRF is specified by a set $\mathbf{N}$ of characteristic central-symmetric voxel neighborhoods $\{\mathbf{n}_\nu : \nu \in \mathbf{N}\}$ on $\mathbf{R}$ shown in Figure 17.3 and a corresponding set $\mathbf{V} = (\mathbf{V}_\nu : \nu \in \mathbf{N})$ of Gibbs potentials, one potential per neighborhood.

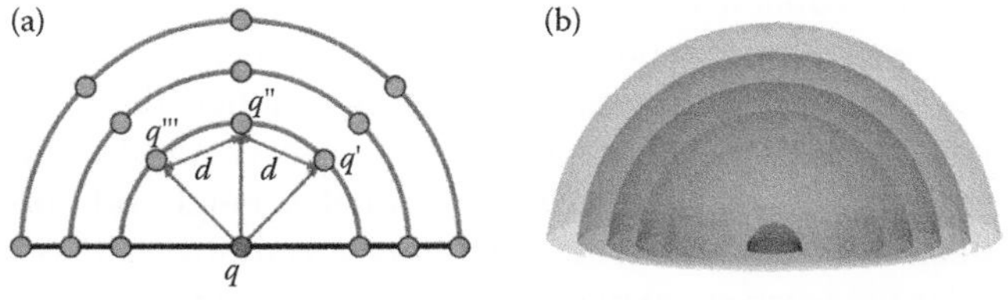

FIGURE 17.3
(See color insert.) Central-symmetric second-order (a) 2D and (b) 3D neighborhood system.

The central-symmetric voxel neighborhood $\mathbf{n}_\nu$ embraces all voxel pairs such that the coordinate offsets between any voxel (x,y,z) and its neighbor (x',y',z') belong to an indexed semiopen interval $[d_{\nu,\min}, d_{\nu,\max}]$; $\nu \in \mathbf{N} \subset \{1,2,3,\ldots\}$ of the intervoxel distances:

$$d_{\nu,\min} \leq \sqrt{(x-x')^2+(y-y')^2+(z-z')^2} \leq d_{\nu,\max} \quad (17.1)$$

Figure 17.3 illustrates the neighborhoods for the distance ranges $d_{\nu,\min} = \nu - 0.5$ and $d_{\nu,\max} = \nu + 0.5$; $\nu \in \mathbf{N} = \{1,\ldots,4\}$.

Each neighborhood $\mathbf{n}_\nu$ has the same potential function $\mathbf{V}_\nu$ of the absolute intensity difference $\Delta = |q - q'|$ between the neighboring voxel pairs: $\mathbf{V}_\nu = (V_\nu(\Delta){:}\ \Delta \in \mathbf{D})$, where $q = g(x,y,z)$; $q' = g(x',y',z')$, and $\mathbf{D} \equiv \mathbf{Q} = \{0,1,\ldots,Q-1\}$. The voxelwise potential function $\mathbf{V}_{\text{vox}} = (V_{\text{vox}}(q) : q \in \mathbf{Q})$ depends on the voxel intensities.

In this chapter, we introduce a new maximum likelihood analytical approach to estimate the potentials of MGRF. The potentials are analytically approximated as

$$V_\nu = \lambda(f_\nu(\Delta) - f_{\text{irf}}(\Delta)); \quad \nu \in \mathbf{N} \quad (17.2)$$

where $f_\nu(\Delta)$ is the empirical probability of the pairwise intensity difference Δ for the voxel pairs corresponding to the neighborhood $\mathbf{n}_\nu$ over the training data set; $f_{\text{irf}}(\Delta)$ denotes the probability of the same difference Δ for the independent random field of equiprobable intensities:

$$f_\nu(\Delta) = \begin{cases} \dfrac{1}{Q} & \text{if } \Delta = 0 \\ \dfrac{2(Q-\Delta)}{Q^2} & \text{otherwise} \end{cases}$$

and the common factor λ is also computed analytically. Below, λ is omitted ($\lambda = 1$) because only relative potentials are used for computing relative energies $E_{\nu,\text{rel}}$ of the neighborhoods.

17.2.1 Neighborhood Selection

The relative energies

$$E_{\nu,\text{rel}} = \sum_{\Delta \in D} f_\nu(\Delta)\left(f_\nu(\Delta) - f_{\text{irf}}(\Delta)\right) \quad (17.3)$$

allow for ranking all the available neighborhoods n° and selecting the characteristic subset N for the prior MGRF appearance model with the potentials of Equation 17.2. Examples of typical 2D axial cross sections of 25 training 3D malignant nodules in Figure 17.4 selected from the 50 malignant nodules used for experiments in Section 17.3 show how the energies of Equation 17.3 vary for the individual central symmetric neighborhoods $\mathbf{n}_\nu$.

To automatically select the characteristic neighbors, an empirical distribution of the relative energies over a large search set of possible neighbors N can be considered as a mixture $P(E) = \pi P_{\text{lo}}(E) + (1 - \pi)P_{\text{hi}}(E)$ of a wide "noncharacteristic" low-energy component and a considerably smaller characteristic high-energy one. Because both the components $P_{\text{lo}}(E)$

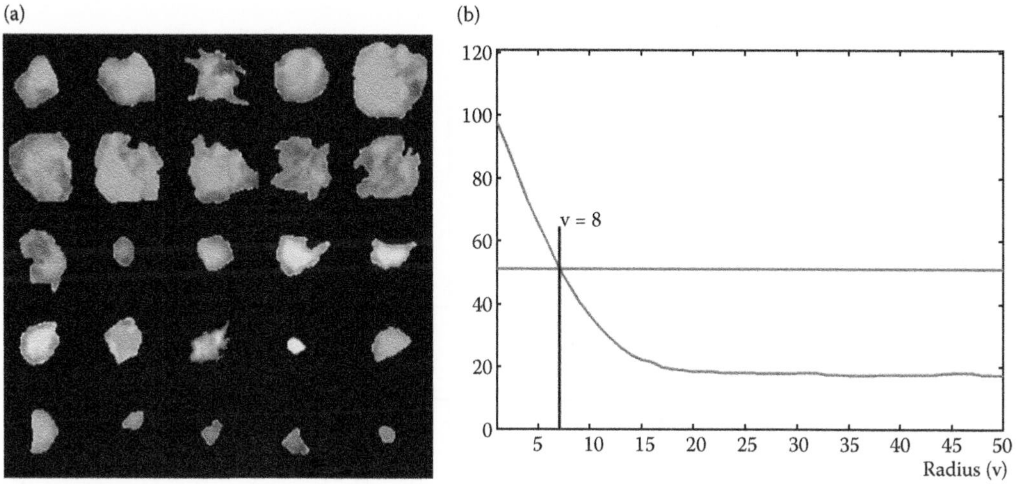

FIGURE 17.4
(a) Selected typical cross sections of the training malignant nodules and (b) the energies of Equation 17.4 for the voxel neighborhoods $N = \{n_\nu : \nu \leq 50\}$ in the training nodules.

and $P_{hi}(E)$ can be of arbitrary shape, their mixture including the prior weight π is closely approximated with two linear combinations of positive and negative discrete Gaussians using efficient expectation-maximization–based algorithms introduced in ref. [10]. Figure 17.5 illustrates the successive approximation steps. The intersection of the estimated weighed mixture components provides an energy threshold θ for selecting the characteristic neighbors: $\mathrm{N} = \{\nu : E_{\nu,\mathrm{rel}} \geq \theta; \nu \in N\}$. This example results in the threshold $\theta = 51$ producing the $|\mathbf{N}| = 8$ characteristic neighbors.

Under the model learned, any nodule image $\mathbf{g}$ is described by its total Gibbs energy

$$E(\mathbf{g}) = \mathbf{V}_{\mathrm{vox}}^{\mathrm{T}}\mathbf{F}_{\mathrm{vox}}(\mathbf{g}) + \sum_{\nu \in \mathbf{N}} \rho_\nu \mathbf{V}_\nu^{\mathrm{T}}\mathbf{F}_\nu(\mathbf{g}) \tag{17.4}$$

where $\mathbf{N}$ is a set of the selected neighbors, $\mathbf{F}_{\mathrm{vox}}(\mathbf{g})$ and $\mathbf{F}_\nu(\mathbf{g})$ are vectors of the empirical probability distributions of intensities and absolute intensity differences collected within the nodule in $\mathbf{g}$, and ρ_ν denotes a relative cardinality of the set of all the voxel pairs corresponding to the neighborhood ν with respect to the lattice cardinality XYZ.

17.3 Experimental Results

To justify the proposed methodology of learning the 3D appearance (i.e., spatial distribution of Hounsfield values) of both malignant and benign nodules after normalizing the image signals, the above appearance analysis was pilot-tested on a database of clinical multislice 3D chest LDCT scans of 109 lung nodules (51 malignant and 58 benign). The scanned CT data sets each have $0.7 \times 0.7 \times 2.0\text{-mm}^3$ voxels, with the diameters of the nodules ranging from 3 to 30 mm.

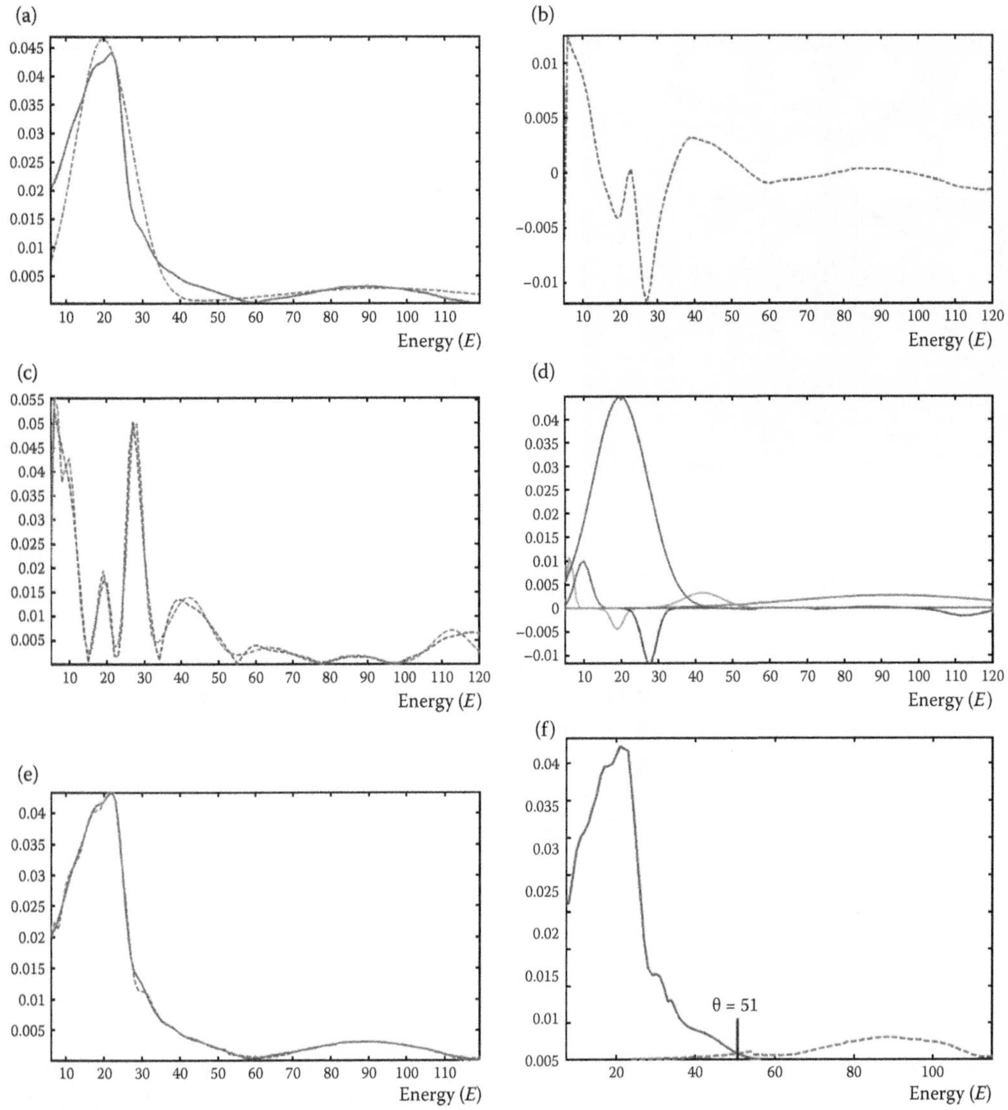

FIGURE 17.5
Steps of calculating the energy threshold in line with ref. [10]: (a) initial approximation of the energy distribution with mixed two dominant Gaussians representing the low and high energies, respectively; (b) sign-alternate and absolute deviations between the empirical and estimated mixtures; (c) the mixture model for the absolute deviations; (d) the resulting positive and negative subordinate components; (e) the final approximation of the empirical distribution, and (f) the two estimated weighed components $\pi P_{\text{lo}}(E)$ and $(1-\pi)P_{\text{hi}}(E)$.

Figures 17.6 and 17.7 show the conditional voxelwise Gibbs energies that are describing the 3D appearance of both malignant and benign lung nodules. It is clear that the Gibbs energy for malignant nodules was higher than the Gibbs energy for benign nodules because slow variations of the voxel intensities for the latter make their absolute differences close to zero. Contrastingly, the intensity variations in the voxels in malignant

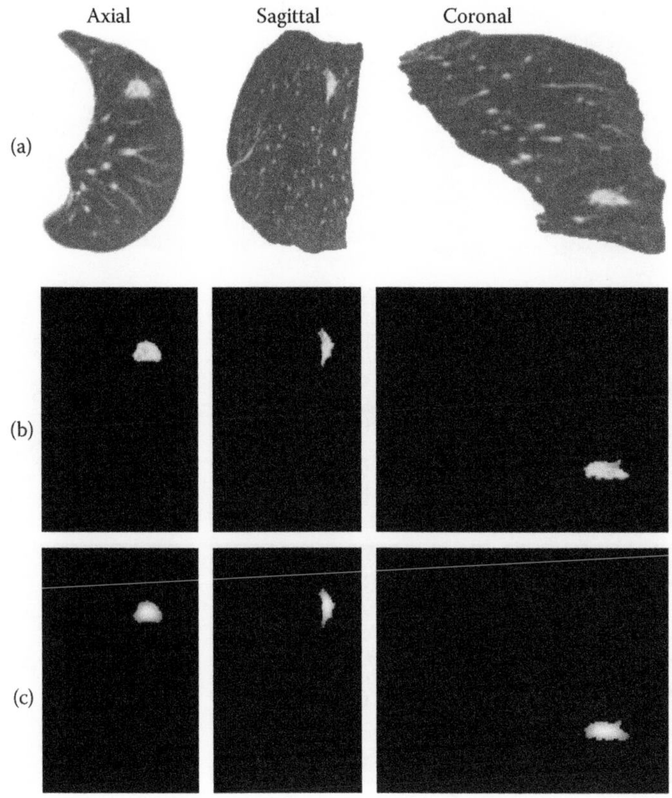

FIGURE 17.6
Appearance analysis of malignant nodules: (a) original LDCT images, (b) nodules segmented with our method in ref. [5], and (c) gray-coded conditional voxelwise Gibbs energies for the learned MGRF model.

nodules make the absolute differences for two neighboring voxels much greater than zero. Shown in Figure 17.8, the probability distributions of the Gibbs energy in Equation 17.4 describing the 3D appearance of 25 malignant and 29 benign nodules were obtained by the close approximation of the empirical mixture using the aforementioned approach in ref. [10].

The training subset for classification (25 malignant and 29 benign nodules) was arbitrarily selected among all the 109 lung nodules (51 malignant and 58 benign nodules). The classification accuracy of a Bayes classifier using the estimated probability models in Figure 17.8 was evaluated using the χ^2 test at three confidence levels—85%, 90%, and 95%—in order to examine significant differences in the Gibbs energy. As expected, the 85% confidence level yielded the best results—the correctly classified 26 out of 26 malignant nodules (100% accuracy) and 29 out of 29 benign nodules (100% accuracy). At the 90% confidence level, 26 out of 26 malignant nodules and 29 out of 29 benign nodules (100% accuracy) were still classified correctly. The 95% confidence level obviously gave smaller accuracy rates for both groups, specifically, 24 out of 26 correct answers for the malignant nodules (92%) and still 29 out of 29 benign nodules (100%). So, the overall accuracy using the proposed 3D appearance-based CAD system for 95% confidence level is 96.4% in the first detection of lung nodules as shown in the first row of Table 17.1.

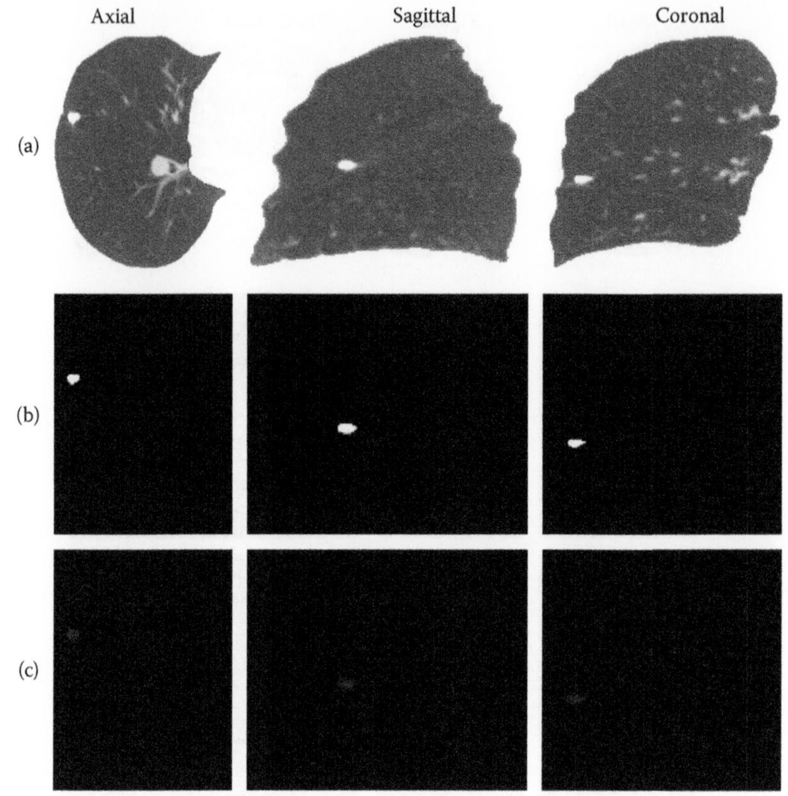

FIGURE 17.7
Appearance analysis of benign nodules: (a) original LDCT images, (b) nodules segmented with our method in ref. [5], and (c) gray-coded conditional voxelwise Gibbs energies for the learned MGRF model.

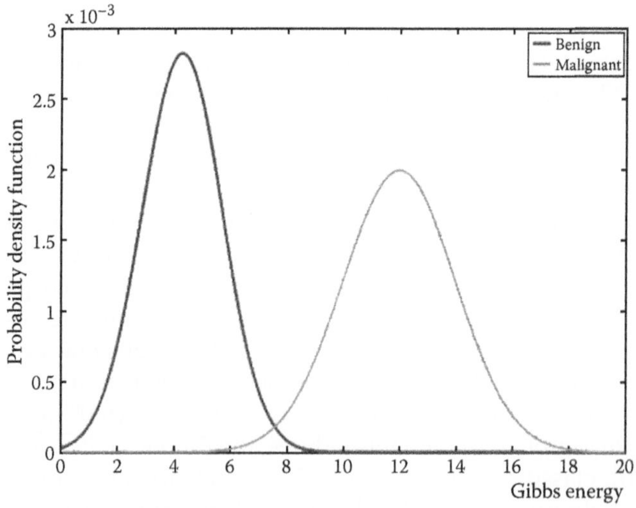

FIGURE 17.8
Energy probability models describing the appearance of 3D malignant and benign nodules (the models are obtained with the mixture learning algorithms in ref. [10]).

TABLE 17.1

Diagnostic Results for 95% Confidence Interval

	Based on Growth Rate			Based on 3D Appearance Analysis		
Diagnostic Results	**M**	**B**	**Accuracy (%)**	**M**	**B**	**Accuracy (%)**
0 month	–	–	–	24/26	29/29	96.4
3 months	9/26	15/29	43.7	24/26	29/29	96.4
6 months	11/26	18/29	52.7	26/26	29/29	100
9 months	19/26	22/29	74.5	26/26	29/29	100
12 months	23/26	26/29	89.9	26/26	29/29	100

Note: M, malignant; B, benign.

The advantages of using the proposed 3D appearance-based CAD system are highlighted by comparing the accuracy of our system to that of the approach proposed by Reeves et al. [11], which was based on the estimation of lung nodule growth rate over a 1-year time frame from the first detection. It has been shown that using the proposed 3D appearance-based CAD system leads to accuracy of 96.36% in the first detection of lung nodules and 100% 6 months after the first detection (Table 17.1). On the other hand, the diagnosis based on estimation of the lung nodules' growth rate lead to an accuracy of 89.9%, only one year after the first detection (Table 17.1).

17.4 Conclusions

The preliminary results shown in this chapter justify further elaboration of the proposed alternative method for diagnosing malignant lung nodules. Its novelty lies in using the appearance of a segmented 3D nodule instead of the more conventional growth rate as a reliable diagnostic feature. The appearance is described in terms of the voxelwise conditional Gibbs energies for a generic rotationally and translationally invariant second-order MGRF model of malignant nodules with analytically estimated characteristic voxel neighborhoods and potentials.

The proposed nodule appearance analysis could lead to more accurate, fast, and clinically useful diagnostics of detected pulmonary nodules without the need for investigating their temporal development on the successive LDCT images of the same subject collected for a relatively long time. The present C++ implementation on the Intel quad processor (3.2 GHz each) with 16-GB memory and 1.5 TB hard drive with the RAID technology takes approximately 5 s for processing 30-mm lung nodules and less than 1 s for processing 5-mm lung nodules.

References

1. H. K.Weir et al., "Annual report to the nation on the status of cancer, 1975–2000," *Journal National Cancer Institute*, vol. 95, no. 17, pp. 1276–1299, 2003.

2. C. Yankelevitz, A. Reeves, W. Kostis, B. Zhao, and C. Henschke, "Small pulmonary nodules: Volumetrically determined growth rates based on CT Evaluation," *Radiology*, vol. 217, no. 1, pp. 251–256, 2000.
3. A. Farag, A. El-Baz, G. Gimelfarb, R. Falk, and S. Hushek, "Automatic detection and recognition of lung abnormalities in helical CT images using deformable templates," *Proceedings of International Conference on Medical Image Computing and Computer-Assisted Intervention (MICCAI'04)*, France, Rennes, Saint-Malo, September 26–29, 2004, vol. II, pp. 856–864.
4. A. Farag, A. El-Baz, and G. Gimel'farb, "Precise segmentation of multi-modal images," *IEEE Transactions on Image Processing*, vol. 15, no. 4, pp. 952–968, April, 2006.
5. A. Farag, A. El-Baz, G. Gimel'farb, R. Falk, M. Abou El-Ghar, T. El-Diasty, and S. Elshazly, "Appearance models for robust segmentation of pulmonary nodules in 3D LDCT chest images," *Proceedings of International Conference on Medical Image Computing and Computer-Assisted Intervention (MICCAI'06)*, Copenhagen, Denmark, October 1–6, 2006, vol. 1, pp. 662–670.
6. R. Gonzalez and R. Woods, *Digital Image Processing*, Addison-Wesley, New York, 1992.
7. J. Maintz and M. Viergever, "A survey of medical image registration," *Journal of Medical Image Analysis*, vol. 2, pp. 1–36, 1998.
8. J. Ko and D. Naidich, "Computer-aided diagnosis and the evaluation of lung disease," *Journal of Thoracic Imaging*, vol. 19, no. 3, pp. 136–155, 2004.
9. W. Kostis, D. Yankelevitz, A. Reeves, S. Fluture, C. Henschke, "Small pulmonary nodules: Reproducibility of three-dimensional volumetric measurement and estimation of time to follow-up CT," *Radiology*, vol. 231, pp. 446–452, May 2004.
10. Authors' publication, 2007.
11. A. Reeves, A. Chan, D. Yankelevitz, C. Henschke, B. Kressler, and W. Kostis, "On measuring the change in size of pulmonary nodules," *IEEE Transactions on Medical Imaging*, vol. 25, no. 4, pp. 435–449, April 2006.

18

Validation of a New Image-Based Approach for the Accurate Estimating of the Growth Rate of Detected Lung Nodules Using Real Computed Tomography Images and Elastic Phantoms Generated by State-of-the-Art Microfluidics Technology

Ayman El-Baz, Palaniappan Sethu, Georgy Gimel'farb, Fahmi Khalifa, Ahmed Elnakib, Robert Falk, Mohamed Abo El-Ghar, and Jasjit Suri

CONTENTS

18.1 Introduction

Lung cancer remains the leading cause of cancer-related death in the United States. In 2006, there were approximately 174,470 new cases of lung cancer and 162,460 related deaths [1]. A pulmonary nodule is the most common manifestation of lung cancer. Lung nodules are approximately spherical regions of relatively high-density tissue that are visible in x-ray images of the lung. Large (generally defined as greater than 2 cm in diameter) malignant nodules can be easily detected with traditional computed tomography (CT) scanning techniques and can be diagnosed by needle biopsy or bronchoscopy techniques. However, the diagnostic options for small indeterminate nodules are limited due to problems associated with accessing small tumors, especially if they are located deep in the tissue or away from large airways; therefore, additional diagnostic and imaging techniques are needed.

One of the most promising techniques for detecting small cancerous nodules relies on characterizing the nodule based on estimating its growth rate over time. The growth rate is estimated by measuring the volumetric change of the detected lung nodules over time. Until now, there has been no accurate approach in the literature to validate proposed techniques for measuring the growth rate of the detected lung nodules. Thus, the objective of this chapter is to present a new way for validating our approach for measuring the growth rate of the detected lung nodules using elastic lung phantoms. They are constructed using state-of-the-art microfluidics technology in order to mimic the contractions and expansions of the lung and nodules seen during normal breathing. In addition, we validate our approach using in vivo data that have been collected from four subjects.

18.1.1 Previous Work

Lung nodule volumetry is used for both nodule diagnosis [2–4] and monitoring the tumor response to therapy [5]. Volume measurement precision and accuracy depends on a number of factors, including the interscan variability, slice selection artifacts, differences in degree of inspiration and scan angles, and performance of nodule segmentation algorithms, which can make comparing serial scans unreliable. This research project aims to address these variations and discrepancies in a way that will make evaluating small lung masses more consistent and allow for more accurate measurement of the growth rates. Below, we provide an overview of the existing work on measuring the growth rate of the detected lung nodules.

Generally, the growth rate of pulmonary nodules is determined by a size-based comparison of different temporal CT scans. Earlier two-dimensional (2D) techniques exploited changes in the maximal transverse diameter of the nodule to estimate the growth rate between the CT scans [5–10]. Unfortunately, these techniques have problems, for example, possible asymmetric growth results not only in minimal changes in the maximal diameter but also in an increase of the overall lesion volume. Hence, alternative three-dimensional (3D) approaches were published for the measurement of the growth rate of small nodules. These volumetric measurements [11–27] have overcome the former 2D limitations.

Yankelevitz et al. [11] used high-resolution CT scans to assess the growth rate of small pulmonary nodules. The region of interest containing the nodule was identified in each image manually by a radiologist. Then it was resampled to obtain an isotropic space using a 3D linear interpolation, thresholded and segmented using a 3D technique to reconstruct the 3D image volume. The number of voxels contained in the resulting volume was counted, and the doubling times were estimated using a simple exponential growth model. This 3D method offered an advantage over the 2D counterpart, which measured the cross-sectional area, but it did not take into account the global motions of the patients due to their movements and the local motions of the whole lung tissues due to breathing and heart beating.

Reeves et al. [14] presented a method for measuring the change in the nodule size from two CT images obtained close in time where the region of interest of each CT scan was selected by hand and resampled to an isotropic space. To make an accurate assessment and facilitate the comparison of the selected regions, a registration process using the 3D rigid-body transformation was performed such that both nodules would have the same position and orientation in the image space. Following the registration stage, an adaptive thresholding technique for segmenting the nodule was applied. A rule-based segmentation adjustment was applied to both nodule segmentations. By comparing the nodule segmentations and the thresholded regions, this rule-based system achieved a more consistent measurement of the nodule volumes by discarding missegmented nodule voxels. The main limitation of this work is that only the global motion of the patient, but not the local motion due to breathing and heart beating, was taken into account. This strongly affects the estimated growth rate, especially for small detected nodules (less than 5 mm in diameter).

Taking into account the difference in inspiration levels, Zhao et al. [9] presented an adaptive doubling time (ADT) measure of the growth rate of the detected lung nodules. The ADT calculation was obtained through nonrigid lung registration that took into account expanding or shrinking of the nodule. This was accomplished by weighting the matching cost of each voxel based on a proposed nodule detection process and a powerful segmentation refinement process. The main limitation of this framework is that the nonrigid registration is applied directly to the segmented nodules. This affects the growth rate estimation because after segmentation of the lung nodules, we can no longer discriminate between the changes due to the true growth rate of the lung nodules and the changes in their shapes that come from breathing and heart beating.

Kawata et al. [15] coregistered the pulmonary nodules by using rigid-body and affine registrations at two different stages. The nodules were segmented using a 3D deformable surface model, and curvature features were calculated to track the temporal evolution of the nodule. The same research group presented an extension of ref. [15] by adding a 3D nonrigid deformable registration stage, and the analysis was performed using a displacement field to quantify areas of the nodule growth over time [16]. Zheng et al. [17] proposed a simultaneous segmentation and registration of the lung to measure the growth rate from serial CT data. They used a nonrigid transformation for lung deformation and rigid structure for the tumor in order to preserve the volume and the shape of the tumor during the registration. Segmentation of the 3D lung and tumor was based on a 2D graph-cut algorithm, and a B-spline–based, nonrigid registration was used. Both these works have the same limitation as the above-mentioned work of Zhao et al. [9].

Jirapatnakul et al. [18] presented a nodule growth measurement method called growth analysis from density. They applied a Gaussian weighting function to the region around the nodule to reduce the influence of structures lying far from the nodule center. Also, some researchers used a number of commercial packages that have been released by the CT vendors for measuring the volume of pulmonary nodules, and a number of studies have evaluated the accuracy and limitations of these software packages. Since the actual volumes of real pulmonary nodules are unknown, such evaluations usually involve either radiologists/experts as the "gold standard" [19–23] or synthetic rigid phantoms for which the volumes of the nodules are known [24–26]. A general limitation of the majority of the volumetric measurement algorithms is that they are only capable of segmenting solid nodules. Moreover, the results from these packages show that the volumetric error depends on the performance of the segmentation algorithms, particularly in the presence of the nodule's vascular and pleural attachments [27]. In summary, the aforementioned existing approaches show the following limitations:

1. Most did not take into account the global motion of the patients due to their movements and the local motions of the whole lung tissues due to breathing and heart beating.
2. Most apply global and local registration directly to the segmented nodule, even though this technique of measuring the growth rate cannot discriminate between the changes due to the true growth of the lung nodules and the changes in the nodule shape that come from breathing and heart beating.

3. Most are not suitable for special types of pulmonary nodules such as cavities and ground-glass nodules.
4. Most require a significant user interaction, which is difficult for a clinical practitioner.
5. All validate their approaches on rigid phantoms without taking into account the effect of breathing and heart beating in estimating the growth rate.

This research chapter aims to address these variations and discrepancies in a way that will make evaluating small lung masses more consistent and allow for a more accurate measurement of the growth rates and shape and appearance analysis of the detected nodules. To the best of our knowledge, this work is the first of its kind that uses elastic phantoms and in vivo data to validate the proposed approach for the growth rate of the detected lung nodules.

18.2 Material and Methods

18.2.1 Materials

Our approach for measuring the growth rate has been validated on elastic lung phantoms constructed using state-of-the-art microfluidics technology and in vivo data that have been collected from a small control study (four subjects). Below, we will illustrate the steps of creating the lung elastic phantoms and colleting the in vivo data.

18.2.1.1 Elastic Phantoms

Elastic lung phantoms were constructed using state-of-the-art microfluidics technology. The models were fabricated out of a flexible transparent polymer, i.e., polydimethylsiloxane (PDMS), a silicone. The motivation for phantom design was to mimic the airway network in a 3D format with individual nodules. By making the phantoms out of a soft polymer, the introduction of compressed air into the network results in deformation due to stretching. This stretching is more significant in the nodules that are larger than in the channels that make up the airway network. Therefore, these phantoms mimic the airway and replicate contractions and expansions of the lung and nodules seen during normal breathing. Two different sets of phantoms were constructed. The first set was designed to replicate differential stretching and consists of two devices with branching microchannels leading to four nodules (5 mm in diameter). The only difference between the two devices was the overall thickness of the devices (Figure 18.1). The second set consists of three devices with branching channels leading to four nodules. Each device had progressively larger diameter (2, 3, and 3.5 mm) nodules (Figure 18.2) and was designed to mimic progressive tumor growth.

The phantoms were fabricated using standard soft-lithography techniques. A layout of the airways and nodules was made using AutoCAD layout software (Autodesk, San Rafael, CA). Masks were fabricated by printing the layout on a transparent sheet at a resolution of 30,000 dpi using a high-resolution printer (Fineline Imaging, Colorado Springs, CO). The masks were then used to define patterns for the airway channels and nodules on silicon wafers coated with a negative photoresist, SU-8 50 (Microchem, Newton, MA).

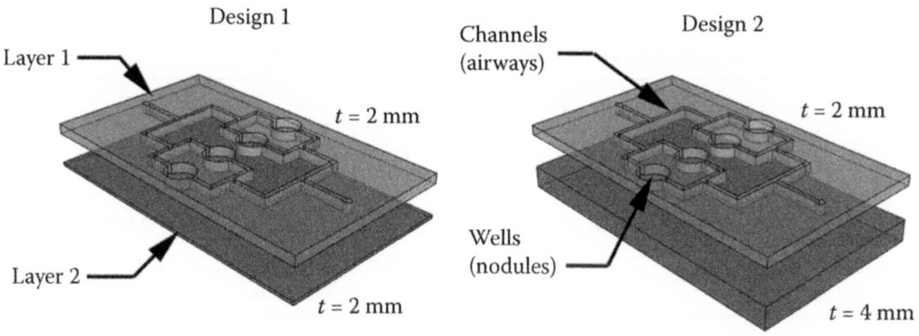

FIGURE 18.1
(See color insert.) The first phantom model consists of two PDMS devices, with channels representing the airways and wells representing the nodules. The only difference between the two devices is the thickness of the bottom layer.

The SU-8 50 was spin-coated at 3000 rpm to yield a thickness of 50 μm and then exposed to an UV light source via the mask. The silicon wafer was then used to mold 2-mm-thick PDMS structures representing the airway and blood vessels. The channel cross sections were 250 × 50 μm, and the lengths were variable. The diameters of the nodules ranged from 2 to 5 mm. Access holes were punched with a blunt 18-gauge needle, and tubing was press-fitted to the holes to supply the compressed air into the network. The molded PDMS piece was then bonded to a blank PDMS piece following exposure to O_2 plasma (March Instruments, Amherst, OH) to seal the channel network. One outlet was closed, and access tubing was inserted into the inlet. A syringe was used to actuate the phantoms.

18.2.1.2 *In Vivo* Data

We performed the control study on four subjects, each of which had multiple nodules. These four subjects were diagnosed by biopsy (ground truth): two out of the four subjects had malignant nodules and the other two had benign nodules. The CT data were collected with the same the following scanning parameters: slice thickness of 2.5 mm reconstructed every 1.5 mm, kilovolt 140, milliampere 100, and FOV 36 cm. The ages, sex, number of detected nodules, and CT scanner manufacturer for each patient are listed in Table 18.1. Table 18.2 shows the type and the maximum diameter for each detected nodule. Table 18.3 shows the axial cross section in one of the detected lung nodules at end-expiration breath and hold (BH) and at end-inspiration BH CT scans.

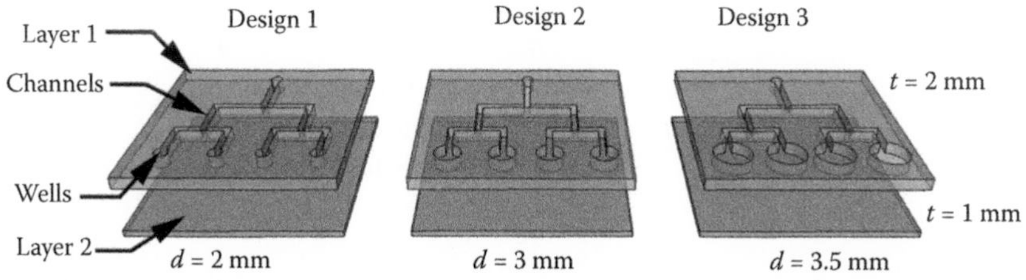

FIGURE 18.2
(See color insert.) The second phantom model mimics tumor progression and is similar in construction to model 1. The only difference among the three designs is the increasing diameter of the nodules.

TABLE 18.1
Information of Subjects Enrolled to the Control Study

	Benign		Malignant	
	Subject 1	**Subject 2**	**Subject 3**	**Subject 4**
Age	60	65	60	48
Sex	Male	Female	Female	Male
No. of nodules	6	13	14	17
CT scanner	Philips	GE	Siemens	GE

18.2.2 Methods

The main steps of our approach for quantifying the volumetric changes (the growth rate) in the detected lung nodules are outlined below.

18.2.2.1 Global Alignment

Basic notation. Let $\mathbf{Q} = \{0,1,\ldots,Q-1\}$; $\mathbf{R} = \{(x,y,z) : x = 0,1,\ldots,X-1; y = 0,1,\ldots,Y-1\}; z = 0,1,\ldots,Z-1$ and $\mathbf{R}_p \subset \mathbf{R}$ be a finite set of scalar image signals (e.g., gray levels), a 3D arithmetic lattice supporting digital LDCT image data $g : \mathbf{R} \to \mathbf{Q}$ and an arbitrary-shaped part of the lattice occupied by the prototype, respectively. Let a finite set $\mathcal{N} = \{(\xi_1,\eta_1,\zeta_1),\ldots\ldots\ldots((\xi_n,\eta_n,\zeta_n)\}$

TABLE 18.2
Maximum Diameter and Type of Each Detected Nodule for the Four Subjects

	Benign Nodules				Malignant Nodules			
	Subject 1		Subject 2		Subject 3		Subject 4	
	Type	*D* (mm)	Type	*D* (mm)	Type	*D* (mm)	Type	*D* (mm)
1	Solid[a]	11.2	Solid	3.7	Solid[b]	12	Solid	3
2	Solid	15.3	Solid[a]	3.5	Solid[a]	11	Solid	5
3	Solid	14.3	Solid[a]	8	Solid[b]	11	Solid[a]	5
4	Solid[a]	8.7	Solid[a]	10	Cavity	11	Solid	8
5	Solid	11.3	Solid	9	Solid[b]	7	Solid[a]	7
6	Solid	17.9	Solid	3.5	Solid[b]	12	Solid	5.5
7			Solid	5	Solid	11	Solid	5
8			Solid[b]	9	Cavity	11	Solid	5
9			Solid[a]	6.5	Solid[b]	16	Solid[b]	5.5
10			Solid[b]	11	Solid	10	Solid	6
11			Solid	5	Solid	9	Solid	4
12			Solid[a]	7	Solid[a]	9.5	Solid[b]	7.5
13			Solid[a]	5	Solid	11	Solid[a]	9
14					Solid	12.5	Solid[b]	5
15							Solid	7
16							Solid	7
17							Solid	7

Note: Note all the detected nodules are noncalcified. *D*, diameter.
[a] Solid juxtapleural nodule.
[b] Solid vascular nodule.

TABLE 18.3

Axial Cross Section of One of the Detected Lung Nodules

	Benign Cases		Malignant Cases	
	Subject 1	**Subject 2**	**Subject 3**	**Subject 4**
End-expiration BHs	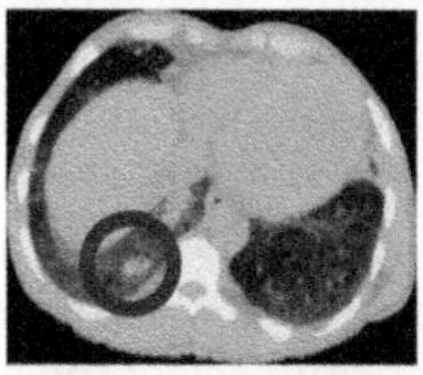	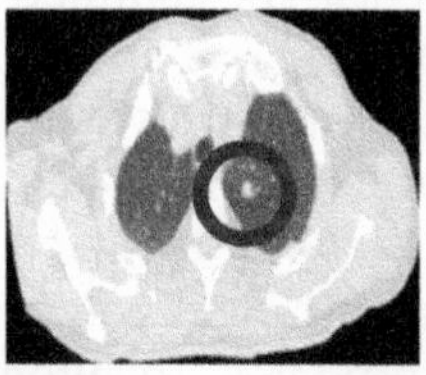	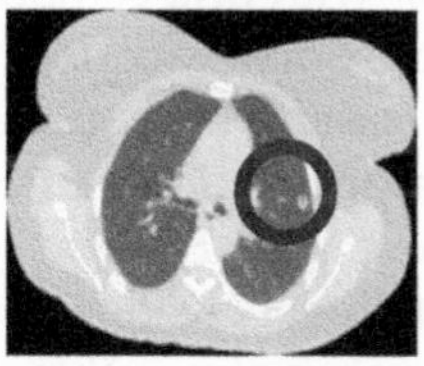	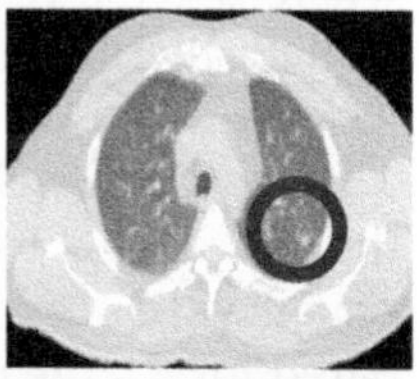
End-inspiration BHs	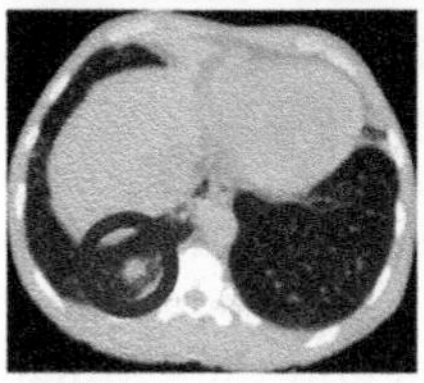	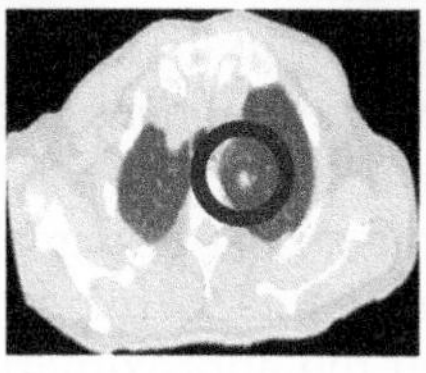	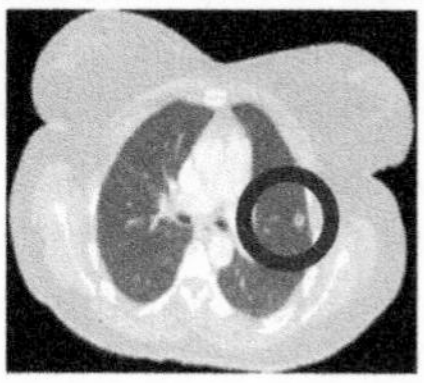	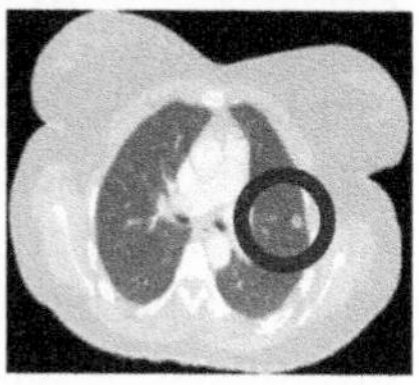

of the (x,y,z)-coordinate offsets define neighboring voxels or neighbors $\{(x + \xi, y + \eta, z + \zeta), (x - \xi, y - \eta, z - \zeta): (\xi,\eta,\zeta) \in \mathcal{N}\} \wedge \mathbf{R}_p$ interacting with each voxel $(x,y,z) \in \mathbf{R}_p$. The set $\mathcal{N}$ yields a 3D neighborhood graph on $\mathbf{R}_p$ that specifies translation invariant pairwise interactions between the voxels with n families $\mathcal{C}_{\xi,\eta,\zeta}$ of second-order cliques $\mathcal{C}_{\xi,\eta,\zeta}(x,y,z) = ((x,y,z),(x + \xi, y + \eta, z + \zeta))$. Interaction strengths are given by a vector $\mathbf{V}^{\mathrm{T}} = \mathbf{V}^{\mathrm{T}}_{\xi,\eta,\zeta} : (\xi,\eta,\zeta) \in \mathcal{N}$ of potentials $\mathbf{V}^{\mathrm{T}}_{\xi,\eta,\zeta} = \mathbf{V}_{\xi,\eta,\zeta}(q,q):(q,q) \in \mathbf{Q}^2$ depending on signal co-occurrences; here, T indicates transposition.

Data normalization: To account for possible monotone (order-preserving) changes of signals (e.g., due to different sensor characteristics), every LDCT data set is equalized using the cumulative empirical probability distribution of its signals.

Markov-Gibbs random field–based appearance model: In a generic Markov-Gibbs random field with multiple pairwise interaction, the Gibbs probability $P(g) \propto Exp(\mathrm{E}(g))$ of an object g aligned with the prototype g° on $\mathbf{R}_p$ is specified with the Gibbs energy $\mathrm{E}(g) = |\mathbf{R}_p|\mathbf{V}^{\mathrm{T}}\mathbf{F}(g)$, where $\mathbf{F}^{\mathrm{T}}(g)$ is the vector of scaled empirical probability distributions of signal co-occurrences over each clique family: $\mathbf{F}^{\mathrm{T}}(g) = \rho_{\xi,\eta,\zeta}\mathbf{F}^{\mathrm{T}}_{\xi,\eta,\zeta} : (\xi,\eta,\zeta) \in \mathcal{N}$, where $\rho_{\xi,\eta,\zeta} = \frac{\mathcal{C}_{\xi,\eta,\zeta}}{|\mathbf{R}_p|}$ is the relative size of the family and $\mathbf{F}_{\xi,\eta,\zeta}(g) = [f_{\xi,\eta,\zeta}(q,q'|g): (q,q') \in \mathbf{Q}^2]^{\mathrm{T}}$; here, $f_{\xi,\eta,\zeta}(q,q\,|g) = \frac{|\mathcal{C}_{\xi,\eta,\zeta;q,q}(g)|}{|\mathcal{C}_{\xi,\eta,\zeta}|}$ are empirical probabilities of signal co-occurrences, and $\mathcal{C}_{\xi,\eta,\zeta;q,q}(g) \quad \mathcal{C}_{\xi,\eta,\zeta}$ is a subfamily of the cliques $\mathcal{C}_{\xi,\eta,\zeta}(x,y,z)$ supporting the co-occurrence $(g_{x,y,z} = q, g_{x+\xi,y+\eta,z+\zeta} = q')$ in g. The co-occurrence distributions and the Gibbs energy for the object are determined over $\mathbf{R}_p$, i.e., within the prototype boundary after an object is affinely aligned with the prototype. To account for the affine transformation, the initial image is resampled to the back-projected $\mathbf{R}_p$ by interpolation. The appearance model consists of the neighborhood $\mathcal{N}$ and the potential $\mathbf{V}$ to be learned from the prototype.

Learning the potentials: The maximum likelihood estimation of $\mathbf{V}$ is proportional in the first approximation to the scaled centered empirical co-occurrence distributions for the prototype:

$$\mathbf{V}_{\xi,\eta,\zeta} = \lambda\rho_{\xi,\eta,\zeta}\ \mathbf{F}_{\xi,\eta,\zeta}\left(g^{o}\right) - \frac{1}{Q^2}\mathbf{U} \quad ; \ (\xi,\eta,\zeta)\in\mathcal{N} \tag{18.1}$$

where **U** is the vector with unit components. The common scaling factor λ is also computed analytically; it is approximately equal to Q^2 if $Q >> 1$ and $\rho_{\xi,\eta,\zeta} \approx 1$ for all $(\xi,\eta,\zeta) \in \mathcal{N}$. In our case, it can be set to $\lambda = 1$ because the registration uses only relative potential values and energies.

Learning the characteristic neighbors: To find the characteristic neighborhood set $\mathcal{N}$, the relative Gibbs energies $E_{\xi,\eta,\zeta}\left(g^{\circ}\right) = \rho_{\xi,\eta,\zeta}\mathbf{V}^{\mathrm{T}}_{\xi,\eta,\zeta}\mathbf{F}_{\xi,\eta,\zeta}\left(g^{\circ}\right)$ for the clique families, i.e., the scaled variances of the corresponding empirical co-occurrence distributions, are compared for a large number of possible candidates. To automatically select the characteristic neighbors, we consider an empirical probability distribution of the energies as a mixture of a large "noncharacteristic" low-energy component and a considerably smaller characteristic high-energy component: $P(E) = \pi P_{\mathrm{lo}}(E) + (1 - \pi)P_{\mathrm{hi}}(E)$. Both the components $P_{\mathrm{lo}}(E)$ and $P_{\mathrm{hi}}(E)$ are of arbitrary shape and thus are approximated with linear combinations of positive and negative discrete Gaussians (efficient expectation–maximization algorithms introduced in ref. [28] are used for both the approximation and the estimation of π). An example of the estimated characteristic neighbors is shown in Figure 18.3.

Appearance-based registration: The desired affine transformation of an object g corresponds to a local maximum of its relative energy $E(g_{\mathrm{a}}) = \mathbf{V}^{\mathrm{T}}\mathbf{F}(g_{\mathrm{a}})$ under the learned appearance model $[\mathcal{N}, \mathbf{V}]$. Here, $g_{\mathbf{a}}$ is the part of the object image reduced to $\mathbf{R}_{\mathrm{p}}$ by the 3D affine transformation $\mathbf{a} = [a_{11},\ldots,a_{23}] : x' = a_{11}x + a_{12}y + a_{13}z + a_{14}; y' = a_{21}x + a_{22}y + a_{23}z + a_{24}; z' = a_{31}x + a_{32}y + a_{33}z + a_{34}$. The initial transformation step is a pure translation with $a_{11} = a_{22} = 1$; $a_{12} = a_{21} = 0$, ensuring the most "energetic" overlap between the object and prototype. In other words, the chosen initial position $(a^*_{14}, a^*_{24}, a^*_{34})$ maximizes the Gibbs energy. Then, the gradient search for the local energy maximum closest to the initialization selects all the 12 parameters **a**. Figure 18.4c and 18.4d shows the results of the global alignment of two segmented lungs. It is clear from Figure 18.4d that the global alignment is not perfect due to local deformation.

18.2.2.2 Local Motion Model

To handle local deformations, we propose to deform the object over evolving closed equispaced surfaces (distance isosurfaces) so that it closely matches the prototype. The evolution is guided by an exponential speed function and intended to minimize distances between corresponding voxel pairs on the isosurfaces in both the images. The normalized

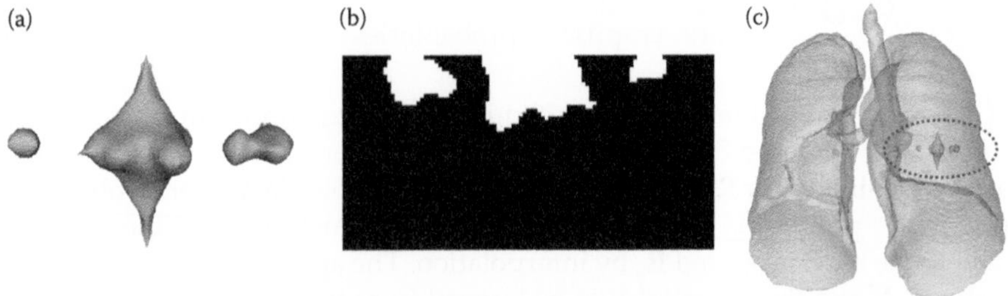

FIGURE 18.3
(See color insert) (a) The 3D neighborhood system estimated for the lung tissues, (b) its 2D cross section in the plane $\zeta = 0$ (in white), and (c) its superposition onto the lungs reconstructed from the LDCT images.

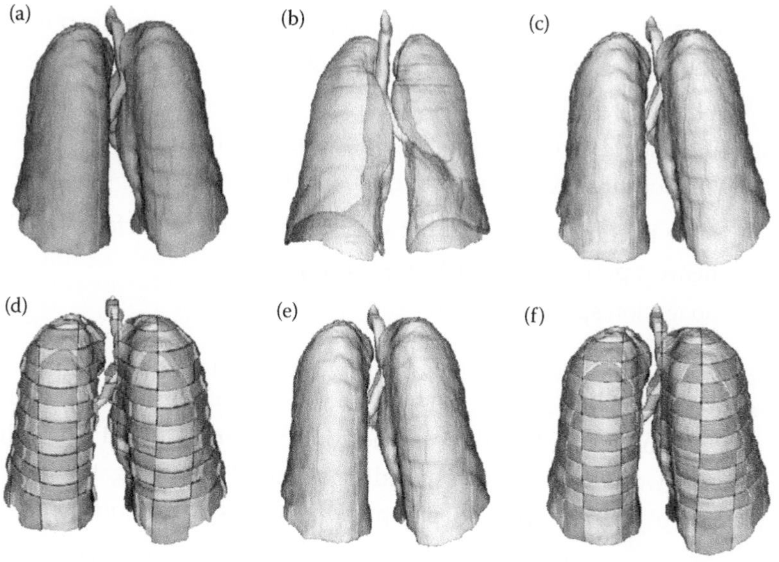

FIGURE 18.4
(See color insert.) 3D global and local registration: (a) reference data, (b) target data, (c) target data after 3D affine transformation, (d) checkerboard visualization to show the motion of lung tissues, (e) results of our nonrigid registration, and (f) checkerboard visualization to show the quality of the proposed local deformation model.

cross-correlation of the Gibbs energy is used to find correspondences between the isosurfaces. Our approach involves the following steps. First, a distance map inside the object is generated using fast marching level sets [29]. Second, the distance map is used to generate isosurfaces (Figure 18.5a). Note that the number of isosurfaces is not necessarily the same for both the images and depends on the accuracy and the speed required by the user. The third step consists of finding correspondences between the isosurfaces using the normalized cross-correlation of the Gibbs energy. Finally, the evolution process deforms the isosurfaces in the first data set (the target image) to match the isosurfaces in the second data set (the prototype).

The following notation is used below for defining the evolution equation:

- $\mathbf{b}^h_{g1} = \mathbf{p}^h_k : k = 1,2,\ldots\ldots\ldots K$: K control points on a surface h on the reference data such that $\mathbf{p}_k = (x_k, y_k, z_k)$ form a circularly connected chain of line segments $(\mathbf{p}_1, \mathbf{p}_2), \ldots,$ $(\mathbf{p}_{K-1}, \mathbf{p}_K)$, $(\mathbf{p}_K, \mathbf{p}_1)$.

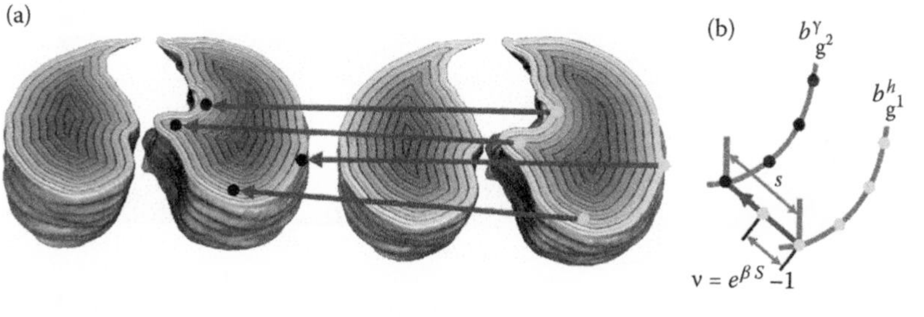

FIGURE 18.5
(a) Equispaced surfaces and (b) the proposed evolution scenario.

- $\mathbf{b}^{\gamma}_{g2} = \mathbf{p}^{\gamma}_{n} : n = 1,2,\ldots\ldots\ldots N$: N control points on a surface h on the reference data such that $\mathbf{p}_n = (x_n, y_n, z_n)$ form a circularly connected chain of line segments $(\mathbf{p}_1, \mathbf{p}_2), \ldots,$ $(\mathbf{p}_{N-1}, \mathbf{p}_N)$, $(\mathbf{p}_N, \mathbf{p}_1)$.
- $\mathbf{S}\left(\mathbf{p}^{h}_{k}, \mathbf{p}^{\gamma}_{n}\right)$: The Euclidean distance between a point on the surface h in the image $\mathbf{g}_1$ and the corresponding point on the surface γ in the image $\mathbf{g}_2$.
- $\mathbf{S}\left(\mathbf{p}^{\gamma}_{n}, \mathbf{p}^{\gamma-1}_{n}\right)$: The Euclidean distance between a point on the surface γ in the image $\mathbf{g}_1$ and the nearest point on the surface $\gamma - 1$ in $\mathbf{g}_1$.
- $\upsilon(\cdot)$: The propagation speed function.

The evolution $\mathbf{b}_\tau \rightarrow \mathbf{b}_{\tau+1}$ of a deformable boundary $\mathbf{b}$ in discrete time, $\tau = 0,1,2,\ldots$, is specified by the system $\mathbf{p}^{\gamma}_{n,\tau+1} = \mathbf{p}^{\gamma}_{n,\tau} + \upsilon\left(\mathbf{p}^{\gamma}_{n,\tau}\right)\mathbf{u}_{n,\tau}$; $n = 1,2,\ldots N$ of difference equations where $\upsilon\left(\mathbf{p}^{\gamma}_{n,\tau}\right)$ is a propagation speed function for the control point $p^{\gamma}_{n,\tau}$ and $u_{n,\tau}$ is the unit vector along the ray between the two corresponding points. The propagation speed function $\upsilon\left(\mathbf{p}^{\gamma}_{n,\tau}\right) = \min\left\{\mathbf{S}\left(\mathbf{p}^{h}_{k}, \mathbf{p}^{\gamma}_{n,\tau}\right), \mathbf{S}\left(\mathbf{p}^{\gamma}_{n,\tau}, \mathbf{p}^{\gamma-1}_{n,\tau}\right), \mathbf{S}\left(\mathbf{p}^{\gamma}_{n,\tau}, \mathbf{p}^{\gamma+1}_{n,\tau}\right)\right\}$ satisfies the condition $\upsilon\left(\mathbf{p}^{\gamma}_{n,\tau}\right) = 0$ if $\mathbf{S}\left(\mathbf{p}^{h}_{k}, \mathbf{p}^{\gamma}_{n,\tau}\right) = 0$ and prevents the current point from cross-passing the closest neighbor surfaces as shown in Figure 18.5b. The latter restriction is known as the smoothness constraint. Again, the checkerboard visualization (Figure 18.4d) of the data set in Figure 18.4a and the aligned data set in Figure 18.4c highlights the effect of the motion of lung tissues. It can be seen that the connections at the lung edges between the two volumes are not smooth when using only the global registration model. This is due to the local deformation that comes from breathing and heartbeats. The connections of the lung edges between the two volumes are considerably smoother when using the proposed local deformation model (Figure 18.4f).

18.3 Results

Our approach for measuring the growth rate of detected lung nodules was validated on elastic synthetic phantoms as well as on a small control study (both introduced in the materials section). Below, we will illustrate our validation results.

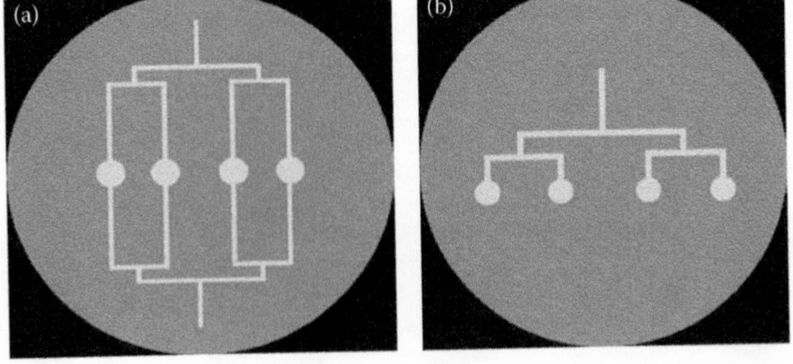

FIGURE 18.6
Typical CT scan slices: (a) from the first set (thick phantom) and (b) from the second set. Note that we inject Optiray 350 (Ioversol injection 74%) inside the channels before pushing the air to make the channels and simulated lung nodules appear with different intensity.

18.3.1 Validating the Proposed Approach on Elastic Phantoms

The five elastic phantoms presented in Section 18.2.1 are scanned twice using high-resolution CT machine. The first scan is done without pushing air inside the channels and nodules to mimic the expiration effect, and the second scan is done after pushing air inside the channels and nodules to mimic the inspiration effect. Both CT scans are collected with the following scanning parameters: KV 140, MA 100, and isotropic voxel resolution 0.075 mm. Figure 18.6 shows an axial cross section in two selected phantoms from the phantoms that are used in this validation study. Table 18.4 visualizes the 3D reconstruction of simulated

TABLE 18.4

3D Visualization of the Simulated Lung Nodules in CT Scans

	Set 1: Simulates No-Growth Rate	
	Mimic Expiration effect	**Mimic Inspiration effect**
Thick phantom	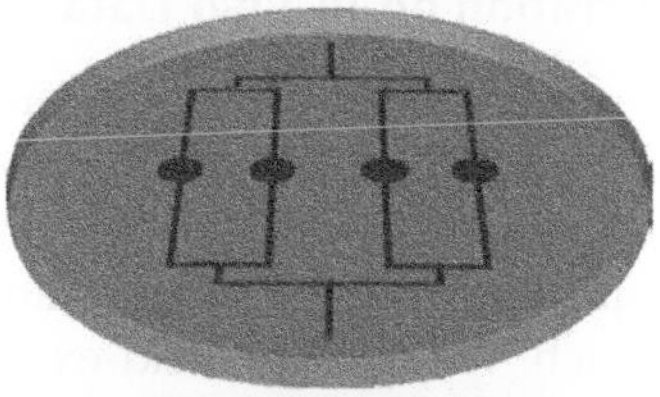	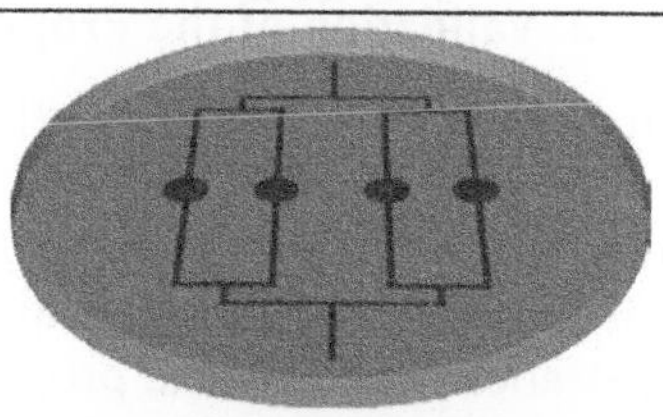
Thin phantom	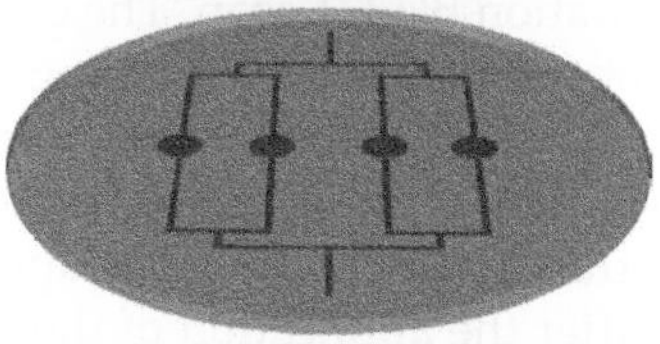	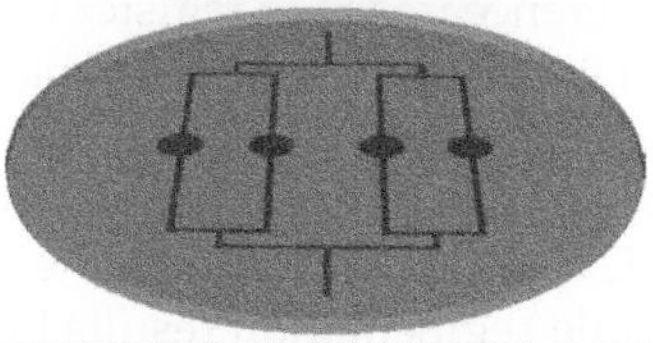
	Set 2: Simulates True Growth Rate	
	Mimic Expiration Effect	**Mimic Inspiration Effect**
2-mm nodule	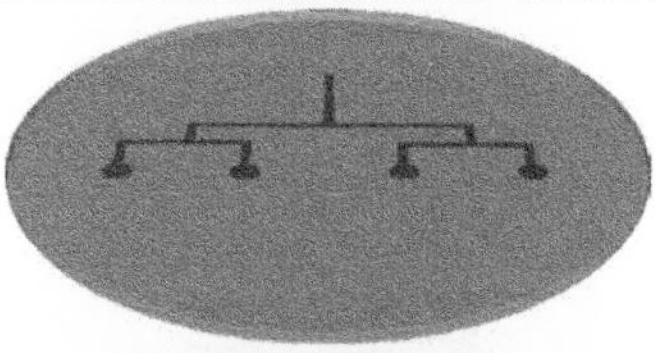	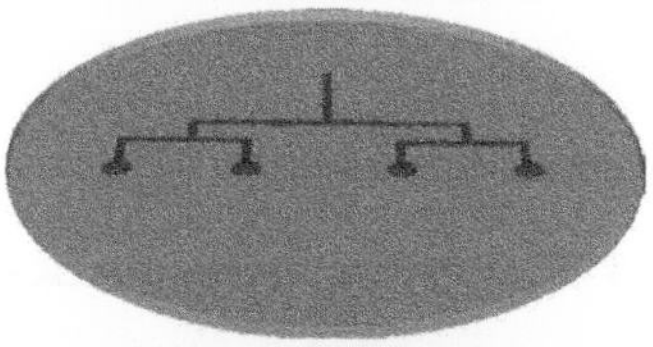
3-mm nodule	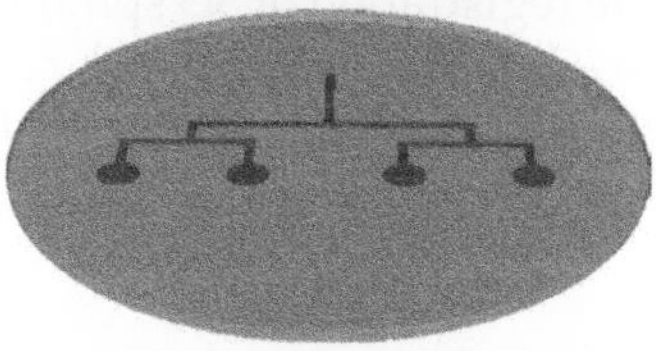	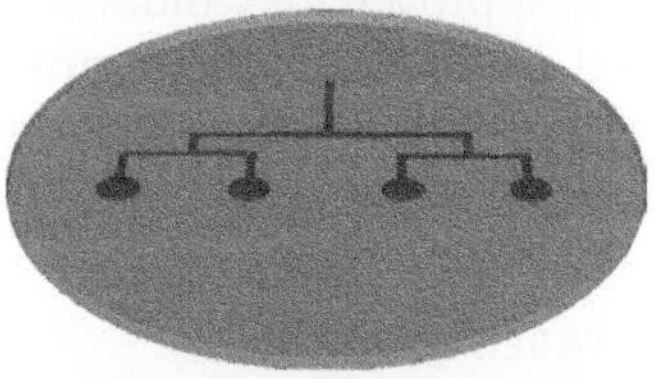
3.5-mm nodule	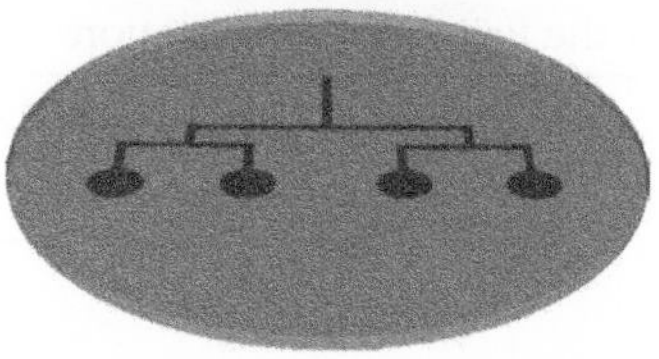	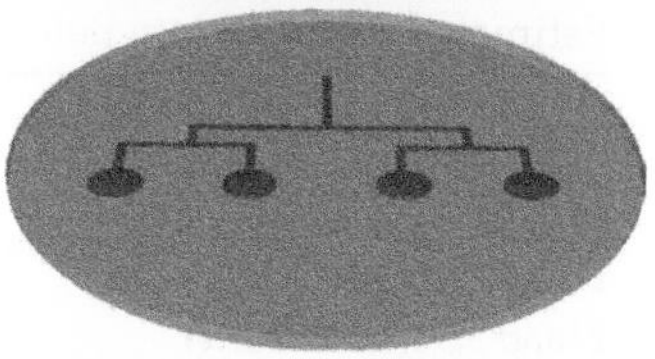

TABLE 18.5
Errors of the Growth Rate Estimated Before and After the Proposed Registration

	Set 1: Simulates No-Growth Rate		
	Before (%)	**After (%)**	**Ground Truth (%)**
Thick Phantom	13.579	0.001	0
Thin Phantom	27.251	0.003	0

lung nodules from CT scans at end-expiration and end-inspiration CT scans. We used the mimic of the end-expiration CT scan as a reference image to register the mimic of the end-inspiration CT scan. Tables 18.5 and 18.6 demonstrate the estimated growth rate before and after the proposed registration. The maximum error in the estimated growth rate after the registration is only 3%, thus highlighting the high registration accuracy of our approach.

18.3.2 Validation of the Proposed Registration on In Vivo Data

Our approach for measuring the growth rate of detected lung nodules was also validated on four control subjects. Each subject had multiple nodules that had been detected by a radiologist as shown in Table 18.7. Also, Table 18.7 visualizes the detected lung nodules in 3D at end-expiration BH and end-inspiration BH CT scans. Table 18.8 illustrates the registration results of the proposed approach. We used the end-expiration BH CT scan as a reference image to register the end-inspiration BH CT scan. The checkerboard visualization in the last column of Table 18.8 demonstrates the quality of registration with the proposed approach. Table 18.9 shows the estimated growth rate before and after the proposed registration. The maximum error in the estimated growth rate after the registration is only 0.072%, thus highlighting the high registration accuracy of our approach. Note that our nodule segmentation results before and after the application of the proposed registration was validated by five radiologists (Dr. R. Falk, Dr. M. Abo El-Ghar, and three junior radiologists at the Department of Radiology at Jewish Hospital, Louisville, KY).

18.4 Concluding Remarks

A new approach for validating the accurate registration of 3D spiral LDCT images is introduced using elastic phantoms and in vivo data. This framework can be used to validate any approach for monitoring the growth rate of detected lung nodules. In this chapter, we validated our approach for monitoring the detected lung nodules, which combines an

TABLE 18.6
Estimated Growth Rate Before and After the Proposed Registration

	Set 2: Simulate True Growth Rate		
	Before (%)	**After (%)**	**Ground Truth (%)**
2- and 3-mm diameter	149.758	127.514	125
2- and 3.5-mm diameter	271.359	209.395	206.25

TABLE 18.7

(See color insert.) 3D Visualization of the Detected Lung Nodules in End-Expiration BH and End-Inspiration BH CT Scans

	Benign Cases		Malignant Cases	
	Subject 1	**Subject 2**	**Subject 3**	**Subject 4**
End-expiration BHs	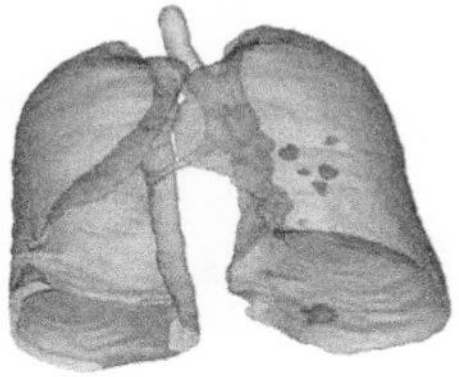	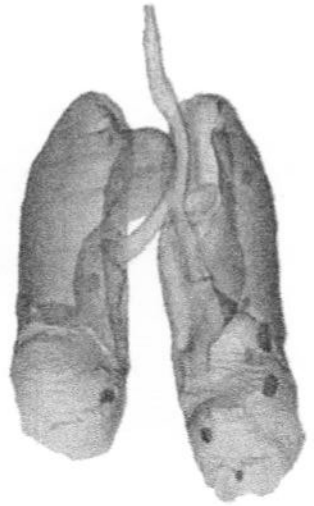	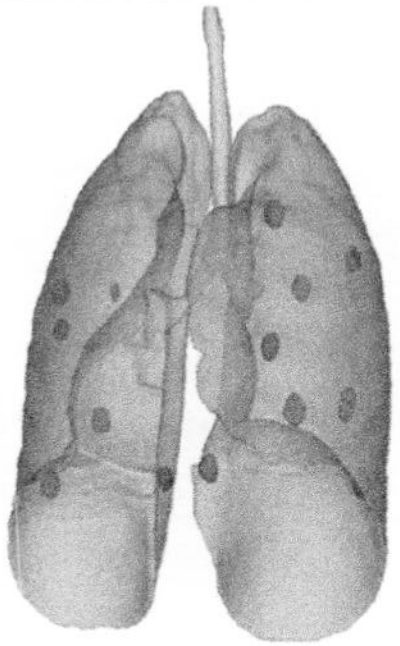	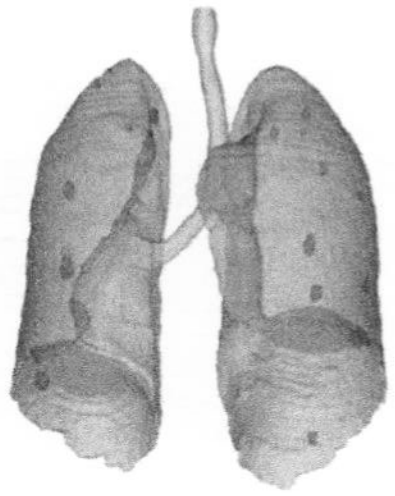
End-inspiration BHs	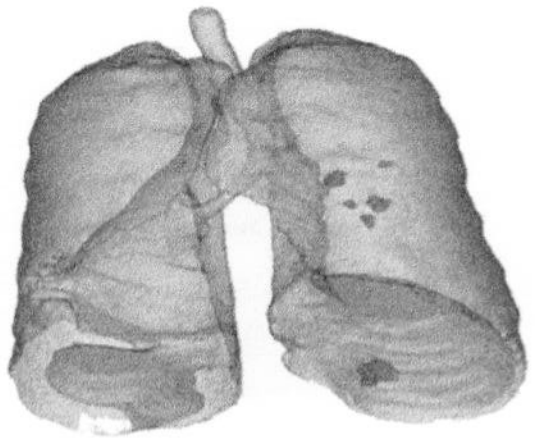	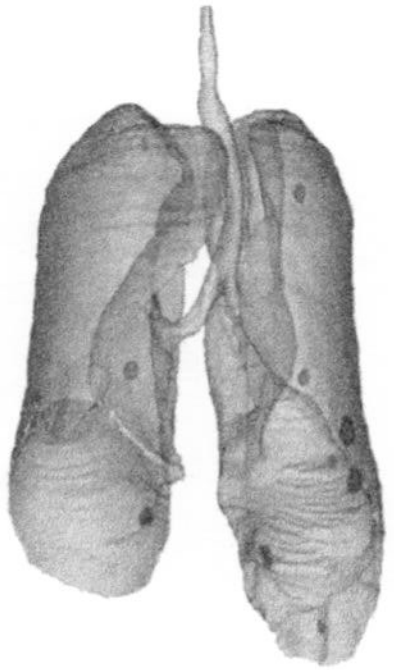	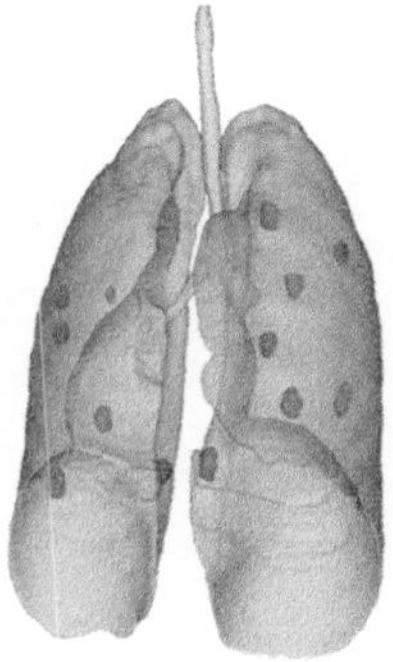	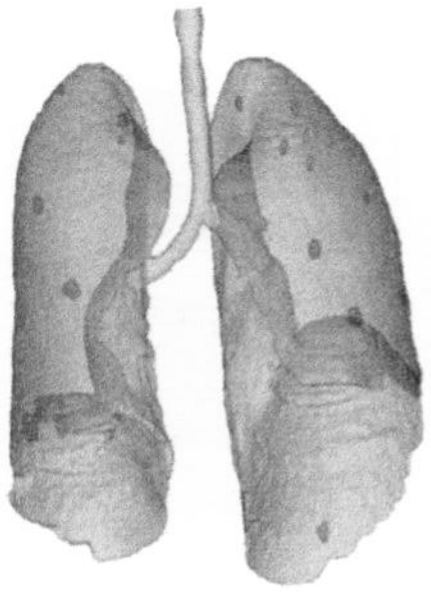

TABLE 18.8

(See color insert.) 3D Illustration of the Registration Results

		End-Expiration BH (Reference)	End-Inspiration BH (Target)	Registration Results	Checkerboard Visualization
Benign cases	Subject 1	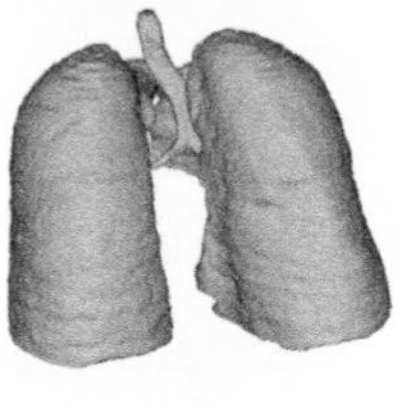	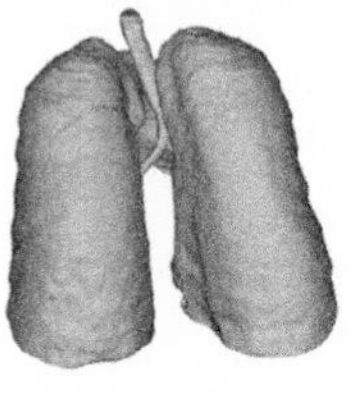	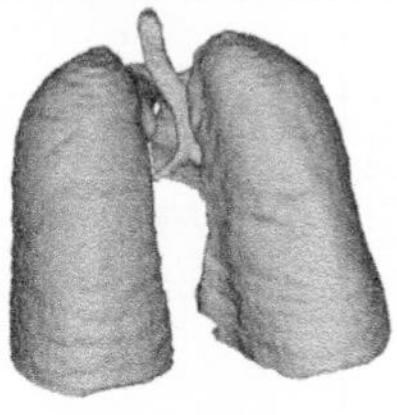	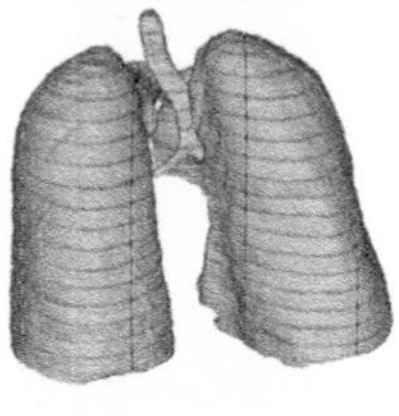
	Subject 2	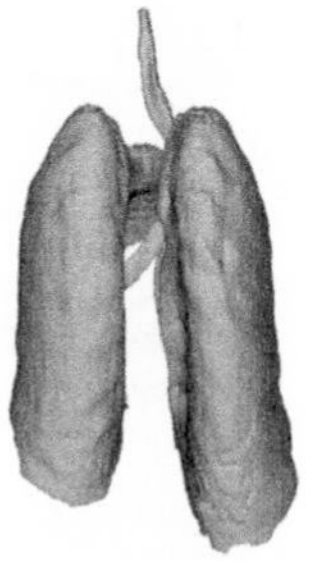	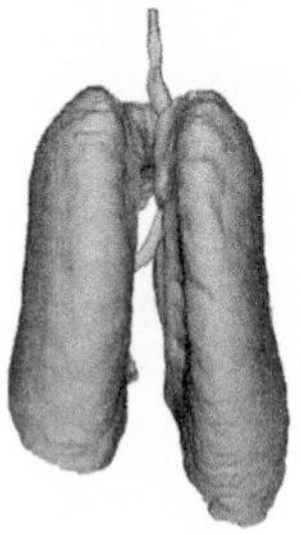	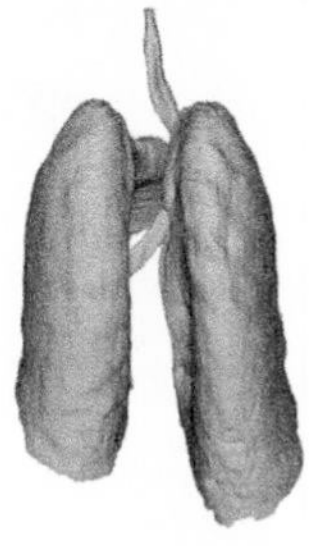	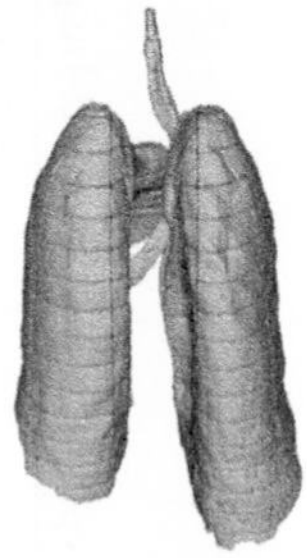
Malignant cases	Subject 3	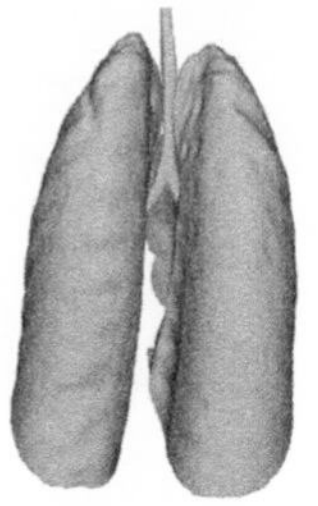	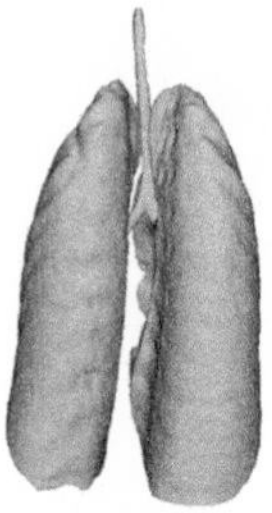	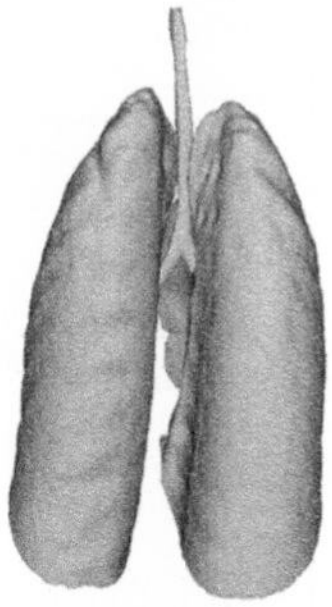	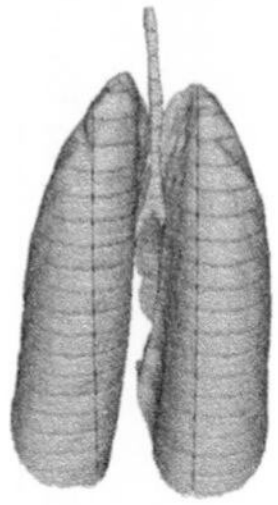
	Subject 4	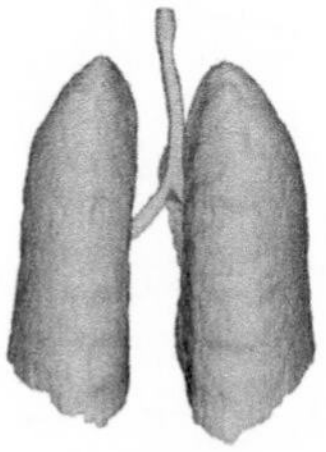	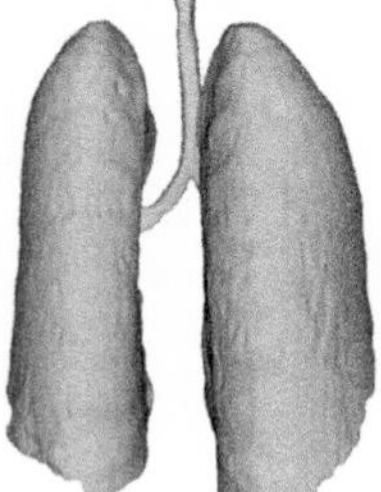	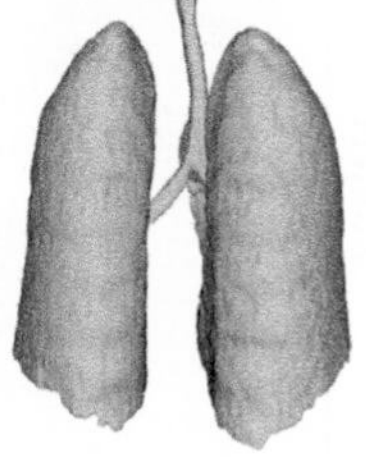	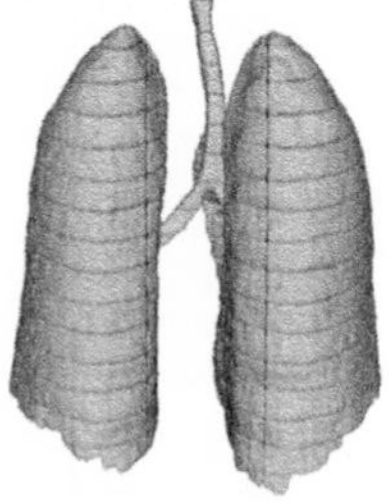

initial global affine alignment of one scan (a target) to another scan (a prototype) using the learned prior appearance model and a subsequent local alignment that accounts for more intricate continuous deformations. Validation results on simulated phantoms and in vivo data showed that the proposed registration could lead to accurate identification of temporal development of detected pulmonary nodules.

References

[1] *American Cancer Society: Cancer Facts and Figures*, 2006.

[2] Libby, D. M., Smith, J. P., Altorki, N. K., Pasmantier, M. W., et al. Managing the small pulmonary nodule discovered by CT. *Chest* 2004, 125, 1522–1530.

[3] Reeves, A. P. Measurement methods for small pulmonary nodules. *Radiology* 2008, 246, 333–334.

[4] Hasegawa, M., Sone, S., Takashima, S., Li, F., et al. Growth rate of small lung cancers detected on mass CT screening. *Br. J. Radiol.* 2000, 73, 1252–1259.

[5] Jaffe, C. C. Measures of response: RECIST, WHO, and new alternatives. *J. Clin. Oncol.* 2006, 24, 3245–3251.

[6] Giger, M. L., Bae, K. T., MacMahon, H. Computerized detection of pulmonary nodules in computed tomography images. *Invest. Radiol.* 1994, 29, 459–465.

[7] Toshioka, S., Kanazawa, K., Niki, N., Satoh, H., et al. Computer aided diagnosis system for lung cancer based on helical CT images. *Int. Soc. Opt. Eng.* 1997, 3034, 975–984.

[8] McNitt-Gray, M. F., Hart, E. M., Wyckoff, N., Sayre, J. W., et al. A pattern classification approach to cha*racterizing solitary* pulmonary nodules imaged on high resolution CT: Preliminary results. *Med. Phys.* 1999, 26, 880–888.

[9] Zhao, B., Yankelevitz, D. F., Reeves, A. P., Henschke, C. I. Two-dimensional multi-criterion segmentation of pulmonary nodules on helical CT images. *Med. Phys.* 1999, 26, 889–895.

[10] Yankelevitz, D. F., Gupta, R., Zhao, B., Henschke, C. I. Small pulmonary nodules: Evaluation with repeat CT—Preliminary experience. *Radiology* 1999, 212, 561–566.

[11] Yankelevitz, D. F., Reeves, A. P., Kostis, W. J., Zhao, B., et al. Small pulmonary nodules: Volumetrically determined growth rates based on CT evaluation. *Radiology* 2000, 217, 251–256.

[12] Kawata,Y., Niki, N., Ohmatsu, H., Eguchi, K., et al. Shape analysis of pulmonary nodules based on thin section CT images. *Int. Soc. Opt. Eng. (Image Process. Med. Imaging)* 1997, 3034, 964–974.

[13] Kostis, W. J., Yankelevitz, D. F., Reeves, A. P., Fluture, S. C., et al. Small pulmonary nodules: Reproducibility of three-dimensional volumetric measurement and estimation of time to follow-up CT. *Radiology* 2004, 231, 446–452.

[14] Reeves, A., Chan, A., Yankelevitz, D., Henschke, C., et al. On Measuring the change in size of pulmonary nodules. *IEEE Trans. Med. Imaging* 2006, 25, 435–449.

[15] Kawata,Y., Niki, N., Omatsu, H., Kusumoto, M., et al. Tracking interval changes of pulmonary nodules using a sequence of three-dimensional thoracic images. *Proc. Int. Soc. Opt. Eng. (Image Process. Med. Imaging)* 2000, 3979, 86–96.

[16] Kawata,Y., Niki, N., Omatsu, H., Kusumoto, M., et al. Analysis of evolving processes in pulmonary nodules using a sequence of three-dimensional thoracic images. *Int. Soc. Opt. Eng. (Image Process. Med. Imaging)* 2001, 4322, 1890–1901.

[17] Zheng, Y., Steiner, K., Bauer, T., Yu, J., et al. Lung nodule growth analysis from 3-D CT data with a coupled segmentation and registration framework. *IEEE Conf. Comput. Vis.* 2009, 1–8.

[18] Jirapatnakul, A. C., Reeves, A. P., Biancardi, A. M., Yankelevitz, D. F., et al. Semi-automated measurement of pulmonary nodule growth without explicit segmentation. *IEEE Int. Symp. BioMed. Imaging (ISBI09)*, 2009, 855–858.

[19] Wormanns, D., Kohl, G., Klotz, E., Marheine, A., et al. Volumetric measurements of pulmonary nodules at multi-row detector CT: In vivo reproducibility. *Eur. Radiol.* 2004,14, 86–92.

[20] Revel, M., Lefort, C., Bissery, A., Bienvenu, M., et al. Pulmonary nodules: Preliminary experience with three-dimensional evaluation. *Radiology* 2004, 231, 459–466.

[21] Winer-Muram, H. T., Jennings, S. G.,Tarver, R. D., Aisen, A. M., et al. Volumetric growth rate of stage I lung cancer prior to treatment: Serial CT scanning. *Radiology* 2002, 223, 798–805.

[22] Jennings, S. G., Winer-Muram, H. T., Tann, M., Ying, J., et al. Distribution of stage I lung cancer growth rates determined with serial volumetric CT measurements. *Radiology* 2006, 241, 554–563.

[23] Marchianò, A., Calabrò, E., Civelli, E., Tolla, G. D., et al. Pulmonary nodules: Volume repeatability at multidetector CT lung cancer screening. *Radiology* 2009, 251, 919–925.
[24] Goo, J., Tongdee, T., Tongdee, R., Yeo, K., et al. Volumetric measurement of synthetic lung nodules with multi-detector row CT: Effect of various image reconstruction parameters and segmentation thresholds on measurement accuracy. *Radiology* 2005, 235, 850–856.
[25] Ko, J., Rusinek, H., Jacobs, E., Babb, J., et al. Small pulmonary nodules: Volume measurement at chest CT-phantom study. *Radiology* 2003, 228, 864–870.
[26] Jiang, H., Kelly, K. Theoretical prediction of lung nodule measurement accuracy under different acquisition and reconstruction conditions. *Int. Soc. Opt. Eng. (Med. Imaging Physiol. Funct. Struct. Med. Images)* 2004, 5369, 406–412.
[27] Gavrielides, M. A., Kinnard, L. M., Myers, K. J., Petrick, N. Noncalcified lung nodules: Volumetric assessment with thoracic CT. *Radiology* 2009, 251, 26–37.
[28] El-Baz, A., Gimel'farb, G. EM based approximation of empirical distributions with linear combinations of discrete Gaussians. *Proc. IEEE Int. Conf. Image Process. (ICIP'07)*, San Antonio, Texas, USA, September 16–19, 2007, IV, 373–376.
[29] Sethian, J. Fast marching level set method for monotonically advancing fronts. *Proc. Natl. Acad. Sci. U.S.A.* 1996, 93, 1591–1595.

19

Three-Dimensional Shape Analysis Using Spherical Harmonics for Early Assessment of Detected Lung Nodules

Ayman El-Baz, Matthew Nitzken, Georgy Gimel'farb, Eric Van Bogaert, Robert Falk, Mohamed Abo El-Ghar, and Jasjit Suri

CONTENTS

19.1 Introduction

Pulmonary nodules are the most common manifestation of lung cancer, which is the principal cause of cancer-related deaths [1]. Fast and accurate classification of the nodules is of major importance for medical computer-aided diagnostic (CAD) systems. A nodule is an approximately spherical volume of higher-density tissue visible in an x-ray lung image. Large malignant nodules (generally defined as greater than 1 cm in diameter) are easily detected with traditional imaging equipment and then diagnosed by needle biopsy or bronchoscopy. However, diagnostic options for small malignant nodules are limited due to difficulties in their accessibility, especially if they are located deep in the tissue or away from the large airways. Therefore, additional imaging and CAD techniques are needed. The popular direction of research in detecting small cancerous nodules is to analyze their growth rate over time. This chapter introduces a new approach to characterize the detected nodules based on their shape.

A great deal of work has been published regarding the usefulness of morphological features for discriminating malignant from benign pulmonary nodules on computed tomography (CT) and to a lesser extent, chest radiographs. Several studies have shown a correlation between different nodule shape characteristics and underlying pathology. For example, Furuya et al. [2] analyzed the margin characteristics of 193 pulmonary nodules on high-resolution CT and subjectively classified them as one of several types, including round, lobulated, densely spiculated, ragged, and halo. They found a high level of malignancy among the lobulated (82%), spiculated (97%), ragged (93%), and halo nodules (100%), while 66% of the round nodules proved to be benign.

Automatically extracted features have also been shown to correlate with underlying malignancy. Kawata et al. [3,4] quantified the surface curvature and degree of surrounding radiating pattern in biopsy-proven benign and malignant nodules and compared the resulting feature maps. Their results showed good separation of the feature maps between the two categories. Their further work [5] extended the curvature analysis method to include internal nodule features, and using this method, which is described in more detail below, they attained similar results. Similarly, fractal analysis has been used to quantify the nodule margin characteristics of benign and malignant nodules. Kido et al. [6] used two- (2D) and three-dimensional (3D) fractal dimensions to analyze the lung–nodule interface in a series of 117 peripheral pulmonary nodules with various underlying pathology including benign hamartomas, tuberculomas, and pneumonias as well as malignant diagnoses including bronchogenic carcinomas. They noted statistically significant differences between the 2D fractal dimensions of hamartomas and all other nodules, as well as differences between the 3D fractal dimensions of pneumonias, tuberculomas, and bronchogenic carcinomas. Although none of these studies directly assessed the accuracy of their methods in predicting a diagnosis, they support the notion that nodule shape can potentially be used by automated systems to distinguish benign from malignant nodules.

Several groups have designed CAD systems with the goal of predicting a diagnosis based on features extracted from CT or chest radiographs. In general, they share common schema, first extracting features from the images, then designing and using an automatic classifier to categorize nodules based on these features, and lastly evaluating the performance of the system with receiver operating characteristics (ROC) analysis. The CAD systems differ in the specific extracted features and the type of classifier used, with linear discriminant classifiers (LDCs) and neural networks (NN) being the most common. First, those systems using LDCs will be discussed followed by NN-based systems and other types of classifiers.

Kawata and colleagues [7] designed a CT-based CAD system that classified pulmonary nodules based on a combination of curvature index and the relationship of the nodules to their surrounding features. The curvature index of a nodule is calculated from a combination of shape index, which describes the surface type (i.e., ridge, saddle, pit, etc.), and curvedness, which describes the degree of curvature. The area surrounding the nodules was assessed for degree of vascular convergence and pleural retraction using vector field analysis. Using an LDC based on these features to evaluate a series of 248 nodules (179 malignant and 69 benign), they found the combination of curvature-based and surrounding features to be most accurate (area under ROC curve (A_z = 0.94) followed by curvature-based (A_z = 0.88) and surround characteristics (A_z = 0.69) alone. Mori et al. [8] also designed a CAD system using curvedness index in combination dynamic contrast-enhanced CT to evaluate temporal change as a possible discriminating feature of benign and malignant nodules. Shape index, curvedness values, and attenuation were calculated at 0, 2, and 4 min after contrast administration, and using these values, a score was generated by an LDC. Attenuation had an A_z value of 0.69 at 2 min postcontrast, the highest of the three time points. Curvedness yielded a maximum A_z of 0.83 at 2 min, and shape index had an

A_z value of 0.90 at 0 and 2 min. The combination of all three features had A_z value of 1.00 at 4 min.

The CAD system developed by McNitt-Gray et al. [9] used a pattern classification approach to determine the malignancy of pulmonary nodules on high-resolution CT (HRCT) in a series of 31 cases (17 malignant and 14 benign). They identified solitary nodules using a semiautomated contouring technique and extracted quantitative measures of the resulting contour related to shape, size, attenuation, distribution of attenuation, and texture. Using a stepwise discriminant analysis, they selected features best able to predict malignancy and used these to design an LDC to characterize the nodules. The selected features predicted malignancy with an accuracy of 90.3% (28/31) cases; however, no A_z value was reported.

Shah et al. [10] designed a CAD system that extracted features from two separate contours, one including only the solid portion of the nodule and one including any ground-glass components. For each contour, 75 features were calculated to measured nodule attenuation, shape, and texture. These features were then input into a feature selection step and four different classifiers to determine if the diagnosis could be predicted from the feature vector. Training and testing were conducted using both resubstitution and leave-one-out methods. With leave-one-out testing methodology the classifiers resulted with A_z ranging from 0.68 to 0.92. When evaluating with resubstitution, A_z ranged from 0.93 to 1.00.

Other LDC-based CAD systems include those developed by Way et al. [11]. They designed a system based on morphological and texture features of pulmonary nodules on CT images using a series of 96 lung nodules, with 44 biopsy- or PET scan–proven malignant nodules and 52 nodules that proved to be benign on biopsy or follow-up CT. The nodules were segmented using 3D active contours guided by a combination of 2D and 3D energies. Next, they extracted several morphological and texture-based features from the segmented nodules. Morphological features included volume, surface area, perimeter, maximum diameter, and maximum and minimum CT value inside the nodule. Using a stepwise method, they selected the most predictive features for use in an LDC. The classifier was trained and tested using a leave-one-out method, and the system achieved A_z of 0.83. More recently, the same group [12] designed a system using the morphological features described above in combination with new measurements of surface characteristics that quantified the smoothness and shape irregularity of the nodule. They calculated ROC statistics for LDCs designed with and without the new surface features and found a significant ($p \leq 0.05$) improvement in performance, with the A_z increasing from 0.821 to 0.857.

One of the early NN-based CAD systems was developed by Gurney and Swensen [13]. They compared two systems, one using a NN-based classifier and one using a Bayesian classifier. Both systems used a combination of subjectively evaluated clinical and radiologic characteristics including border smoothness, spiculation, and lobulation. The Bayesian system showed a significantly ($p \leq 0.05$) higher level of performance ($A_z = 0.894$) than the NN-based system ($A_z = 0.871$). Another NN-based system using subjectively extracted features was developed by Matsuki et al. [14]. Radiologic features included shape-based parameters such as border definition, spiculation, and concavity as well as other associated features such as blood vessel involvement, lymphadenopathy, and emphysematous changes. From a series of 155 nodules found on HRCT (99 malignant and 56 benign), features were extracted by attending radiologists using subjective rating scales and used to train the NN. The NN alone showed a high level of performance ($A_z = 0.951$)

and significantly increased the radiologists' performance, increasing the A_z value from 0.831 to 0.959.

Other CAD systems have been designed to automatically define and extract features as well as classify nodules. For example, Henschke et al. [15] adapted the S-MODALS NN, originally designed for tactical and strategic reconnaissance, to the task of nodule classification. Features were automatically selected from the example image using an NN clustering technique with operator-defined selection parameters including spatial separation of features and the degrees of similarity and dissimilarity that grouped features in to clusters. The system was tested on a series of 28 biopsy-proven nodules (14 malignant and 14 benign), and all but three benign nodules were correctly classified. Another NN using automatically extracted features was designed by Lo et al. [16] and used a combination of radiographic parameters including vascularity, CT density distribution, and shape indices including aspect ratio, circularity, irregularity, extent, compactness, and convexity. Nodules were segmented using an automatic thresholding method, and the resulting 3D volumes were automatically smoothed and pruned of vasculature. The vascular index was calculated during this smoothing process, and shape indices were calculated from the resulting volume. Using a leave-one-out method, they trained the NN on a series of 48 nodules (24 malignant and 24 benign). The results yielded an A_z value of 0.89, and they found that they most predictive features were vascular index, size, compactness, and difference entropy of the CT density.

Nakamura et al. [17] compared the performance of two separate networks, one trained on subjective features rated by radiologists and the other trained on features automatically extracted from chest radiographs. Both sets included shape-based features including margin irregularity, spiculation, lobulation, and nodule shape as well measures of homogeneity and CT density. The network based on objective features demonstrated the highest level of performance ($A_z = 0.854$) followed by the subjective feature network ($A_z = 0.761$) and the radiologists ($A_z = 0.752$).

Iwano et al. [18] developed a system to automatically classify pulmonary nodules detected on HRCT into different shape categories and compared the performance to radiologists. The nodules were extracted from a series of 102 CT images without prior diagnosis of malignancy and classified into different shape categories based on quantitative measures of aspect ratio, circularity, and second central moment. The results were compared with the subjective classification by the radiologists, and they found that the automated system classified the nodules as accurately as the radiologists. Although no direct attempt at automatic diagnosis was carried out, they concluded that system had the potential to aid radiologists in classifying nodules as malignant or benign based on the correlation between certain shape categories and underlying pathology.

Matsukoa et al. [19] analyzed the differences nodule appearance on HRCT images from emphysematous and nonemphysematous patients based on subjective and quantitative measures of nodule appearance. Using a series of 41 emphysematous patients (21 malignant and 20 benign nodules) and 40 nonemphysematous patients (20 malignant and 20 benign nodules), two radiologists, who were blinded the diagnosis, independently evaluated the appearance of the nodule and classified nodules as being either malignant or benign. The fractal dimensions of the nodule interfaces and circularity of the nodule shape were calculated, and the percentage of the nodule surrounded by emphysema was obtained. In patients with emphysema, there were no significant differences in fractal dimension, circularity, or frequency of lobulation or spiculation between malignant and benign nodules. Of all the nodules in patients with emphysema, 63% were correctly diagnosed. Thirteen benign nodules (65%) were misdiagnosed as malignant in patients with emphysema. Of the nodules in nonemphysematous lungs, 93% were correctly diagnosed. The mean percentage of emphysematous tissue around the nodule was greater for misdiagnosed nodules than for correctly diagnosed nodules ($P < 0.003$), indicating that its presence complicates the diagnosis of pulmonary nodules.

In summary, the aforementioned existing approaches show the following limitations:

- Most of them classify the lung nodules based on extracted 2D features (e.g., round, lobulated, ragged, and halo) and they did not take into account the 3D features of lung nodules.
- Most of them did not provide a quantitative measure that has the ability to describe the shape complexity of detected lung nodules.
- Most of the existing features (e.g., curvature, round) depend on the accuracy of the used nodule segmentation algorithm, which makes it difficult for clinical practitioners to use.

This work aims to address these variations and discrepancies in a way that will make evaluating small lung masses more consistent and allow for a more accurate description of the shape complexity of the detected lung nodules.

19.2 Methods

In this work, we propose a novel shape-based approach for the analysis of lung nodule variability between malignant and benign nodules (see Figure 19.1). In this chapter, we will focus on steps 2 to 5, and the first step is shown in detail in Chapter 1. Segmentation of lung nodules is presented in detail in Chapter 3, but for completeness, this section will briefly describe this algorithm, too.

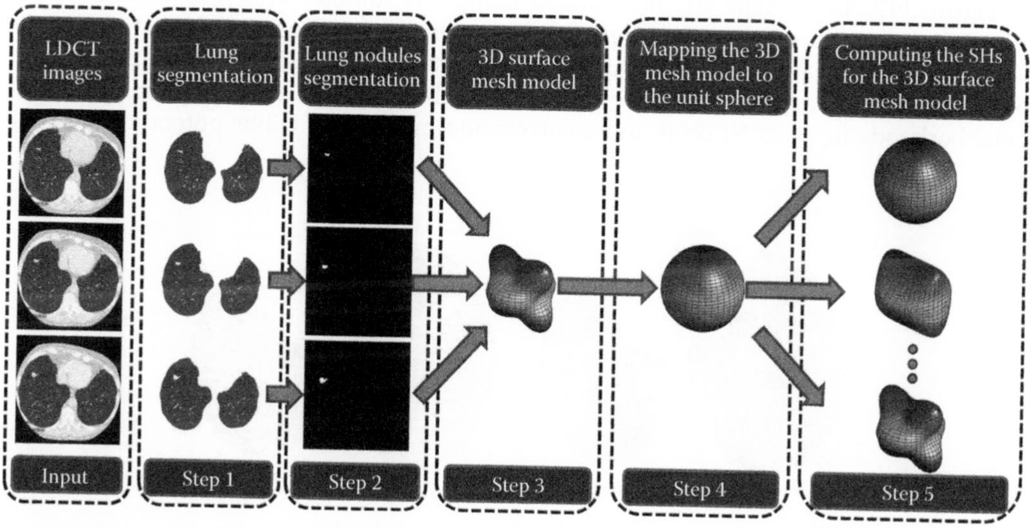

FIGURE 19.1
Proposed shape-based system for early diagnosis of malignant nodules.

19.2.1 Lung Nodules Segmentation

Accurate lung nodule segmentation from a 3D LDCT images is a challenging problem because intensities of the lung nodules and surrounding tissues (e.g., blood vessels, chest) are not clearly distinguishable. To overcome this problem, we use a conventional 3D parametric deformable boundary [13] but control its evolution with two probabilistic visual appearance models, namely, a learned lung nodule appearance prior and a current appearance model of the image to be segmented. The prior is a 3D Markov-Gibbs random field (MGRF) model of the lung nodules intensities, with translation- and rotation-invariant pairwise voxel interaction being learned analytically from training data in accord with ref. [15]. The current appearance is modeled by a mixed marginal distribution of the voxel intensities in both the lung nodule and surrounding tissues. To extract the voxelwise model of the current nodule appearance, the mixture is precisely approximated with a linear combination of discrete Gaussians (LCDGs) [14] and automatically separated into the lung nodule and background LCDG models.

Let (x,y,z) be Cartesian 3D point coordinates. A conventional parametric deformable surface, $\mathbf{B}(\mathbf{P}_1,\ldots\ldots,\mathbf{P}_K)$, specified by K control vertices $\mathbf{P}_k = (x_k,y_k,z_k)$, evolves in the directions that minimize its energy, E, depending on internal, $\zeta_{\text{int}}(\mathbf{B})$, and external, $\zeta_{\text{ext}}(\mathbf{B})$, forces [20]:

$$E = E_{e\text{int}} + E_{\text{ext}} = \int_{\mathbf{B}} \left(\zeta_{\text{int}t}\left(\mathbf{B}\right) + \zeta_{\text{ext}}\left(\mathbf{B}\right)\right) d\mathbf{B} \tag{19.1}$$

As demonstrated in Chapter 3, we used a new type of external energy that depends on both the learned prior and the current (ongoing) appearance model.

Let $\mathbf{Q} = \{0,1,\ldots,Q-1\}$ and $L = \{\text{nl},\text{bg}\}$ be finite sets of image intensities (gray values) and region labels, respectively. Let a finite 3D arithmetic lattice $\mathbf{R} = [(x,y,z) : x = 0,\ldots X; y = 0,\ldots Y; z = 0,\ldots Z]$ support a 3D image $\mathbf{g} : \mathbf{R} \to \mathbf{Q}$ and its region map $\mathbf{m} : \mathbf{R} \to \mathbf{L}$. The label, $m_{x,y,z}$, associates the voxel $g_{x,y,z}$ with the lung nodule or background. To reduce impacts of global contrast and offset deviations of intensities due to different sensors, each input 3D image is normalized by mapping its signal range $[q_{\min},q_{\max}]$ to the maximal range of [0,255] as in Figure 19.2. To consider the normalized images as samples of a prior MGRF model but exclude any image alignment before the segmentation, we use a generic translation- and rotation-invariant MGRF with only voxelwise and central-symmetric pairwise voxel interaction. The latter is specified by a set $\mathbf{N}$ of characteristic central-symmetric voxel neighborhoods $\{\mathbf{n}_\nu : \nu \in \mathbf{N}\}$ on $\mathbf{R}$ and a corresponding set $\mathbf{V}$ of Gibbs potentials, one per

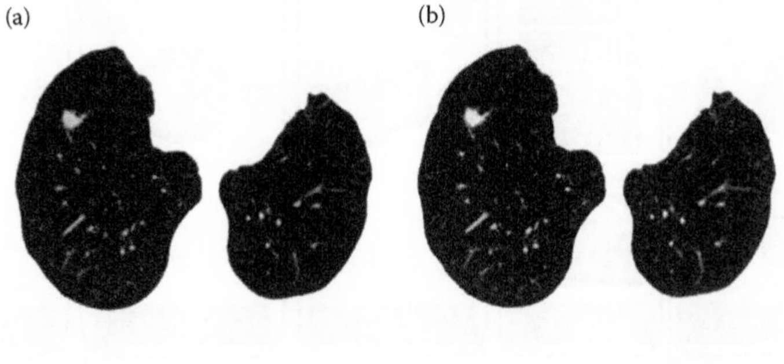

FIGURE 19.2
(a) Initial and (b) normalized LDCT images.

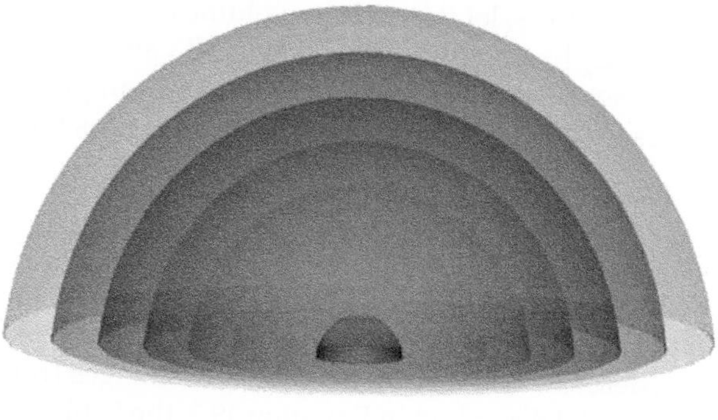

FIGURE 19.3
Eight central-symmetric 3D neighborhoods.

neighborhood. A central-symmetric neighborhood $\mathbf{n}_\nu$ embraces all voxel pairs such that the (x,y,z)- coordinate offsets between any voxel (x,y,z) and its neighbor (x',y',z') belong to an indexed semiopen interval $(d_{\nu,\min}, d_{\nu,\max})$; $\nu \in \mathbf{N} \subset \{1,2,3,\ldots\}$ of the intervoxel distances: $d_{\nu,\min} \le \sqrt{(x-x')^2+(y-y')^2+(z-z')^2} \le d_{\nu,\max}$. Figure 19.3 illustrates the neighborhoods $\mathbf{n}_\nu$ for the uniform distance ranges $(\nu - 0.5, \nu + 0.5)$; $\nu \in \mathbf{N} = \{1,\ldots,8\}$.

19.2.1.1 Learning the Appearance Prior

Let $\mathbf{S} = \{(g_t, m_t) : t = 1,\ldots,T\}$ be a training set of 3D images with known region maps. Let $\mathbf{R}_t = \{(x,y,z) : (x,y,z) \in \mathbf{R} \wedge m_{t;x,y,z} = \text{nl}\}$ denote the part of $\mathbf{R}$ supporting lung nodule in the t-th training pair (g_t, m_t); $t = 1,\ldots,T$. Let $\mathbf{C}_{\nu,t}$ be a family of voxel pairs in $\mathbf{R}_t^2$ with the coordinate offset $(\xi,\eta,\gamma) \in \mathbf{n}_\nu$ in a particular neighborhood. Let $\mathbf{F}_{\text{vx},t}$ and $\mathbf{F}_{\nu,t}$ be an empirical marginal probability distribution of voxel intensities and of intensity co-occurrences, respectively, in the training lung nodule from $\mathbf{g}_t : \mathbf{F}_{\text{vx},t} = f_{\text{vx},t}(q) = \frac{|\mathbf{R}_{t,q}|}{|\mathbf{R}_t|} : q \in \mathbf{Q}$ and $\mathbf{F}_{\nu,t} = f_{\nu,t}(q,q') = \frac{|\mathbf{C}_{\nu,t;q,q'}|}{|\mathbf{C}_{\nu,t}|} : (q,q') \in \mathbf{Q}^2$, where $\mathbf{R}_{t,q} = \{(x,y,z) : (x,y,z) \in \mathbf{R}_t \wedge g_{x,y,z} = q\}$ is a subset of voxels supporting the intensity q and $\mathbf{C}_{\nu,t;q,q'}$ is a subset of the voxel pairs $\mathbf{c}_{\xi,\eta,\gamma}(x,y,z) = \big((x,y,z),(x+\xi, y+\eta, z+\gamma)\big) \in \mathbf{R}_t^2$ supporting the intensity co-occurrence (q,q') in the training lung nodules from g_t. Let $\mathbf{V}_{\text{vx}} = [\mathbf{V}_{\text{vx}}(q) : q \in \mathbf{Q}]$ be a potential function of voxel intensities that describes the voxelwise interaction. Let $\mathbf{V}_\nu = [\mathbf{V}_\nu(q,q') : (q,q') \in \mathbf{Q}^2]$ be a potential function of intensity co-occurrences in the neighboring voxel pairs that describes the pairwise interaction in the neighborhood $\mathbf{n}_\nu$; $\nu \in \mathbf{N}$.

The MGRF prior model of the t-th training pair is specified by the joint Gibbs probability distribution on the sublattice $\mathbf{R}_t$:

$$P_t = \frac{1}{Z_t}\exp |\mathbf{R}_t|(\mathbf{V}_{\text{vx}}^{\mathrm{T}}\mathbf{F}_{\text{vx},t} + \sum_{\nu \in \mathbf{N}} \rho_{\nu,t}\mathbf{V}_{\nu,t}^{\mathrm{T}}\mathbf{F}_{\nu,t}) \tag{19.2}$$

where $\rho_{\nu,t} = \frac{|\mathbf{C}_{\nu,t}|}{|\mathbf{R}_t|}$ is the average cardinality of $\mathbf{n}_\nu$ with respect to $\mathbf{R}_t$.

To simplify the learning process, let the nodules volumes in the training images be similar, so that $|\mathbf{R}_t| \approx R_{\text{nl}}$ and $|\mathbf{C}_{\nu,t}| \approx C_{\nu,\text{nl}}$ for $t = 1,\ldots,T$. Here, R_{nl} and $C_{\nu,\text{nl}}$ are the average cardinalities over the training set **S**. Assuming the independent samples, the joint probability distribution of intensities for all the training nodules images is as follows:

$$P_{\mathrm{S}} = \frac{1}{Z} \exp\ TR_{\text{cortex}}(\mathbf{V}_{\text{vox}}^{\mathrm{T}} \mathbf{F}_{\text{vox}} + \sum_{\nu \in \mathbf{N}} \rho_\nu \mathbf{V}_\nu^{\mathrm{T}} \mathbf{F}_\nu) \tag{19.3}$$

where $\rho_\nu = C_{\nu,\text{nl}}/R_{\text{nl}}$, and the marginal empirical distributions of intensities $\mathbf{F}_{\text{vx,nl}}$ and intensity co-occurrences $\mathbf{F}_{\nu,\text{nl}}$ describe now all the lung nodules images from the training set.

To identify the MGRF model described in Equation 19.3, the Gibbs potentials are approximated analytically (see ref. [21]): for $q \in \mathbf{Q}$

$$V_{\text{vx,nl}}(q) = \log f_{\text{vx,nl}}(q) - \frac{1}{Q} \sum_{q \in \mathbf{Q}} \log f_{\text{vx,nl}}(q) \tag{19.4}$$

and for $(q,q') \in \mathbf{Q}^2$ and all $\nu \in \mathbf{N}$

$$V_{\nu,\text{nl}}(q,q') = \lambda \rho_\nu (f_{\nu,\text{nl}}(q) - f_{\text{vx,nl}}(q) f_{\text{vx,nl}}(q')) \tag{19.5}$$

where the common factor λ is also computed analytically.

19.2.1.2 LCDG Models of Current Appearance

Nonlinear intensity variations in a data acquisition system due to a scanner type and scanning parameters affect the visual appearance of lung nodules in each data set g to be segmented. Thus, in addition to the learned appearance prior, an ongoing lung nodule appearance within a current position of the evolving boundary **B** in **g** is modeled with its marginal intensity distribution. The whole marginal distribution of the voxel intensities within the boundary is considered as a dynamic mixture of two probability models that characterize the lung nodule and its background, respectively. The mixture is partitioned into these two LCDG models by using the EM-based approach detailed in ref. [22].

19.2.1.3 Boundary Evolution under the Two Appearance Models

Let $p_{\text{vx,nl}}(q)$ be the marginal probability of the intensity q in the estimated current LCDG model for the lung nodule. To guide the boundary evolution, we combine in the external energy term of Equation 19.1 both the learned prior and the ongoing nodule appearance model as follows:

$$\zeta_{\text{ext}}(\mathbf{P} = (x,y,z)) = -p_{\text{vx,nl}}(g_{x,y,z}) \pi_{\mathrm{p}}(g_{x,y,z} | \mathbf{S}) \tag{19.6}$$

Here, $\pi_{\mathrm{p}}(q|\mathbf{S})$ is the prior conditional probability of q, given the fixed current intensities in the characteristic central-symmetric neighborhood of **P** for the MGRF prior model of Equation 19.3:

$$\pi_{\mathbf{P}}(g_{x,y,z} | \mathbf{S}) = \frac{\exp\left(E_{\mathbf{P}}(g_{x,y,z} | \mathbf{S})\right)}{\sum_{q \in \mathbf{Q}} \exp\left(E_{\mathbf{P}}(g_{x,y,z} | \mathbf{S})\right)}$$

where $E_p(q|\mathbf{S})$ is the conditional Gibbs energy of pairwise interaction for the voxel **P** provided that an intensity q is assigned to the lung nodule while the other current intensities in all its neighboring voxels over the characteristic neighborhoods $\mathbf{n}_\nu$; $\nu \in \mathbf{N}$ remains fixed:

$$E_P(q|S) = V_{vx,nl}(q) + \sum_{\nu \in N} \sum_{(\xi,\eta,\gamma) \in n_\nu} V_{\nu,nl}(g_{x-\xi,y-\eta,z-\gamma}, q) + V_{\nu,nl}(q, g_{x+\xi,y+\eta,z+\gamma})$$

After changing the total energy $E_\mathbf{B}$ of the 3D region $\mathbf{R}_\mathbf{B} \subset \mathbf{R}$ inside the boundary **B**

$$E_\mathbf{B} = \sum_{\forall \mathbf{P}=(x,y,z) \in \mathbf{R}_\mathbf{B}} E_\mathbf{P}(g_{x,y,z}|\mathbf{S}) \tag{19.7}$$

stops, the evolution terminates.

19.2.2 Spherical Harmonic Shape Analysis

Spectral spherical harmonics (SH) analysis [23] considers 3D surface data as a linear combination of specific basis functions. In our case, the surface of the segmented lung nodule is approximated first by a triangulated 3D mesh (see Figure 19.4) built with an algorithm by Fang and Boas [24]. Second, the lung nodule surface for each subject is mapped for the SH decomposition to the unit sphere. We propose a novel mapping approach, called "attraction–repulsion" that calls for all the mesh nodes to meet two conditions: (i) the unit distance of each node from the lung nodule center as shown in Figure 19.5 and (ii) an equal distance of each node from all of its nearest neighbors as shown in Figure 19.6. To detail our attraction–repulsion algorithm (see its summary in Algorithm 1), let τ denote the iteration index, I be the total number of the mesh nodes (in all the experiments below $I = 4896$ nodes), and $\mathbf{P}_{\tau,i}$ be the Cartesian coordinates of the surface node i at iteration τ; $i = 1,\ldots,I$. Let J be the number of the neighbors for a mesh node (see, e.g., Figure 19.6) and $d_{\tau,ij}$ denote the Euclidean distance between the surface nodes i and j at iteration τ (as shown in Figure 19.6b), where $i = 1,\ldots,I$ and $j = 1,\ldots,J$. Let $\Delta_{\tau,ij} = \mathbf{P}_{\tau,j} - \mathbf{P}_{\tau,i}$ denote the displacement between the nodes j and i at iteration τ . Let $C_{A,1}$, $C_{A,2}$, C_R be the attraction and repulsion constants, respectively, that control the displacement of each surface node.

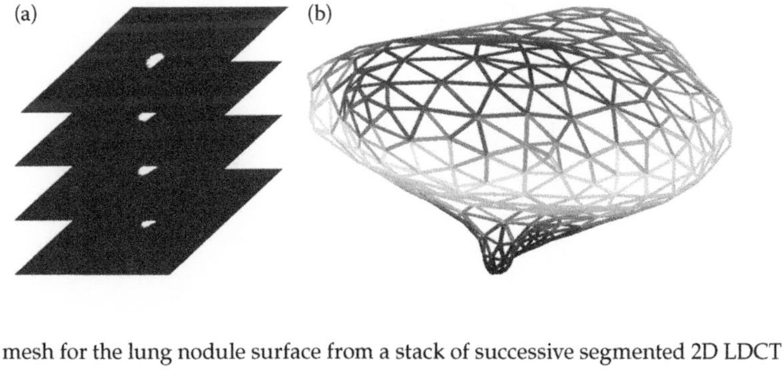

FIGURE 19.4
Generating a 3D mesh for the lung nodule surface from a stack of successive segmented 2D LDCT slices.

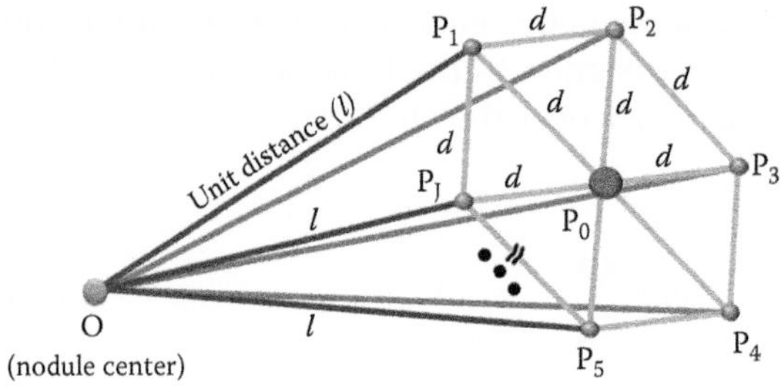

FIGURE 19.5
3D illustration of the unit distance from all surface nodes to the center of the lung nodule.

The starting attraction step of the proposed mapping tends to center each node $\mathbf{P}_i$; $i = 1,\ldots,I$, with respect to its neighbors by adjusting iteratively its location:

$$\mathbf{P}_{\tau,i} = \mathbf{P}_{\tau,i} + C_{A,1} \sum_{j=1;j\neq i}^{J} \Delta_{\tau,ij} d_{\tau,ij}^2 + C_{A,2} \frac{\Delta_{\tau,ij}}{d_{\tau,ij}} \tag{19.8}$$

where the factor $C_{A,2}$ keeps the tightly packed nodes from collision and also pushes the adjusted nodes away from their neighbors if a certain neighbor is much closer than the others.

The subsequent repulsion step inflates the whole mesh by pushing all the nodes outwards to become evenly spaced after their final back-projection onto the unit sphere along the rays from the center of the sphere. To ensure that the nodes that have not been shifted will not collide with the altered node, the location of each node $\mathbf{P}_i$; $i = 1,\ldots,I$, is updated before the back-projection as follows:

$$\mathbf{P}^{\circ}_{\tau+1,i} = \mathbf{P}_{\tau,i} + C_R \sum_{j=1;j\neq i}^{J} \frac{\Delta_{\tau,ij}}{\left|\Delta_{\tau,ij}\right|^2} \tag{19.9}$$

where a repulsion constant C_R controls the displacement of each surface node and establishes a balance between the processing time and accuracy (e.g., a smaller C_R values guarantees that the node faces will not become crossed during the iterations at the expense of

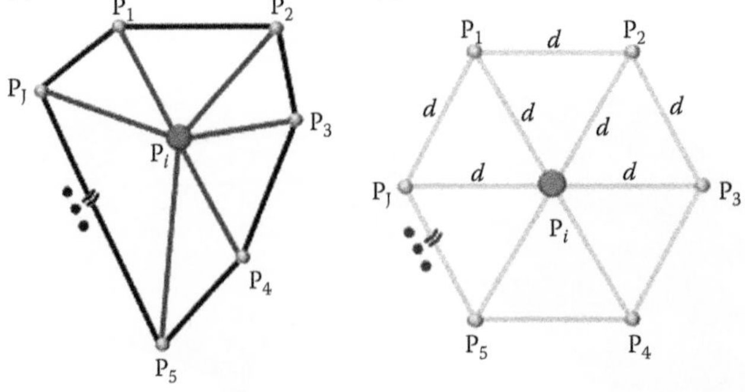

FIGURE 19.6
2D illustration of the neighbor rearrangement: (a) initial versus (b) final equidistant locations in all the directions.

the increased processing time). All the experiments below are obtained with $0.3 \le C_R \le 0.7$. Figure 19.7 demonstrate a step-by-step illustration of the output of attraction–repulsion algorithm at different iterations.

ALGORITHM 1: ATTRACTION–REPULSION ALGORITHM

Initialization

1. Construct the 3D lung nodule mesh (Figure 19.8a).
2. Smooth it by the Laplacian filtering (Figure 19.8b). Application of attraction–repulsion algorithm for node positioning refinement on expanded mesh.
3. Initialize the mapping of the smoothed mesh to the unit sphere.

Repeat

4. For $i = 1 \rightarrow I$
   a. Attraction
      i. Select a node to process.
      ii. Update the node using Equation 19.8.
   b. Repulsion
      i. Update the node using Equation 19.9.
   c. End (all nodes in the mesh are shifted and back-projected onto the unit sphere).

While changes in the node positions occur (Figure 19.8c).

The original lung nodule mapped to the unit sphere with the proposed attraction–repulsion algorithm is approximated by a linear combination of SHs, the lower-order harmonics being sufficient to represent more generic information, while the finer details requiring the higher-order ones. The SHs are generated by the solving an isotropic heat equation for the nodule surface on the unit sphere. Let $S : \mathbf{M} \rightarrow \mathbf{U}$ denote the mapping of a nodule mesh $\mathbf{M}$ to the unit sphere $\mathbf{U}$. Each node $\mathbf{P} = (x,y,z) \in \mathbf{M}$ mapped to the spherical position $\mathbf{u} = S(\mathbf{P})$ is represented by the spherical coordinates $\mathbf{u} = (\sin\theta\cos\varphi, \sin\theta\sin\varphi, \cos\theta)$ where $\theta \in [0,\pi]$ and $\varphi \in [0,\pi]$ are the polar and azimuth angles, respectively. The SH $Y_{\alpha\beta}$ of degree α and order β is defined as [25]:

$$Y_{\alpha\beta} = \begin{cases} c_{\alpha\beta} G_\alpha^{|\beta|}(\cos\theta)\sin(|\beta|\,) & -\alpha \le \beta \le -1 \\ \dfrac{c_{\alpha\beta}}{\sqrt{2}} G_\alpha^{|\beta|}(\cos\theta) & \beta = 0 \\ c_{\alpha\beta} G_\alpha^{|\beta|}(\cos\theta)\cos(|\beta|\,) & 1 \le \beta \le \alpha \end{cases} \tag{19.10}$$

where $c_{\alpha\beta} = \sqrt{\dfrac{2\alpha+1}{2\pi}\dfrac{(\alpha-|\beta|)!}{(\alpha+|\beta|)!}}$ and $G_\alpha^{|\beta|}$ is the associated Legendre polynomial of degree α and order β. For the fixed α, the polynomials G_α^{β} are orthogonal over the range [–1,1]. As shown in ref. [26], the Legendre polynomials are effective in calculating SHs, and this is the main motivation behind their use in this work.

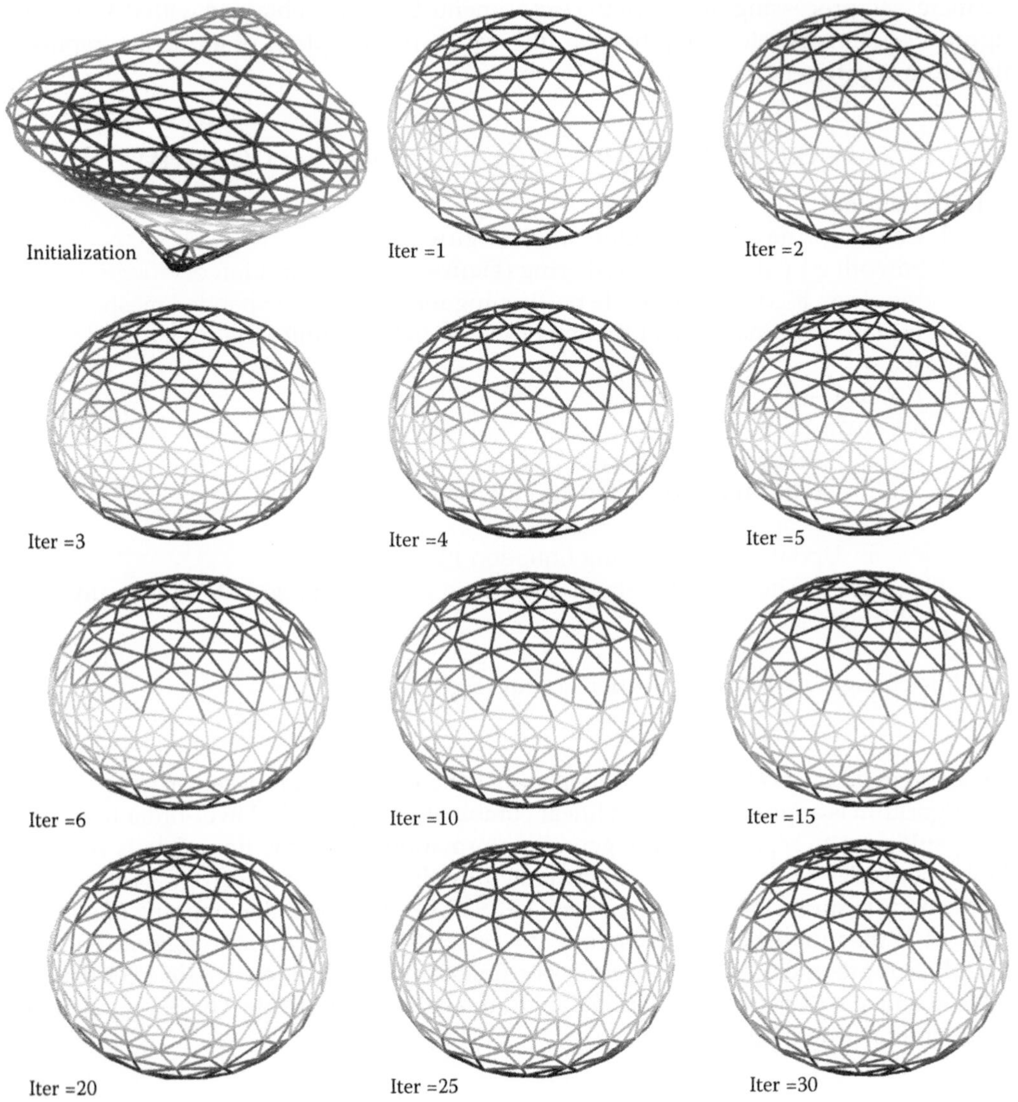

FIGURE 19.7
(See color insert.) A step-by-step illustration of the output of attraction–repulsion algorithm at different iterations.

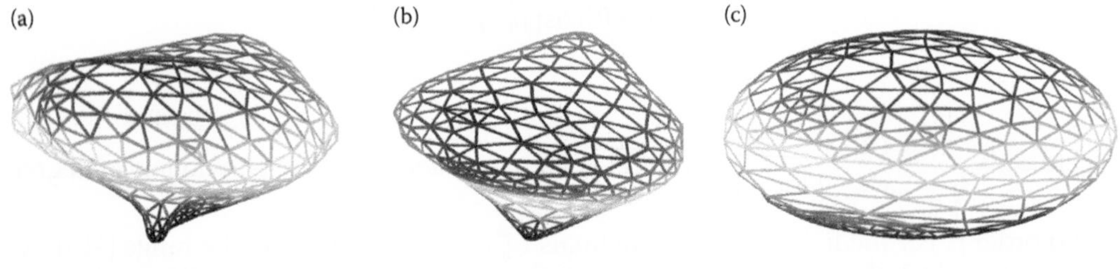

FIGURE 19.8
(a) Lung nodule mesh, (b) its smoothed version, and the (c) attraction–repulsion mapping to the unit sphere.

Finally, the lung nodule is reconstructed from the SHs of Equation 19.10. In the case of the SHs expansion, the standard least square fitting does not model accurately the 3D shape of the lung nodule and can miss some of the shape details that discriminate between the malignant and benign lung nodules. To circumvent this problem, we used the iterative residual fitting by Shen et al. [27] that accurately approximates 3D shape of malignant and benign lung nodules (Figure 19.9). As demonstrated in Figure 19.10, the model

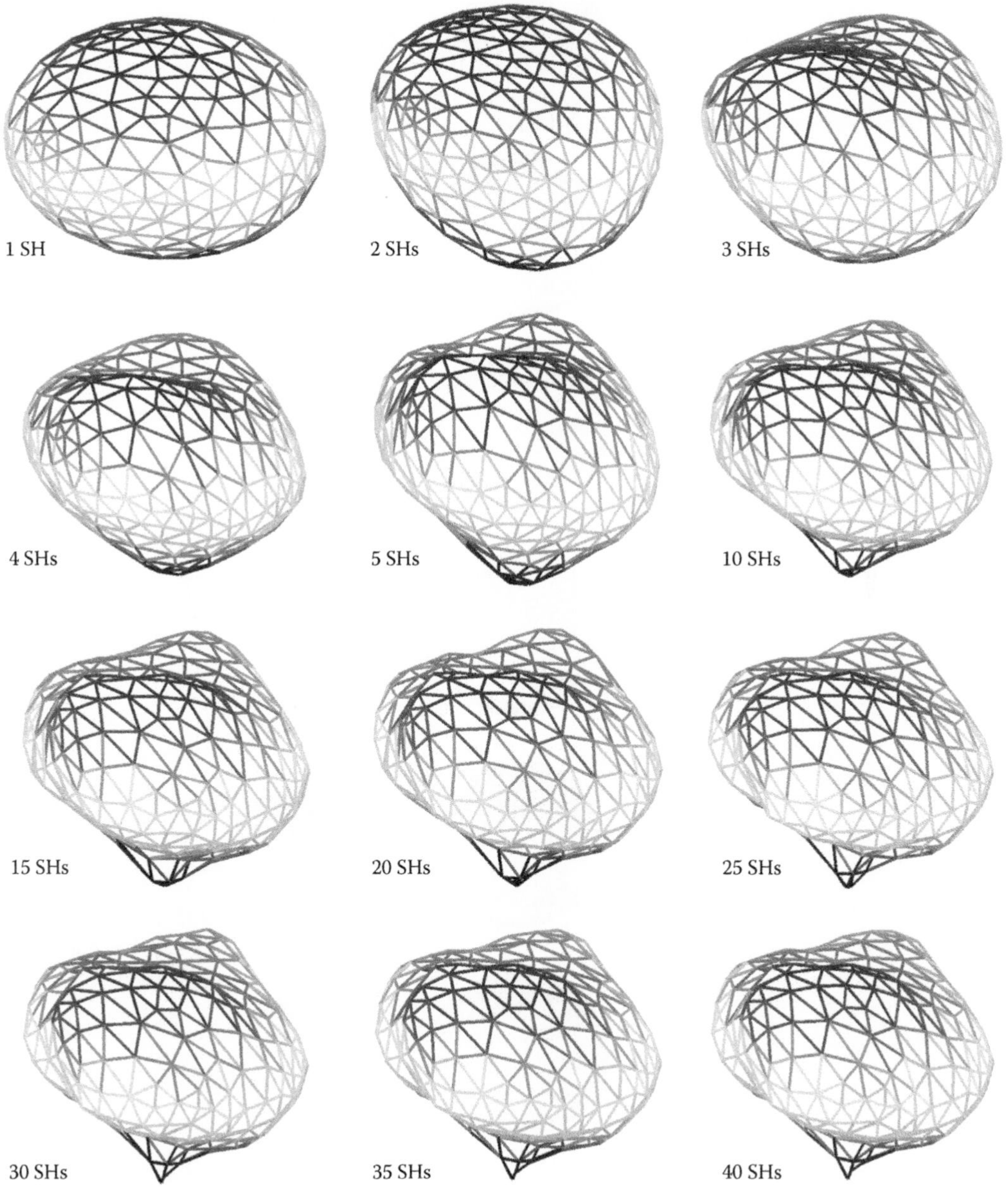

FIGURE 19.9
(See color insert.) A step-by-step lung nodule surface reconstruction using SHs.

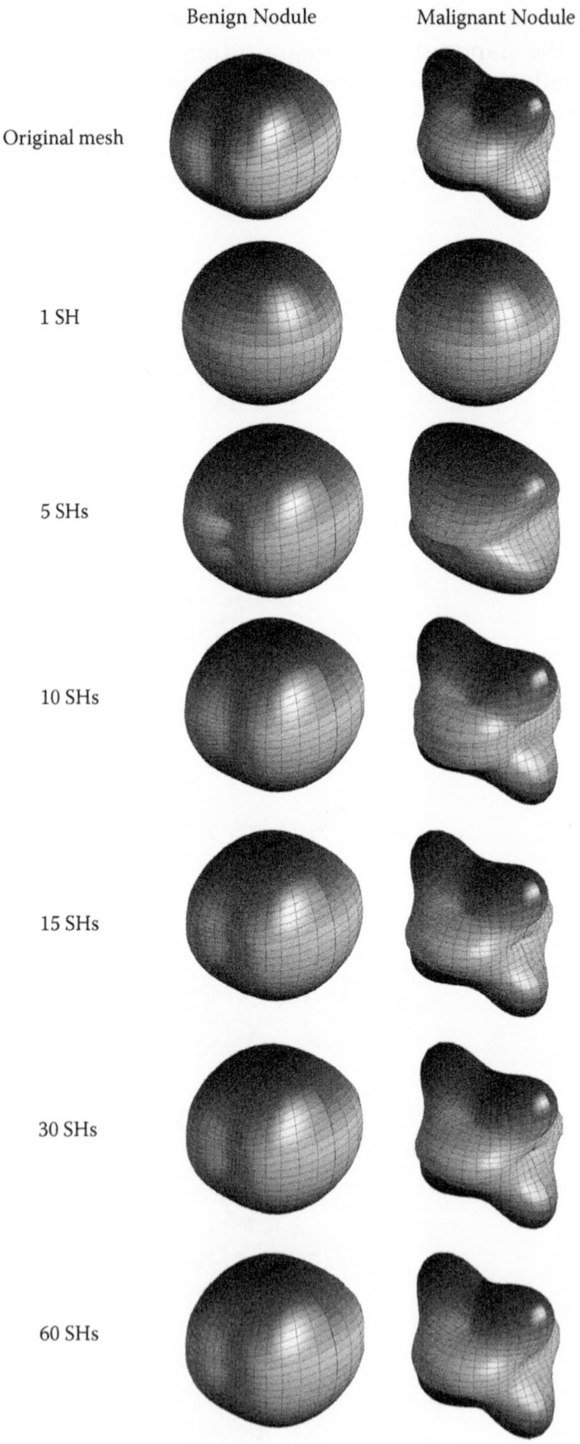

FIGURE 19.10
(See color insert.) Approximation of the 3D shape for malignant and benign lung nodules.

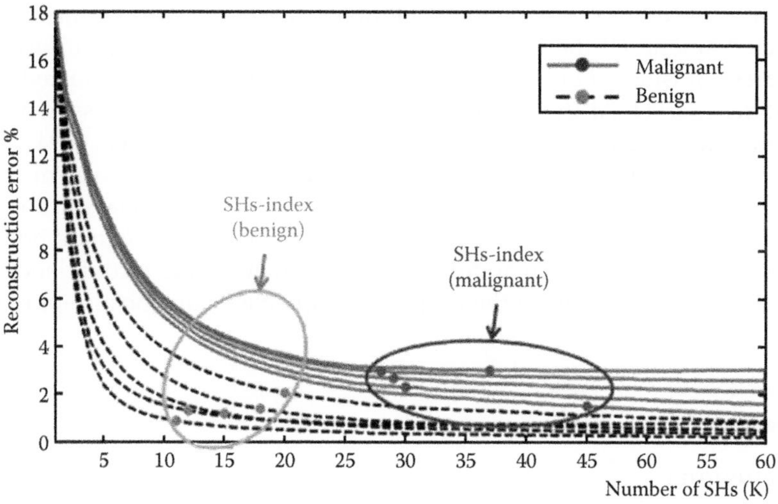

FIGURE 19.11
Estimation of the shape index from the total nodule approximation error for malignant and benign nodules.

accuracy does not significantly change for the benign nodule from the 15 to 60 SHs, while it continues to increase for the malignant nodule.

19.2.3 Quantitative Lung Nodule Shape Analysis

Our main hypothesis is that the shape of malignant nodules is more complicated (e.g., with spiculation) if it is compared with the shape of benign nodules, which is simpler (smoothed shape, as in Figure 19.7), so that more SHs have to be used for accurate approximation of the shape of malignant lung nodule. Therefore, the number of the SHs after which there are no significant changes in the approximations can be used as a new shape index quantifying the shape complexity of the detected lung nodules. Due to the unit sphere mapping, the original mesh for each nodule is inherently aligned with the mesh for the approximate shape, and the sum of the Euclidean distances between the corresponding nodes gives the total error between both the mesh models. As shown in Figure 19.11, the total error curves for the increasing number κ of the SHs can be statistically analyzed to differentiate between the subjects.

19.3 Experimental Results

To justify the proposed methodology of analysis the 3D shape of both malignant and benign nodules, the above-proposed shape analysis framework was pilot-tested on a database of clinical multislice 3D chest LDCT scans of 109 lung nodules (51 malignant and 58 benign). The scanned CT data sets each have $0{:}7 \times 0{:}7 \times 2{:}0\text{-mm}^3$ voxels, with the diameters of the nodules ranging from 3 to 30 mm.

The training subset for classification (10 lung nodules shown in Figure 19.9) was arbitrarily selected among all the 109 lung nodules. The accuracy of classification based on using *K*-nearest classifier of both the training and test subjects was evaluated using χ^2 test at 95% confidence level. At the 95% confidence level, the correctly classified 47 out of 51 malignant nodules (a 92.1% accuracy) and 55 out of 58 control subjects (a 94.8% accuracy). So, the overall accuracy using the proposed 3D shape-based CAD system for 95% confidence level is 94.4% in the first detection of lung nodules. The classification based on traditional growth rate approach [28] over 1 year is 29 out of 51 malignant nodules (56.9% accuracy) and 49 out of 58 benign nodules (84.4% accuracy) at a 95% confidence level, these results highlight the advantage of the proposed shape-based diagnostic approach.

19.4 Conclusions

As demonstrated in this chapter, the preliminary results justify further elaboration of the proposed alternative method for diagnosing malignant lung nodules. Its novelty lies in using the shape of a segmented 3D nodule instead of the more conventional growth rate as a reliable diagnostic feature. The shape is described in terms of a linear combination of SHs.

The proposed nodule shape analysis could lead to more accurate, fast, and clinically useful diagnostics of detected pulmonary nodules without the need for investigating their temporal development on the successive LDCT images of the same subject collected for a relatively long time. The present C++ implementation on the Intel quad processor (3.2 GHz each) with 16-GB memory and 1.5-TB hard drive with RAID technology takes approximately 7 s for processing 30-mm lung nodules and less than 3 s for processing 5-mm lung nodules.

References

1. B. Edwards, E. Ward, B. Kohler, C. Eheman, A. Zauber, R. Anderson, A. Jemal, M. Schymura, I. Lansdorp-Vogelaar, L. Seeff, M. Van Ballegooijen, S. Goede, and L. Ries, "Annual report to the nation on the status of cancer, 1975–2000," *Journal National Cancer Institute*, vol. 95, no. 17, pp. 1276–1299, 2003.
2. K. Furuya, S. Murayama, H. Soeda, J. Murakami, Y. Ichinose, H. Yabuuchi, Y. Katsuda, M. Koga, and K. Masuda, "New classification of small pulmonary nodules by margin characteristics on high-resolution CT," *Acta Radiologica*, 1999, vol. 40, no. 5, pp. 496–504.
3. Y. Kawata, N. Niki, H. Ohmatsu, R. Kakinuma, K. Eguchi, M. Kaneko, and N. Moriyama, "Classification of pulmonary nodules in thin-section CT images based on shape characterization," *Proceedings of the International Conference on Image Processing*, vol. 3, pp. 528–530, 1997.
4. Y. Kawata, N. Niki, H. Ohmatsu, R. Kakinuma, K. Eguchi, M. Kaneko, and N. Moriyama, "Quantitative surface characterization of pulmonary nodules based on thin-section CT images," *IEEE Transactions on Nuclear Science*, vol. 45, no. 4, pp. 2132–2138, 1998.
5. Y. Kawata, M. Kaneko, K. Eguchi, R. Kakinuma, N. Moriyama, N. Niki, and H. Ohmatsu, "Curvature based analysis of pulmonary nodules using thin-section CT images," *Proceedings of the International Conference on Pattern Recognition*, vol. I, pp. 361–363. 1998.

6. S. Kido, K. Kuriyama, M. Higashiyama, T. Kasugai, and C. Kuroda, "Fractal analysis of small peripheral pulmonary nodules in thin-section CT: Evaluation of the lung-nodule interfaces," *Journal of Computer Assisted Tomography*, vol. 26, no. 4, pp. 573–578, 2002.
7. Y. Kawata, N. Niki, H. Ohmatsu, M. Kusumoto, R. Kakinuma, K. Mori, H. Nishiyama, K. Eguchi, M. Kaneko, and N. Moriyama, "Computerized analysis of 3-D pulmonary nodule images in surrounding and internal structure feature spaces," *Proceedings of the International Conference on Image Processing*, vol. 2, pp. 889–892, 2001.
8. K. Mori, N. Niki, T. Kondo, Y. Kamiyama, T. Kodama, Y. Kawada, and N. Moriyama, "Development of a novel computer-aided diagnosis system for automatic discrimination of malignant from benign solitary pulmonary nodules on thin-section dynamic computed tomography," *Journal of computer assisted tomography*, vol. 29, no. 2, pp. 215–222.
9. M. McNitt-Gray, E. Hart, N. Wyckoff, J. Sayre, J. Goldin, and D. Aberle, "A pattern classification approach to characterizing solitary pulmonary nodules imaged on high resolution CT: Preliminary results," *Medical Physics*, vol. 26, no. 6, pp. 880–888, 1999.
10. S. Shah, M. McNitt-Gray, S. Rogers, J. Goldin, R. Suh, J. Sayre, I. Petkovska, H. Kim, and D. Aberle, "Computer-aided diagnosis of the solitary pulmonary nodule," *Academic Radiology*, vol. 12, no. 5, pp. 570–575, 2005.
11. T. Way, L. Hadjiiski, B. Sahiner, H. Chan, P. Cascade, E. Kazerooni, N. Bogot, and C. Zhou, "Computer-aided diagnosis of pulmonary nodules on CT scans: Segmentation and classification using 3D active contours," *Medical Physics*, vol. 33, no. 7, pp. 2323–2337, 2006.
12. T. Way, B. Sahiner, H. Chan, L. Hadjiiski, P. Cascade, A. Chughtai, N. Bogot, and E. Kazerooni, "Computer-aided diagnosis of pulmonary nodules on CT scans: Improvement of classification performance with nodule surface features," *Medical physics*, vol. 36, no. 7, pp. 3086–3098, 2009.
13. W. Gurney and S. Swensen, "Solitary pulmonary nodules: Determining the likelihood of malignancy with neural network analysis," *Radiology*, vol. 196, no. 3, pp. 823–829, 1995.
14. Y. Matsuki, K. Nakamura, H. Watanabe, T. Aoki, H. Nakata, S. Katsuragawa, and K. Doi, "Usefulness of an artificial neural network for differentiating benign from malignant pulmonary nodules on high-resolution CT: Evaluation with receiver operating characteristic analysis," *American Roentgen Ray Society*, vol. 178, no. 3, pp. 657–663, 2002.
15. C. Henschke, D. Yankelevitz, I. Mateescu, D. Brettle, T. Rainey, and F. Weingard, "Neural networks for the analysis of small pulmonary nodules," *Clincal Imaging*, vol. 21, pp. 390–399, 1997.
16. S. Lo, L. Hsu, M. Freedman, Y. Lure, and H. Zhao, "Classification of lung nodules in diagnostic CT: An approach based on 3D vascular features, nodule density distribution, and shape features," *Proceedings of the SPIE, Medical Imaging 2003: Image Processing*, vol. 5032, pp. 183–189, 2003.
17. K. Nakamura, H. Yoshida, R. Engelmann, H. MacMahon, S. Katsuragawa, T. Ishida, K. Ashizawa, and K. Doi, "Computerized analysis of the likelihood of malignancy in solitary pulmonary nodules with use of artificial neural networks," *Radiology*, vol. 214, no. 3, pp. 823–830, 2000.
18. S. Iwano, T. Nakamura, Y. Kamioka, and T. Ishigaki, "Computer-aided diagnosis: A shape classification of pulmonary nodules imaged by high-resolution CT," *Computerized Medical Imaging and Graphics*, vol. 29, no. 7, pp. 565–570, 2005.
19. S. Matsuoka, Y. Kurihara, K. Yagihashi, H. Niimi, and Y. Nakajima, "Peripheral solitary pulmonary nodule: CT findings in patients with pulmonary emphysema," *Radiology*, vol. 235, no. 1, pp. 266–273, 2005.
20. A. El-Baz, G. Gimelfarb, R. Falk, M. Abou El-Ghar, Holland, and T. Shaffer, "A new stochastic framework for accurate lung segmentation," *Proceedings of International Conference on Medical Image Computing and Computer-Assisted Intervention (MICCAI'08)*, New York, September 6–10, 2008, pp. 322–330.
21. M. Kass, A. Witkin, and D. Terzopoulos, "Snakes: Active contour models," *International Journal of Computer Vision*, vol. 1, pp. 321–331, 1987.
22. G. Gimel'farb, *Image Textures and Gibbs Random Fields*, Kluwer Academic, Dordrecht, 1999.

23. A. El-Baz and G. Gimel'farb, "EM based approximation of empirical distributions with linear combinations of discrete Gaussians," *Proceedings of IEEE International Conference on Image Processing (ICIP'07)*, San Antonio, TX, September 16–19, 2007, vol. IV, pp. 373–376.
24. M. K. Chung, K. M. Dalton, L. Shen, , A. C. Evans, and R. J. Davidson, "Weighted Fourier series representation and its application to quantifying the amount of gray matter," *IEEE Transactions on Medical Imaging*, vol. 26, pp. 566–581, 2007.
25. Q. Fang and D. Boas, "Tetrahedral mesh generation from volumetric binary and gray-scale images," *IEEE International Symposium on Biomedical Imaging (ISBI'09).*
26. R. Courant and D. Hilbert, *Methods of Mathematical Physics*, Vol. II. Interscience, New York, 1953.
27. L. Shen and M. K. Chung, "Large-scale modeling of parametric surfaces using spherical harmonics," *Proceedings of the 3rd International Symposiun on 3D Data Processing and Visualization Transmission*, Chapel Hill, NC, June 14–16, 2006, pp. 294–301.
28. A. Reeves, A. Chan, D. Yankelevitz, C. Henschke, B. Kressler, and W. Kostis, "On measuring the change in size of pulmonary nodules," *IEEE Transactions on Medical Imaging*, vol. 25, no. 4, pp. 435449, April 2006.

20

Review on Computer-Aided Detection, Diagnosis, and Characterization of Pulmonary Nodules: A Clinical Perspective

Luca Saba and Jasjit Suri

CONTENTS

"Science is an imaginative adventure of the mind seeking truth in a world of mystery."

Sir Cyril Herman Hinshelwood (1897–1967)
English chemist. Nobel Prize 1956

20.1 Introduction

Lung cancer is the leading cause of cancer death among men and women in the United States, and it is responsible for 1.3 million deaths worldwide annually. Extrathoracic and thoracic malignancies frequently metastasize to the lung parenchyma as pulmonary nodules, and their detection is extremely important in order to plan a correct therapeutical approach. The sensitivity of a chest radiograph is quite low, and this exam may not reveal the cancerous mass; computed tomography (CT) represents one of the most sensitive diagnostic imaging modalities for detecting lung neoplasm and, in particular, lung nodules. The introduction of multidetector-row systems allowed an exquisite anatomical detail that is achieved at the expense of large data volumes (1000 or more images), with the consequence of a massive explosion of data whose interpretation is very time consuming. Computer-aided detection (CAD) systems serve as a useful second opinion when physicians examine patients at lung cancer screening, and CAD will have a major impact on medical imaging and diagnostic radiology in the field of lung cancer in the near future.

20.2 Clinical Setting and Imaging Approach

Nowadays, lung cancer is the leading cause of cancer death among men and women in the United States, and it is responsible for 1.3 million deaths worldwide annually. The overall 5-year survival rate with lung cancer is 14%[1]. However, patients with early-stage disease, who undergo curative resection, have 5-year survival rates of 40% to 70%[2,3]. The most common cause of lung cancer is long-term exposure to tobacco smoke; in fact, the occurrence of lung cancer in nonsmokers accounts for as many as 15% of cases, and it is often attributed to a combination of genetic factors, radon gas, and air pollution, including second-hand smoke[4–11]. Lung cancers are classified according to histological type, and this classification has important implications for clinical management and prognosis of the disease. The vast majority of lung cancers are carcinomas—malignancies that arise from epithelial cells. The two most prevalent histological types of lung carcinoma, categorized by the size and the appearance of the malignant cells seen, are nonsmall-cell lung carcinoma (NSCLC) and small-cell lung carcinoma (SCLC). This distinction is important because the treatment varies; NSCLC is usually treated with surgery, whereas SCLC usually responds better to chemotherapy and radiation.

Extrathoracic and thoracic malignancies frequently metastasize to the lung parenchyma as pulmonary nodules, and their detection is extremely important in order to plan a correct therapeutical approach. The identification of a small pulmonary metastasis is also extremely important; in fact, pulmonary metastasectomy has been an established treatment in selected patients with lung metastases from various solid tumors. Many studies have reported improved survival benefits of pulmonary metastasectomy in selected patients.

In the detection and characterization of pulmonary pathology, it is important to underline that pulmonary nodules are a common (incidental) finding in imaging studies, and many nodules, even if advanced imaging techniques have improved the characterization of the nodules, helping to differentiate from benign to malignant, remain indeterminate and require temporal characterization to confirm stability or invasive assessment for a definitive diagnosis. Classically a "pulmonary nodule" is defined as "round opacity, at least moderately well marginated and no greater than 3 cm in maximum diameter"[12]. A pulmonary nodule can be caused by a variety of malignant or benign disorders[13–16]. CT is more sensitive than standard radiograph in the detection of pulmonary nodules, and with the multidetector-row CT (MDCT) systems, nodules smaller than 1 cm are detected with an increased frequency. As a result, small lesions that would otherwise have been invisible on radiographs can now be detected, and it is reported that 11% of incidental nodules were eventually diagnosed as lung cancer, with the majority being stage I.

Performing a chest radiograph is the first step when a patient reports symptoms that may suggest lung cancer. Although less sensitive and specific, the chest CT radiography often reveals nodules of the chest. It is interesting to understand that usually the small nodules detected on radiography are calcified. Ketai et al.[17] reported that 77% of nodules that are smaller than 7 mm visualized on a chest radiograph are calcified. Very small nodules that are visible on radiographs therefore have a higher probability of representing calcified granulomas.

The detection of a pulmonary nodule on radiography is limited by the number of overlapping structures and low contrast of the nodule on radiography in comparison with CT. Missed nodules on the frontal radiograph include those at the apices and lung bases as well as centrally located lesions[18–20]. Failure to diagnose a nodule can relate to an inadequate or incomplete visual survey or to interpretative failures[21–23]. A systematic approach toward the interpretation of the radiograph improves the detection of abnormalities.

For chest radiography, dual-energy radiography and temporal-subtraction radiography show significant potential for enhanced detection of subtle and often overlooked lung lesions on radiographs[23–25]. Dual-energy chest radiography exploits the difference in the energy-dependent attenuation between bone and soft tissues to produce tissue-selective images. By more clearly depicting calcification, the technique greatly aids in characterizing pulmonary nodules as benign. By reducing anatomic noise from overlying bones, the technique also has improved sensitivity for noncalcified lung nodules.

The sensitivity of a chest radiograph, however, is considered suboptimal. Nowadays CT represents one of the most sensitive diagnostic imaging modalities for detecting lung neoplasm and, in particular, lung nodules.

CT is more sensitive than projectional radiography in the detection of metastatic lung nodules, particularly small nodules[26–30]. When metastatic disease to the lung is discovered, precise quantitative and reproducible analysis is required[30] to better assess disease progression or regression with therapy. There has been no technological advance for imaging of the thorax with as profound impact as MDCT on the way data are visualized, diagnosed, and managed. Fast acquisition times and higher resolution have forever changed imaging of the lung, an organ whose dynamic nature demands rapid acquisition and whose complex anatomy demands isotropic resolution for fine anatomic detail and true three-dimensional (3D) analysis. MDCT allows routinely acquiring data sets with high spatial resolution, detecting a consistent number of nodules and micronodules. It also allows shorter breath holds and therefore fewer breathing and motion artifacts. With MDCT, the chest can be surveyed in one suspended breath hold with high in-plane resolution, narrow collimation, and narrow reconstruction intervals[30]. This technique produces the degree of anatomic precision that is necessary to computerized systems to discriminate accurately between micronodular lung cancers and in normally branching the anatomy of other types of benign lesions that can appear as small nodules. The rapid uptake of MDCT scanners in the clinical marketplace is an indication of their significant technological advance. The uptake of MDCT scanners in the United States increased exponentially and between 1998 and 2004 had a compound annual growth rate of 160%. This dramatic increase is due likely to the increased clinical value provided with a faster, higher resolution scanner.

However, anatomic detail is achieved at the expense of large data volumes[28,29]. The use of thinner sections and overlapping reconstruction intervals improves the longitudinal resolution, but it requires larger data sets (1000 or more images) to be generated[30] with the consequence of a massive explosion of data whose interpretation is very time consuming. Therefore, while the increase in resolution of data and acquisition speeds brings greater interpretative potential and variety of applications capable of being performed with CT, the enormity of the acquired image volume has resulted in significant workflow challenges to the radiologist.

It is interesting to note that this increase in generated data also comes at a time when radiology departments are increasingly resource constrained. In fact, availability of radiologists increased just 3% in 2000, whereas CT procedures increased 19.4% in that same year. Therefore, the demand for alternative image reading techniques emerged to reliably assess the increasing amount of data in a reasonable amount of time. In this context, the detection of pulmonary nodules is one example of a repetitive process performed multiple times during the daily routine of a radiologist.

A significant drawback that a radiologist can suffer may be represented by the well-known "satisfaction-of-search" effect, in which unrelated findings take away the radiologist's attention from the cancer's detection[31]. It has been demonstrated how double reading by two observers improves the detection of nodules (this was demonstrated also in lung and breast cancer on chest radiographs and mammograms, respectively)[32].

Nevertheless, the high cost of interpretation when two readers are employed in double reading, and the high time needed, has motivated the development of CAD[32] as a possible tool that helps radiologists have a "second look" (Figure 20.1). Similarly, several software packages that help radiologists in other organ analyses have been created such as the automated vascular analysis (Figure 20.2).

One of the first works about the CAD system for pulmonary nodule detection was proposed by Bae et al.[33] in 1991, and many other papers have been published since then. The earlier CAD system algorithms for nodule detection were based on two-dimensional morphologic features on each section and/or limited 3D structural information; recent CAD systems have been reported to use 3D algorithms that take advantage of thin section volumetric CT data[34]. Another problem radiologists face in clinical practice is the necessity to diagnose a pulmonary nodule as benign or malignant. Sometimes this kind of decision is not simple, and it has motivated the development of CAD software. This is the second area in which CAD can assist a physician; in fact, only a fraction of the pulmonary nodules are malignant carcinomas from lung cancer or metastasis from cancer in other organs. CAD

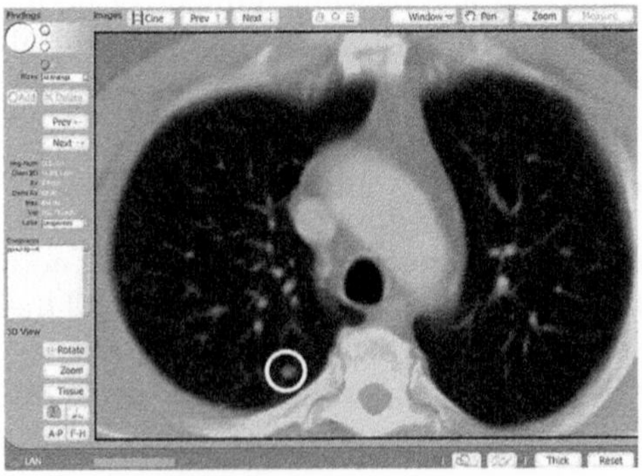

FIGURE 20.1
CT axial image demonstrating a pulmonary nodule (white circle).

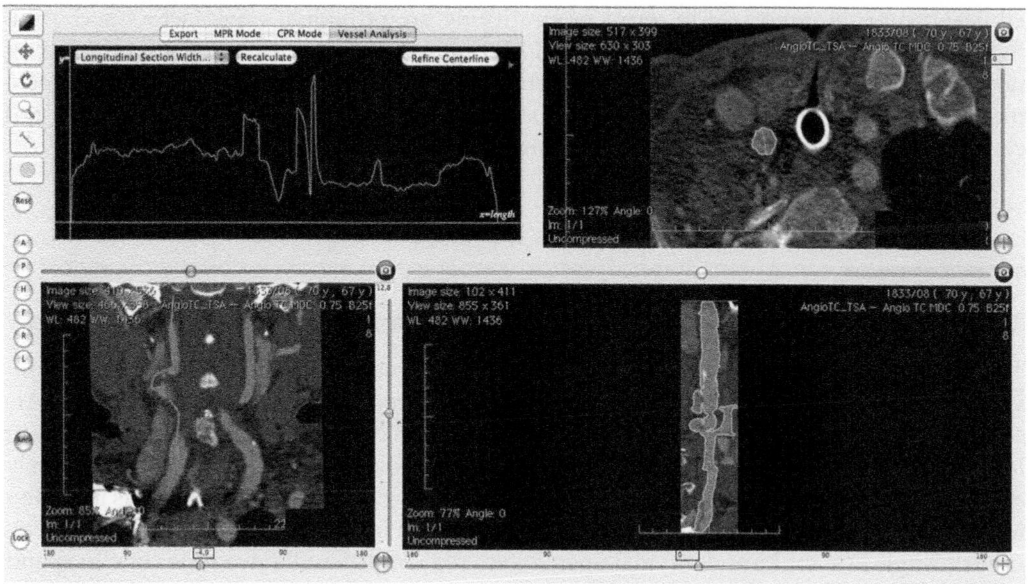

FIGURE 20.2
Vascular analysis software—Osirix™.

has the potential to improve a radiologist's diagnostic accuracy in distinguishing small benign nodules from malignant nodules.

20.3 Management of the Pulmonary Nodule

The management of a patient with a pulmonary nodule requires a case-by-case evaluation of both radiological features and clinical factors. Consideration of patient age, smoking history, and history of malignancy is particularly important. The availability of prior imaging studies is extremely useful for solid nodules because stability over time may lead to consideration of a conservative approach given the lower likelihood of malignancy. Larger nodules greater than 7 mm are amenable to noninvasive and invasive characterization. For solid nodules, lack of enhancement and low metabolic activity are reassuring for a benign lesion, although low-grade neoplasia, such as carcinoid, remains a consideration. Subsolid nodules are unsuitable for nodule enhancement studies and have been associated with low metabolic activity on positron emission tomography (PET). Alternatively, positive nodule enhancement studies and PET scans should also be interpreted in the clinical context because of the overlap with inflammatory conditions. Biopsy can often confirm that a nodule is malignant or infectious, although the diagnosis of a noninfectious benign lesion is less successfully achieved. Management of the pulmonary nodule requires the expertise and collaboration of a range of specialists including the referring clinician, diagnostic and interventional radiologists, the bronchoscopist, the surgeon, and the pathologist. The clinical context is important in terms of stratifying an individual's risk factors and guiding subsequent management. MDCT and PET improve the detection and surveillance of nodules and have enabled physiologic information to be obtained. Advances in these techniques and the potential contribution of fast magnetic resonance imaging sequences and computer applications should continue to impact our evaluation of the pulmonary nodule.

20.4 CAD Technology, Potential Application, and Application in Workflow

The potential impact of CAD in thoracic radiology is immense. CAD techniques aim to provide a method of assisting interpretation by means of computerized image analysis. CAD schemes have been reported to improve reader detection of lung nodules on radiographs in large-scale observer tests for both radiologists and radiologists in training[35,36]. It is widely accepted that one measure of effective computer assistance in radiological exams is its ability to focus radiologists' valuable time on the interpretation of images. With an increasing volume of single and multimodality data generated, radiologists will have little time to spend on each examination and will need to focus their attention and interpretation. CAD has the potential to take the time-consuming tasks of radiologists and minimize their involvement in those areas where their expertise is not required. CAD has been developed primarily to serve as a second reader. A number of studies lend support to this idea of CAD as a second interpreter, providing improved radiologist sensitivity for nodule detection with the assistance of CAD. CAD can accomplish this point by directing the radiologist's review and automatically generate quantitative information about the finding for faster interpretation. Another measure of the effectiveness is the consistency and repeatability of the CAD system to identify patterns that indicate abnormalities. When this consistency is synergized with the variability of the human observation, the accuracy of the radiologist can increase and may increase at different rates for the same observation depending on environmental conditions. The CAD schemes so far have primarily concentrated on the frontal radiograph, although more recently, investigation has addressed the lateral radiograph. A large amount of CAD research has been devoted to nodule detection on CT. The evolution in computer-assisted technology has been in part driven by the increasing use of MDCT, rendering smaller abnormalities apparent, yet generating a larger amount of image data for review. CAD can potentially take advantage of the benefits of thin-section images, although the amount of image data that the radiologist addresses is kept within reason so that the usual approach to interpretation is not hindered. Sensitivity and specificity vary widely among CAD systems relative to the diversity of algorithms, CT input, and varying populations of nodules in which CAD has been studied. The need for increased sensitivity, however, is offset by the desire to minimize the number of false-positive detections, which are often significant in number, particularly when lower size criteria for nodules are used. Clinical use of CAD will likely be hindered unless false-positive detections are minimized. CAD has been shown to identify clinically significant nodules that were overlooked by radiologists.

CAD systems are usually used for automatic detection in medical images and are currently used as a second review for radiologists. They target the problem of improved accuracy of clinical detection and provide other analysis tools to aid clinical interpretation. Given a consistent set of patterns, CAD systems can identify potential abnormalities, but the diagnosis of the finding remains the responsibility of the radiologist. However, some authors proposed CAD systems that also may potentially assist the radiologist in terms of the estimation of malignancy[37,38]. CAD systems that integrate both CT and PET information may also improve characterization of lung nodules in the future. Nie et al.[39] studied a semiautomatic computer-aided method using features from both PET and CT scans. The scheme was able to differentiate benign from malignant nodules better than those based on either PET or CT data alone. CAD methods can aid the assessment of nodule size and volume, attenuation, and enhancement characteristics by performing global analysis of high-resolution MDCT data of the entire nodule while minimizing the need for user intervention. Computer techniques can also decrease the tedium involved in the temporal characterization of nodules, particularly when the nodules are multiple and imaged at many time points. Such techniques can automatically identify the corresponding CT sections for a particular nodule, decreasing reader interpretation time. The use of CAD to improve textural characterization may, in time, prove beneficial for assessing textural change within subsolid lesions in which increased solid elements may indicate transformation to a more malignant histological grade[40]. For CAD technology to be fully used in all aspects of nodule evaluation, the integration of multifunctional CAD platforms into pulmonary artery catheters is necessary to enable easy accessibility for the user during reading interpretation. In previous studies, it was adequately demonstrated that CT offers major information in comparison with plain radiograph in the definition of pulmonary nodules. With the introduction of spiral CT and, in particular, with the newer multidetector-row CT, radiologists and chest physicians obtained an impressive number of information about pulmonary pathology and, in particular, in detecting pulmonary nodules. On the other hand, such information overload, produced by a huge CT data set, may lead to paradox cases in which the pulmonary nodule was retrospectively visible but at the first examination could not be detected by radiologists because of hundreds of CT images acquired for each patient[41–43]. In the Anti-Lung Cancer association screening program, 32% of lung cancers with diameter ranging from 4 to 13 mm were initially missed and were diagnosed only retrospectively at follow-up with CT imaging[41,42]. In a study by Swensen et al.[43], nodules were missed in 26% of the patients. It has been demonstrated that double reading by two trained observers improves the detection of pulmonary nodule, so consensus or double reading may help in reducing the error, but it is a time-consuming procedure. Considering these problems, the necessity to have a "second look" that may help radiologists in the correct evaluation of the CT data set is derived. CAD algorithms have been introduced to decrease diagnostic error and can be successfully integrated into clinical imaging as a second reader. Several vendors offer CAD systems that use proprietary CAD algorithms to examine the CT study in three dimensions, automatically and accurately highlighting potential actionable lung nodules and quickly computing measurements of detected regions. Among these CAD software packages, there are Visia™ CT lung nodule CAD and Philips Lung Care™ CAD systems. There are many different mathematical models for the CAD of pulmonary nodules. At the base of the CAD system are the automatic detection algorithms that detect regions consistent with suspicion of disease. CAD can be broadly divided into two groups: density-based CAD and geometric model–based CAD. The principle of the density-based system uses the high density interval between the nodule and the pulmonary parenchyma by using several techniques such as fuzzy clustering, multiple thresholding, region growing, and locally adaptative thresholding in combination with region growing[44]. The geometric model uses the nodule shape to create a model for nodule identification by adopting several approaches such as "N-Quoit filter," object-based deformation, template matching, and anatomy-based generic models. It is evident that the comparison between these different methodologies, in order to obtain homogeneous data, is problematic because of different algorithms used and because no standardized nodule databases were employed[45].

The integration of CAD into the current radiological environment of MDCT is extremely important because CAD is in a position to facilitate the change; in fact, by using a CAD system, a nodule can be automatically detected, the contour is generated, and automatically two-dimensional and volumetric measurement of the nodule is calculated. These measures can be saved and tracked over time to automatically evaluate nodule progression or regression. Once the nodule is automatically detected, these workflow enhancements are available to the user. This kind of approach can help in the pulmonary nodule management; in fact, these automatically generated measurements could save time and produce more repeatable results than human interaction. CAD therefore has immediate potential to focus a radiologist's energy on the interpretation of images and increase the efficiency of a radiologist in an MDCT environment. The observer performance of CAD for the detection of lung nodules is not developed well enough to determine its effect on clinical outcome. When these systems become available for routine clinical use, these data will become more readily available.

20.5 CAD Sensitivity

A wide variation in CAD sensitivity for detection of pulmonary nodules according to the different kind of CAD software and different types of scanner and acquisition parameters is present. Measuring stand-alone CAD performance for lung nodule detection is not easy, and in fact, biopsy of nodules as small as 3 to 4 mm in diameter is not common; therefore, a database of small cancers is difficult, but it is likely that smaller abnormalities pose a larger detection problem. Another reason is that detection algorithms designed to detect lung nodules as an abnormality are not designed to detect malignancies since not all nodules are malignant, but may nonetheless be important clinical findings. Generally gold standard algorithms for the detection of lung nodules are defined by consensus panels but, by their very nature, are a more subjective standard than biopsy. Getting a repeatable reference data set with consensus panels relies on a very tight definition of the reference measurement. One method of producing a repeatable reference data set is through the insertion of artificial nodules with properties similar to the true nodules into the original imaging database: this tighter standard may prove to be valuable in the evaluation of stand-alone performance in CAD systems. In the literature, the CAD sensitivity ranged from 38% in a study by Wormanns et al.[47] to 95% in a study by Bae et al.[34], and if we considered subrange > 3 mm, Brown et al.[29] reported a 100% sensitivity. Sensitivity is, in fact, a parameter affected by various factors, in particular, slice thickness, dimension, and nodule position. The detection of pulmonary nodules at CT is influenced substantially by the method of image data acquisition.

Another point is that pulmonary nodules may be easily detected by the CAD system if the nodule is solid. Actually, in a study by Yuan et al.[48], the detection sensitivity of solid pulmonary nodules was 80% (448 of 561 nodules) for CAD and 81% for the radiologist (455 of 561), but the overall values in detecting nodules (solid and nonsolid) were 73% (456 of 628) for CAD and 82% (518 of 628) for the radiologist. This fact is probably due to the software architecture that easily identifies as "nodule" groups of voxel with a high HU difference with the near, normal pulmonary parenchyma. We can define as "solid nodule" a solid, spherical, or more irregular, complex structure that displays a density CT^{peak} greater than –100 HU to calcific density[45,49]. In an interesting study by Armato et al.[50], where CAD algorithms were applied to 31 patients in whom lung cancers were initially missed by the radiologist, the automated detection method identified missed cancer in 26 (84%) out of 31 patients.

20.6 CAD Sensitivity Plus Radiologist

The use of CAD may help a radiologist as a second reader; therefore, the evaluation of the diagnostic impact of CAD should be evaluated. In comparison with a data set with CAD sensitivity and with CAD plus radiologist sensitivity, it was observed that values were higher by using this second option. The value was 92%. In the work of Rubin et al.[32], it was clearly demonstrated that CAD plus radiologist has higher sensitivity because it detected additional lesions. This is not surprising because of the high interobserver variability. In another study[44], a poor interobserver agreement was present between CAD and readers together with the contemporary presence of significant improvement in pulmonary nodule detection. Awai et al.[51] studied the CAD sensitivity in detecting pulmonary nodules in 50 patients by comparing five board-certified radiologists and five residents (with 2.8 years of experience) with and without employing a CAD system. In this study, the authors compared the observers' performance in detecting pulmonary nodules by using the area under each alternative free-response receiver operating characteristic curve (A_z). They observed that in the board-certified radiologist group, the values obtained with and without CAD indicated a significant difference (A_z without CAD = 0.63 ± 0.08; with CAD = 0.66 ± 0.09; $p < .01$). In the resident group, the values obtained with and without CAD also indicated a significant difference (A_z without CAD = 0.66 ± 0.04; with CAD = 0.68 ± 0.04; $p = .02$). The results of the study by Awai et al.[51] evidenced that the CAD system led to improved performances in the detection of pulmonary nodules at chest CT for both board-certified radiologists and the radiology residents. The difference in detecting pulmonary nodules between the board-certified radiologist group and the resident group was not significant. The author stated that radiologist performance in detecting pulmonary nodules probably depends more on how attentively each observer reads CT images than on his/her experience, and, in this condition, the use of CAD is expected to improve the radiologist's detection performance, irrespective of the knowledge or experience of each observer. In their work, Marten et al.[45] produced different results. They compared the performance of two board-certified radiologists and two residents, and they observed that experienced readers significantly outperformed inexperienced readers. Moreover, agreement between experienced readers was very good (weighted kappa value $k_w = 0.81$, 95% confidence interval = 0.65–0.97), but agreement between the inexperienced readers was poor (weighted kappa value $k_w = 0.30$, 95% confidence interval = 0.19–0.39). This difference in the study by Awai et al.[51] and Marten et al.[45] can be partially explained because the authors recruited residents with different experience (2.8 years and 6 months, respectively). Another difference was that Awai et al. used a 7.5-mm-thick slice excluding 4-mm nodules or lesser by giving also information to readers about numbers and the size of the nodules. In the study by Marten et al.[45], the performance of experienced readers was always not substantially altered by consensus of one experienced with one inexperienced reader, but consensus reading of the experienced readers and inexperienced readers with CAD significantly improved both readers' performances. Therefore, it is derived from this study that the use of a CAD system by an experienced radiologist for evaluation of pulmonary nodules produces optimal results. The efficacy of the lung nodule CAD as a second reader was confirmed also in a multicentric study published in 2008 by White et al.[72] where CAD software was shown to be effective as a second reader by improving the sensitivity of the radiologist in detecting pulmonary nodules.

20.7 Technical Parameters

Radiation dose is a critical problem for correct diagnostic planning, in particular, in patients that perform long-time follow-up. In the subgroup that undergoes CT examination many times, radiation exposure may be very high. The introduction of low dose, which may guarantee optimal results although lower radiation doses were given, may represent an optimal choice. In the studies in which a low-dose protocol was used[44–48,52–54], the results of sensitivity and sensibility were not affected by the use of this parameter with the exclusion of Goo et al.[54], where the CAD sensitivity reported was 65%. This value is lower when compared with other studies if we consider, moreover, that the nodules included in the analysis were 5 mm or larger. A classical protocol for normal dose is when the tube potential is 120 kVp or higher, and the tube current is 100 mA or higher. A typical "low-dose" protocol is when the tube potential is 120 kVp or lesser, and the tube current is lesser than 80 milliampere/second (mAs) (in the study by Goo et al.[54], 120 kilovolt (kV) and 38 mAs were used; in the study by Armato et al.[50], 120 kV and 25–50 mAs were used). The "low-dose" issue and the radiation exposure issue are related with the section thickness problem because routine acquisition of thin sections for lung CT exam may increase the radiation exposure to the patient. When an MDCT is used, this concern is spurious for several reasons. A 16-detector-row CT scanner cannot be used to acquire raw projection data in section thickness larger than 1 or 1.5 mm. For this reason, the reconstruction of thicker sections is simply the result of the weighted addition of raw projection data acquired with narrow detector widths[32]. Therefore, the radiation exposure for 1-mm section thickness is equal to the radiation exposure for the thicker reconstruction.

20.7.1 Nodule Dimension

The dimension of the pulmonary nodule represents a fundamental parameter. Generally, sensitivity for nodule detection increases with increasing nodule size. In a study by Ko et al.[53], the CAD sensitivity was 86%, but if we consider only the group larger than 3 mm, the sensitivity increased up to 91%. Brown et al.[29] reported 100% sensitivity for nodules with dimension larger than 3 mm and 70% for nodules lesser than 3 mm. In a study by Austin et al.[12], the sensitivity was 97.2% for nodules 5 mm or larger and 95.1% for nodules 3 mm or larger. It is important that the performance of radiologists in the detection of nodules lesser than 3 mm is lower than in the detection of larger nodules, and the relative contribution of CAD to improve radiologists' performance is higher than that for the detection of larger nodules.[12] Recently, in a study by Das et al.[46], they have compared the effects of two CAD systems in the detection of *small* pulmonary nodules (average diameter of 3.4 mm; average volume of 32.05 mm^3) by using 1–2 mm section thickness, and they observed that the overall sensitivity was 73%–75%. The use of CAD systems improved the reader's performance by 11%, 12%, and 3%, respectively.

20.7.2 Section Thickness

Nowadays the section thickness represents a secondary parameter in the CAD assessment because most of the scanners are multidetector row with the capacity of producing isotropic voxels. However, it is important to understand the application of the slice thickness in the lung nodule CAD analysis, and we will discuss about this point in this paragraph. In a recently published meta-analysis[72], CAD sensitivity with the use of thin-section and thick-section protocols was compared (thin section if < 2 mm and thick section if > 2 mm), and an 80% sensitivity was obtained by considering the thin-section protocols: but when the authors excluded the study by Yuan et al.[48], where they used a low-dose protocol, and where other studies were performed with normal dose, the obtained sensitivity was 90%. The average sensitivity observed by using thick-section methods was 74%. From these data, it is possible to hypothesize that section thickness changes CAD sensitivity in detecting pulmonary nodules. In previous studies, it was demonstrated that the use of thin sections in the evaluation of CT images for lung nodules substantially improves the detection of the nodules[56,57]: in the work of Fischbach et al.[57], the number of nodules that were observed by two radiologists on 5-mm-thick CT images was 86%–88% of the nodules that were identified by using 1.25-mm-thick CT images. The overall sensitivity of conventional CT with the use of 8- to 10-mm-thick sections in detecting pulmonary metastases ranged from 58% to 78%[58–60]. In the CAD studies, some authors used thick CT images, such as Armato et al.[61] and Ko et al.[53], and other authors used thin CT images, such as Brown et al.[29], Bae et al.[34], Yuan et al.[48], and Rubin et al.[32] Unfortunately, in these studies, it is not possible to define the effects produced by using different CT thickness because of different techniques (mAs, kV) and types of CAD tools used. In a study by Kim et al.[62], it was clearly demonstrated that the effect produced by using a thinner slice is important: in the *thin group*, CAD showed a sensitivity of 95.2%, and in the *thick group*, the sensitivity was 88.6%. Marten et al.[44] evaluated CAD sensitivity by using 4-, 2-, and 0.75-mm section thickness and obtained statistically significant results by using the lesser thickness. The use of a thick or thin slice also modified the false positive (FP); in the same study[30], the use of a thin slice produced 5.4 false-positive nodules for the data set, and the use of a thick slice produced 23.6 false-positive nodules for the data set. Therefore, in the CAD algorithms, the use of a thin slice is important because it affects substantially the sensitivity and the false-positive rate. In our opinion, it may be interesting to observe that Brown et al.[29] obtained 100% sensitivity in detecting long nodules > 3 mm by using thin-section CT images. Therefore, the performance of the CAD system appears to be highly associated with the section thickness and appears to be better on thin-section than on thick-section CT images. In the study by Rubin et al.[32], it was demonstrated that it is possible to develop a CAD algorithm that has sensitivity that is comparable with that of radiologists with only a small number of false-positive detections, when thin-section multidetector-row scanners are used.

20.7.3 False Positive

In the meta-analysis by Saba et al.[63], it was observed that the absolute number of false-positive nodules ranged from 0.55[64] to 74.4[65] for each patient (Figures 20.3–20.6). Usually CAD software shows high false-positive values, and this situation is derived from the inclusion of nonnodule structures. This fact is probably due to the difficulties, during the segmentation phases, in making a distinction between nodules and other structures. In particular, if we observe the "type" of false positive, the higher number of FP is due to vascular structures (over 62% in a study[32]).

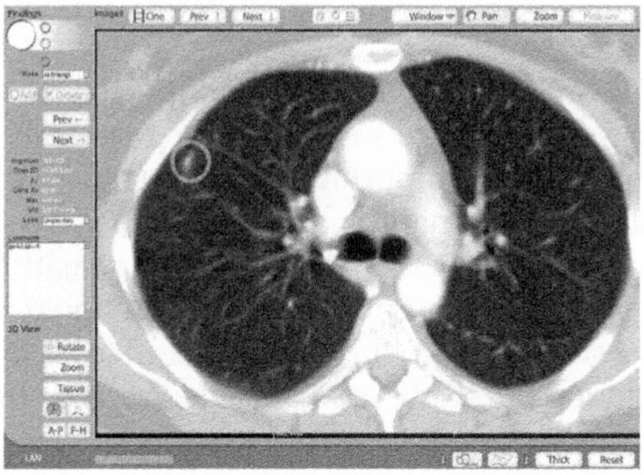

FIGURE 20.3
CT axial image demonstrating a false positive. The CAD classified this parenchymal alteration as pulmonary nodule (white circle).

Vascular tree, in its spatial development, produces in single axial images a nodule-like appearance when the vessel course is along the *z*-axis. Radiologists, by using their experience and logical pathways, exclude the pulmonary vessel by comparing it with other axial images. The CAD algorithms, to exclude vascular structure, have to operate segmentation where a 3D reconstruction of a pulmonary vessel is made. If the spatial position of the suspected nodule in the volumetric segmented reconstruction is included, the nodule is then consequently excluded. These systems are not perfect, and a great number of vascular-like nodule structures could be included as nodules. A second pitfall that produces FP in the CAD is that the segmentation algorithm only recognizes nodules entirely surrounded by lung parenchyma, and unfortunately, the pulmonary vessel often appears likewise.

The majority of vascular FP detection appears to be small peripheral vessels, most commonly branch points. There are many other causes that may produce false-positive nodules, although vessels are the most important: parenchymal disease (areas of parenchymal disease resulted in ground glass, reticular, or airspace attenuation)[7] and fragmented airway walls (some airway walls were fragmented as a result of volume averaging). In the study

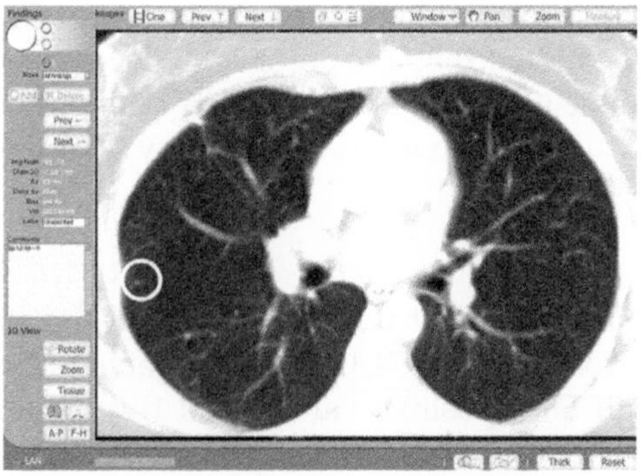

FIGURE 20.4
CT axial image demonstrating a false positive. The CAD classified this truncated vessel as pulmonary nodule (white circle).

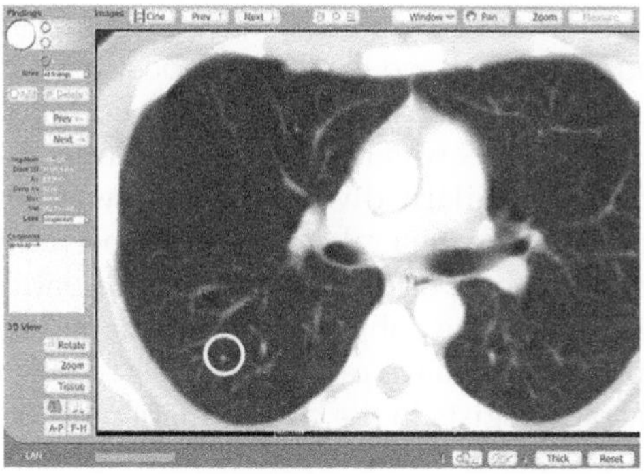

FIGURE 20.5
CT axial image demonstrating a false positive. The CAD classified this fragmented blood vessel as pulmonary nodule (white circle).

by Rubin et al.[32], five types of false-positive nodules were described: peripheral vessel, central vessel, airway wall, amorphous parenchymal opacity, and artifact.

If we observe the *trend* in the years about the false-positive nodules in the CAD tools, the number of false-positive nodules appears markedly lower in the years 2005–2006 than in the previous ones: the number of false-positive nodules for patients studied in 2001–2004 was 30.5, and in the years 2005–2006, the number was 3.7. These data about false-positive nodules for each patient suffer from multiple bias that is derived from the different type of the CT acquisition data set (low dose or not, section thickness, increment, reconstruction interval) and the different type of CAD software. From 2005 to 2009, published papers showed reduced FP rates.

An ideal CAD system would show no false-positive nodules and would show all the true-positive nodules, but it is a well-known issue that as the true-positive nodules approach 100%, the false-positive percentage also tends to increase.[51]

While there is ongoing research into reducing false-positive detections by CAD systems, studies have not yet addressed the fact that readers surprisingly tend to reject some

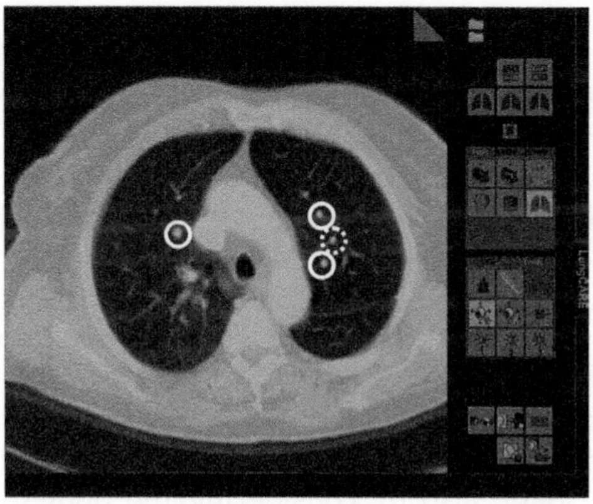

FIGURE 20.6
CT axial image demonstrating several false-positive cases (white circles) and a pulmonary nodule (open white circle).

true-positive CAD nodules and thus potentially reduce the benefit of CAD. In a study by Roos et al.[66], the first reader rejected one in two true-positive CAD nodules, and the second reader only rejected one in seven true-positive CAD nodules. This diversity in acceptance of true-positive CAD nodules was responsible for the variable benefit that readers achieved from the use of CAD. Similarly diverse behavior was observed in the acceptance of false-positive CAD detections. In general, good reader performance during free search did not automatically ensure good performance when evaluating the CAD output. One explanation for this variability is the subjectivity of readers' decisions when classifying pulmonary findings. Armato et al.[67] have recently described substantial variability across very experienced thoracic radiologists in the determination of "truth" for the first 30 cases of the Lung Nodule Database Consortium.

20.7.4 False Negative

Another important problem in evaluating the CAD is the false-negative rate. The high false-negative rate limits CAD application as a stand-alone technique[48]. Near one fourth of the pulmonary nodules were not detected by CAD in the study by Yuan et al.[48] Missing true nodules by CAD may be due to various factors such as attenuation, size, shape, location, and error in segmentation algorithm. Several missed nodules were located in pleural or subpleural position, and they were excluded because of segmentation errors[34,38].

20.7.5 Nodule Position

An important point to understand CAD sensitivity is its relationship to the position of the "suspected nodules." As evidenced by Yuan et al.[48], CAD shows higher sensitivity in detecting hilar nodules, which are prone to be misinterpreted as vessels by radiologists. On the other hand, radiologists have higher sensitivity in detecting subpleural and peripheral nodules, even if these nodules are small, because there is no vessel of similar size near the pleural surface. The CAD sensitivity in detecting hilar nodules is near 100%; in detecting central nodules, the CAD sensitivity is 84%, and in detecting subpleural nodules, it is 61%[27]. Similar results were described in the study by Ko et al.[53] and Wormanns et al.[47], and in a study by Peldschus et al.[69] wherein they reported that most of the missed lesions by radiologists that were detected by CAD were located in the central areas of the lung in close proximity to adjacent vessels. This may be easily understood by thinking that radiologists usually make diagnosis by analyzing axial images. In the axial images, isolated nodules can be frequently identified without the need for comparison of adjacent sections because these isolated nodules are dissimilar to adjacent blood vessels and have good tissue contrast from the surrounding much-lower-attenuation pulmonary parenchyma[34]. Juxtavascular nodules that are closely associated or attached to adjacent blood vessels may not be easily detected. Some vessels, perpendicular to the imaging plane, may appear in fact as nodules, and volumetric evaluation (3D) is important. In the study by Bae et al.[34], the CAD sensitivity for detecting nodules according to position was 97.4% for isolated nodules, 92.3% for juxtapleural nodules, and 94.1% for juxtavascular nodules. These results are different from the others previously described; this may be due to the different CAD system used, where different bidimensional and tridimensional algorithms are combined. However, it is clearly evident, also by considering the poor interobserver agreements between radiologists and CAD systems, underlined in several studies[32,44,45], that CAD and radiologists detect different groups of nodules, and when they work together, it increases markedly the sensitivity rates.

20.8 About Pulmonary Nodules Missed by Radiologists but Detected by CAD

Radiologists may commit two types of errors during the interpretation of imaging studies: classification error and perception error[63,39]. In the first type of mistake, the radiologist does not report a detected lesion because he/she does not attribute adequate clinical importance to the detected nodules. In the second type of error, the reader does not see an abnormality that is possible to see retrospectively. This situation may occur from many causes: distraction, inexperience, satisfaction search effect, huge workload, and, last but not least, because of a particular position of the lesion. Missing lesion at thoracic CT is a well-recognized phenomenon, and it is possible to fail in detecting nodules even in specialized academic departments. In the important study by Peldschus et al.[69], 100 patients were analyzed where the radiologist excluded nodules and the CAD system detected 53 nodules in 33 patients: in this situation, CAD clearly demonstrated itself as an effective tool because lung nodules missed at the clinical interpretation can be detected if CAD is used as an additional reader. Moreover, in the study by Marten et al.[45], the CAD system detected 84% of the nodules, which were not previously detected in patients with biopsy-proved lung cancer. In a recent study by Roos et al.[66], the potential of CAD to improve radiologists' diagnostic performance in the detection of pulmonary nodules on chest MDCT has been confirmed. However, the magnitude of the performance increase with the use of CAD is influenced by the quality of the reader interpretation of CAD output as well as by the inherent properties of the algorithm. The diagnostic performance of CAD evaluation was variable among readers and did not follow the patterns of reader performance during free search.

20.9 Contrast Material

The use of contrast material is not absolutely necessary to detect a lung nodule, in particular, when its dimension is less than 1 cm. In the literature, some authors described the use of iodinated contrast material[32,44,45,53,66], whereas others did not use such material[50,51]. Contrast material administration appears not to affect sensitivity, specificity, and false-positive rate. On the contrary, the administration of contrast material may be useful in the characterization of lung nodules to distinguish them from benign to malignant lesion.

20.10 Reference Standard in the Evaluation of CAD Systems

A common limitation in these studies is the lack of an absolute reference standard. The majority of the authors of these papers used a consensus of two or three experts to establish the nodule presence, because histological findings are rarely available for comparison with lung CT scans. Often the reference standard of nodules has been defined by means of consensus reading; however, determining whether they accurately identified a true nodule is problematic. This is a primary problem because it may reduce markedly the value of a study; this was previously marked by Gur et al.[70] It was reported by Kang et al.[71] that more than 20% of additional nodules can be detected by manual palpation than by preoperative chest scan: these data clearly explain the poor value of the means by consensus reading. For in-depth evaluation of sensitivity, specificity, and false-positive and false-negative values, it would be necessary that authors of CAD studies follow up data as the gold standard. Armato et al.[50] studied CAD performance in 31 patients in whom lung cancers were initially missed by the radiologist and were later all biopsy-confirmed as "missed cancers." In the meta-analysis by Saba et al.[63], in the majority of the studied papers, the CT cases did not contain areas of complex parenchymal disease[34], such as ground-glass areas or honeycomb regions, or severe pulmonary fibrosis, diffuse bronchiectasis, extensive inflammatory scars,[51] areas of atelectasis or consolidation, and interstitial lung disease[45]. If these parenchymal diseases are present, it is necessary to improve the detection methods in order to first exclude these areas and to detect the possible nodules. In the CAD systems, the presence of artifacts, primarily motion artifacts, could also be possible: this one reflects the patient's movements during the CT scans or from the pulsation of the heart and great vessels. The presence of artifacts may determine the failure of the CAD algorithms because the continuity of tubular structures (vessel) in the z-direction is disrupted, producing many FP results[47].

20.11 Consideration and Conclusion

The CAD system serves as a useful second opinion when physicians examine patients at lung cancer screening, and CAD will have a major impact on medical imaging and diagnostic radiology in the field of lung cancer in the near future. The CAD system for analysis of pulmonary nodules has the following advantages: (1) great speed of numerical calculation, allowing precise, quantitative, and reproducible measurements; (2) an ever-increasing knowledge base to provide diagnostic information; and (3) no susceptibility to fatigues. CAD may be an effective tool in the diagnosis of pulmonary nodules, and the use of CAD plus radiologist gives better results than the use of only a radiologist's analysis. In particular, CAD shows its best potentialities in detecting nodules located in the central areas of the lungs, where, moreover, a radiologist shows a lack of efficacy. CAD has the potential to equalize performance among readers by reducing individual detection errors of lung nodules on chest CT. Analysis of CAD-dependent temporal variations in performance may facilitate the establishment of optimized thresholds for the duration of CAD interaction. It is important, however, that other studies are included to evaluate what number of false-positive detection would be acceptable with CAD in the routine clinical practice. Although the false-positive rate is still a drawback, CAD showed an increased sensitivity that expenses the low specificity: reduction of the number of false-positive findings will be an important focus of ongoing developments. The high false-positive rate of CAD requires radiologists to look for each "suspected nodule" to confirm it as a "true nodule," but the trend is in reducing the FP rates, providing better information; however, radiologists would be able to delete correctly false-positive detections. CAD tools are useful in supporting a radiologist's detection performance, but all suspected lesions detected by CAD must always be interpreted by a radiologist to rule out false positives.

References

1. Fry WA, Menck HR, Winchester DP. The National Cancer Data Base report on lung cancer. *Cancer* 1996;77:1947–1955.
2. Martini N, Bains MS, Burt ME, et al. Incidence of local recurrence and second primary tumors in resected stage I lung cancer. *J Thorac Cardiovasc Surg* 1995;109:120–129.
3. Flehinger BJ, Kimmel M, Melamed M. The effect of surgical treatment on survival from early lung cancer. *Chest* 1992;101:1013–1018.
4. Thun, MJ, Hannan LM, Adams-Campbell LL, et al. Lung cancer occurrence in never-smokers: An analysis of 13 cohorts and 22 cancer registry studies. *PLoS Med* 2008;5:e185–189.
5. Gorlova, OY, Weng SF, Zhang Y, et al. Aggregation of cancer among relatives of never-smoking lung cancer patients. *Int J Cancer* 2007;121:111–118.
6. Hackshaw, AK, Law MR, Wald NJ. The accumulated evidence on lung cancer and environmental tobacco smoke. *Br Med J* 1997;315:980–988.
7. Catelinois O, Rogel A, Laurier D, et al. Lung cancer attributable to indoor radon exposure in France: Impact of the risk models and uncertainty analysis. *Environ Health Perspect* 2010;114:1361–1366.
8. O'Reilly, KM, Mclaughlin AM, Beckett WS, Sime PJ. Asbestos-related lung disease. *Am Fam Phys* 2007;75:683–688.
9. Kabir, Z, Bennett K, Clancy L. Lung cancer and urban air-pollution in Dublin: A temporal association? *Irish Med J* 2007;100:367–369.
10. Coyle, YM, Minahjuddin AT, Hynan LS, Minna JD. An ecological study of the association of metal air pollutants with lung cancer incidence in Texas. *J Thoracic Oncol* 2006;1:654–661.
11. Chiu, HF, Cheng MH, Tsai SS, et al. Outdoor air pollution and female lung cancer in Taiwan. *Inhalation Toxicol* 2006;18:1025–1031.
12. Austin JH, Muller NL, Friedman PJ, et al. Glossary of terms for CT of the lungs: Recommendations of the Nomenclature Committee of the Fleischner Society. *Radiology* 1996;200:327–331.
13. Osada H, Takahashi T. Molecular pathogenesis of lung cancer [in Japanese]. *Nippon Rinsho* 2000;58:1012–1016.
14. Oshiro Y, Kusumoto M, Moriyama N, et al. Intrapulmonary lymph nodes: Thin-section CT features of 19 nodules. *J Comput Assist Tomogr* 2002;26:553–557.
15. Zwirewich CV, Vedal S, Miller RR, Müller NL. Solitary pulmonary nodule: High-resolution CT and radiologic–pathologic correlation. *Radiology* 1991;179:469–476.
16. Zerhouni EA, Stitik FP, Siegelman SS, et al. CT of the pulmonary nodule: A cooperative study. *Radiology* 1986;160:319–327.
17. Ketai L, Malby M, Jordan K, Meholic A, Locken J. Small nodules detected on chest radiography: Does size predict calcification? *Chest* 2000;118:610–614.
18. Shah PK, Austin JH, White CS, et al. Missed non-small cell lung cancer: Radiographic findings of potentially resectable lesions evident only in retrospect. *Radiology* 2003;226:235–241.
19. Austin JH, Romney BM, Goldsmith LS. Missed bronchogenic carcinoma: Radiographic findings in 27 patients with a potentially resectable lesion evident in retrospect. *Radiology* 1992;182:115–122.
20. Samei E, Flynn MJ, Peterson E, Eyler WR. Subtle lung nodules: Influence of local anatomic variations on detection. *Radiology* 2003;228:76–84.
21. Berbaum KS, Franken EA Jr, Dorfman DD, et al. Role of faulty visual search in the satisfaction of search effect in chest radiography. *Acad Radiol* 1998;5:9–19.
22. Kundel HL, Nodine CF, Krupinski EA. Searching for lung nodules: Visual dwell indicates locations of false-positive and false-negative decisions. *Invest Radiol* 1989;24:472–478.
23. Samuel S, Kundel H, Nodine C, Toto L. Mechanism of satisfaction of search: Eye position recordings in the reading of chest radiographs. *Radiology* 1995;194:895–902.
24. MacMahon H. Improvement in detection of pulmonary nodules: Digital image processing and computer-aided diagnosis. *RadioGraphics* 2000;20:1169–1177.

25. Abe H, MacMahon H, Shiraishi J, Li Q, Engelmann R, Doi K. Computer-aided diagnosis in chest radiology. *Semin Ultrasound CT MR* 2004;25:432–437.
26. Henschke CI, McCauley DI, Yankelovitz DF, et al. Early lung cancer action project: Overall design and findings from baseline screening. *Lancet* 1999;354:99–105.
27. Kalender WA, Polacin A, Suss C. A comparison of conventional and spiral CT: An experimental study on the detection of spherical lesions. *J Comput Assist Tomogr* 1994;18:167–176.
28. Remy-Jardin M, Remy J, Giraud F, Marquette CH. Pulmonary nodules: Detection with thick-section spiral CT versus conventional CT. *Radiology* 1993;187:513–520.
29. Brown MS, Goldin JG, Suh RD, et al. Lung micronodules: Automated method for detection at thin section CT-initial experience. *Radiology* 2003;226:256–262.
30. Naidich DP. Helical computed tomography of the thorax: Clinical applications. *Radiol Clin North Am* 1994;32:759–774.
31. White CS, Romney BM, Mason AC, Austin JH, Miller BH, Protopapas Z. Primary carcinoma of the lung overlooked at CT: Analysis of findings in 14 patients. *Radiology* 1996;199:109–115.
32. Rubin GD, Lyo JK, Paik DS, et al. Pulmonary nodules on multi detector row CT scans: Performance comparison of radiologist and computer aided detection. *Radiology* 2005;234:274–284.
33. Bae KT, Giger M, MacMahon H, Doi K. Computer-aided detection of pulmonary nodules in CT images. *Radiology* 1991;181(P):144.
34. Bae KT, Kim JS, Na YH, et al. Pulmonary nodules: Automated detection on CT images with morphologic matching algorithm preliminary result. *Radiology* 2005;236:286–294.
35. Schilham AMR, van Ginneken B, Loog M. A computer-aided diagnosis system for detection of lung nodules in chest radiographs with an evaluation on a public database. *Med Image Anal* 2006;10:258.
36. Abe H, MacMahon H, Engelmann R, et al. Computer-aided diagnosis in chest radiography: Results of large-scale observer tests at the 1996–2001 RSNA scientific assemblies. *RadioGraphics* 2003;23:255–265.
37. Awai K, Murao K, Ozawa A, et al. Pulmonary nodules: Estimation of malignancy at thin-section helical CT-effect of computer-aided diagnosis on performance of radiologists. *Radiology* 2006;239:276–284.
38. Li F, Aoyama M, Shiraishi J, et al. Radiologists' performance for differentiating benign from malignant lung nodules on high-resolution CT using computer-estimated likelihood of malignancy. *AJR* 2004;183:1209–1215.
39. Nie Y, Li Q, Li F, Pu Y, Appelbaum D, Doi K. Integrating PET and CT information to improve diagnostic accuracy for lung nodules: a semiautomatic computer-aided method. *J Nucl Med* 2006;47:1075–1080.
40. Suzuki K, Kusumoto M, Watanabe S, Tsuchiya R, Asamura H. Radiologic classification of small adenocarcinoma of the lung: Radiologic–pathologic correlation and its prognostic impact. *Ann Thorac Surg* 2006;81:413–419.
41. Kaneko M, Eguchi K, Ohmatsu H, et al. Peripheral lung cancer: Screening and detection with low-dose spiral CT versus radiography. *Radiology* 1996;201:798–802.
42. Kakinuma R, Ohmatsu H, Kaneko M, et al. Detection failures in spiral CT screening for lung cancer: Analysis of CT findings. *Radiology* 1999;212:61–66.
43. Swensen SJ, Jett JR, Sloan JA, et al. Screening for lung cancer with low-dose spiral computed tomography. *Am J Respir Crit Care Med* 2002;165:508–513.
44. Marten K, Grillhosl A, Seyfarth T, et al. Computer assisted detection of pulmonary nodules: Evaluation of diagnostic performance using an expert-knowledge-based detection system with variable reconstruction slice thickness settings. *Eur Radiol* 2005;15:203–212.
45. Marten K, Seyfarth T, Auer F, et al. Computer-assisted detection of pulmonary nodules: Performance evaluation of an expert knowledge based detection system in consensus reading with experienced and inexperienced chest radiologists. *Eur Radiol* 2004;1930–1938.
46. Das M, Muhlenbruch G, Mahnken A, et al. Small pulmonary nodules: Effect of two computer-aided-detection systems on radiologist performance. *Radiology* 2006;241:564–571.

47. Wormanns D, Fiebich M, Saidi M, et al. Automatic detection of pulmonary nodules at spiral CT: Clinical application of a computer-aided diagnosis system. *Eur Radiol* 2002;12:1052–1057.
48. Yuan R, Vos PM, Cooperberg PL. Computer aided detection in screening CT for pulmonary nodules. *AJR* 2006;186:1280–1287.
49. Miller D, Burns R, Schneider A, et al. A Multi-reader, multi case ROC study demonstrating improved performance detecting lung nodules using computer-aided-detection (CAD) in multi-slice CT (MSCT) of the chest. *Proc RSNA* 2003:479.
50. Armato SG, Giger ML, MacMahon H, et al. Lung cancer: Performance of automated lung nodule detection applied to cancers missed in a CT screening program. *Radiology* 2002;225:685–692.
51. Awai K, Murao K, Ozawa A, et al. Pulmonary nodules at chest CT: Effect of computer-aided diagnosis on radiologists' detection performance. *Radiology* 2004;230:347–352.
52. Fraioli F, Catalano C, Almberger M, et al. Evaluation of effectiveness of a computer system (CAD) in the identification of lung nodules with low dose MSCT: Scanning techniques and preliminary results. *Radiol Med* 2004;109:40–49.
53. Ko JP, Betke M. Chest CT: Automated Nodule detection and assessment of change over time—Preliminary experience. *Radiology* 2001;218:267–273.
54. Goo JM, Lee JW, Lee HJ, et al. Automated lung nodule detection at low dose CT: Preliminary experience. *Korean J Radiol* 2003;4:211–216.
55. Saba L, Caddeo G, Mallarini G. Computer-aided-detection of pulmonary nodules in computed tomography: Analysis and review of the literature. *J Comput Assist Tomogr* 2007;31:611–619.
56. Paranjpe DV, Bergin CJ. Spiral CT of the lungs: Optimal technique and resolution compared with conventional CT. *AJR Am J Roentgenol* 1994;162:561–567.
57. Fischbach F, Knollmann F, Griesshaber V, et al. Detection of pulmonary nodules by multislice computed tomography: Improved detection rate with reduced slice thickness. *Eur Radiol* 2003;13:2378–2383.
58. Chang AE, Schaner EG, Conkle DM, et al. Evaluation of computed tomography in the detection of pulmonary metastases: A prospective study. *Cancer* 1979;43:913–916.
59. McCormack PM, Ginsberg KB, Bains MS, et al. Accuracy of lung imaging in metastases with implications for the role of thoracoscopy. *Ann Thorac Surg* 1993;56:863–865; discussion 865–866.
60. Peuchot M, Libshitz HI. Pulmonary metastatic disease: Radiologic–surgical correlation. *Radiology* 1987;164:719–722.
61. Armato SG 3rd, Giger ML, MacMahon H. Automated detection of lung nodules in CT scans: Preliminary results. *Med Phys* 2001;28:1552–1561.
62. Kim JS, Kim JH, Cho G, Bae KT. Automated detection of pulmonary nodules on CT images: Effect of section thickness and reconstruction interval—Initial results. *Radiology* 2005;236:295–299.
63. Saba L, Caddeo G, Mallarini G. Computer-aided-detection of pulmonary nodules in computed tomography: Analysis and review of the literature. *J Comput Assist Tomogr* 2007;31:611–619.
64. Marten K, Engelke C, Seyfarth T, et al. Computer-aided detection of pulmonary nodules: Influence of nodule characteristic on detection performance. *Clin Radiol* 2005;60:196–206.
65. Gurcan MN, Sahiner B, Petrick N, et al. Lung nodule detection on thoracic computed tomography images: Preliminary evaluation of a computer-aided diagnosis system. *Med Phys* 2002;29:2552–2558.
66. Roos JE, Paik D, Olsen D, et al. Computer-aided detection (CAD) of lung nodules in CT scans: Radiologist performance and reading time with incremental CAD assistance. *Eur Radiol* 2010;20:549–557.
67. Armato SG 3rd, McNitt-Gray MF, Reeves AP, Meyer CR, McLennan G, Aberle DR, Kazerooni EA, MacMahon H, van Beek EJ, Yankelevitz D, Hoffman EA, Henschke CI, Roberts RY, Brown MS, Engelmann RM, Pais RC, Piker CW, Qing D, Kocherginsky M, Croft BY, Clarke LP. The Lung Image Database Consortium (LIDC): An evaluation of radiologist variability in the identification of lung nodules on CT scans. *Acad Radiol* 2007;14:1409–1421.
68. Lee IJ, Gamsu G, Czum G, et al. Lung nodule detection on Chest CT: Evaluation of a computer-aided system. *Korean J Radiol* 2005;6:89–93.

69. Peldschus K, Herzog P, Wood SA, et al. Computer-aided diagnosis as a second reader. *Chest* 2005;128:1517–1523.
70. Gur D, Zheng B, Fuhrman CR, Hardesty L. On the testing and reporting of computer-aided detection results for lung cancer detection. *Radiology* 2004;232:5–6.
71. Kang MC, Hang CH, Lee HJ, Goo JM, Kim YT, Kim JH. Accuracy of 16-channel multi-detector-row chest computed tomography with thin sections in the detection of metastatic pulmonary nodules. *Eur J Cardiothorac Surg* 200;33:473–479.
72. White CS, Pugatch R, Koonce T, Rust SW, Dharaiya E. Lung nodule CAD software as a second reader: A multicentre study. *Acad Radiol* 2008;15:326–333.

Index

Page numbers followed by f and t indicate figures and tables, respectively.

M

R

U

V

W

Printed and bound by CPI Group (UK) Ltd, Croydon, CR0 4YY
18/10/2024
01776249-0012